T0329681

Global Epidemiology of Cancer

Global Epidemiology of Cancer

Diagnosis and Treatment

Jahangir Moini, MD, MPH
Professor of Science and Health (retired)
Eastern Florida State College
Florida, USA

Nicholas G. Avgeropoulos, MD
Director of the Brain and Spine Tumor Center, and
Medical Director of Neuro-Oncology
Orlando Health / UF Health Center
Florida, USA

Craig Badolato, MD
Medical Oncologist
US Oncology
Florida, USA

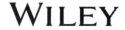

This edition first published 2022
© 2022 John Wiley and Sons Ltd

The right of Jahangir Moini, Nicholas G. Avgeropoulos, and Craig Badolato to be identified as the authors of this work has been asserted in accordance with law.

Registered Offices
John Wiley & Sons, Inc., 111 River Street, Hoboken, NJ 07030, USA
John Wiley & Sons Ltd, The Atrium, Southern Gate, Chichester, West Sussex, PO19 8SQ, UK

Editorial Office
9600 Garsington Road, Oxford, OX4 2DQ, UK

For details of our global editorial offices, customer services, and more information about Wiley products visit us at www.wiley.com.

Wiley also publishes its books in a variety of electronic formats and by print-on-demand. Some content that appears in standard print versions of this book may not be available in other formats.

Library of Congress Cataloging-in-Publication Data
Names: Moini, Jahangir, 1942- author. | Avgeropoulos, Nicholas G., author. |
  Badolato, Craig, author.
Title: Global epidemiology of cancer : diagnosis and treatment / Jahangir
  Moini, MD, MPH, Professor of Science and Health (retired), Eastern
  Florida State College, Florida, USA, Nicholas G. Avgeropoulos, MD,
  Director of the Brain and Spine Tumor Center and Medical Director of
  Neuro-Oncology, Orlando Health / UF Health Center, Florida, USA, Craig
  Badolato, MD, Medical Oncologist, US Oncology, Florida, USA.
Description: Hoboken, NJ : John Wiley & Sons, 2022. | Includes
  bibliographical references and index.
Identifiers: LCCN 2021045156 (print) | LCCN 2021045157 (ebook) | ISBN
  9781119817444 (hardback) | ISBN 9781119817178 (pdf) | ISBN 9781119817185
  (epub) | ISBN 9781119817192 (ebook)
Subjects: LCSH: Cancer–Epidemiology. | World health.
Classification: LCC RA645.C3 M58 2022 (print) | LCC RA645.C3 (ebook) |
  DDC 614.5/999–dc23/eng/20211103
LC record available at https://lccn.loc.gov/2021045156
LC ebook record available at https://lccn.loc.gov/2021045157

Cover image: © By Siberian Art, Lightspring, peterschreiber.media
Cover design by Wiley

Set in 9.5/12.5pt STIXTwoText by Integra Software Services Pvt. Ltd, Pondicherry,
IndiaPrinted and bound by CPI Group (UK) Ltd, Croydon, CR0 4YY

C9781119817444_0303022

Dr. Moini
To the memory of my parents, who taught me the value of perseverance and hard work. To my wife Hengameh, my daughters Mahkameh and Morvarid, and also my precious granddaughters, Laila and Anabelle, thanks for your understanding and tremendous support.

Dr. Avgeropoulos
I would like to dedicate this effort to the man I admire most, his namesake, and my namesake who followed after that. May we all relentlessly seek to separate what we believe from what we know; in doing so, may we ever implement knowledge that brings forth change for good.

Dr. Badolato
I dedicate my work to the patients who have entrusted their care to me for over 30 years.

Contents

About the Authors

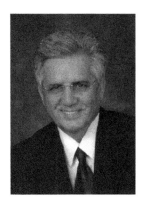

Dr. Jahangir Moini was assistant professor at Tehran University, Medical School, Department of Epidemiology and Preventive Medicine, for nine years. For 18 years, he was the director of epidemiology for the Brevard County Health Department. For 15 years, he was the director of science and health for Everest University in Melbourne, Florida. He was also professor of science and health at Everest for a total of 24 years. For 6 years, he was professor of science and health at Eastern Florida State College, but is now retired. Dr. Moini has been actively teaching for 39 years, and for 21 years, he has been an international author of 47 books. His *Anatomy & Physiology for Health Professionals* has been translated into the Japanese and Korean languages.

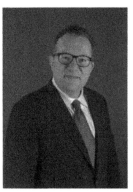

Dr. Nicholas G. Avgeropoulos is director of the Brain and Spine Tumor Center at Orlando Health/UF Health Cancer Center where he also serves as medical director of neuro-oncology. He is board certified in neurology and medical neuro-oncology and has been in clinical practice for over 20 years, with particular focus on clinical research. His current research affiliation is with the Brain Tumor Trials Collaborative, a National Cancer Institute centered consortium. Dr. Avgeropoulos has received fellowship training in neurovirology/neuroimmunology at the Medical University of South Carolina, in neuropathology at Yale New Haven Hospital, and in neuro-oncology at Massachusetts General Hospital.

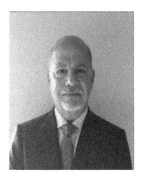

Craig Badolato, MD is a medical oncologist with US Oncology in Melbourne, Florida. Dr. Badolato is board certified in internal medicine, hematology, and medical oncology. He is a graduate from LaSalle University and Hahnemann University, both in Philadelphia.

Preface

The authors welcome you to this first edition of *Global Epidemiology of Cancer (Diagnosis and Treatment)*. Since cancer is a leading cause of death globally and the second highest cause of death in the United States, our goals are to discuss the global epidemiology of cancer, with detailed focus on diagnosis and treatment. The book will meet the needs of readers by providing solid information about epidemiology, etiology, risk factors, pathophysiology, clinical manifestations, diagnosis, treatment, prevention, early detection, and prognosis. It has been written to provide logical, step-by-step information on a large variety of cancers in different organs. The chapters are formatted to include keywords, significant points, clinical cases with questions and answers, key terms, and references. Tables summarize information into easy-to-remember topics throughout the chapters. The book has 18 chapters, organized into three parts. It is designed for graduate and postgraduate students, including medical students; residents in internal medicine and oncology; and nurses, nurse practitioners, and physician assistants.

Acknowledgments

The authors appreciate the contributions of everyone who assisted in the creation of this book, especially Andrew Harrison, Mandy Collison, and Greg Vadimsky.

Part I

Introduction

1

Pathogenesis of Cancer

<table>
<tr><td>OUTLINE</td></tr>
<tr><td>

The Origin of Cancer
Cancer Biology
Genetics and Cancer
Cell Division
Cell Cycle
Carcinogenesis
Mutation and Cancer
Metastasis
Key Terms
Bibliography
</td></tr>
</table>

The Origin of Cancer

Cancers are often named after tissues or cell types they originate from. For example, *carcinomas* are cancers that originate from epithelial cells covering the skin surface and internal organs (see Figure 1.1). They are derived from the embryonic **ectoderm** and **endoderm**. *Sarcomas* are cancers that arise from bone, connective tissue, fat, or muscle cells derived from the embryonic **mesoderm**. *Gliomas* arise from glial cells (nerve cells) that have become altered. *Myeloma* is a type of blood cancer arising in the bone marrow, from altered plasma cells that produce many abnormal antibodies. *Leukemia* arises from malignant white blood cells (leukocytes). Since cells of various embryonic origins become differentiated in dissimilar ways, their growth and biochemistry are also different. Even though cancer consists of different diseases, all of them have similar neoplasia, anaplasia, and metastasis.

Cancer often originates from agents outside of the human body, illustrated by some cancers occurring in people with similar genetic backgrounds that develop different cancers and live in different countries. A good example is the high incidence of stomach cancer in Japan. If a Japanese person moves to the United States, where stomach cancer rates are low, he or she becomes much less likely to develop the disease. This shows that outside factors are involved, including diet and lifestyle. However, for all people in all countries, the likelihood of older people to develop cancer is higher than for younger people. A 65-year-old person has 10 times higher chances of developing cancer than an adult that is 40 years old. This shows that the development of cancer is a progressive process. Multiple, random changes accumulate with aging, and may be of two types: genetic or epigenetic.

Genetic changes are DNA nucleotide gene sequence mutations or alterations. This affects

Global Epidemiology of Cancer: Diagnosis and Treatment, First Edition. Jahangir Moini, Nicholas G. Avgeropoulos, and Craig Badolato.
© 2022 John Wiley & Sons Ltd. Published 2022 by John Wiley & Sons Ltd.

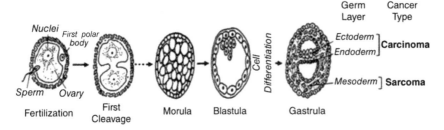

Figure 1.1 Early stages of embryo development and differentiation, leading to the formation of carcinomas and sarcomas. *Source*: Stein and Luebbers [36].

the structure and function of proteins encoded by the affected genes. Mutations may be only changes in one DNA base pair of a gene, known as a **point mutation**. They can also involve a large portion of a chromosome that contains multiple genes being deleted, inserted, duplicated, or translocated. Mutations are either hereditary (familial) or acquired (somatic). Hereditary mutations are also called **germline mutations**. They are inherited from the parents and exist in mostly every body cell. Acquired mutations occur during life, and can be seen only in *some* body cells.

Epigenetic changes influence gene activity and expression, but do not alter the DNA nucleotide sequence. This means that epigenetic changes are not mutations. The two main examples of epigenetic changes are as follows:

- Chemical modification of histones – this means the acetylation, deacetylation, and methylation of special proteins that join with genomic DNA to form chromatin
- Hypomethylation and hypermethylation of cytosine residues in DNA

These epigenetic changes affect the structure and function of **chromatin**, which in turn affects gene expression. If there is histone deacetylation or DNA methylation, chromatin can be condensed. It is then inaccessible for transcription factors required for gene expression. Histone hypoacetylation or DNA hypermethylation can stop the expression of tumor suppressor genes. These genes then cannot prevent the growth and proliferation of cells. This means that carcinogenesis is able to occur.

Every day, we are exposed to carcinogens in the environment that are able to cause both genetic and epigenetic changes (see Figure 1.2). There are three primary categories of carcinogens, as follows:

- Chemical carcinogens – tobacco, alcohol, poor quality foods, arsenic, benzene, beryllium, cadmium, chromium, nickel, radon, vinyl chloride, asbestos
- Biological carcinogens – bacterial or viral infections
- Physical carcinogens – ionizing radiation and ultraviolet radiation

Less often, age-related changes in the immune system and imbalances of hormones contribute to carcinogenesis, and familial genes are also linked to the origin of cancer.

Chemical carcinogens are estimated to cause 80% or more of all cancers. Smoking is a proven cause of lung, oral, pharyngeal, laryngeal, esophageal, colorectal, renal, bladder, hepatic, and cervical cancers, along with acute myeloid leukemia. Tobacco smoke has more than 50 different carcinogenic agents. These include acetaldehyde, benzopyrene, arsenic, and benzene. Chewing tobacco or other smokeless tobacco products increases risks for oral, esophageal, and pancreatic cancers.

The consumption of alcohol is linked to oral, pharyngeal, laryngeal, esophageal, colorectal, hepatic, and breast cancers. Alcohol is thought to increase cancer risks in a variety of ways, which include:

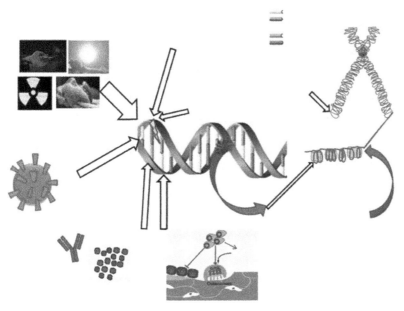

Figure 1.2 The causes of cancer, with mutations due to many different factors. DNA mutations result from the environment, lifestyle choices, epigenetic alterations, viruses, cell microenvironments, heredity, inflammation, and telomere shortening. *Source*: Stein and Luebbers [36].

- Metabolizing ethanol (ethyl alcohol) to acetaldehyde – this is a strong agent with high DNA-damaging characteristics
- Forming reactive oxygen species – via oxidation, these can damage DNA, lipids, and proteins
- Increasing blood levels of estrogen – which is linked to increased risks for breast cancer

Combining alcohol with tobacco smoking results in a much higher risk for a variety of cancers. Asbestos exposure is linked to higher risks for lung cancer and mesothelioma, which is cancer of the pleura lining the chest and abdomen. Asbestos contains six natural fibrous materials. If they enter the deeper lung tissues, they can cause irritation and fibrotic scarring, which has a proven connection with cancer. Therefore, exposure to asbestos eventually results in full-blown lung cancer. Asbestos is released as the brake linings of our cars wear out, and as tires wear down. Asbestos fibers that are inhaled by a smoker increase the risk of developing lung cancer.

About 30% of all types of cancer in the United States and other Westernized countries is related to poor diet. Breast, colorectal, and prostate cancers are highly linked with excessive meat consumption. Animal meat contains proteins, saturated fat, and sometimes, carcinogenic compounds. These include heterocyclic amines as well as polycyclic aromatic hydrocarbons that form as meat is being processed and cooked. Bile acids from the gall bladder chemically alter meat fats inside the intestine, so that the fats can be absorbed. However, bacteria convert the bile acids into *secondary bile acids*, which are carcinogen-promoting agents. High fat content in meat and other animal food sources increases the production of hormones such as estrogen and testosterone, increasing risks for breast and prostate cancers. Many chemicals must be changed inside cells to become carcinogenic. Certain foods and drugs change the enzyme systems that activate carcinogens. For example, phenobarbital stimulates the **P450 enzyme** system, which activates benzopyrene and other carcinogens. Therefore, cancer origination is linked to combinations of dietary and environmental agents.

Coal tar products such as benzopyrene and dibenzanthracene are carcinogens. Benzopyrene is also a hydrocarbon that is converted via oxidation to extremely reactive compounds such as epoxides. The reactions mainly occur by enzyme-driven catalysis in the liver. The activated carcinogens can then affect other body cells.

Bacterial and viral infections are linked to about 15–20% of all cancers. Chronic infection of the stomach wall with *Helicobacter pylori* is implicated in stomach cancer, and *Chlamydia pneumonia*, in lung cancer. Chronic inflammation from bacterial infections is related to the origin of cancer. Inflammation due to parasites is also related. In developing countries, the parasitic flatworm *Schistosomiasis haematobium* is prevalent, and infestation is linked to bladder cancer. In Asia, *Schistosomiasis japonicum* is linked to colorectal cancer. In relation to viruses, two terms that should be understood are *tumor viruses* and *oncoviruses*. There are five DNA tumor viruses. These include Epstein–Barr virus (EBV), hepatitis B virus (HBV), human herpesvirus 8 (HHV8), human papillomavirus (HPV), and Merkel cell polyomavirus (MCV). There are also 2 RNA viruses linked to cancer, which include hepatitis C virus (HCV) and human T lymphotrophic virus type I (HTLV-1). These viruses cause cancer via the introduction of their genetic material into normal host cells.

In a DNA virus, the genetic material that is used is the DNA. In an RNA virus, the genetic material is the RNA that is reverse-transcribed into the DNA. Either way, the amount of DNA needed to cause cancer is only in one tiny part of the virus genome, and is enough to code for one or several proteins. A viral infection alone is usually not enough to cause cancer, so events such as immunosuppression, genetic disposition, exposure to carcinogens, or somatic mutations are also needed. With acquired immune deficiency syndrome (AIDS), the human immunodeficiency virus (HIV) cannot cause cancer directly. However, HIV damages cellular immunity so much that the individual is more likely to be infected with a tumor virus such as HHV8, causing cancer. Therefore, carcinogenesis requires multiple steps, of which a virus is only one.

Physical carcinogens, such as radiation of various types, are all around us. The X-rays and gamma rays that come from outer space, radioactive portions of the earth, or nuclear power plants are all strong carcinogens. These rays are examples of high-frequency ionizing radiation that can contact DNA molecules in cells and result in direct damage. Ionizing radiation can also produce free radicals that react with and damage DNA. When only low doses of this radiation are present, human cells are able to undergo repair, and will survive. All of us are continually exposed to low levels of ionizing radiation from natural sources. However, dosages of X-rays as used in diagnostic equipment, as well as in the body scanners that are used at airports, need to be kept as low as possible.

Ultraviolet radiation from the sun consists of UVA and UVB rays. The DNA of our skin absorbs UVB more easily than UVA. However, both types of UV rays are able to cause cancer. Melanoma is a common skin cancer caused by UV rays. When UVB is absorbed by DNA, it bonds with nearby thymine base pairs in genetic sequence, forming **pyrimidine dimers**. These dimers are normally removed when DNA is repaired, but if the process becomes defective, the cells survive but have been altered by radiation. They can now develop into cancers. The UV radiation from sunlamps and tanning booths is also carcinogenic.

Significant Point

Some of the earliest evidence of cancer was found in fossilized bone tumor, human mummies from ancient Egypt, and in very old manuscripts. The actual oldest description of cancer, though the term was not yet used, was found in Egypt and dated back to approximately 3000 BC. The *Edwin Smith Papyrus* described eight cases of tumors or ulcers of the breast removed by an early method of cauterization. The papyrus described the disease as being otherwise untreatable.

Cancer Biology

Cancer cell biology is controlled by signaling pathways and molecular components. The cells are able to proliferate, avoid attrition, and invade body tissues. Today we know more than ever about the alterations of cancer cells, and these alterations may help us develop better-targeted therapies against the disease. Each type of cancer is different in phenotypes and heterogeneity created from different types of cells, as well as genetic or epigenetic differences. The two common forms of cancer development include *clonal evolution* and the development of the *cancer stem cell* – both of which influence the ability of cancer to metastasize. Another proposed method of cancer development is *plasticity* between non-cancer stem cells and cancer stem cells (CSCs) – the possibility that non-CSCs are able to reacquire a CSC phenotype. Also, there is a theory about cancer development as a result of inflammation.

The clonal evolution of cancer begins with just one cell. The first mutations that occur result in an ability to proliferate spontaneously, without any need for external cytokines, growth factors, or hormones that are usually required for proliferation. The next generations of the cells are predisposed to acquire more mutations, which continually change cellular behavior. Tumor growth and progression occur because of selective growth of cells after multiple mutations (see Figure 1.3). The steps of cancer progression include *initiation* events during the early stages and *promotion* events that signify obvious neoplasia. There may be months to years in between initiation and promotion. Mutagens are agents that cause initiation. They include benzopyrene, found in tobacco smoke, that causes DNA damage. Once damaged, a cell must multiply to become cancerous, which is a process aided by an irritant that acts as a promoter. Examples of irritants include asbestos and **phorbol esters**, which are uncommon products that come from plants. These and other promoters cause DNA-damaged cells to rearrange their chromosomes during multiplication. This causes even more gene changes. Cancer may develop even when there is a lot of time between the exposures to initiators and promoters.

With the retinoblastoma (Rb) gene mutation, we can see that one genetic defect alone is not enough to cause the development of cancer. Additional genetic changes are required, even though the familial Rb mutation does predispose the individual to cancer. The further genetic or epigenetic changes, from continued exposure to chemicals, hormones, or viruses alter the regulating factors that normally control cell proliferation, differentiation, and cell death.

Since stem cells survive much longer than normal cells, there is an increased chance that they may accumulate genetic mutations. It could take just a few mutations for a stem cell to lose control, potentially becoming a source for cancer. CSCs are a rare subset that can self-renew, differentiate into defined daughter cells, and then initiate and sustain tumor growth in vivo. They have distinctive capacities for self-renewal, proliferation, and

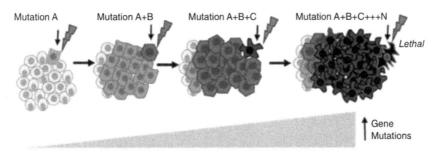

Time to cancer progression (in months and years)

Figure 1.3 The clonal origin of cancer, from one cell, through multiple gene mutations. *Source*: Stein and Luebbers [36].

differentiation. The CSCs are believed to play an important role in cancer initiation, maintenance, progression, resistance to drugs, recurrence, and metastasis. These cells were first identified in leukemia patients during the experimental technique called *xenotransplantation*, and since have been identified in many other malignancies. Treatment failure may be partly due to the ability of CSCs to resist therapy. If they are intrinsically more resistant than other tumor cells, treatments are likely to *increase* the percentage of CSCs in comparison with the percentage before treatment. In a recent study of colon cancer xenografts, the *CD44 + ESA + cells*, which is the population containing colon CSCs, were much greater after treatment with cyclophosphamide.

During cancer progression, tumor cells experience molecular and phenotypic changes. These changes are known as **cellular plasticity**. They are caused by microenvironmental factors, genetic and epigenetic changes, and treatment-related factors. These causes contribute to tumor heterogeneity and resistance to therapy. The most common example of tumor cell plasticity is epithelial–mesenchymal plasticity. The condition of cellular plasticity influences premalignant progression, evolution of tumors, and adaptations to treatments. Changes in cell identity are common at various stages of tumor progression, and it is clear that cellular plasticity is a strong mediator of tumor progression as well as **chemoresistance**. When we understand the mechanisms of cellular plasticity, we may develop new methods of targeting the most lethal aspects – metastasis and resistance to treatment.

Chronic inflammatory processes can develop from infections that are not resolved, abnormal immune reactions to normal tissues, and even obesity. Chronic inflammation leads to DNA damage, and therefore, an increased likelihood of developing cancer. As far back as 1863, an observation was made that cancer often developed at the sites of chronic inflammation. People with chronic inflammatory bowel diseases such as ulcerative colitis and Crohn's disease have an increased risk of colon cancer. As many as 20% of all cancers may be caused or influenced by chronic inflammation. Cytokines are produced, which stimulate the growth of blood vessels that carry nutrients and oxygen to tumors. Free radicals may be generated, causing further DNA damage. Basically, anything that causes inflammation causes DNA to replicate more quickly. The higher the speed of replication, the higher chance of developing cancer. Inflammatory pancreatitis increases risks for pancreatic cancer, and hepatitis increases risks for liver cancer. Chronic inflammation from a *Helicobacter pylori* infection increases risks for stomach cancer. Chronic lung inflammation from asbestos exposure increases risks for mesothelioma. There are many studies investigating the use of anti-inflammatory medications, including aspirin and non-steroidal anti-inflammatory drugs, as a method of reducing the risks for cancer. Inflammation may be the initiator for cancer metastasis as well, by producing chemicals that help tumor cells infiltrate tissues. Table 1.1 summarizes the links between chronic inflammation and cancer.

Table 1.1 Chronic inflammation and various types of cancer.

Inflammatory condition	Causative agents	Types of cancer
Hashimoto thyroiditis, Sjögren syndrome	————	MALT lymphoma
Barrett esophagus, reflux esophagitis	Gastric acid	Esophageal carcinoma
Silicosis, asbestosis	Silica particles, asbestos fibers	Lung carcinoma, mesothelioma
Gastritis, ulcers	*Helicobacter pylori*	Gastric adenocarcinoma, MALT lymphoma

(Continued)

Table 1.1 (Continued)

Inflammatory condition	Causative agents	Types of cancer
Pancreatitis	Alcoholism, germ line mutations, such as of the trypsinogen gene	Pancreatic carcinoma
Chronic cholecystitis	Bacteria, bile acids, gallbladder stones	Gallbladder cancer
Hepatitis	Hepatitis B or C virus	Hepatocellular carcinoma
Cholangitis, opisthorchis	Liver flukes (*Opisthorchis viverrini*)	Cholangiocarcinoma, colon carcinoma
Inflammatory bowel disease	————	Colorectal carcinoma
Osteomyelitis	Bacterial infection	Carcinoma in draining sinuses
Chronic cystitis	Schistosomiasis	Bladder carcinoma
Lichen sclerosis	————	Vulvar squamous cell carcinoma
Chronic cervicitis	Human papillomavirus	Cervical carcinoma

Significant Point

Unlike normal cells, cancer cells grow out of control. They ignore signals that "tell" them to stop dividing, to differentiate, or to die. Cancer cells do not recognize their own boundaries and can spread to other sites in the body. Several genes mutate in cancer cells and their function becomes defective. Abnormal cell division occurs when active oncogenes are expressed, or when tumor suppressor genes are lost.

Genetics and Cancer

There are genetic conditions that make the development of cancer more likely, though they do not actually cause it. Familial polyposis is one example, in which there are polyps or other small growths in the intestinal tract. These can easily transform into cancer. When a person has such a genetic defect, the chance of developing cancer is higher because the DNA is not repaired very well. Conditions that involve inherited defects of the DNA repair system include **Bloom syndrome, Fanconi anemia**, and **Werner syndrome**. Mutations of the DNA repair genes *breast cancer 1 (BRCA1), breast cancer 2 (BRCA2), tumor protein p53*, and *retinoblastoma (Rb)* are linked to inherited breast, ovarian, pancreatic, and prostate cancers. These particular genes are also described as *tumor suppressor genes*. To avoid the development of cancer, it is crucial that damaged DNA can be correctly repaired. Even so, a large number of cancers are not inherited. Generally, inherited mutations are present in about 7.5% of all cancers. Today, there is ongoing study about hereditary genetic mutations that increase the likelihood of cancer development, to use this information for the surveillance and prevention of cancer. Table 1.2 illustrates specific cancer genes with inherited predisposition for specific cancerous conditions.

Genetic tests for hereditary cancer syndromes can detect if a person from a family that shows the signs of a syndrome has a suspected gene mutation. The tests also show if family members with no obvious signs of disease have the same gene mutation. Genetic testing is often recommended when there is a personal or family

Table 1.2 Specific cancer genes with inherited predispositions for cancer.

Cancer genes	Inherited predisposition
Autosomal dominant cancer syndromes	
APC	Familial adenomatous polyposis/colon cancer
BRCA1, BRCA2	Breast and ovarian tumors
CDKN2A	Melanoma
MEN1, RET	Multiple endocrine neoplasia 1 and 2
MLH1, MSH2, MSH6	Hereditary nonpolyposis colon cancer
NF1, NF2	Neurofibromatosis 1 and 2
PTCH1	Nevoid basal cell carcinoma syndrome
RB	Retinoblastoma
TP53	Li–Fraumeni syndrome, with various tumors
Autosomal recessive syndromes, with defective DNA repair	
ATM	Ataxia-telangiectasia
BLM	Bloom syndrome
Various genes involved in DNA cross-link repair	Fanconi anemia
Various genes involved in nucleotide excision repair	Xeroderma pigmentosum

history suggesting an inherited cancer risk condition. This type of testing is often very helpful in guiding future medical treatments. If a cancer susceptibility variant is present in a family, not everyone who inherits the variant automatically develops cancer. This is influenced by **penetrance**. When not everyone carrying the variant develops the disease related to the variant, it is said to have *incomplete* or *reduced* penetrance. Hereditary cancer syndromes also vary in expressivity. This means that those with the variant may be different in the extent that they exhibit signs and symptoms of the syndrome. Disease expression is also influenced by lifestyle and environment. An extended list of hereditary cancer syndromes includes the following:

- BRCA1 hereditary breast and ovarian cancer syndrome – also called familial susceptibility to breast/ovarian cancer 1 or BROVCA1
- BRCA2 hereditary breast and ovarian cancer syndrome – also called familial susceptibility to breast/ovarian cancer 2 or BROVCA2
- Cowden syndrome – also called Cowden disease
- Diaphyseal medullary stenosis with malignant fibrous histiocytoma – also called bone dysplasia with medullary fibrosarcoma
- Duodenal carcinoid syndrome
- Endolymphatic sac tumor
- Familial adenomatous polyposis
- Familial isolated pituitary adenoma
- Gardner syndrome
- Hereditary diffuse gastric cancer
- Hirschsprung disease ganglioneuroblastoma
- Li–Fraumeni syndrome
- Lynch syndrome
- Multiple endocrine neoplasia type 1 (MEN1)

- Multiple endocrine neoplasia type 2A (MEN2A)
- Multiple endocrine neoplasia type 2B (MEN2B), and formerly, multiple endocrine neoplasia type 3
- Perlman syndrome
- Pheochromocytoma
- Stewart Treves syndrome
- Von Hippel–Lindau disease

Significant Point

Though nearly every family has members that have had cancer, this does not generally mean they have a hereditary predisposition. Most cases of cancer originate from a combination of external influences such as environmental and lifestyle factors, along with a small genetic component. Only a genetic defect can be inherited – in other words, a genetic predisposition, but not cancer itself.

Cell Division

Complicated regulatory networks cause cells to proliferate and maintain homeostasis in tissues or organs that they originated in. The circuits within these networks are made up of enzymes and proteins. Their expression as well as activity is linked to mitogenic signals from cytokines, growth factors, and other extracellular molecules in the surrounding tissues. Random gene mutations encoding the enzymes and proteins disrupt activation and expression, allowing cells to change in function, increasing the likelihood of cancer. All types of cancer need the following six characteristics to progress to metastatic cancer:

- Proliferative autonomy
- Resistance to anti-proliferative signals
- Evasion of **apoptosis**
- Unlimited ability to replicate
- Tumor neovascularization
- Invasion and metastasis

Cell division occurs step by step, through four unique phases or periods (see Figure 1.4). The steps are described as follows:

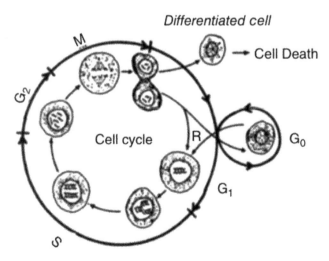

Figure 1.4 The cell cycle and differentiation, in which each division will result in two daughter cells being generated. Note that cancer cells stay in the cycle without differentiating or entering G0, regardless of any improper conditions. *Source*: Stein and Luebbers [36].

- Gap 1 (G1) – A biochemically active period involving synthesis of protein and RNA as the cells grow before dividing; this lasts until the start of DNA synthesis
- Synthesis (S) – The cells start to duplicate genetic material
- Gap 2 (G2) – Newly replicated chromatin is condensed, forming chromosomes
- Mitosis (M) – Duplicated chromosomes separate, and cell division begins; if there is a lack of enough nutrients or growth factors, cells exit their cycle to enter a resting state known as quiescence or G0; if conditions become favorable again, the cells can reenter the cell cycle; the "decision" to remain in the cycle or go into quiescence is made during G1

Also, after mitosis (M), cells can exit the cycle and differentiate, performing different variations of normal functions. For example, nerve cells can conduct impulses and muscle cells can cause contraction.

Significant Point

In 2020, it was reported that the protein LEM2 was discovered to have two important functions during cell division. The protein first creates "seals" in the protective coating of nuclei that are forming, keeping the two sets of DNA from being damaged. Next, LEM2 recruits factors that disassemble the "machinery" of fibers that are responsible for separating the DNA sets. Scientists devised a method that allowed them to actually view this process in the laboratory.

Cell Cycle

The events in the cell cycle are regulated by proteins, such as cyclins and cyclin-dependent kinases (CDKs). This means that the cells will only divide when necessary, when circumstances are adequate. Normal cells need the mitogenic signals from external growth factors. These growth factors include the following:

- Epidermal growth factor (EGF)
- Fibroblast growth factor (FGF)
- Platelet-derived growth factor (PDGF)
- Insulin-like growth factor (IGF)

These growth factors help the cells to move from the G0 state into active proliferation. Growth factors bind to similar transmembrane receptors. They transmit mitogenic signals required for G0 or G1 phase cells to grow and conduct proper DNA synthesis. When growth factors are not present, normal cells stop dividing. However, cancer cells are different, continuing to divide regardless of whether growth factors are present. This is proliferative autonomy, occurring because of genetic or epigenetic changes that may change the structure of growth factor receptors, or cause extreme overexpression of the growth factors. In some breast cancers, shortened EGF receptor (EGFR) continually sends signals that stimulate growth even when there is no EGF binding. In various other breast cancers, *human epidermal growth factor receptor 2 (HER2)/neural (neu)* receptor overexpression causes cells to be over-responsive to low levels of growth factor, which usually would be insufficient to cause cell division.

Cells also contain integrins, which are transmembrane receptors that can promote the active cell cycle. Integrin receptors are heterodimer proteins. They attach the cytoskeletons of cells to extracellular matrix, which makes up about 30% of the tissue in each organ. The extracellular matrix is noncellular material consisting of a "mesh" of glycoproteins, proteins, proteoglycans, and polysaccharides. These substances provide structure and biochemical activity, along with being needed for chemical signaling. There are 24 or more heterodimer integrin receptors. They are formed by 18 alpha-subunits combining with 8 beta-subunits, and have specific binding to certain protein portions on the extracellular matrix. Integrin receptors are activated to generate signals in cells that influence their proliferation, survival, migration, and invasion. In cancer, integrin heterodimers that favor growth and proliferation are significantly upregulated.

Proliferative autonomy is also due to changes in fundamentals of downstream effector proteins. These proteins receive and process signals from ligand-activated growth factor receptors as well as integrin receptors. Proliferative signaling in normal tissues is opposed by many anti-proliferative signals, which result in cellular quiescence. Tissue homeostasis requires this delicate balance. Anti-proliferative signals come from growth inhibitory molecules on the surface of contacted nearby cells, or within the extracellular matrix. The signals also come from soluble growth inhibitory factors.

Growth and proliferation of normal cells are regulated via interactions between growth factor signaling, nutrient availability, and cell density. Normal cells require a minimum area of space that they can spread in, for normal growth. Cells that are widely spaced grow and divide, eventually covering all available space. With increased cell density, the cells touch each other. Movements are restricted, and growth stops even though there are enough nutrients and growth factors. This is called *density dependent* or *contact inhibition* of cell growth and proliferation. This is needed to regulate normal tissue growth, differentiation, and development. Contact inhibition regulates the size of each organ as it develops. When tissues are injured, it also plays a role. If the liver is partially resected, the hepatocytes become mobilized for rapid division so that the organ can regenerate. Upon reaching its normal size, the liver stops growing – controlled by the hepatocytes to prevent overgrowth. Most cancer cells do not behave in this manner – continuing to grow and proliferate regardless.

Programmed cell death, or apoptosis, is a genetically controlled type of cell death that occurs naturally, often initiated by the Fas ligand and tumor necrosis factor (see Figure 1.5). Dysfunctional or unneeded cells within tissues self-destruct, known as *cellular suicide*. This occurs in what appear to be normal physiological conditions. Over 10 billion cells self-destruct every day in the human body, balancing the production of new cells from stem cells. Apoptosis is needed for tissue homeostasis, immune tolerance, and embryogenesis. It stops unwanted cell proliferation, which could lead to tumorigenesis. If apoptosis becomes dysregulated, there can be one of two conditions:

- Tissue outgrowth – cells die slower than they can divide, as in cancer
- Tissue atrophy – cells die faster than they can divide, as in neurodegenerative diseases

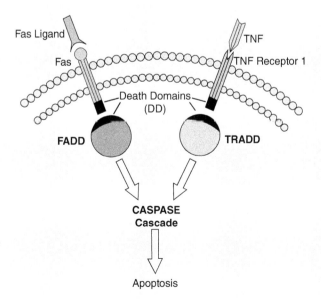

Figure 1.5 Apoptosis, as related to the effects of the Fas ligand and tumor necrosis factor (TNF). *Source:* Israels and Israels [18].

Carcinogenesis

Cancer cells, to continue proliferating, must acquire *replicative immortality*. For carcinogenesis, the cells must overcome *replicative senescence*. **Telomeres** are structures of DNA protein at the ends of chromosomes. They are the primary determinant of replicative potentials of cells. They protect the ends of linear chromosomes from fusing together, which maintains genome function, integrity, and stability. Telomeres have several **kilobase pairs** of double-stranded DNA. The pairs are made of hexanucleotides sequence repeats. The **end replication problem** is caused by a limitation of the DNA polymerases to completely replicate the ends of chromosome DNA duplexes. Therefore, the DNA polymerase that duplicates chromosomal DNA leaves 50–200 base pairs in the ends of telomeric DNA strands unreplicated. This causes telomere shortening after each round of DNA replication. Since most somatic cells do not express telomerase, their telomeres are progressively shortened, reaching a dangerously short length as telomeres become dysfunctional. Cells that do not enter senescence die from p53-controlled apoptosis. Senescence and apoptosis help prevent proliferation of cells that are at risk of genome instability, which may lead to neoplastic transformation. Just one in 10

million cells that survive experience genome instability, acquiring gene mutations. They can develop unlimited proliferative potential, known as **immortalization**, from additional genetic or epigenetic changes. The catalytic subunit of telomerase (*telomerase reverse transcriptase*) is expressed. It activates telomerase, stabilizing telomeres for continued proliferation. Nearly all (90%) of cancer cells need telomerase for stability of the telomeres. The other 10% experience *alternative lengthening of telomeres*. So, telomere dysfunction and genome instability, without normal senescence or an apoptotic response with telomere stabilization, allow cells to have unlimited proliferation.

The p53 protein is usually mutated late during tumorigenesis in the majority of organs, but primarily the bladder, colon, pancreas, and prostate. However, p53 mutation is also found in ductal cell carcinoma in situ, which is a *premalignant* lesion of the breast. Also, p53 is lost or mutated early in tumorigenesis of astrocytomas and esophageal adenocarcinomas. In liver cancer, p53 as well as pRb may be eliminated early during tumorigenesis. Germline p53 mutations are linked to carcinomas of the adrenal cortex, breast, gastrointestinal tract, lungs, sarcomas of soft tissues and bone, and lymphomas – but at much earlier ages than expected. Germline pRb mutations are linked to childhood retinoblastoma, plus a predisposition for osteosarcoma. There appears to be a strong relationship between loss of pRb and lack of functional p53 in different tumors. Loss of function of both p53 and pRb is needed for cancer cells to have replicative immortality and to become tumorigenic.

Tumor cells, like normal cells, need a good supply of nutrients and oxygen, plus ways to discharge carbon dioxide and metabolic waste. Primary sources for this are the blood vessels and lymphatic vessels. During pre-malignancy, tumors are separated from vascularized peritumoral tissue by a basal lamina. This does not allow blood vessels to infiltrate the tumors. Without vasculature, tumors stop growing past about 1–2 mm in diameter, becoming necrotic or apoptotic. Tumors must have neovascularization that can deliver blood to intratumoral spaces for survival and transformation into a fully malignant form. Neovascularization is mostly achieved via angiogenesis, in which new blood vessels develop from preexisting vessels.

Angiogenesis starts as vascular endothelial cells being to proliferate, as a response to angiogenic stimuli. They then acquire an angiogenic phenotype. In adults, endothelial cells of mature blood vessels are mostly dormant and only divide once per every 1,000 days. Endothelial cell growth and proliferation initiates angiogenesis. Hypoxia or oncogene activation causes the cells of quickly growing tumors to secrete vascular endothelial growth factor (VEGF) and basic fibroblast growth factor. These factors diffuse through nearby tissues, binding to similar receptors on endothelial cells of preexisting blood vessels. The endothelial cells are stimulated to secrete proteases such as **matrix metalloproteases** (MMPs). These degrade the basement membrane and the peri-vascular extracellular matrix. Proliferating endothelial cells can then escape and migrate toward the source of the angiogenic stimulus. *Primary sprouts* are formed, and extending sprouts have two distinct forms of endothelial cells: *tip cells* and *stalk cells.*

Tip cells only proliferate slightly, but allow breakdown of the extracellular matrix around preexisting blood vessels. There is growth of new sprouts toward tumor cells secreting angiogenic factors. The stalk cells have active proliferation, extending sprouts and promoting the formation of the vascular lumen. The endothelial cells stabilize the vasculature via secretion of the platelet-derived growth factor. This attracts pericytes and smooth muscle cells, forming a basement membrane around new vesicles. Without the basement membrane, the new vessels are unstable and often regress. The formed blood vessels bring blood to the tumors and sustain the proliferating tumor cells.

Antiangiogenic molecules also regulate angiogenesis. Proangiogenic factors must be accompanied with downregulation of antiangiogenic molecules that restrict vascular growth. The most prevalent proangiogenic factor is VEGF. The levels of angiogenic factors and their receptors are prognostic about the state of cancer progression. Expression of the VEGF family of angiogenic factors is linked to the progression of breast, colon, head and neck, lung, stomach, and uterine cancers. The amount of neovascularization between these cancers is varied, however. Highly aggressive pancreatic ductal carcinomas are largely avascular, while renal and pancreatic neuroendocrine carcinomas are highly vascularized. This is because some tumors form and progress by using preexisting vessels without angiogenesis.

Natural antiangiogenic factors include **angiostatin**, thrombospondin-1 (TSP-1), endostatin, interferon, and metalloprotease inhibitors. They can cause apoptosis in tumor cells and endothelial cells. They also block migration and formation of lumens in sprouting endothelial cells. The factors are often downregulated in tumors, from loss of function of tumor suppressor genes. Synthetic inhibitors of angiogenesis include sorafenib, sunitinib, and temsirolimus. They are being studied in combination with chemotherapies to treat various aggressive cancers. Antiangiogenic drugs may improve the delivery of chemotherapy to tumors by normalizing tumor blood vessels. New vessels in tumors are both structurally and functionally abnormal. The blood vessels are immature, and leakage occurs. Such abnormalities affect the delivery of chemotherapies to tumors. Because of excessive proangiogenic stimuli, antiangiogenic drugs may normalize tumor vessels by neutralizing angiogenic stimuli. However, antiangiogenic drugs interfere with blood pressure, wound healing, clotting, and kidney function – increasing risks for heart attacks and strokes. Newer antiangiogenic drugs with selective effects on tumor vessels are needed to treat aggressive cancers.

Significant Point

The basics of carcinogenesis include oncogenes – the genes that are activated in tumors – acting at key stages of proliferation, differentiation, and programmed apoptosis, gene mutations that lead to cells no longer responding to external regulation, and combined disorders of several oncogenes that lead to malignant transformation.

Mutation and Cancer

Gene mutations related to cancer can be extremely varied. **Driver mutations** are those that change the function of cancer genes, directly contributing to the disease's development and progression. Driver mutations are usually acquired and less often inherited. **Passenger mutations** are acquired and do not affect cellular behavior. They occur randomly, throughout the entire genome, while driver mutations are usually clustered tightly in cancer genes. In cancers caused by carcinogen exposure, such as lung cancer and melanoma, there are many more passenger mutations than driver mutations. The carcinogens that a person is exposed to directly cause most genomic damage. Passenger mutations create genetic variants that may give tumor cells an advantage over normal cells. There may be mutations that result in drug resistance. It appears that the effects of treatment convert neutral passenger mutations *into* driver mutations, making the cancer more difficult to cure or treat.

Point mutations activate or inactivate protein production by affected genes, based on position and strength. These mutations, when converting proto-oncogenes into oncogenes usually produce a gain or function. They do this by changing amino acid residues in part of the microenvironment that usually keeps the protein's activity controlled. A good example is with the proteins that convert the RAS gene into a cancer gene. Oppositely, point mutations in tumor suppressor genes limit or stop functions of the encoded proteins. The TP53 gene is often affected by point mutations.

Gene rearrangements may be caused by chromosomal inversions or translocations. These occurrences are greatly linked with neoplasms that are derived from hematopoietic and other mesenchymal cells. There are two ways that gene rearrangements activate proto-oncogenes, as follows:

- Removing proto-oncogenes from normal regulatory elements – the rearrangements place them under the control of a highly active enhancer or promoter, as occurs with B cell lymphomas. In over 90% of patients with Burkitt lymphoma, there is a translocation, usually between chromosomes 8 and 14. This results in overexpression of the MYC gene on chromosome 8, via juxtaposition with regulatory elements of the immunoglobulin heavy chain gene on chromosome 14. With follicular lymphomas, there is a reciprocating translocation between chromosomes 14 and 18. This results in the overexpression of BCL2 on chromosome 18, and is also controlled by immunoglobulin gene regulatory elements.

- Creation of fusion genes that encode certain chimeric proteins – for example, with the Philadelphia chromosome in chronic myeloid leukemia, there is a balanced, reciprocal translocation between chromosomes 9 and 22. Therefore, the Philadelphia chromosome (22) appears smaller than usual. This change occurs in over 90% of chronic myeloid leukemia cases. It causes fusion of parts of the BCR gene on chromosome 22, and of the ABL gene on chromosome 9. The small amounts of Philadelphia chromosome-negative cases have a cytogenetically silent BCR-ABL fusion gene. Its presence is the essential component of chronic myeloid leukemia.

Chromosomal translocations have two modes of alteration. They can break initially, followed by more mobility of their broken ends, resulting in juxtaposition. The second mode is when they contact each other initially, suffering breaks, and then juxtaposition – see Figure 1.6.

   Deletions are also common, in which specific chromosomal regions are removed, which can cause the loss of certain tumor suppressor genes. There is often an inactivating point mutation in one allele. This is then followed by the deletion of the other allele, even though it is not mutated. **Gene amplifications** convert proto-oncogenes to oncogenes, with resulting overexpression and hyperactivity of proteins that would otherwise be normal. There can be several hundred copies of the gene, with either multiple small, extrachromosomal structures known as **double minutes**, or *homogenously staining regions*. Important examples of gene amplifications include the NMYC gene (neuroblastoma) and the HER2 gene (breast cancer). **Aneuploidy** is the number of chromosomes that is not a multiple of 23, which is often linked to cancer.

Significant Point

Usually, several gene mutations are needed before a cell becomes malignant. Most cancers begin because of acquired gene mutations over time. Sometimes the mutations are caused by external factors such as tobacco use or exposure to sunlight, but they can also be random events that happen without any understood cause. Genetic testing is indicated if one or more family members already have a known gene mutation.

Metastasis

Metastasis is the deadliest occurrence related to cancer. Tumor cells invade nearby tissues and use the blood or lymphatic vessels to spread, when conditions for this are favorable. Whether a blood or lymphatic vessel is entered is based on the amount and easiness of accessibility of the

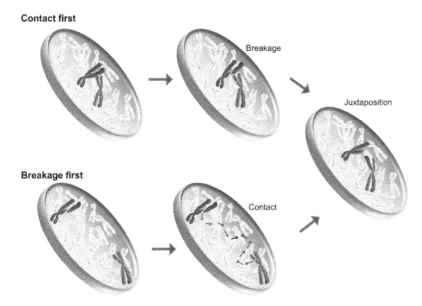

Figure 1.6 The two modes of alteration in chromosomal translocations. *Source*: Javadekar and Raghavan [19].

vessels. A vasculature network formed by angiogenesis means that cancer cells are more accessible to blood vessels than lymphatic vessels. Often, lymphatic vessels within tumors are not as highly functional as those formed outside of tumors. Tumor cells must then invade through nearby connective tissues to enter functional lymphatic vessels. So, most tumor cells utilize the bloodstream for invasion and metastasis. Those that enter the lymphatic vessels often eventually also enter the blood vessels, since the lymphatic vessels drain into the venous blood as they join the large thoracic duct. On the way to the thoracic duct, a series of lymph nodes can be encountered. They are often the first sites of tumor cell metastasis. The tumor cells can also invade localized lymph nodes directly via penetration through nearby connective tissue. This is why lymph nodes closer to a primary tumor are evaluated for tumor cells, as an early indicator of metastasis.

Metastasis involves migration (invasion) of tumor cells at the initial site into surrounding normal tissues to reach blood or lymphatic vessels. The cells must **intravasate** the endothelial barrier to enter the circulation. They must **extravasate** from a distant capillary bed so that they can colonize (grow) at a secondary location (see Figure 1.7).

Invasion is the first step in metastasis, involving migration of tumor cells toward the blood or lymphatic vessels. Solid tumor cells must cross the basement membrane, an extracellular matrix made of collagen and many other cell types. Metastasizing cells then migrate through the extracellular matrix to reach the blood or lymphatic vessels. For motility, cancer cells develop morphological and migratory characteristics; due to changes in the expression of oncogenes and tumor suppressor genes. These cells usually have increased contractility, migrating individually or in a stream of cells. However, cells with a mesenchymal phenotype have lower contractility, migrating in clusters of at least five cells – such as with breast and colorectal tumors.

Tumor cells must use genes involved in embryonic development to develop factors needed for them to invade and metastasize. Tumor cells acquire an epithelial–mesenchymal transition (EMT)-regulated mesenchymal phenotype during invasion. However, they later change to the epithelial phenotype in metastasized tumors at a secondary location. They are similar, both

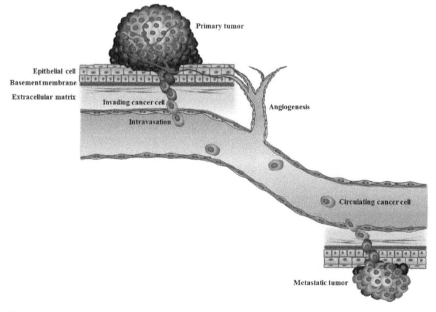

Figure 1.7 Biological processes linked to cancer spread from a primary site to other body organs. *Source:* Courtesy: "From Invasion to Metastasis".

histopathologically and morphologically, to cells in primary tumors before EMT. Therefore, the mesenchymal phenotype is only temporary, during invasion and metastasis. Returning to an epithelial phenotype requires a reversal of the EMT process, called *mesenchymal–epithelial transition* (MET). The metastasized cells become noninvasive so that they can grow and colonize at the secondary location. These transitions are still not fully understood.

Intravasation, the entry of cancer cells into the blood or lymphatic vessels, determines the amount of tumor cells that will metastasize, and the likelihood of tumor formation at another body site. Intravasation occurs naturally as part of embryonic development, wound healing, and to fight infections. The ability of cancer cells to intravasate the vessels is not as efficient as it is in these processes. Tumor cells can intravasate lymphatic vessels more easily, since cell–cell junctions of endothelial cells in peripheral lymphatic walls have spaces of about 3 μm – large enough for cancer cells to squeeze through. In the blood vessels, the junctions are much tighter, and endothelial cells are also supported by a basement membrane stabilized with **pericytes**. To cross, the cancer cells must experience cytoskeletal changes as well as upregulate integrins and other adhesion molecules. Also, macrophages exiting blood vessels produce the EGF, which guides cancer cells to them. Cancer cells with the mesenchymal phenotype may be able to move with endothelial cells to enter blood vessels at locations where the macrophages exit. Cancer cells can also passively enter the circulation via **tumor neovasculature**. Usually, the vasculature of tumors is disorganized and leaky. The looser vascular basement membrane plus endothelial cells and pericytes create holes that are about 2.5 μm in size, allowing cancer cells to move through. Growing tumors push cells against the blood vessels, forcing them through the holes. Entry of cancer cells in this way does not greatly disrupt the basement membrane.

In the bloodstream, there are damaging mechanical forces, including those from blood flow itself. **Shear stress** is so extreme that more than 99.9% of cancer cells die in a few minutes. Cytoskeletons are fragmented, and the cells become microparticles absorbed by myeloid cells. However, the cells can be shielded if they aggregate along with platelets and coagulation factors into **cell pellets**. The cancer cells in the center can survive. Also, single cancer cells with an amoeboid-like morphology usually survive by attaching to the substratum, and developing more contractility.

Circulating tumor cells also have to evade the immune system. Cells in solid tumors are protected by the strong immunosuppressive microenvironment within the tumors. Once a tumor cell is in the bloodstream, they are exposed to aggressive antitumor activity and destruction. Natural killer (NK) cells are the biggest threat. They contain *NK group 2d (NKG2D)* receptors able to recognize *major histocompatibility complex (MHC)* class 1 polypeptide-related sequences A and B, also known as *MICA* and *MICB*. These are expressed on malignant cell surfaces. *Cytolytic granzyme B* and **perforin** are secreted, which destroy tumor cells.

Colonization of tumor cells at secondary sites is the least efficient part of the metastatic process. Most tumor cells that infiltrate distant organs are unable to develop overt metastasis. They must colonize the tissues, which of course sometimes occurs. The most likely sites in which this occurs include the bones and liver. Tumor cells must *seed* or colonize, and some organs allow them to do this with much greater ease than other organs. Effective colonization is also based on tumor cells' intrinsic ability to survive hostile tissue environments. Infiltrated tumor cells express specific genes in various organs that encourage metastatic growth.

Transendothelial migration is better in the liver and bones, compared with the brain and lungs. In the liver and bones, there are sinusoidal capillaries consisting of discontinuous basal lamina and fenestrated endothelial cells. These allow extravasation and a higher incidence of metastasis. In the lungs, the tight endothelial junctions are not as conducive for extravasation. Brain capillary walls are also strengthened by **astrocytes** and pericytes that make up the blood–brain barrier.

<table>
<tr><td>

Significant Point

When cancer metastasizes, there can be some signs and symptoms that may resemble those of a variety of other diseases. These include progressive

</td><td>

headaches, weakness, seizures, balance problems, pain, bone fractures, dizziness, shortness of breath, jaundice, and inflammation in body areas related to the type of cancer. In some patients, metastatic cancer causes no symptoms, and is discovered incidentally.

</td></tr>
</table>

Key Terms

Aneuploidy
Angiostatin
Apoptosis
Astrocytes
Bloom syndrome
Cell pellets
Cellular plasticity
Chemoresistance
Chromatin
Deletions
Double minutes
Driver mutations
Ectoderm
Endoderm
End replication problem
Epigenetic
Extravasate
Fanconi anemia
Gene amplifications
Gene rearrangements
Germline mutations

Immortalization
Intravasate
Intravasation
Invasion
Kilobase pairs
Matrix metalloproteases
Mesoderm
Metastasis
P450 enzyme
Passenger mutations
Penetrance
Perforin
Pericytes
Phorbol esters
Point mutation
Pyrimidine dimers
Shear stress
Telomeres
Tumor neovasculature
Werner syndrome

Bibliography

1 Ahmad, A. (2016). *Introduction to Cancer Metastasis*. Cambridge: Academic Press.

2 Armstrong, S. (2014). *P53: The Gene that Cracked the Cancer Code*. London: Bloomsbury Sigma.

3 Banfalvi, G. (2017). *Cell Cycle Synchronization: Methods and Protocols (Methods in Molecular Biology, 1524)*, 2nd Edition. Totowa: Humana Press.

4 Bunz, F. (2016). *Principles of Cancer Genetics*, 2nd Edition. New York: Springer.

5 Chen, G.G. and Lai, P.B.S. (2009). *Apoptosis in Carcinogenesis and Chemotherapy (Apoptosis in Cancer)*. New York: Springer.

6 Compton, C. (2020). *Cancer: The Enemy from Within: A Comprehensive Textbook of Cancer's Causes, Complexities and Consequences*. New York: Springer.

7 DeVita, V.T., Jr., Lawrence, T.S., and Rosenberg, S.A. (2020). *Cancer: Principles and Practice of Oncology: Primer of the Molecular Biology of Cancer*, 3rd Edition. Philadelphia: Lippincott, Williams, and Wilkins.

8 Evens, A.M. and Blum, K.A. (2016). *Non-Hodgkin Lymphoma: Pathology, Imaging, and Current Therapy, Indexed in PubMed/Medline (Cancer Treatment and Research)*. New York: Springer.

9 Fang, D. and Han, J. (2020). *Histone Mutations and Cancer (Advances in Experimental Medicine and Biology, 1283)*. New York: Springer.

10 Frank, D.A. (2012). *Signaling Pathways in Cancer Pathogenesis and Therapy*. New York: Springer.

11 Gerstman, B.S. (2020). *The Physics of Cancer: Research Advances*. Singapore: World Scientific Publishing Company Pte. Ltd.

12 Gilkes, D.M. (2019). *Hypoxia and Cancer Metastasis (Advances in Experimental Medicine and Biology, 1136)*. New York: Springer.

13 Giordano, A. and Galderisi, U. (2010). *Cell Cycle Regulation and Differentiation in Cardiovascular and Neural Systems*. New York: Springer.

14 Gotta, M. and Meraldi, P. (2017). *Cell Division Machinery and Disease (Advances in Experimental Medicine and Biology, 1002)*. New York: Springer.

15 Gregory, C.D. (2016). *Apoptosis in Cancer Pathogenesis and Anti-cancer Therapy: New Perspectives and Opportunities (Advances in Experimental Medicine and Biology, 930)*. New York: Springer.

16 Grundman, E. (2012). *Current Topics in Pathology, 67: Carcinogenesis*. New York: Springer.

17 Heim, S. and Mitelman, F. (2015). *Cancer Cytogenetic: Chromosomal and Molecular Genetic Aberrations of Tumor Cells*, 4th Edition. Hoboken: Wiley-Blackwell.

18 Israels, L.G. and Israels, E.D. (2009). *Stem Cells Journals Volume 17, Issue 5, P. 306–313 Special Feature: Apoptosis*. Durham: AlphaMed Press. Figure 4.

19 Javadekar, S.M. and Raghavan, S.C. (2015). *The FEBS Journal Volume 282, Issue 14, P. 2627–2645 Review Article: Snaps and Mends: DNA Breaks and Chromosomal Translocations*. Cambridge: Federation of European Biochemical Societies. Figure 6.

20 Juan, H.F. and Huang, H.C. (2018). *A Practical Guide to Cancer Systems Biology*. Singapore: World Scientific Publishing Company Pte. Ltd.

21 Kleinsmith, L. (2005). *Principles of Cancer Biology*. Upper Saddle River: Pearson.

22 Lyden, D., Welch, D.R., and Psaila, B. (2011). *Cancer Metastasis: Biologic Basis and Therapeutics*. Cambridge: Cambridge University Press.

23 Martin, T.A. and Jiang, W.G. (2013). *Tight Junctions in Cancer Metastasis (Cancer Metastasis – Biology and Treatment, 19)*. New York: Springer.

24 Maxwell, C. and Roskelley, C. (2015). *Genomic Instability and Cancer Metastasis: Mechanisms, Emerging Themes, and Novel Therapeutic Strategies (Cancer Metastasis – Biology and Treatment, 20)*. New York: Springer.

25 McIntosh, J.R. (2019). *Understanding Cancer: An Introduction to the Biology, Medicine, and Societal Implications of This Disease*. New York: Garland Science.

26 Mercier, I., Jasmin, J.F., and Lisanti, M.P. (2012). *Caveolins in Cancer Pathogenesis, Prevention and Therapy (Current Cancer Research)*. New York: Springer.

27 Morgan, D.O. (2006). *The Cell Cycle: Principles of Control (Primers in Biology)*. Sunderland: Sinauer Associates, Inc.

28 Nikiforov, Y.E., Biddinger, P.W., and Thompson, L.D.R. (2019). *Diagnostic Pathology and Molecular Genetics of the Thyroid: A Comprehensive Guide for Practicing Thyroid Pathology*, 3rd Edition. Philadelphia: Lippincott, Williams, and Wilkins.

29 Noguchi, E. and Gadaleta, M.C. (2014). *Cell Cycle Control: Mechanisms and Protocols (Methods in Molecular Biology, 1170)*, 2nd Edition. Totowa: Humana Press.

30 Pecorino, L. (2016). *Molecular Biology of Cancer: Mechanisms, Targets, and*

Therapeutics, 4th Edition. Oxford: Oxford University Press.

31 Pezzella, F., Tavassoli, M., and Kerr, D. (2019). *Oxford Textbook of Cancer Biology (Oxford Textbooks in Oncology)*. Oxford: Oxford University Press.

32 Poirier, M.C. (2018). *Carcinogens, DNA Damage and Cancer Risk: Mechanisms of Chemical Carcinogenesis*. Singapore: World Scientific Publishing Pte. Ltd.

33 Prodi, G., Liotta, L.A., Lollini, P.L., Garbisa, S., Gorini, S., and Hellmann, K. (2013). *Cancer Metastasis: Biological and Biochemical Mechanisms and Clinical Aspects (Advances in Experimental Medicine and Biology)*. *Volume*. 233, New York: Springer.

34 Seyfried, T. (2012). *Cancer as a Metabolic Disease: On the Origin, Management, and Prevention of Cancer*. Hoboken: Wiley.

35 Sompayrac, L. (2004). *How Cancer Works*. Burlington: Jones & Bartlett Learning.

36 Stein, G.S. and Luebbers, K.P. (2019). *Cancer: Prevention, Early Detection, Treatment and Recovery*, 2nd Edition. Hoboken: Wiley-Blackwell. Figure 2 from Page 17, Figure 1 from Page 54, Figure 3 from Page 23, Figure 4 from Page 25, Figure 10 from Page 41.

37 Tassan, J.P. and Kubiak, J.Z. (2017). *Asymmetric Cell Division in Development, Differentiation and Cancer (Results and Problems in Cell Differentiation, 61)*. New York: Springer.

38 Weinberg, R.A. (2013). *The Biology of Cancer*, 2nd Edition. New York: W.W. Norton & Company.

2

Global Epidemiology of Cancer

OUTLINE
Incidence Prevalence Survival Distribution of Cancer by Gender, Race, and Age Global Burden of Cancer in Men and Women Global Trends in Cancer Global Prevalence of Cancer Global Incidence and Mortality Mortality due to Cancer in the United States Risk Factors for Cancer Development Years of Life Lost Disability-Adjusted Life Years Global Cancer Prevention Key Terms Bibliography

Incidence

Incidence is a measurement of the likelihood that a specific medical condition will occur in a selected population, within a certain period of time. It focuses on new cases within a certain time period. According to the International Agency for Research on Cancer, part of the World Health Organization, in 2020, there were 19.3 million new cases, and 10 million deaths related to cancer. Table 2.1 summarizes the top 20 most common types of cancer, as of 2018 – the most recent year this list was updated.

In the United States alone, there were 1.8 million new cases of cancer, and nearly 607,000 related deaths in 2020. According to the American Cancer Society, the following were the most common types of cancer:

- Breast cancer (female) – 276,480 cases and 42,170 deaths
- Lung cancer, including bronchial cancer – 228,820 cases and 135,720 deaths
- Prostate cancer – 191,930 cases and 33,330 deaths
- Colorectal cancer – 147,950 cases and 53,200 deaths
- Melanoma – 100,350 cases and 6,850 deaths
- Bladder cancer – 81,400 cases and 17,980 deaths
- Non-Hodgkin lymphoma (NHL) – 77,240 cases and 19,940 deaths
- Kidney cancer – 73,750 cases and 14,830 deaths
- Endometrial cancer – 65,620 cases and 12,590 deaths

Global Epidemiology of Cancer: Diagnosis and Treatment, First Edition. Jahangir Moini, Nicholas G. Avgeropoulos, and Craig Badolato.
© 2022 John Wiley & Sons Ltd. Published 2022 by John Wiley & Sons Ltd.

Table 2.1 Top 20 most common types of cancer, globally, 2018.

Rank	Type	New cases, 2018
1	Lung	2,093,876
2	Breast	2,088,849
3	Colorectal	1,800,977
4	Prostate	1,276,106
5	Stomach	1,033,701
6	Liver	841,080
7	Esophagus	572,034
8	Cervical	569,847
9	Thyroid	567,233
10	Bladder	549,393
11	Non-Hodgkin lymphoma	509,590
12	Pancreas	458,918
13	Leukemia	437,033
14	Kidney	403,262
15	Uterus	382,069
16	Lip/mouth	354,864
17	Brain/spine	296,851
18	Ovaries	295,414
19	Skin (melanoma)	287,723
20	Gallbladder	219,420

- Leukemia (all types) – 60,530 cases and 23,100 deaths
- Pancreatic cancer – 57,600 cases and 47,050 deaths
- Thyroid cancer – 52,890 cases and 2,180 deaths
- Liver and intrahepatic bile duct cancer – 42,810 cases and 30,160 deaths
- Brain or spinal cord cancer – 24,530 cases and 18,600 deaths

Prevalence

Prevalence is defined as the proportion of any population affected at a *specific* time by a certain disease, and includes incidence (new cases) as well as preexisting cases. Prevalence compares the number of people affected to the total number of people studied. It is commonly expressed as a fraction, based on the number of cases per 10,000 or more people. It is used in health planning, allocation of resources, and to estimate cancer survivorship. It is important to understand that prevalence does *not* include the number of people who may develop cancer during their lifetimes. Prevalence counts are the highest for the most common cancers that have the longest survival times. A common cancer with a shorter survival time may have a lower prevalence count than a less common cancer that has a longer survival time. For example, lung cancer is extremely common in both men and women. Even so, its prevalence count is lower than the prevalence count for non-Hodgkin lymphoma, which is a much less common type of cancer because people diagnosed with non-Hodgkin lymphoma survive for a longer time than people with lung cancer. This means that there are more people surviving after being diagnosed with non-Hodgkin lymphoma than after being diagnosed with lung cancer.

According to the organization called *Our World in Data*, the global prevalence of cancer is lower than in the United States. The overall combined global prevalence of cancer was 1.3% of the total population in 2017. Figure 2.1 shows the countries with the highest and lowest rates of cancer, with the color black used for the countries with the highest prevalence (6% of their populations), and various shades of gray, indicating prevalence between 1% and 6%. The color white is shown for countries either with rates lower than 1% or if no accurate data could be obtained.

When broken down by the type of cancer, breast cancer is the most prevalent form, globally, followed by prostate and colorectal cancer. There were an estimated 17 million cases of breast cancer throughout the world. Figure 2.2 breaks down the most common cancers globally in 2017 and lists the percentage of the population affected. Any cancers not listed affected 0.01%, or less, of the global population.

In the United States, according to the American Cancer Society's *Cancer Treatment and Survivorship Facts & Figures (2019 to 2021)*, 10 prevalence counts are listed below. Note that these counts do not include noninvasive cancer of any sites except the urinary bladder, and also

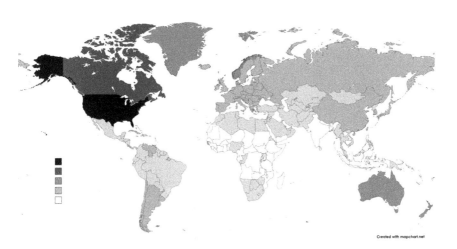

Figure 2.1 Varying prevalence of cancer throughout the world, 2017.

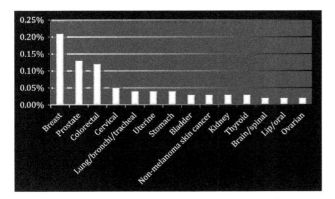

Figure 2.2 Percentages of the global population with various cancers, 2017.

do not include basal cell or squamous cell skin cancers. The top 10 prevalence counts are as follows:

- Males – all types of cancer – 8,138,790 cases

  - Prostate cancer – 3,650,030 (45%)
  - Colorectal cancer – 776,120 (10%)
  - Melanoma – 684,470 (8%)
  - Urinary bladder cancer – 624,490 (8%)
  - NHL – 400,070 (5%)
  - Kidney cancer – 342,060 (4%)
  - Testicular cancer – 287,780 (4%)
  - Lung and bronchial cancer – 258,200 (3%)
  - Leukemia – 256,790 (3%)
  - Oral cavity and pharyngeal cancer – 249,330 (3%)

- Females – all types of cancer – 8,781,580 cases

  - Breast cancer – 3,861,520 (44%)
  - Uterine corpus cancer – 807,860 (9%)
  - Colorectal cancer – 768,650 (9%)
  - Thyroid cancer – 705,050 (8%)
  - Melanoma – 672,140 (8%)
  - NHL – 357,650 (4%)
  - Lung and bronchial cancer – 313,140 (4%)
  - Cervical cancer – 283,120 (3%)
  - Ovarian cancer – 249,230 (3%)
  - Kidney cancer – 227,510 (3%)

To understand prevalence further, 67% of cancer survivors were diagnosed five or more years previously. Only 18% of cancer survivors were diagnosed 20 or more years previously. Nearly 64% of cancer survivors are age 65 or older.

Significant Point

In 2020, cancers of the prostate, colorectum, and skin melanoma were the three most *prevalent* types of cancer among males. Cancers of the breast, uterine corpus, and colorectum were the most prevalent types among females. It is important to compare prevalence with *incidence* of these cancers to fully understand the differences.

Survival

The world population is aging rapidly, and humans are living longer due to healthier lifestyles and better medical diagnosis and treatments. Average life expectancy in the United States and many other countries is higher now than during any other time in history. According to the United Nations, individuals that are 65 years and older used to make up 8% of the total population in 1950. In 2000, this percentage increased to 12% of the total population. It is expected to increase to 20% by 2050, and will probably continue to rise. These changes are primarily due to large improvements in health care, investment into medical research, and better health insurance availability. Less people are dying from diseases such as cancer.

According to the World Health Organization, there will soon be more elderly people than children, and more people at *extreme old age* than ever in history. Chronic diseases such as cancer and cardiovascular disease began to increase in prevalence during the twentieth century, and public health departments began to identify risk factors for many chronic diseases. Interventions were then developed, which reduced mortality. Cancer is an example of a noncommunicable disease. It is a noninfectious health condition that cannot be spread from person to person, lasts for a long period of time, and is also referred to as a *chronic disease*. A combination of environmental, genetic, lifestyle, and physiological factors can cause cancer. Risk factors include unhealthy diets, lack of physical activity, smoking, and excessive use of alcohol.

Life expectancy is also called *longevity*, and is calculated by creating a **life table**, which records deaths and survivors of illnesses in a specific year, for successive life span intervals. Deaths, survivors, and **age-specific death rates** are established for various age groups. A second life table is created that represents the total mortality rates from birth to death, per 100,000 live births. Age-specific death rates in the population are studied for a chosen year, and life expectancy is calculated as the average *life years* for all members of the population, since birth. Life expectancy = total years of life for all members of the life table, divided by the total number of people, at birth. *Longevity at birth* describes the *mean years of life*, based only on age-specific death rates for the population and the year of interest.

The "oldest old" are people 85 or older, who make up 8% of the global elderly population. Odds of living to age 100 have risen from one of every 20 million people to *one of every 50 people* – with this figure being for females in low-mortality countries such as Japan and Sweden. The term *elderly* is defined as age 65 or older. The elderly make up 12% of the populations of more developed countries, and 6% of less developed countries. Less developed countries have generally earlier mortality, because of unemployment, lower standards of living, malnutrition, unsafe or contaminated food, poor quality housing, and lack of protection from the climate. The countries with the oldest populations include: Monaco, Japan, Germany, Italy, Greece, Sweden, Spain, Austria, Bulgaria, and Estonia. In Monaco, 22.8% of the population is age 65 or older. Women generally live longer than men. Reasons for this include faster development in utero, less risky behaviors, development of heart disease later in life, reduced stress levels due to better social interactions, and better self-management of their own health care.

According to the Centers for Disease Control and Prevention in 2020, life expectancy at birth for Americans, combining males and females, was 77.8 years. Today, 10% of females will live past the age of 100 years, and almost 5% of males will live past 100. For some reason, individual statistics for males and females are listed as being from 2018, with life expectancy for females being 81.2 years. For males, it was 76.2 years. In 2019, 13.1% of the United States' population was age 65 or older. Though it should be understood that some cancers have an extremely poor survival rate, such as pancreatic cancer (9% survival over five years), it is estimated by the American Cancer Society that the population of cancer survivors will increase to over 22.1 million people in the United States by 2030. The National Cancer Institute's estimated number of United States cancer survivors, by gender and years since diagnosis, is described as follows:

- Males
  - 0–5 years since diagnosis – 2,921,800 (36%)
  - 5–10 years since diagnosis – 1,957,220 (24%)
  - 10–15 years since diagnosis – 1,323,430 (16%)
  - 15–20 years since diagnosis – 843,970 (10%)
- Females
  - 0–5 years since diagnosis – 2,605,620 (30%)
  - 5–10 years since diagnosis – 1,844,830 (21%)
  - 10–15 years since diagnosis – 1,361,190 (16%)
  - 15–20 years since diagnosis – 1,011,810 (12%)

Figure 2.3 illustrates the five-year survival percentages for a variety of different cancers.

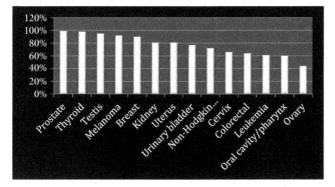

Figure 2.3 The five-year survival percentages for different cancers.

The term *relative cancer survival* describes the percentage of patients alive at various times after diagnosis, adjusted for normal life expectancy. The five-year relative survival discussed above is the most conventionally used method of prognosis. However, this does not identify the proportion of patients eventually cured, since some cancer deaths will occur after more than five years since diagnosis. For most types of cancer, five-year relative survival has improved over the past several decades. Along with the actual type of cancer that is present, factors that influence survival times include the patient's age, stage of the cancer upon diagnosis, treatment options that are available, being insured, financial resources, and any other serious health conditions. Obviously, access to high-quality cancer treatments increases a person's chances of survival, and also improves quality of life. A good example is shown when an uninsured patient is diagnosed with stage I colorectal cancer. Statistics show that for such a person, there is a lower survival rate than for a person that has health insurance and is diagnosed with stage II colorectal cancer. Therefore, cancer survival is affected by disparities that include socioeconomic status and ethnic or racial factors.

Significant Point

Globally, humans are living longer than any time previously in history, with the oldest average combined life expectancy (males and females) being 83.7 years, in Japan. Switzerland and Singapore rank second and third. The United States is ranked 31st. The three lowest average life expectancies are Sierra Leone (50.1 years), Angola (52.4 years), and Central African Republic (52.5 years).

Distribution of Cancer by Gender, Race, and Age

Globally, as of 2018, the most common cancers between men and women were slightly varied. Table 2.2 compares the cases of cancer, globally, between men and women.

Cancer also has some disparities when different racial or ethnic groups are compared. Generally, cancer of all types affects racial or ethnic groups in differing amounts. The following list shows the rate of new cases of cancer per 100,000 people by race and ethnicity. Note that there are also some disparities between males and females:

- Black males – 515.1 new cases/100,000 – with 221.1 deaths
- Non-Hispanic males – 497.0 – with 190.7 deaths
- Caucasian males – 485.5 – with 185.9 deaths
- Caucasian females – 432.0 – with 134.3 deaths
- Non-Hispanic females – 431.5 – with 137.6 deaths
- Black females – 390.7 – with 150.5 deaths
- Hispanic males – 370.4 – with 134.0 deaths
- Hispanic females – 339.5 – with 94.6 deaths
- American Indian/Alaska Native males – 321.0 – with 169.3 deaths
- American Indian/Alaska Native females – 305.9 – with 120.1 deaths
- Asian/Pacific Islander females – 304.7 – with 84.6 deaths
- Asian/Pacific Islander males – 304.4 – with 114.6 deaths

By age, the majority of cancers occur, globally, in older people. About 70% of cancers occur in people over age 50. In 2017, Our World in Data calculated the global cases of cancer. This is shown in Figure 2.4.

On breaking down these statistics further, the following age groups experience various cancers in higher rates in comparison with other age groups:

- Age 50 or older – breast, prostate, colorectal, and lung cancers
- Age 40–49 – breast and thyroid cancer, and melanoma
- Age 30–39 – breast and thyroid cancer, leukemia, lymphoma, and melanoma
- Age 20–29 – thyroid cancer, leukemia, lymphoma, melanoma, and germ cell tumors
- From birth to age 19 – leukemia, lymphoma, and brain or spinal tumors

Table 2.2 Global cases of different cancers, between men and women.

Type of cancer	Cases in men	Cases in women
Lung cancer	1,368,524	725,352
Breast cancer	23,100	2,088,849
Prostate cancer	1,276,106	N/A
Colorectal cancer	1,006,019	794,958
Stomach cancer	683,754	349,947
Liver cancer	596,574	244,506
Cervical cancer	N/A	569,847
Thyroid cancer	130,889	436,344
Bladder cancer	424,082	125,311
Uterine (corpus) cancer	N/A	382,069
Esophageal cancer	399,699	172,335
Ovarian cancer	N/A	295,414
Non-Hodgkin lymphoma	284,713	224,877
Kidney cancer	254,507	148,755
Leukemia	249,454	187,579
Lip, oral cavity cancer	246,420	108,444
Pancreatic cancer	243,033	215,885
Brain, central nervous system cancer	162,534	134,317
Laryngeal cancer	154,977	22,445
Melanoma of the skin	150,698	137,025
Gallbladder cancer	97,396	122,024
Nasopharyngeal cancer	93,416	35,663
Multiple myeloma	89,897	70,088
Oropharyngeal cancer	74,472	18,415
Testicular cancer	71,105	N/A
Hypopharyngeal cancer	67,496	13,112
Hodgkin lymphoma	46,559	33,431
Cancer of the vulva	N/A	44,235
Salivary gland cancer	29,256	23,543
Anal cancer	20,196	28,345
Kaposi sarcoma	28,248	13,551
Mesothelioma	21,662	8,781
Vaginal cancer	N/A	17,600

Global Burden of Cancer

The majority of the global cancer burden is in low- and middle-income countries, with about 70% of cancer-related deaths occurring in these countries.

The sub-Saharan region of Africa is projected to have above an 85% increase in cancer incidence by 2030. The global population is growing and aging. Low- and middle-income countries often have great difficulty responding to challenges posed by

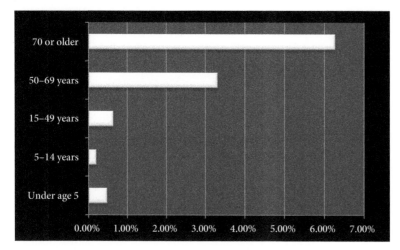

Figure 2.4 Global cancers, in various age groups, 2017.

cancer. More people are diagnosed late in the disease course, resulting in more deaths. By 2040, the global burden of cancer is estimated to be at 28.4 million new cases, an increase of 47% from 2020, and 16.3 million cancer deaths. It is likely that the future burden will be even larger, because risk factors are increasing in prevalence, and include smoking, physical inactivity, poor diet, and fewer childbirths. A larger increase in cancer cases is expected in low- and middle-income countries (64% to as much as 95%) compared with high-income countries (32–56%).

However, the cancer burden is also expanding in countries with higher-income levels. Along with morbidity and mortality, cancer carries a huge economic burden. Direct costs include the costs of treatment, while indirect costs include loss of income or productivity because of the disease. While the exact global economic burden of cancer is unknown, data is available from some countries. In the European Union (EU), health-care spending was 57.3 billion euros in 2017 alone. Productivity losses from morbidity were 10.6 billion euros, and losses from premature deaths totaled 47.9 billion euros. Informal health-care costs were at 26.1 billion euros, and the total cancer burden increased to 141.8 billion euros, which was 1.07% of the gross domestic product (GDP). A further breakdown of cancer burden in various countries is as follows:

- Germany – 39.5 billion euros
- France – 19.0 billion euros
- Italy – 18.5 billion euros
- United Kingdom – 16.2 billion euros
- Spain – 10.1 billion euros
- The Netherlands – 7.1 billion euros
- Belgium – 3.6 billion euros
- Czechia – 1.5 billion euros

The cost of cancer in EU countries is widely varied based on population size and age, available health care, employment, and the rates of cancer incidence and mortality. The economic burden of lost productivity is almost 60% of the total economic burden associated with cancer. In the United States, in 2017, estimated costs of cancer were at $161.2 billion, with losses, because of morbidity at $30.3 billion, and losses due to

Significant Point

For cancer patients, the cost of chemotherapy alone varies widely, based on the drug used, how it is administered, and the number of treatments needed. Costs for surgery also are varied. Countries such as India offer lower-cost surgeries for many cancers compared with the costs in countries such as the United States, United Kingdom, and Canada.

premature deaths at $150.7 billion. These figures are equivalent to 1.8% of the GDP.

Global Trends in Cancer

Global trends in cancer involve research into many new drugs and other forms of treatment. In 2018, 15 new therapeutic drugs were launched – a record number for a single year. More than half of these drugs are given orally, have designations as orphan drugs, or are labeled with a predictive biomarker. Immuno-oncology therapies have doubled in availability since 2017. Treatment with new cyclin-dependent kinase (CDK) 4/6 inhibitors for human epidermal growth factor receptor 2 (HER-2) negative breast cancer has greatly increased. Drugs in late-stage development expanded by 19% in 2018, and have expanded 63% since 2013. The largest focus is on almost 450 immunotherapies that have over 60 different mechanisms of action. A total of 98 cell, gene, and nucleotide therapies – formally referred to as *Next-Generation Biotherapeutics* – are under clinical study.

However, the field of oncology is highly challenging, with many treatment failures and long periods of drug development. The overall success of oncology trials has improved by 22% since 2010 but is still much lower than trials for non-cancer therapies. The spending for new cancer drugs, which was nearly $150 billion in 2018, usually increases by double-digit percentages every year. Average annual cost of new drugs is increasing, though there are occasional drops in cost. Nearly 33% of approved indications over the past five years have been for hematologic cancers. Out of all solid tumors, lung cancer has 12 indications, followed by breast cancer and melanoma. Spending on cancer drugs will reach almost $240 billion through 2023, which shows a growth of approximately 12%.

Lung cancer rates among men are slightly trending downward over most of the planet, but they remained high in countries such as the Czech Republic and Slovakia, as well as in the African-American population in the United States. Rates of lung cancer in women are increasing in many countries, including France, Germany, Norway, Canada, Denmark, and the Netherlands. Breast cancer rates are increasing in women of many countries. For unknown reasons, rates of breast cancer are increasing in premenopausal women of higher-income countries, and increasing in postmenopausal women of lower-income countries. Nearly 50% of breast cancer cases and 58% of deaths from the disease occur in lower-income countries, according to the *World Journal of Surgical Oncology*. About 47% of women diagnosed with premenopausal breast cancer in these countries will die from the disease. In the most developed countries, this same situation is only fatal in 11%. In lower-income countries, postmenopausal breast cancer is fatal in 56% of cases, but only 21% in higher-income countries. Early diagnosis and access to treatment is desperately needed in lower-income countries.

Globally, colorectal cancer is expected to increase by 60%, to over 2.2 million new cases and 1.1 million deaths by 2030. Colorectal cancer is increasing rapidly in many low-income and middle-income countries. In developed countries, cases of colorectal cancer in elderly people are dropping, while they are increasing in younger age groups. The decrease in colorectal cancer in elderly people is likely due to better screening methods, including colonoscopy, to achieve earlier diagnoses. As of 2020, 12% of colorectal cancers are diagnosed in people under age 50. Rates have also been increasing in adults between 20 and 54 years, though younger adults have the highest rate of increase. In people 65 and older, the decrease in colorectal cancer is documented at 3% per year between 2011 and 2016. For those aged 50–64, rates increased by 1% per year during this same period, and in those under 50, the rates increased by 2.2% per year. Overall, colorectal cancer is the third most common type of cancer in men and women. Death rates from this cancer declined by 3% per year in those 65 or older, but increased by 1.3% in those younger than age 50.

Age-adjusted rates of prostate cancer have increased greatly, mostly because of increased screening for prostate-specific antigen (PSA). Stomach cancer has been significantly declining worldwide, but is still a significant cause of death. The reduction in cases may be related to the lower prevalence of **Helicobacter pylori** infection. However, stomach cancer is still relatively common in Eastern Asia and more common in Latin America than in well-developed countries. Incidence in Latin America is not likely to decline greatly over the coming decades because there is a high prevalence of *H. pylori* infections in younger people in that area.

Global Prevalence of Cancer

Globally, the six most prevalent cancers include lung (2.09 million cases), breast (2.09 million), colorectal (1.80 million), prostate (1.28 million), non-melanomas of the skin (1.04 million), and stomach cancers (1.03 million). The next most common cancers include liver, esophageal, cervical, thyroid, and bladder cancers. Approximately one of every six deaths is due to cancer. About 70% of deaths from cancer occur in low- and middle-income countries. Globally, in children less than 15 years of age, brain tumors are second only to acute lymphoblastic leukemia as the most common form of cancer. Better diagnostic technology and access to health care, including clinical specialization, is related to the increased prevalence of brain tumors. The highest rates of brain tumors are in the United States, Canada, Australia, and the United Kingdom. In the United Kingdom, CNS tumors are the ninth most common cancer, with about 10,600 diagnoses every year. These tumors are also the eighth most common cause of cancer death, with about 5,200 fatalities.

The World Health Organization reported in 2018 about various global areas and the prevalence of cancer there. Though 48.4% of the total world cancer cases occurred in Asia, it must be remembered that 60% of the global population lives there. To understand further, the number of cases and percentage of total cases should be examined. Cancer prevalence throughout the world are: Asia – 48.4%; Europe – 23.4%; North,

Central, and South America – 21.0%; Africa – 5.8%; and Oceania – 1.4% (see Figure 2.5).

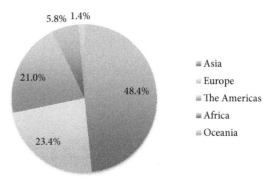

Figure 2.5 Cancer prevalence throughout the world.

Global Incidence and Mortality

The global incidence of cancer in 2018 included 20 types of cancer that made up more than 1% of all new cases. These types include the following, which are also shown in Figure 2.6:

- Lung cancer – 12.3% of all types of cancer
- Breast cancer – 12.3%
- Colorectal cancer – 10.6%
- Prostate cancer – 7.5%
- Stomach cancer – 6.1%
- Liver cancer – 5.0%
- Esophageal cancer – 3.4%
- Cervical cancer – 3.3%
- Thyroid cancer – 3.3%
- Bladder cancer – 3.2%
- NHL – 3.0%
- Pancreatic cancer – 2.7%
- Leukemia – 2.6%
- Kidney cancer – 2.4%
- Uterine corpus cancer – 2.2%
- Lip and oral cavity cancers – 2.1%
- Brain and spinal cancer – 1.7%
- Ovarian cancer – 1.7%
- Melanoma of the skin – 1.7%
- Gallbladder cancer – 1.3%

Mortality is the primary indicator of health status of populations. Basically, mortality is expressed by *mortality rate* and *case fatality ratio*. The mortality rate is the number of deaths in a

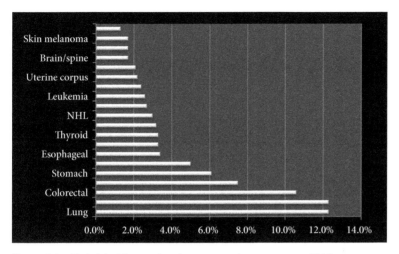

Figure 2.6 Global incidence of various cancers by percentage, 2018.

specific population over a certain time period. The case fatality ratio is the proportion of people with a disease who die from that disease, at any time, unless specified. The mortality rate is equal to the case fatality ratio multiplied by the incidence rate of disease within the population. The most common causes of global deaths from cancer are as follows, according to 2018 statistics:

- Lung cancer – 1.76 million deaths
- Colorectal cancer – 862,000 deaths
- Stomach cancer – 783,000 deaths
- Liver cancer – 782,000 deaths
- Breast cancer – 627,000 deaths

It should be noted that the top five global causes of cancer deaths do not exactly match the top five most common types of cancer throughout the world. This demonstrates the varying *lethality* of the various types. After breast cancer, the next most lethal types of cancer include: pancreatic, esophageal, and prostate cancers, leukemia, and then cervical, brain/spinal, bladder, lip/oral cavity, ovarian, and gallbladder/biliary tract cancers.

Mortality due to Cancer in the United States

Each type of cancer has its own unique mortality rates. In the United States, people diagnosed with breast or prostate cancer have a general prognosis that is much better than those diagnosed with, for example, lung or stomach cancer. Age is implicated in mortality rates, since many older adults die from a large number of cancers, while younger people survive them. According to the National Cancer Institute, the five-year and ten-year survival rates for all cancers are 71.1% and 52.0%, respectively. However, a breakdown of the various types indicates large variations in mortality – see Table 2.3.

All other types of cancer in the United States have a less than 50% survival rate over five years, and an even poorer rate over 10 years. These cancers include: non-lymphoma lymph node cancer; ovarian, hypopharyngeal, brain, stomach, and uterine cancers; leukemia (acute myelomonocytic); liver and bile duct cancer; esophageal, gallbladder, lung, and heart cancers; mesothelioma; pancreatic cancers; glioblastoma; and the worst of all – diffuse intrinsic pontine glioma of the brain stem, which has less than 1% survival over five years and 0% survival over 10 years. Brain tumors account for 2% of all adult cancer deaths, and incidence is slightly higher in males. About 6 of every 100,000 adults die from brain tumor, and about 1 of every 100,000 children as well. Caucasians generally have a higher rate of brain cancer mortality than other ethnic groups. According to the *Central Brain Tumor Registry of the United States (CBTRUS)*, the average annual mortality rate in the United States is

Table 2.3 Cancer mortality rates in the United States.

Type of cancer	Five-year survival	Ten-year survival
Breast cancer in situ	100%	100%
Prostate cancer	98.6%	91%
Thyroid cancer	98.2%	94.6%
Testicular cancer	95.1%	87%
Skin cancer (except for basal and squamous)	91.7%	90%
Lip cancer	91%	89%
Breast cancer	89.7%	81%
Appendix cancer	88%	81%
Hodgkin lymphoma	86.4%	76%
Leukemia (chronic lymphocytic)	83.2%	69%
Ocular cancer	82.7%	79.7%
Bladder cancer	77.3%	71%
Kidney cancer	74.1%	69%
Non-Hodgkin lymphoma	71%	52%
Leukemia (acute lymphocytic)	68.2%	51%
Bone cancer	67.7%	56%
Small intestine cancer	67.5%	63%
Cervical cancer	67.1%	61%
Leukemia (chronic myeloid)	66.9%	50%
Colorectal cancer	64.9%	59%
Soft tissue cancers (not otherwise specified)	64.4%	62%
Pancreatic neuroendocrine tumor	61%	50%
Laryngeal cancer	60.7%	60%
Oral cancer	60%	50%
Tracheal cancer	52.9%	50%
Multiple myeloma	52%	18%

about 4.37 per 100,000 people, with 77,375 deaths attributed to primary malignant brain and spinal tumors. In 2018, there were approximately 16,830 deaths from these tumors, of which 9,490 were males and 7,340 were females.

Risk Factors for Cancer Development

Most risk factors for cancer development are first identified in epidemiological studies. Scientists monitor large groups of people, comparing those with cancer to those without. The studies may reveal that people with cancer behave in specific ways, or are exposed to certain substances, that are different from people without cancer. The most well-known or suspected risk factors for cancer include the following. Some of these can be avoided, reducing cancer risks, but some cannot:

- Aging – advanced age is the most important overall risk factor for cancer, and the median age of cancer diagnoses is 66 years. About 25% of new cancer diagnoses occur in people from age 65 to 74. Median ages of diagnosis differ slightly between certain cancers. The median ages are 61 years for breast cancer, 66 years for prostate cancer, 68 years for colorectal cancer, and 70 years for lung cancer, though cancer occurs in people of all ages. Bone cancer is most diagnosed in people less than 20 years of age, and over 25% of cases occur in this age group. While only 1% of overall cancers are diagnosed in individuals below age 20, that age group experiences 10% of all leukemias. Cancers such as neuroblastomas are more common in people under age 20, however.

- Alcohol use – drinking alcohol increases risks for oral, pharyngeal, esophageal, laryngeal, liver, and breast cancers. Risks are increased with the more alcohol that is consumed. Also, for those who drink alcohol as well as smoke, the risks are extremely increased. Moderate alcohol use is one drink per day for women and two drinks per day for men.
- Carcinogens – these include chemicals in tobacco smoke, ground water, certain foods, and workplace substances. Also, carcinogens are found in polluted air. The carcinogens that most commonly harm humans include: aflatoxins, aristolochic acids, arsenic, asbestos, benzene, benzidine, beryllium, 1,3-butadiene, cadmium, coal tar and coal-tar pitch, coke-oven emissions, crystalline silica, erionite, ethylene oxide, formaldehyde, hexavalent chromium compounds, indoor emissions from coal combustion, untreated or mildly treated mineral oils, nickel compounds, radon, secondhand tobacco smoke, soot from chimneys or furnaces, strong inorganic acid mists that contain sulfuric acid, thorium, trichloroethylene, vinyl chloride, and wood dust.
- Chronic inflammation – caused by persistent infections, abnormal immune reactions, and other conditions such as obesity. Chronic inflammation leads to DNA damage, and an increased risk of cancer. Examples of chronic inflammatory conditions include Crohn disease and ulcerative colitis, which increases the risk of developing colon cancer.

- Diet – food sources that are potentially related to cancer are those that contain acrylamide, artificial sweeteners, excessive calcium, charred meat, **glucosinolates**, excessive fluoride, and excessive vitamin D.
- Hormones – excessive estrogen, excessive progesterone.
- Immunosuppression – from immunosuppressants after organ transplantation.
- Infectious agents – HIV, Epstein–Barr virus, HBV, HCV, human herpesvirus 8, Kaposi sarcoma-associated herpesvirus, human papillomaviruses, human T cell leukemia/lymphoma virus type 1, Merkel cell polyomavirus, *H. pylori, Schistosoma hematobium.*
- Obesity – this increases risks for postmenopausal breast cancer, colon cancer, rectal cancer, and endometrial cancer of the uterus, esophageal cancer, kidney cancer, pancreatic cancer, and gallbladder cancer.
- Radiation (ionizing) – radon, X-rays, gamma rays, and other high-energy radiation. Radon increases risks for lung cancer. Aside from the small amounts of radiation used in medical imaging procedures, high-energy radiation can come from nuclear power plants and atomic weapons.
- Tobacco use – the leading cause of cancer and death from cancer. Tobacco use is linked to many cancers, including lung, laryngeal, oral, esophageal, pharyngeal, urinary bladder, kidney, liver, stomach, pancreatic, colorectal, and cervical cancers, as well as acute myeloid leukemia. Tobacco does not have to be smoked to be dangerous. Snuff or chewing tobacco increases risks for oral, esophageal, and pancreatic cancers. No level of tobacco use is safe.
- Ultraviolet radiation – may come from the sun, tanning booths or beds, and sun lamps. Exposure to UV radiation causes early skin aging and damage that may result in skin cancer. All people, regardless of skin color, must limit the amount of exposure to ultraviolet radiation. Regarding the sun, the worst times

to be outdoors for long periods of time are between 10:00 a.m. and 3:00 p.m.

Years of Life Lost

According to the National Cancer Institute in 2018, the average years of life lost (YLL) to cancer was 15.3 years; YLL is calculated following early death from a particular cause or disease. It is measured as the difference between the actual ages based on the disease and the expected age of death due to the disease. This is estimated by using life table data to each death of a person of a specific age and gender. Life tables allow for the determination of the extra years an average person of that age, gender, and even racial group would have been expected to live. The average YLL listed above is for males and females, but separately, the 2018 estimates state that males have an average of 14.3 YLL to cancer, and females have an average of 16.4 YLL. The average death rate for all cancers combined is 149.1 per 100,000 people per year. According to the American Association for Cancer Research, the largest number of YLLs is due to cancers of the lungs or bronchi, followed by colorectal cancer, and then breast cancer.

Disability-Adjusted Life Years

Disability-adjusted life years (DALYs) link information about disease occurrence with health outcomes. They are calculated by adding YLL with the **years of life lived with a disability** (YLD). One lost DALY = one lost year of healthy life, as a result of premature death from the disease, or from disease-related illnesses or disability. Disability weights represent a value preference scaling the disease from "full health" (zero) to "death" (1). Since the *Global Burden of Disease Study* in 2010, age weighting is no longer a default value choice for DALYs. Today, DALY values can be calculated with or without using age weighting, and also with or without discounting the rates for future life. Options for calculation include the following:

- Using age weights as well as discounting
- Using either age weights or discounting
- Using neither age weights nor discounting

Another consideration is *healthy life years lost per 1,000 populations per year (HeaLY)*. This differs from DALYs. The start point for HeaLY is the beginning of a disease. It is the loss of healthy life based on the natural disease history, modified by interventions. When disease incidence changes, the DALY calculation may not fully explain the actual disease situation. Both HeaLY and DALY calculations measure *health gaps*. They are nearly the same if the disease in question is constant over time, if age weighting is not applied, or if the same measures of disability are used.

In 2017, cancer caused 233.5 million DALYs throughout the world. Out of this number, 97% came from YLL and 3% came from YLD. The odds of developing cancer were one of every three men and one of every four women. The most common causes of death and DALYs for men were lung, bronchus, tracheal, liver, and stomach cancers. The most common causes of death and DALYs for women were breast, lung, bronchus, tracheal, and colorectal cancers. Breaking down DALYs by cancer type, the following information is obtained:

- Lung, bronchus, and tracheal cancer – 40.9 million DALYs
- Liver cancer – 20.8 million
- Stomach cancer – 19.1 million
- Colorectal cancer – 19.0 million
- Breast cancer – 17.7 million
- Cervical cancer – 8.1 million
- Prostate cancer – 7.1 million
- NHL – 7.0 million
- Bladder cancer – 3.6 million
- Non-melanoma skin cancer – 1.3 million

Global Cancer Prevention

According to the American Cancer Society, which works with global organizations to prevent cancer, the following two methods are of significant focus, especially in low- and middle-income countries, which have the highest burden of cancer deaths:

- Tobacco taxation – making tobacco products more expensive is very effective in reducing tobacco use and cancer death.
- Human papillomavirus (HPV) vaccination – countries that are already benefiting from HPV vaccinations include Colombia, India, Kenya, and Uganda.

Both of these interventions are based on detailed evidence and present an opportunity to greatly reduce the development of cancer. However, they are not well used in many of these countries, partly because people are unaware of their life-saving abilities. Also, both interventions are extremely effective for teenagers, who are often overlooked regarding cancer prevention – even though this helps prevent later adulthood disease.

According to the World Health Organization, between 30% and 50% of all cancers can be prevented by avoiding risk factors and using evidence-based prevention methods. Cancer can also be reduced via early detection and treatment, and many cancers are highly curable if diagnosed early and treated sufficiently. Risk factors that can be modified or avoided include the following:

- Cigarettes, cigars, pipes, and smokeless tobacco
- Overuse of alcohol
- Being overweight or obese
- Eating a poor diet, with insufficient quantities of fruits and vegetables
- Indoor smoke from using solid fuels in the home
- Insufficient physical activity
- Ionizing and ultraviolet radiation
- Viral hepatitis
- Sexually transmitted human papillomavirus infection
- Air pollution

Other prevention strategies include controlling occupational hazards and being vaccinated against the hepatitis B virus. Early diagnosis of cancer requires awareness and access to care, clinical evaluation, diagnosis, staging, and access to treatment. Screening methods include examples such as:

- Human papillomavirus testing for cervical cancer
- PAP cytology testing for cervical cancer, in middle- and high-income countries
- Visual inspection with acetic acid (VIA), for cervical cancer, in low-income countries
- Mammography screening for breast cancer, in countries with strong or intermediately strong health systems
- Colonoscopy is now recommended for people with a familial history of colon polyps below the age of 40, and also for anyone after age 50, usually every 10 years
- To prevent prostate cancer, the PSA test should be performed beginning at age 50, every year afterward; a rectal examination to assess the prostate gland is also required
- To prevent testicular cancer, which is more common in young men, self-examinations must be performed monthly, starting at age 15 and continuing to age 35
- The prevention of skin cancers requires avoiding excessive sun exposure, and exposure to tanning beds and other forms of ultraviolet light

---

Significant Point

Smoking is the most critical factor in the prevention of cancer. The relationship between smoking, cancer, and death in adults aged 30 or older, is significant for many forms of the disease. Smoking is implicated in 82% of lung cancers, 74% of laryngeal cancers, 50% of esophageal cancers, 49% of oral/pharyngeal/nasal/paranasal sinus cancers, and 47% of bladder cancers.

Key Terms

Age-specific death rates

Disability-adjusted life years

Glucosinolates

Helicobacter pylori

Life expectancy

Incidence

Life table

Prevalence

Years of life lived with a disability

Years of life lost

Bibliography

1 Adami, H.O., Hunter, D.J., Lagiou, P., and Mucci, L. (2018). *Textbook of Cancer Epidemiology*, 3rd Edition. Oxford: Oxford University Press.

2 Al Moustafa, A.E. (2017). *Development of Oral Cancer: Risk Factors and Prevention Strategies*. New York: Springer.

3 American Association for Cancer Research. (2020). *Lung cancer*. https://www.aacr.org/patients-caregivers/cancer/lung-cance. Accessed 2021.

4 American Cancer Society. (2020). *Cancer facts & figures 2020 (from American Cancer Society Journal, CA: A Cancer Journal for Clinicians)*. https://www.cancer.org/research/cancer-facts-statistics/all-cancer-facts-figures/cancer-facts-figures-2020.html Accessed 2021.

5 American Cancer Society. (2021). *Cancer Treatment & Survivorship Facts & Figures 2019–2021*. https://www.cancer.org/research/cancer-facts-statistics/survivor-facts-figures.html Accessed 2021.

6 American Cancer Society. (2021). *Global Cancer Prevention (GCP) Tax & Vacs*. https://www.cancer.org/health-care-professionals/our-global-health-work/global-cancer-initiatives/cancer-prevention-tobacco-control.html Accessed 2021.

7 Anttila, S. and Boffetta, P. (2020). *Occupational Cancers*, 2nd Edition. New York: Springer.

8 Balogh, E., Patlak, M., and Nass, S.J., National Cancer Policy Forum, Board on Health Care Services, and Institute of Medicine.(2013). *Reducing Tobacco-Related Cancer Incidence and Mortality: Workshop Summary*. Washington: National Academies Press.

9 Banerjee, D. (2020). *Enduring Cancer: Life, Death, and Diagnosis in Delhi (Critical Global Health: Evidence, Efficacy, Ethnography)*. Durham: Duke University Press Books.

10 Bhullar, M.D. and Singh, J. (2014). *Gastric Cancer: Risk Factors, Treatment and Clinical Outcomes*. Hauppauge: Nova Science Publishers, Inc.

11 Boffetta, P., Boccia, S., and La Vecchia, C. (2014). *A Quick Guide to Cancer Epidemiology (Briefs in Cancer Research)*. New York: Springer.

12 Bollinger, T. (2015). *The Truth About Cancer: A Global Quest – 9 Episodes – Complete Transcripts*. Portland: TTAC Publishing.

13 Centers for Disease Control and Prevention, NVSS Vital Statistics Rapid Release. (2021). *Provisional Life Expectancy Estimates for January through June, 2020 (Report No. 010)*. U.S. Department of Health and Human Services, Centers for Disease Control and Prevention, National Center for Health Statistics, National Vital Statistics System. https://www.cdc.gov/nchs/data/vsrr/VSRR10-508.pdf Accessed 2021.

14 Central Brain Tumor Registry of the United States. (2018). *2018 CBTRUS fact sheet*. https://www.cbtrus.org/www.cbtrus.org/factsheet/factsheet.html Accessed 2021.

15 Compton, C. (2020). *Cancer: The Enemy from Within: A Comprehensive Textbook of Cancer's Causes, Complexities and Consequences*. New York: Springer.

16 DeVita, V.T., Jr., Lawrence, T.S., and Rosenberg, S.A. (2018). *DeVita, Hellman, and Rosenberg's Cancer: Principles & Practice of*

Oncology, 11th Edition. Philadelphia: Lippincott, Williams, and Wilkins.

17 El-Mazny, A. (2020). *Cervical Cancer: Risk Factors and Screening*. Scotts Valley: CreateSpace Independent Publishing Platform.

18 Harris, R.E. (2015). *Global Epidemiology of Cancer*. Burlington: Jones & Bartlett Learning.

19 Mason, T.J. and Riggan, W.B. (2006). *U.S. Cancer Mortality Rates and Trends 1950–1979. Volume* II. Houston: Two Sixty Press.

20 Matemba, T. (2020). *Understanding Prostate Cancer Risk Factors, Diagnosis, Treatment Options, and Prevention*. St. Petersburg: Compass Publishing.

21 Nasca, P.C. and Pastides, H. (2008). *Fundamentals of Cancer Epidemiology*, 2nd Edition. Burlington: Jones & Bartlett Learning.

22 National Cancer Institute: Surveillance, Epidemiology, and End Results Program. (2020). *Cancer Stat Facts: Cancer of Any Site*. U.S. Department of Health and Human Services, National Institutes of Health, National Cancer Institute, USA.gov. https://seer.cancer.gov/statfacts/html/all.html Accessed 2021.

23 National Cancer Institute: Cancer Trends Progress Report. (2020) *Online Summary of Trends in US Cancer Control Measures*. U.S. Department of Health and Human Services, National Institutes of Health, National Cancer Institute, USA.gov. https://www.progressreport.cancer.gov/end/life_lost Accessed 2021.

24 National Institutes of Health. (2020). *Screening Mammography & Breast Cancer Mortality: Meta-Analysis of Quasi-Experimental Studies*. Bethesda: National Institutes of Health.

25 Roser, M. and Ritchie, H. (2017). *Cancer*. Our World in Data. https://ourworldindata.org/cancer Accessed 2021.

26 Schottenfeld, D. and Fraumeni, J.F., Jr. (2006). *Cancer Epidemiology and Prevention*, 3rd Edition. Oxford: Oxford University Press.

27 Shaikh, K., Krishnan, S., and Thanki, R. (2020). *Artificial Intelligence in Breast Cancer – Early Detection and Diagnosis*. New York: Springer.

28 Shetty, M.K. (2013). *Breast and Gynecological Cancers: An Integrated Approach for Screening and Early Diagnosis in Developing Countries*. New York: Springer.

29 Srivastava, S. (2017). *Biomarkers in Cancer Screening and Early Detection (Translational Oncology)*. Hoboken: Wiley-Blackwell.

30 Tabar, L. and Tot, T. (2011). *Casting Type Calcifications: Sign of a Subtype with Deceptive Features (Breast Cancer – Early Detection with Mammography)*. Stuttgart: Thieme.

31. Thun, M., Linet, M.S., Cerhan, J.R., Haiman, C.A., and Schottenfeld, D. (2017). *Cancer Epidemiology and Prevention*, 4th Edition. Oxford: Oxford University Press.

32 United Nations Department of Economic and Social Affairs. (2019). *World Population Ageing 2019*. https://www.un.org/en/development/desa/population/publications/pdf/ageing/WorldPopulationAgeing2019-Highlights.pdf Accessed 2021.

33 Verma, M. (2018). *Cancer Epidemiology Volume 2, Modifiable Factors (Methods in Molecular Biology 472, Springer Protocols)*. Totowa: Humana Press.

34 WHO Classification of Tumours Editorial Board. (2019). *Breast Tumours: WHO Classification of Tumors (Medicine)*, 5th Edition. Geneva: World Health Organization.

35 World Cancer Research Fund, American Institute for Cancer Research. (2007). *Food, Nutrition, Physical Activity, and the Prevention of Cancer: A Global Perspective*. Arlington: American Institute for Cancer Research.

36 World Health Organization. (2021). *Breast cancer now most common form of cancer: WHO taking action*. https://www.who.int/news/item/03-02-2021-breast-cancer-now-most-common-form-of-cancer-who-taking-action. Accessed 2021.

37 World Health Organization, National Institute on Aging, National Institutes of Health, U.S. Department of Health and Human Services.

(2011). *Global health and aging.* https://www.who.int/ageing/publications/global_health.pdf Accessed 2021.

38 World Health Organization. (2021). *Cancer.* https://www.who.int/news-room/fact-sheets/detail/cancer Accessed 2021.

39 World Journal of Surgical Oncology. (2015). *Breast cancer survival experiences at a tertiary hospital in sub-Saharan Africa: A cohort study.* V. 13, PMC4506617. 220. https://www.ncbi.nlm.nih.gov/pmc/articles/PMC4506617 Accessed 2021.

Part II

Cancers of the Body Systems

3

Brain and Spine Tumors

OUTLINE

Benign / Low-Grade Tumors

Benign tumors of the brain usually develop into cell masses that, under a microscope, do not have the characteristic appearance of an aggressive cancer. The benign brain tumors may be discovered incidentally during MRI or CT scans. They grow slowly, do not metastasize, and often have an identifiable edge or border. The benign tumors can be removed or potentially irradiated, and usually do not recur. However, benign brain tumors may be life-threatening since they can compress adjacent critical structures and can cause symptoms including vision, hearing, and balance loss; changes in mental ability; seizures or muscle jerking; changes in smell perception; nausea or vomiting; facial paralysis; headaches; and/or numbness in the extremities. The most commonly diagnosed benign brain tumors include meningiomas, schwannomas, and pituitary adenomas. Treatments for benign tumors of the brain are similar to those performed for malignant tumors, except that chemotherapy is rarely employed. There are situations where low-grade tumors may be genetically driven and susceptible to targeted therapy, however.

Global Epidemiology of Cancer: Diagnosis and Treatment, First Edition. Jahangir Moini,
Nicholas G. Avgeropoulos, and Craig Badolato.

Meningioma

A **meningioma** is a slow-growing, benign tumor of the meninges. It is usually derived from meningothelial cells in the arachnoid layer and villi. The tumor may compress nearby brain tissue. Meningiomas have three primary grades, each with specific biological pathologies. Most meningiomas are grade I. Some subtypes have worse outcomes, and are graded as II or III tumors. They can occur in any part of the skull, because they originate from the arachnoid villi. Meningioma was one of the first solid tumors discovered with cytogenetic changes – usually in monosomy 22.

Epidemiology

Meningiomas are the most common intracranial tumors, and account for about 11% of all brain tumors. According to the American Society of Clinical Oncology and the Brain Science Foundation, meningiomas make up 36% of all *primary* brain tumors, in different ages. Malignant meningiomas make up 2–3% of all meningiomas. They are more common in females than males. For females, the prevalence is 10.5 cases per 100,000, while males have 5 cases per 100,000. The incidence of meningiomas is 14.45% of the overall population. For both genders, risks for meningioma increase with age. The peak of meningioma cases is in the sixth and seventh decades of life. The incidence of non-malignant meningiomas increased greatly for every 5-year age group, from ages 65 to 69 (23.85 cases per 100,000), to people aged 85 and over (50.34 cases per 100,000). In children, meningiomas make up just 2.8% of all *primary* brain tumors. These tumors also often occur in pre-menopausal women. Females between 35 and 45 years are three times more likely to develop a meningioma than males in the same age group.

Over 90% of meningiomas are single tumors. About 81.1% are grade I (typical), 16.9% of meningiomas are grade II tumors (atypical), and 1.7% are grade III anaplastic. The grade III tumors are more common in males. The significant racial breakdown for meningiomas is as follows (and illustrated in Figure 3.1):

- 9 cases per 100,000 occur in African Americans
- 7.5 cases per 100,000 occur in Caucasians
- 5 cases per 100,000 occur in Asian-Americans/ Pacific Islanders

Incidence rate is between 1.3 and 7.8 cases per 100,000 population, based on population-based registries, according to global studies done by the National Center for Biotechnology Information. The incidence rates are higher in Northern

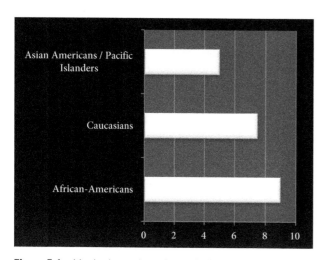

Figure 3.1 Meningiomas in various ethnic groups (cases per 100,000 population).

European countries and in Canada, and lowest in Asia and India. As in the United States, meningiomas throughout the world are most common in the sixth and seventh decades of life, and are also nearly twice as common in women. However, according to the *African Health Sciences Journal*, one study revealed that the mean age of female patients was 47 years, and the female-to-male ratio was much higher, at 3.8:1. The mean age of male patients was 39 years. However, the peak age range was in the fifth decade of life. The highest frequency was in black Africans (75%) compared with other ethnicities.

Etiology and Risk Factors

The actual cause of meningiomas is unknown; however, an environmental risk factor is ionizing radiation, particularly during childhood. High doses of therapeutic radiation to the head have also been implicated, though lower doses of radiation are also related to meningiomas. There is a confirmed genetic susceptibility to meningioma after ionizing radiation exposure. Hormones may also have a role to cause meningiomas, supporting the higher incidence in women. Meningiomas sometimes contain progesterone receptors, which may indicate slightly higher risks from the use of various hormones. Speaking to this point, there is a decreased risk if breastfeeding occurs for at least six months. Women who have had breast cancer, endometriosis, or uterine fibroids also have a higher risk of later development of meningiomas. Risks for meningiomas are also related to smoking and obesity.

Clinical Manifestations

Clinical manifestations depend on the brain area compressed by the tumor. Neurological manifestations may develop from compression of brain tissues, particularly with grade 2 or 3 meningioma, with deficits based on tumor location. Headaches and seizures are common symptoms, but are non-specific. Cranial neuropathies include loss of smell, taste, vision, and hemiparesis. In elderly patients, meningiomas can cause dementia without many focal neurologic problems. Other symptoms may include chronic low back pain and bilateral absence of pathological reflexes.

Pathology

Meningiomas can occur in all layers of the meninges. The tumors can develop in the olfactory grooves, optic nerve sheath, and sphenoid ridges. They are attached to the dura mater, and arise in the intracranial cavity, spinal cavity. Grade 1 meningiomas compress the brain parenchyma but do not invade it. Histologies vary, but they all develop similarly, and sometimes become malignant. Many patients have little or no edema, even after the tumors have become very large. This differs from high-grade gliomas and other brain tumors, in which edema is very common. Benign meningiomas usually occupy the dura and nearby structures, though this is usually slight in comparison with the more aggressive forms. As a result, meningiomas can cause significant morbidity and mortality.

Diagnosis

CT and/or MRI, particularly using a paramagnetic contrast agent, may detect the presence of meningioma. In CT scan or plain X-rays, boney remodeling may appear, potentially along with intratumoral calcifications. On CT scan, meningiomas are well-defined extra-axial masses, sometimes with brain displacement instead of invasion (see Figure 3.2). Neuroimaging is not totally diagnostic, and does not accurately predict tumor pathology or exclude differential diagnoses. It is difficult to distinguish between grades I, II, and III meningiomas on imaging alone, although clues such as invasive tumor, presence of vasogenic edema, and necrosis may direct one to consider more malignant possibilities. Definite diagnosis of meningiomas requires histology and molecular analysis.

Macroscopically, meningiomas are often firm or rubbery, with spots of different colors. The tumors may be round and lobulated. Meningiomas can encase or attach to cerebral arteries. Nearby brain tissues are usually

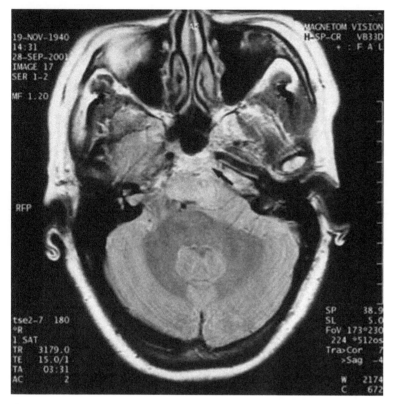

Figure 3.2 CT scan showing a meningioma. *Source:* Soo, M. Y., et. al. (2004).

compressed, but only rarely invaded. Some have a gritty appearance, related to many psammoma bodies that are present. Atypical and anaplastic meningiomas are usually larger, with necrosis. Microscopically, meningiomas usually have a sharp border between the brain and tumor tissues. Cytoplasm is abundant, but feather-like in appearance. The cell borders are indistinct. Psammoma bodies and meningothelial whorls are common.

Treatment

Excision or radiation therapy may be applied to enlarging or symptomatic meningiomas. Neuroimaging is often helpful for monitoring of asymptomatic small meningiomas, particularly in older adults or persons with multiple systemic comorbidities. Surgery is preferred if the meningioma is large, unless the tumor is close to the brainstem or other critical areas. Sometimes, **stereotactic radiosurgery** is prescribed for

surgically inaccessible meningiomas. This method may be used when there is residual tumor tissue after surgical excision, or if the patient is elderly, as applicable, and according to the best standard of care. Various radiation modalities including proton and fractionated treatment plans are frequently employed treatments.

Prevention and Early Detection

There is no known prevention for meningiomas, but a recent study of upregulation of inflammatory cyclooxygenase in these tumors may have a potential for evaluating the use of anti-inflammatory drugs for prevention. In the hereditable tumor suppressor gene condition Neurofibromatosis Type 2 (NF2) or in pediatric patients who have received cranial radiation, there is a greater likelihood of meningioma to appear. As such, proactive surveillance is usually part of the anticipatory follow-up for these conditions. Otherwise, the usual slow growth rate of meningiomas complicates early detection and prediction of tumor progression. Radiation exposure risks of screening CT head imaging and potential renal or pulmonary complications associated with gadolinium contrast agent of MRI head screening procedures, in addition to low-cost effectiveness of these studies related to incidence make preventive screening unfeasible.

Prognosis

Most meningiomas are asymptomatic, and do not require surgery. With complete removal of the tumor, 80% of patients can survive for 10 years. Only 22% of totally resected benign meningiomas recur with 20 years. Recurrence is mostly depending on the extent of resection or invasion, location, attachment to intracranial structures, and surgical familiarity with the tumor type (Simpson Grading of resection). Benign meningiomas have recurrence rates of about 7%, but atypical meningiomas recur in 30–50% of cases. Anaplastic meningiomas recur in 70% of cases. Over 10 years, recurrence is 14% for completely resected tumors, and 34% for subtotal resections. Grade II meningiomas recur in an average of five years, while grade III tumors recurred in an average of two years. As such, it is common standard of care practice to irradiate grade 2 or grade 3 meningiomas post-operatively to consolidate treatment rather than to wait for regrowth.

Significant Point

A meningioma is a primary central nervous system tumor, manifesting in the brain or spinal cord. It is the overall most common type of primary brain tumor, though higher-grade meningiomas are very rare. The most common subtype is grade I, in which the tumor cells grow slowly. Grade II meningiomas include the choroid and clear cell forms. Grade III meningiomas include the papillary and rhabdoid histologies.

Clinical Cases

Clinical Case 1

1. How prevalent are meningiomas in females?
2. What are the risk factors for meningiomas?
3. What are the primary treatments for meningiomas?

An 82-year-old woman was examined because of increasingly severe headaches and progressive visual loss that had occurred over one year. The radiographic diagnosis was of a presumptive meningioma surrounding the optic chiasm and compressing the pituitary gland. The tumor was considered inoperable due to its location. The patient had a past medical history of arthritis, and had been treated with prednisolone for two years. The steroid was increased in dosage after discovery of the meningioma and tapered after radiation therapy was initiated. With 10 days, the headaches had disappeared, and her vision improved. An MRI was ordered after radiation therapy was completed, and the tumor did not remain stable in size. It was followed up sequentially with imaging, ophthalmologic, endocrine, and neurological examinations with reduction in the size of the tumor over time noted on imaging. The patient was able to resume her activities of daily living.

Answers:

1. **For females, the prevalence of meningiomas is 10.5 cases per 100,000. Risks increase with age, and the peak of meningioma cases in the sixth and seventh decades of life. The incidence of meningiomas in females increases substantially between ages 65–85. These tumors often occur in pre-menopausal women. In fact, females between 35 and 45 years are three times more likely to develop a meningioma than males in the same age group.**
2. **An environmental risk factor for meningioma is therapeutic ionizing radiation,**

particularly during childhood, utilized for the treatment of another childhood tumor. Hormones may also have a role in causing or precipitating meningiomas, supporting the higher incidence in women. Meningiomas sometimes contain progesterone receptors, which may indicate slightly higher risks from the use of various hormones. Breast cancer, endometriosis, or uterine fibroids are also related to a higher risk of later development of meningiomas. Further associations between smoking, obesity and meningioma have been described. NF2, a genetic condition, is also associated with meningiomas but not relevant to this 82-year-old patient.

3. Maximum feasible surgical resection is recommended for tumors that are symptomatic and appropriately surgically accessible. Extent of resection for this tumor type makes a difference in recurrence rates and outcomes. Other considerations factoring into the decision to approach the case surgically would include other medical comorbidities that might make the risk–benefit ratio less favorable for the patient. Radiation is an important treatment modality that can be used to control difficult to resect meningiomas, or grade 2 or grade 3 meningiomas as an adjunct to surgery as applicable.

Hemangioma

A **hemangioma** is a benign, vascular tumor that may manifest in different sizes and locations in the CNS. Most are primary bone lesions that affect the CNS secondarily. In the CNS they mostly occur in the brainstem, cerebellum, and spinal cord. Hemangioma may be referenced as a family of *congenital hemangioma, cavernous hemangiomas, or cerebral cavernous malformations.*

Epidemiology

Brain hemangiomas are relatively rare, affecting only 0.4% of the overall population of the United States. About 12.5% of all brain hemangiomas occur after intracerebral hemorrhage. The prevalence of these tumors is very low because they are often asymptomatic and therefore undiagnosed while the patient is alive. The incidence is estimated at 0.3 and 0.5 cases per 100,000 people. Hemangiomas often are seen in children, and more commonly so in girls than boys. Congenital hemangiomas are less common than *infantile hemangiomas.* Cavernous hemangiomas usually occur in the third to fourth decade of life, with no gender preference. The overall age range for intracranial hemangiomas has been documented as between 14 months and 61 years, though they are more common in adults over 40 years. Cavernous hemangiomas that cause vision problems are more prevalent in females, between 20 and 40 years of age, than in males of the same age group. Generally speaking, intracranial hemangiomas are just slightly more common in women than in men. For cavernous hemangiomas, for unknown reasons, about 50% of Hispanic patients have a familial link. This occurs in 15% of cases in Caucasians. However, the general consensus is that intracranial hemangiomas show no predilection for any particular race or ethnicity.

Cerebral cavernous malformations are present in 0.5% of the overall global population, with about 40% of those affected having symptoms. Asymptomatic patients may develop the malformation sporadically, while symptomatic people usually have an inherited genetic mutation. According to the World Health Organization, there are about 0.3 cases in every 100,000 people throughout the world. About 25% of cases are in children and 75% of cases are in adults. There is no satisfactory data to provide an adequate estimate of life expectancy. Hemangiomas occur in all areas of the world, with no racial or ethnic predilection.

Etiology and Risk Factors

A majority of hemangiomas have a congenital link, but they may also develop over an individual's lifetime. However, the cause is unknown. Cerebral cavernous malformations are inherited as an autosomal dominant disorder, in 20% of cases, yet most cases are sporadic. Inherited cerebral cavernous malformation pathogenesis involves biallelic somatic and germline mutations, within one of the cerebral cavernous malformation genes. Radiation treatment for other medical conditions is a commonly noted cause of cavernous malformations, particularly years after the exposure. There are no known risk factors for hemangiomas.

Clinical Manifestations

Cavernous hemangiomas may cause intraparenchymal hemorrhage, loss of memory, seizures, decreased level of consciousness, double vision, language difficulties, and incidental hydrocephalus. Less severe symptoms include weakness, limb numbness, headaches, and ataxia. If the tumor extends to the eyes, proptosis may occur. As might be expected, location and rate of lesion expansion dictate symptoms for the most part.

Pathology

Hemangiomas often grow from capillary blood supplies, but also from arteriovenous blood supplies. Infantile hemangiomas are usually positive for *glucose transporter 1 (GLUT1)*, which helps distinguish these tumors from arteriovenous malformations in extracranial locations. Hemangiomas often grow quickly in a few months. Cavernous hemangiomas are reddish-brown and sponge-like in appearance. Cerebral

cavernous malformations differ from other cavernous hemangiomas in that there is no tissue within the malformation, and the borders are not encapsulated. This means that they can change in size and quantity.

Diagnosis

Gradient-echo T2-weighted magnetic resonance imaging is one of the more sensitive sequences for the detection of cavernous hemangiomas along with susceptibility imaging. Radiographic images reveal a "popcorn"-shaped tumor (see Figure 3.3). CT scans are not specific, and angiography may be used to rule out other diagnoses if there is any question of the differential diagnosis. Biopsies may be obtained from the tumor tissue for examination, and correct diagnosis is important because these lesions are less aggressive than tumors such as **angiosarcomas**. Biopsies are not common pressure today because of the accuracy of the MRI imaging for these tumors.

Treatment

Total surgical excision (gross total resection) is often done as possible, particularly when the tumor is destroying surrounding tissues and causing major symptoms. Complications of surgery can be hemorrhage, stroke, or death. Treatments such as radiosurgery or microsurgery

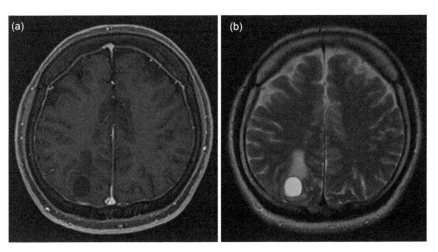

Figure 3.3 MRI of a cavernous hemangioma, seen in (A) T1-weighted imaging and (B) T2-weighted imaging. *Source*: Takamori et al. (2020).

may be applicable, based on the tumor site, size, and symptoms. Microsurgery is preferred if the tumor is superficial within the CNS, or risks of damage to surrounding tissues from radiation therapy are too high. Other indications for microsurgery are large hemorrhages, seizures, or a coma. The preferred radiation technique is stereotactic radiosurgery, either single dose or fractionated, directing a precise radiation dose to the hemangioma. After surgery, some patients experience transient diabetes insipidus, weakness due to injury to the hypothalamus, and somnolence. These symptoms usually resolve over a few months.

Prevention and Early Detection

There is no prevention strategy currently applicable for hemangiomas. Both MRI and CT are crucial for detection and to consider the differential diagnosis of hemangiomas. Once an enhancing mass has been found, appropriate MRI/CT imaging for detailed visualization of any associated changes to adjacent structures is implemented.

Prognosis

Cavernous hemangiomas may result in a serious outlook since they may cause bleeding and seizures. Patients who have experienced previous brain bleeding from these tumors have a higher risk of subsequent bleeding. Fortunately, once these tumors are completely excised there is minimal risk of growth or rebleeding.

Significant Point

With cavernous hemangiomas, there is abnormal tissue that causes slowed blood flow through the caverns (cavities) of the brain. The leakage of blood causes many different symptoms. Asymptomatic individuals have usually developed the malformation sporadically, but symptomatic individuals frequently carry a genetic mutation.

Clinical Case 2

1. Discuss epidemiological statistics regarding cavernous hemangiomas.
2. Describe relevant pathology of cavernous hemangiomas.
3. What is the preferred therapeutic technique for cavernous hemangiomas?

A 40-year-old woman presented to the emergency department after experiencing a sudden decreased level of consciousness accompanied by change in vision. Brain imaging revealed a hemorrhagic popcorn-shaped mass in the third ventricle, and the woman was hospitalized and scheduled for surgery. The lesion involved the foramen of Monroe and the hypothalamus. The lesion was completely removed and diagnosed as a cavernous hemangioma. In a few days, the patient had transient diabetes insipidus, somnolence, and weakness because of hypothalamic injury, but within two months, had recovered normal function.

Answers:

1. **Cavernous hemangiomas usually present in the third to fourth decade, with no gender preference. Cavernous hemangiomas that cause vision problems are more prevalent in females, between 20 and 40 years of age, than in males of the same age group. For reasons yet to be elucidated, about 50% of Hispanic patients with cavernous hemangiomas have a familial link, but this occurs in 15% of cases in Caucasians.**
2. **Cavernous hemangiomas are grossly reddish-brown and sponge-like in appearance. Cerebral cavernous malformations differ from other cavernous hemangiomas in that there is no tissue within the malformation, and the borders are not encapsulated. This means that they can change in size, geometry, and quantity.**
3. **The preferred targeted/locoregional technique is stereotactic radiosurgery, directing a precise radiation dose to the hemangioma.**

Neurofibroma

A **neurofibroma** is a fibrous nerve tissue tumor of abnormal proliferation of Schwann cells. It is benign and well differentiated. Neurofibromas consist of neoplastic Schwann cells, mixed with mast cells, and non-neoplastic fibroblasts forming a matrix. Multiple and plexiform neurofibromas are usually linked to neurofibromatous type 1 (NF1). Even so, sporadic neurofibromas are encountered regularly. Neurofibromas are usually intimately cutaneous tumors, occurring in any body area.

Epidemiology

Neurofibromas are common peripherally, but do not typically occur in the brain, and may be sporadic. There may be single, multiple, or numerous lesions, the latter mostly related to NF1. Neurofibromas are the most prevalent type of benign peripheral nerve sheath tumor. Solitary neurofibromas are sporadic in 90% of cases and inherited in the remaining 10%. The prevalence of skin neurofibromas is 1 in every 2,600 to 3,000 people, which is really quite common, but there is little information about the prevalence of brain neurofibromas. Over 100,000 people are affected by skin neurofibromas in the United States. Incidence of brain neurofibromas has not been determined. Age of onset is widely varied, but neurofibromas are most common in adults between 20 and 40. They affect men and women equally in a 1:1 ratio, and have no racial or ethnic predisposition. Globally, the statistics are nearly identical, according to the World Health Organization.

Etiology and Risk Factors

The cause of neurofibroma involves genetics, cell signaling, the cell cycle, and histology. Non-myelinating Schwann cells make up the neoplastic factor in neurofibromas. The tumors arise from non-myelinating Schwann cells, which only express the inactive version of the NF1 gene. This results in complete loss of expression of functional neurofibromin. Most neurofibromas are sporadic, with a very low risk of malignant transformation. There are no definite risk factors for sporadic neurofibromas developing outside of the context of NF1.

Clinical Manifestations

Neurofibromas are usually not painful and manifest simply as masses. If they are deeper, such as the paraspinal form, they may cause motor and sensory deficits related to the nerve from which they form. Neurofibroma is often a skin nodule, known as a *cutaneous neurofibroma* (see Figure 3.4). Less commonly, they occur in a peripheral nerve, or as a plexiform mass in a major nerve plexus or trunk. There may be extensive or massive effects on soft tissues, known as *localized gigantism* or **elephantiasis neuromatosa**. Neurofibroma rarely involves spinal roots sporadically, but often involves these roots if the patient has NF1. When this occurs, there are multiple, bilateral tumors often linked to scoliosis. These rarely affect the cranial nerves. Multiple neurofibromas are characteristic of NF1, along with other common manifestations.

Pathology

The World Health Organization classifies neurofibromas as grade I tumors. Macroscopically, cutaneous neurofibromas are nodular to polyploid in appearance. Neurofibromas involve the skin and subcutaneous fat tissues. Fat and other normal structures may be entrapped in the tumors. Diffuse neurofibromas can be in different sizes, but are often large. There is a good amount of dermal and subcutaneous thickening. Plexiform neurofibromas have multinodular, twisted structures that resemble a "bag of worms" when they involve trunks of a neural plexus. However, they resemble rope-like lesions, such as the sciatic nerve. Cut surfaces appear glistening, pale, and grayish-tan.

Microscopically, neurofibromas have neoplastic Schwann cells with thin, lengthened, and curved nuclei, with a little cytoplasm. Encapsulation is absent. The nuclei are much smaller than those of schwannomas. Formation of stromal collagen is greatly different.

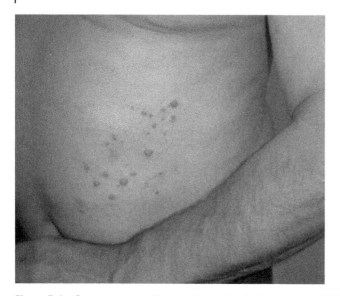

Figure 3.4 Cutaneous neurofibroma. *Source*: García-Romero et al. (2015).

Intraneural neurofibromas are usually fixed to a nerve and surrounded by its thickened epineurium. However, tumors that start in smaller cutaneous nerves often show diffuse spread into the adjacent dermis and soft tissues.

Diagnosis

The diagnosis of neurofibroma is confirmed by skin biopsy, which will reveal a non-encapsulated tumor made up of fascicles of slender, spindle-shaped cells. The surrounding matrix is stains with a pale appearance, with thin, wavy collagen. Neurofibromas have large numbers of mast cells, and stain positively for the S100 protein. A neurofibroma can also diagnose via a blood test for protein melanoma inhibitory activity (MIA). *Melanoma-derived growth regulatory protein* is encoded by the *MIA gene*, and is a marker for malignant melanoma. Subcutaneous and plexiform neurofibromas are usually encapsulated, and surrounded by epineurium or perineurium. They contain many large nerve fascicles in a cellular matrix of collagen, fibroblasts, mucin, and Schwann cells. To determine involvement of plexiform neurofibromas, an MRI may be required. If suspected, but with no clinical criteria, genetic testing for NF1

is available. Differential diagnoses for cutaneous neurofibromas include **acrochordon**, dermal melanocytic nevus, fibroma, lipoma, and neuroma.

Treatment

The treatment of cutaneous neurofibromas relieves symptoms such as bleeding, itching, pain, irritation caused by clothing, and to address cosmetic appearance. For large numbers of lesions related to NF1, carbon dioxide laser vaporization and electrosurgical excision have been successful interventions. For solitary neurofibromas, a simple excision via shave biopsy is performed. Multiple lesions can also be removed by simple excision. For diffuse neurofibromas, treatment is partial or complete surgical excision. However, these tumors can recur due to their infiltrative growth patterns. For some patients, complete excision is not successful with extensive surgery, which sometimes causes permanent scarring. Diffuse neurofibromas require follow-up every year. Plexiform neurofibromas are infiltrative, meaning that they are harder to be completely removed, and often recur. An MRI must be conducted before surgical excision to determine the extent of each lesion and the chances for successful removal. Major risks include hemorrhage and permanent nerve damage. The medical treatment of plexiform neurofibromas may include interferon-alpha, vincristine, methotrexate, or more recently approved targeted therapies such as selumetinib.

Prevention and Early Detection

There is no known prevention for neurofibromas. Early detection is the best preventive method to reduce recurrence. Regular follow-up is required to assess areas of resection and detect early growth or nodule formation. The entire body should be screened to rule out new neurofibromas. This reduces chances of further complications and provides for early care.

Prognosis

The prognosis of neurofibroma is based on the subtype, and the presence of NF1 or NF2. Neurofibromas on the skin occur more often with aging, resulting in cosmetic issues with secondary emotional consequence to be discriminated from cognitive impact from different etiology. Quick diagnosis and treatments can greatly affect the overall prognosis. Patients with NF1 may have a reduced life expectancy of up to 15 years. Prognosis for those with NF2 is based on the numbers and locations of tumors.

Significant Point

The central nervous system manifestations of neurofibromas, in relation to neurofibromatosis type 1 (NF1) include cognitive disabilities, visual disturbances, precocious puberty, acute hemiplegia, and focal neurological deficits. Other related types of tumors involved in this tumor suppressor gene condition include malignant peripheral nerve sheath tumors, gliomas, and gangliogliomas.

Schwannoma

A **schwannoma** is a benign tumor composed entirely of well-differentiated Schwann cells, and grows slowly. It is encapsulated, affecting the myelin nerve sheaths covering the peripheral nerves. Schwannomas can also emerge from the optic and olfactory nerves, which lack myelin sheaths. They are attached to the cranial or spinal nerves from which they originate.

Epidemiology

The prevalence and incidence of schwannomas of the central nervous system are not well documented. Intracranial schwannomas, unlike other schwannomas, are more common in older adults, within the fourth to sixth decades. However, patients may be of any age, but pediatric cases are rare. There is a female predominance of nearly twice compared with males. However, cerebral intraparenchymal schwannomas have a male predominance and occur in younger people. There is no racial or ethnic predilection, and the global statistics are identical to those of the United States.

Etiology and Risk Factors

The causes of schwannomas are unknown. Family history may suggest a genetic link. Exposure to radiation is a possible cause. No identified risk factors exist for schwannomas outside of the context of NF2.

Clinical Manifestations

The clinical findings of peripherally located schwannomas depend on their shape, location, and rate of growth. They can be asymptomatic paraspinal tumors, or spinal nerve tumors that cause **radicular pain** and signs of nerve root or spinal cord compression. Schwannomas usually present with painless swelling. Symptoms are primarily based on the location of the tumor. There may be tingling and numbness along the involved nerve. Lower back pain or partial leg paralysis may be related to a lumbosacral tumor. Schwannomas may involve cranial nerve, with symptoms of hearing loss or tinnitus. Sometimes there is difficulty walking, nausea, vomiting, horizontal nystagmus, slow corneal reflexes, or vertigo. Clinical finding may be linked to trigeminal nerve dysfunction, causing numbness, **neurasthenia**, or neuralgia. When schwannoma affects the nose, there may be nosebleeds, difficulty breathing, and dysphasia. There are no specific signs, symptoms for intracerebral schwannoma. It may result in increased intracranial pressure, local neurological dysfunction, or seizures.

Pathology

By definition, schwannomas themselves arise outside the CNS, in the peripheral nerves of the skin and subcutaneous tissue. Similarly, schwannomas can occur along cranial nerves. They may also arise from the cervical or brachial plexuses, although rare. Less than 5% of upper extremity schwannomas develop from the cervical plexus. The cochlear peripheral nerve division can be affected resulting in enlargement of the internal auditory meatus; as such, auditory screening and neuroimaging easily detect and diagnose them. Central nervous system schwannomas are not always linked to a specific nerve. There have been roughly only 70 cases of spinal intramedullary schwannomas and 40 additional cases of intraventricular or cerebral parenchymal schwannomas reported in the literature. Peripheral nerve schwannomas are often attached to nerve trunks, commonly involving the head and neck. About 90% of all schwannomas are solitary and sporadic. However, less than 1% of all intracranial schwannomas are intracerebral. They are usually **supratentorial**, in the superficial sections of the brain parenchyma or near the ventricle. Almost 45% of schwannomas occur in the head and neck area. Less than 1% of schwannomas become malignant, and degenerate into **neurofibrosarcomas**. Schwannomas occur in the frontal and temporal lobes, cerebellar hemisphere, cerebellar vermis, and fourth ventricle.

Neurofibromatosis type 2 is an autosomal dominant syndrome that results from mutations in the *NF2* tumor suppressor gene, merlin (moesin-ezrin-radixin-like protein, also known as schwannomin, located on chromosome 22q. Half of patients inherit a germline mutation from an affected parent and the remainder acquires a de novo mutation for neurofibromatosis type 2. Patients develop nervous system tumors including bilateral vestibular schwannomas and cutaneous lesions described above.

Diagnosis

MRI is preferred for the diagnosis of schwannoma. There is often an abnormal cystic signal and nodular shadows above the cystic wall, in the parenchyma. A vestibular schwannoma often has an "ice cream cone" shape, with a tapered intraosseous "cone" emerging from the internal auditory canal. The cone expands out into a circular cerebellopontine angled mass. In MRI images, an intracranial schwannoma has high contrast resolution, and a detailed view of brain structures. This allows for precise tumor localization. Differential diagnoses include acoustic schwannoma, meningioma, chondrosarcoma, or ependymoma. If the tumor is only within the **Meckel's cave**, and is small, the differential diagnoses additionally include pituitary adenoma, and aneurysm. Paraspinal tumors may be shaped like a "dumbbell," with a point of constriction at the neural exit foramen. Lumbosacral schwannomas are solid, and well enhanced compared with other lesions. They cannot be diagnosed only via physical examination. Although an MRI scan with contrast is helpful, a histopathological examination is absolute. Many times, sequential imaging and the tincture of time with palliative symptom management may help the clinician better understand the indolent nature of the tumor's biology. Macroscopically, schwannomas are globoid in shape, and less than 10 mm in size. They are encapsulated, except for tumors of bone, skin, and the intraparenchymal CNS sites. A cut tumor surface usually reveals hemorrhages and glistening tissue of a light tan color, with bright yellow areas.

Treatment

To treat schwannoma, corticosteroid injections into the joints may be administered, along with local anesthetics to decrease pain. If the tumor is small and not causing any extreme problems, it may only be monitored for signs of growth or change. Schwannomas are surgically resected, and they can often be scraped off of nerves without any permanent nerve damage. Based on tumor size and location, recovery length and remaining symptoms are varied. If it is cancerous or there are coexisting conditions making surgery dangerous, *stereotactic radiosurgery* may be done. A high dose of radiation is provided directly to the tumor, with the goal of shrinking it over time. This method has fewer adverse effects than traditional radiation, which uses smaller doses of radiation over a longer period. Chemotherapy and immunotherapy medications are also sometimes used. For lumbosacral schwannomas, treatment can include complete excision, sacrificing the nerve root. Results are usually good, but surgical trauma may cause neurological deficits in some cases.

Prevention and Early Detection

There is no known prevention for schwannomas. Early detection outside the context of NF2 is sometimes difficult since the symptoms may be slight, and may not appear in the beginning stages of growth. For vestibular schwannomas, MRI scans, genetic testing, and auditory testing are critical.

Prognosis

The prognosis for schwannomas is mostly based on tumor location, size, geometry, and whether it is benign or malignant. Since majority of schwannomas are benign and never produce symptoms, overall prognosis is excellent. Monitoring of all changes in symptoms to improve outcomes is important.

Significant Point

Schwannoma is a benign, slow-growing tumor that arises from the Schwann cells. This type of tumor can occur on any peripheral nerve that is surrounded by Schwann cells. This includes the cranial nerves, which pass information between the brain and areas of the head and neck. Schwannomas are most common on cranial nerve VIII (the vestibulo-cochlear nerve). Neurofibromatosis Type 2 is almost categorically related to the formation of schwannomas, although the converse is not true.

Astrocytoma

Astrocytomas are diffuse, primary, infiltrative, and intrinsic tumors that may arise in the brain or spinal cord. These tumors develop from cells called astrocytes, which support neurons as part of a family of glial cells. They may be indolent in their grade 1 subtype, but for the most part they range from low-grade to malignant tumors with an extremely high propensity for recurrence or upgrading to a more malignant form. The most common type of grade I astrocytomas are *pilocytic astrocytomas*, and these usually affect children and younger adults. They may develop in optic pathways, hypothalamus, third ventricle, cerebellum, and the spinal cord. *Subependymal giant cell astrocytoma* is also a grade 1 astrocytoma and occurs in younger patients who have *tuberous sclerosis*, a spontaneous or autosomal dominant condition caused by mutations in the *TSC1* or *TSC2* gene. Other grades of astrocytomas include *low-grade astrocytoma (grade 2), anaplastic astrocytoma (grade 3)*, and *glioblastoma (grade 4)*. Glioblastoma is very aggressive and the deadliest of all primary brain tumors.

Epidemiology

Astrocytomas are the most common type of glial cell tumor, accounting for 5% of all glioma diagnoses. Epidemiology of astrocytomas depends upon their classification. Grade I astrocytomas are most common children and teenagers, while g rade II astrocytomas are mostly seen in adults. Grade III astrocytomas are most common in slightly older adults, males, and account for 4% of all brain tumors. *Subependymal giant cell* tumors affect 5–20% of patients with tuberous sclerosis and are only occasionally found in people over age 20. Low-grade astrocytomas usually occur in adults between the ages of 20 and 50. In the United States, *anaplastic astrocytoma* has an incidence rate of 0.44 per every 100,000 people, occurring slightly more often in men.

Glioblastomas are malignant type tumors that mostly affect children and adults of all ages but highest in prevalence between ages 55 and 85 and is the most common intraparenchymal adult primary brain tumor. In adults, glioblastoma is the second most common type of intracranial neoplasm. Glioblastomas, as is the case for all astrocytoma grades, are more common in Caucasians than in other races, and for all tumor grades, are slightly more common in males than in females. Primary glioblastomas are 1.33 times more common in males than females, but secondary glioblastomas (mutating from lower grade as opposed to *de novo*) are 0.65 times as common in males than females. Overall, glioblastomas are the third most common cancer between ages 15 and 34, and the fourth most common cancer between ages 35 and 54. For children in the United States, there are 0.14 new cases per 100,000, annually. Global statistics are not well documented.

Etiology and Risk Factors

Astrocytomas, for the most part, are sporadic and with uncertain causality. They originate in star-shaped cerebral cells called *astrocytes*. Aging is a risk factor for all forms of astrocytomas, along with **Li-Fraumeni syndrome**, neurofibromatosis, **tuberous sclerosis**, **Turcot syndrome**, and previous radiation therapy. Additional risk factors include exposure to pesticides, smoking, and work in a petroleum refining or rubber manufacturing facility.

Clinical Manifestations

The initial symptoms of astrocytomas include behavioral changes, headaches, loss of memory, and seizures. If the posterior fossa is affected, signs include incoordination, neck stiffness, and tilting of the head. In children, a pilocytic astrocytoma may cause difficulty coordinating movements, headache, irritability, lack of normal weight gain, weight loss, nausea and vomiting, torticollis, and visual problems, such as nystagmus. Symptoms are different based on the tumor's location and size. The most common symptoms are due to increased intracranial pressure because of the size of the neoplasm. When symptoms appear after incomplete surgical resection, they may be related to the concurrent presence of a cyst, as it continues to enlarge, and not the solid tissue mass.

Pathology

Pilocytic astrocytomas are most common in the frontal lobes, cerebellum, and cerebral hemispheres. They occur less often in the spinal cord, or manifest as **drop metastases**. Regional effects are caused by compression, invasion, and destruction of brain parenchyma. Pilocytic astrocytomas account for 0.6–5.1% of all intracranial neoplasms, are the most common primary brain tumors in children, and constitute 77% of all cerebellar astrocytomas. *Low-grade astrocytomas* are relatively uncommon and they make up about 10% of all gliomas. *Anaplastic astrocytomas* make up 7.5% of all gliomas, and 5% of all primary brain tumors. *Glioblastomas* cause 15% of all intracranial neoplasms and constitute about 45–50% of all primary malignant brain tumors. Astrocytomas may cause arterial and venous hypoxia. They compete for nutrients, and release metabolic end products such as free radicals, altered electrolytes, and neurotransmitters. They also release **cytokines** and other cellular mediators, which disrupt parenchymal functions. When the tumors are solid, there is a significantly circumscribed appearance, which lays in contradistinction with their diffuse and infiltrative microscopic nature.

Cerebellar pilocytic astrocytomas are many times hemispheric, made up of a large cyst filled with fluid, along with an enhancing mural nodule. If within the hypothalamus or optic nerve, the tumor is usually solid. Within the optic nerve, they look like a focal segmental nerve swelling. Unilateral and bilateral optic nerve tumors are among the most commonly occurring. The dense areas have hair-like or bipolar astrocytes, plus long, spindle-shaped processes, usually with **Rosenthal fibers** (see Figure 3.5). There is a fusiform or corkscrew shape and a hyaline-like appearance.

Diagnosis

Pathology confirmation of astrocytomas often requires three to six months after onset of clinical manifestations since the patient often does not realize the cause of symptoms. Pilocytic astrocytomas are well circumscribed in imaging studies. They are usually cystic and enhanced when **gadolinium contrast** is used, and are near the ventricle or subarachnoid space (see Figure 3.6). Often, there is no surrounding edema, which is a very common feature of higher-grade astrocytomas. Malignant transformation is rare. Astrocytomas are usually diagnosed with clinical,

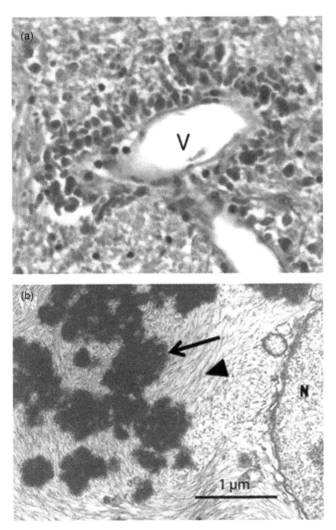

Figure 3.5 Rosenthal fibers, (a) among the astrocytes surrounding a blood vessel (labeled "V"); (b) an arrow indicating the Rosenthal fibers surrounded by intermediate filaments (arrowhead). *Source*: Messing et al. (2012).

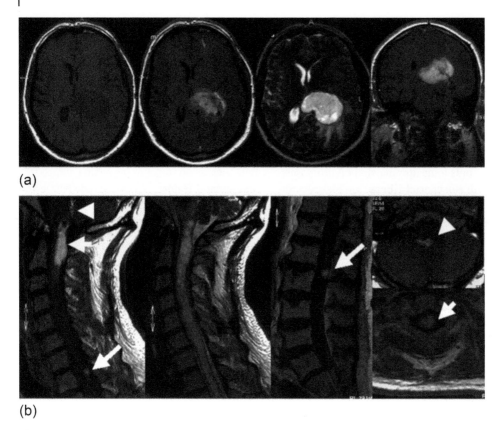

(a)

(b)

Figure 3.6 Pilocytic astrocytoma, (a) from left to right: T1-weighted axial MRI before and after administration of contrast medium, plus T2-weighted images showing perifocal edema; (b) from left to right: T1-weighted sagittal MRI with contrast of the craniocervical junction and cervical spine, with arrowhead indicating subarachnoid spread in the fourth ventricle; the small arrow indicates intramedullary tumor growth in the upper cervical cord; the large arrow indicates leptomeningeal metastasis at the level of the first thoracic segment. In the third image, the large arrow indicates another leptomeningeal metastasis at the level of the first and second lumbar segments. In the fourth image, the arrowhead indicates subependymal growth in the fourth ventricle, and the small arrow indicates the intramedullary tumor. *Source*: Stüer et al. (2007).

neurological, and ophthalmological examinations, along with CT scan or MRI. Contrasted imaging studies are easily able to identify tumor characteristics. Astrocytoma may be biopsied before surgical resection. Microscopically, these tumors appear to be made up of bipolar cells with long, hair-like processes, which are related to the term "pilocytic," since it means "fiber-like." There are usually eosinophilic granular bodies, microcysts, and Rosenthal fibers. **Myxoid foci** and oligodendroglioma-like cells may be present, but are non-specific. Lesions that have existed for a long time may have calcifications, and macrophages filled with hemosiderin.

Treatment

Maximum feasible surgical resection is usually the initial required approach for diagnosis, cytoreduction, and possible relief of symptoms. Contingent on the geometry, location, grading, and biological or genetic nature of the astrocytoma, various modalities of intervention may be applied. These include but are not limited to observation, radiation, biochemotherapy, alternating electrical fields, or other clinical trials that may use immune or cellular therapies. The treatment algorithms are usually multidisciplinary, complex, and must consider the patient's neurological functionality and concurrent illnesses as well as the performance status of the patient.

Prevention and Early Detection

There is no current way to prevent or reduce risks of developing astrocytoma beyond awareness of genetic syndromes such as NF1 to be aware to screen for them. Routine screening outside of this context with MRI studies is not cost-effective. Routine healthy person examinations that include neurological review of systems and examination can help detect findings of which the patient was unaware and initiate an imaging study that would have otherwise waited.

Prognosis

For pilocytic astrocytoma, overall survival over 15 years is 80%. For completely resected tumors in the cerebellum, the 15-year survival rate is 95%. After surgical resection of pilocytic astrocytoma, the 25-year survival rate is 50–94%. Malignant transformation is exceedingly rare. For grades 2–4 astrocytoma, the range of survival with optimal therapy and appropriate genomic profiling, can range from over a decade to 18–24 months, for glioblastoma.

Significant Point

Astrocytomas are likely to have diffuse growth patterns, invading nearby tissues, then locally progressing to other brain structures and adjacent tissues. Over time, they may become very large, ironically if they are slower growing. Pilocytic astrocytomas are the most common brain tumors in children. They usually affect the cerebellum and brainstem, with the pons being the area most commonly involved. Astrocytomas grades 2–4 are graded based on histology and genomic profiling and are increasingly on a spectrum of malignant/aggressive biological behavior. For grades 2–4 astrocytoma, the range of survival with optimal therapy and appropriate genomic profiling, can range from over a decade to 18–24 months, for glioblastoma.

Pituitary Adenoma

A **pituitary adenoma** is a generally benign type of pituitary tumor. In some cases, they can become invasive or develop as carcinomas. Tumors more than 1 cm in size are called macroadenomas, while those smaller than this size are called microadenomas. The majority of pituitary adenomas are microadenomas. They are also classified as *intrasellar* or *extrasellar* based on their proclivity and propensity to expand beyond the anatomic sella turcica.

Epidemiology

Pituitary adenomas make up 10–25% of all intracranial neoplasms. A study of 1,120 patients for sellar masses, 91% had a pituitary adenoma. Invasive pituitary adenomas occur in 35% of all pituitary adenoma cases, and only 0.1–0.2% are carcinomas. Pituitary adenomas represent 10–25% of all intracranial neoplasms. Most of them are being classified as *microadenomas*, of a diameter less than 10 mm. The prevalence rate of pituitary adenomas in the United States is approximately 17%. They are found 22.5% of the time in radiologic studies, and 14.5% of the time in autopsy studies. Overall, pituitary adenomas affect about one of every six people in the general population. However, *clinically active* pituitary adenomas affect about one of every 1,000 in the general population. In one study of 2,598 patients who underwent an MRI, pituitary adenomas made up 82% of all visible lesions. In the United States, the incidence has increased from 2.52 per 100,000 populations to 3.13 per 100,000, between the years 2004 and 2009.

In older people, most adenomas have an equivalent male-to-female ratio. For **prolactinomas**, the peak occurrence is in the second to fifth decades of life. However, for endocrine-inactive adenomas, the peak occurrence or discovery is in the fourth to eighth decades of life. The GH-releasing, ACTH-releasing, and TSH-releasing adenomas are more evenly distributed through adult life span. Prolactinomas, ACTH-releasing adenomas, and TSH-releasing adenomas are most common in females. Endocrine-inactive and GH-releasing adenomas occur mostly in males. African Americans have the highest rates of pituitary adenomas. The following tumors occur in varying percentages, as illustrated in Figure 3.7:

- Prolactinomas (57%)
- Nonfunctioning adenomas (28%)
- Growth hormone (GH)-secreting adenomas (11%)
- Cushing's adenomas (2%).

The global prevalence of pituitary adenomas is also about 17% of the total population, but incidence varies by country. In the United Kingdom, there were 64 pituitary adenomas out of 89,434 individuals. In Japan, 16% of 28,428 cases were confirmed to be pituitary adenomas. Prolactinomas are the most common secretory pituitary tumors, with an annual incidence of about 30 per 100,000 people. For *microprolactinomas*, females are diagnosed 20 times more than males, but for *macroprolactinomas*, the ratio is nearly equivalent. People from African countries/heritage have the highest rates of these tumors.

Etiology and Risk Factors

The exact cause of adenomas is unknown, but inherited genetic mutations are suspected to be contributory. Some sporadic pituitary adenomas have acquired mutations of the *acute intermittent porphyria (AIP) gene.* Many growth-hormone-secreting adenomas have an acquired *guanine nucleotide alpha stimulating* mutation. Risk factors for pituitary adenomas include multiple endocrine neoplasia 1 (MEN1), Carney complex, and familial isolated pituitary adenoma.

Clinical Manifestations

Pituitary adenomas are the most common cause of *hyperpituitarism*, with specific manifestations based on the type of hormone secretion. Some of these tumors secrete more than one hormone (usually growth hormone plus prolactin), resulting in unexpected bone growth and lactation – in men as well as women. There may be visual field defects, most often **bitemporal hemianopsia**, due to the tumor compressing the optic nerve. Specifically, the tumor compresses the *optic chiasma*, producing a defect in the temporal visual field on both sides because of the crossed nature of roughly half the retinal input neurons through this area. If the adenoma laterally expands, and the **abducens nerve** is also compressed, there will be *lateral rectus muscles palsy*. Pituitary adenomas may increase intracranial pressure with its related symptoms. Psychiatric symptoms may include anxiety, depression, apathy, emotional instability, and easy irritability or hostility for varying reasons relating to the size of the pituitary tumor as well as what it is or is not secreting.

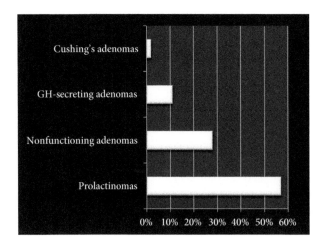

Figure 3.7 Percentages of various subtypes of pituitary adenomas.

About 95% of cases of **acromegaly** come from a pituitary adenoma, causing the anterior pituitary gland to produce excessive growth hormone. This is most common in middle-aged adults. Acromegaly may result in stereotypical orthopedic disfigurement, sleep apnea, heart problems, type 2 diabetes mellitus, colon polyps, and premature death. Acromegaly is often missed for many years, until changes in the soft tissue enlargement and widening and thickening of skeletal bones in the face, jaw, hands, and feet. (see Figure 3.8).

Cushing's disease can result in excessive adrenocorticotropic hormone (ACTH) secretion. Signs and symptoms of Cushing's disease include central upper body obesity with supraclavicular fat accumulation, thin arms and legs, a moon-shaped face. Other signs and symptoms include acne or skin infections, purple striae on the skin and thinning of the skin, easy bruising, backache, bone pain or tenderness, a buffalo

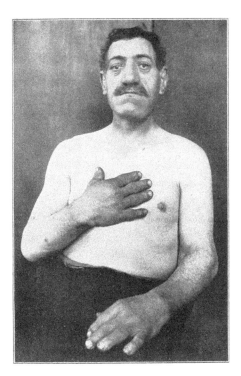

Figure 3.8 An individual with acromegaly.
Source: Sajous's analytical cyclopædia of practical medicine" (1904) / Flicker / Public Domain.

hump of fat on the back between the shoulders, plus bone and muscle weakening. Additional complications include **pituitary apoplexy** and central diabetes insipidus.

Pathology

Though in most cases pituitary adenomas are benign and noninvasive, an invasive adenoma may enter the dura mater, and sphenoid bone. When the tumor reaches 1 cm in diameter, visual manifestations more often appear. Pituitary adenomas are classified based on their anatomical, histological, and functional criteria. Cell differentiation, driven by transcription factors, lead to the acidophilic, gonadotrophic, and corticotrophic cell lineages.

Diagnosis

Diagnosis is confirmed by blood testing hormone levels, and via radiographic imaging of the pituitary – usually MRI, or CT if MRI is contraindicated in some way or to better investigate boney windows. The radiographic classifications of pituitary adenomas include five different categories:

- 0 – Normal appearance of the pituitary
- I – Enclosed in the sella turcica, microadenoma; smaller than 10 mm
- II – Enclosed in the sella turcica, macroadenoma; 10 mm or more
- III – Invasive, locally, into the sella
- IV – Invasive, diffusely, into the sella

Classification is based on which type of hormone is secreted by the tumor. Functional classification is based on endocrine activity, determined by serum hormone levels, and immunohistochemical staining to detect pituitary tissue cellular hormone secretion.

Treatment

Treatments are based on the type of pituitary adenoma and its size. Prolactinomas are usually treated with the dopamine agonists called cabergoline or quinagolide. They decrease the size of the tumor. Serial imaging is used to detect any increases in size. If the tumor is large, radiation therapy, stereotactic radiosurgery (e.g. proton, IMRT, other), or surgery can be used – usually with good results. Progesterone antagonists have been tried in the treatment of prolactinomas without success. Somatotrophic adenomas often respond to the long-acting somatostatin analog called octreotide. Thyrotrophic adenomas usually do not respond well to treatment with dopamine agonists. For surgery, the most common approach is **transsphenoidal** adenectomy, which usually removes the tumor and leaves the brain and optic nerves unaffected. Transsphenoidal surgery is performed through the sphenoid sinus. Many neurosurgeons use a direct transnasal approach. An incision is made in the back wall of the nose, and the sphenoid sinus is entered directly. Another method is to make an incision along the front of the nasal septum, and create a tunnel back to the sphenoid sinus. The final option is to make an incision under the lip and approach through the upper gum, entering the nasal cavity, and then the sphenoid sinus. Other surgical approaches include endoscopic surgery, which is usually **endonasal**, and craniotomy for rare, invasive, suprasellar masses that extend into the frontal or middle cranial fossa, optic nerves, or for significant posterior **clival** invasion.

Pituitary radiation can also be used, in which high-energy ionizing radiation is delivered to the deep tissues using ionizing megavoltage. Today, this is much more effective and safer than in previous decades. Radiation can be administered in multiple fractions over five to six weeks, or in a single radiobiologic equivalent dose. Complications of stereotactic radiosurgery include worsened hypopituitarism, thyroid problems, cortisol abnormalities, cranial nerve (especially visual) dysfunction, GH abnormalities, gonadotropin abnormalities, additional required debridement surgery, additional tumor growth, and diabetes insipidus. Use of radiation is extremely individualized per patient. Generally, radiation is used for persistent hormone hypersecretion or residual mass effects following surgery, or when a surgical procedure is contraindicated or when medical management is insufficiently effective. Mostly, radiation is adjuvant to surgery. Adverse effects of radiation include hypopituitarism, secondary brain tumors, cerebrovascular disease, visual damage, and brain necrosis.

Prevention and Early Detection

There is no known prevention for pituitary adenomas. The disease is difficult to diagnose in its early stages, and is often missed for many years until changes in external features begin to occur. The non-secreting adenomas are undetected for a long time since no obvious abnormalities are seen. No imaging tests or blood tests are recommended to screen for pituitary adenomas in people that are not at any increased risk. For members of families known to be at an increased risk due to a genetic syndrome, regular blood testing of pituitary hormone levels is usually recommended. Eventual detection is via immunohistochemical staining of pituitary tissue cellular hormone secretion.

Prognosis

The prognosis for pituitary adenomas is based on virulence of hormonal imbalance as well as the size and type of these tumors. When treatment is successful in destroying adenomas, most patients resume full and normal lives, providing that longitudinal multidisciplinary management is possible to include an endocrinologist, ophthalmologist, neurosurgeon, and radiation oncologist as applicable. These tumors do recur however, resulting in the need for more treatment. In these cases, the tumors are (as might be expected) usually non-functional or prolactinomas.

Malignant Tumors

Malignant tumors of the brain grow quickly, spreading to other areas of the brain and also to the spine. They are generally graded from III to IV, based on their behaviors of growth and recurrence. The majority of malignant brain tumors are secondary cancers that spread to the

Significant Point

The treatment of choice for asymptomatic pituitary adenomas, except for prolactinomas, is surgical removal via the endoscopic endonasal approach. Over 90% of pituitary adenomas are benign, slow-growing tumors, with about 5–10% being atypical, and more aggressive. Via autopsy studies and MRI, we now know that up to 20% of the general population has a reasonable likelihood of harboring a pituitary adenoma, albeit indolent, asymptomatic, and discovered by serendipity.

brain from another body area. The majorities of malignant brain tumors develop from glial tissue and are referred to as *gliomas*.

Pituitary Carcinoma

Pituitary carcinoma is a very rare tumor of the adenohypophyseal cells. It metastasizes craniospinally from a primary sellar tumor, and also to distant sites. The most common subtype secretes prolactin, followed by the corticotrophic pituitary carcinomas. Unfortunately, most pituitary carcinomas have already metastasized by the time they are discovered.

Epidemiology

Pituitary carcinoma makes up only 0.12% of all adenohypophyseal tumors, according to the *German Pituitary Tumor Registry*. According to the American Cancer Society, there have only been a few hundred cases of pituitary carcinomas ever described. This means that the incidence of pituitary carcinomas is less than 0.2% of the population. Though these tumors have been documented between the ages of 12 and 70 years, most patients diagnosed with pituitary carcinomas are in their sixth decade of life. Clinically non-functional tumors occur at younger ages in comparison with benign brain

tumors of the pituitary. The *Surveillance, Epidemiology, and End Results (SEER) program* describes these tumors as having a 1.33:1 female-to-male ratio. More than 70% of cases are of the lactotroph and corticotroph forms. There is no predilection for any racial or ethnic group. Globally, pituitary carcinomas are just as rare in their prevalence and incidence. The same ages are affected as in the United States, as well as genders, and there is no racial or ethnic predilection.

Etiology and Risk Factors

The etiology of pituitary carcinomas is unknown. Radiation appears not to play a role in the development of a pituitary carcinoma from a benign adenoma. Risk factors for these tumors include Carney complex, familial acromegaly, and MEN1. No predisposition has been identified. However, a slow-growing adenoma may transform into an invasive adenoma, and then into a carcinoma. Less commonly, a carcinoma develops from a normal gland or a common adenoma. The genetic factor is still not fully understood.

Clinical Manifestations

Malignant brain tumors differ in their symptoms based on size and location, but common symptoms include drowsiness, headaches, mental or behavioral changes, progressive weakness or paralysis on one side of the body, seizures, nausea and vomiting, speech problems, and vision abnormalities. When a metastasis is hormonally inactive, manifestations are based on their location. If the bones are involved, pain and fractures are common. The patient may be asymptomatic for a long period of time, or the metastasis may only be found during autopsy. Lactotroph carcinomas usually resist dopamine agonists, before and after metastases. Resistance may be present when they form, or can develop as treatments progress.

Primary pituitary carcinomas usually do not affect pituitary endocrine function. Prolactin-secreting carcinomas and elevated serum prolactin result in typical PRL-mediated symptoms of erectile dysfunction in males, and in amenorrhea and galactorrhea in females. Serum PRL levels are often similar to values measured in PRL-secreting macroadenomas. For corticotrophic pituitary carcinomas, typical features of hypercortisolism are seen. Growth hormone-secreting pituitary carcinomas have symptoms closely resembling those of GH-secreting adenomas. Gonadotrophic or thyrotrophic pituitary carcinomas are very rare, usually causing male impotence and oligomenorrhea in females.

Pathology
Primary pituitary carcinomas in the sellar region are invasive macroadenomas. Two cases of ectopic adenomas have evolved to multiple metastases in the brain and subarachnoid space. A few recorded tumors have bound to the sella turcica. Metastasis often occurs within the craniospinal axis, via dissemination within the subarachnoid space. Deeper deposits in the parenchyma usually reach the cerebral cortex and cerebellum. Intra-axial and systemic metastases are similar to deposits from other solid cancers. Systemic metastases usually reach the lymph nodes, bones, liver, and lungs. Dural metastases, especially with slow growth, may be identical to meningiomas during imaging. Primary lesions and their metastases are very similar to common adenomas. No method exists to determine if an invasive adenoma will become a carcinoma; however, genomic profiling and appearance of histology as well as sequential imaging are apt to reflect the biology of the tumor.

Diagnosis
Pituitary carcinoma is diagnosed only when there is a tumor that is non-contiguous with the sella turcica. Diagnosis is complicated, causing delays that can negatively affect treatment and prognosis. Neuronal differentiation is rare, and approximately 75% of cases are diagnosed only at autopsy. Aggressive tumor phenotypes may result in unresponsiveness or escalating serum prolactin levels, along with tumor growth, despite dopamine agonist treatments. Pituitary carcinoma is often a diagnosis of exclusion.

Differential diagnosis is *metastasis to the pituitary gland*. Fine-needle aspiration may be helpful to diagnose extra-CNS metastases, and it is nearly as effective as frozen sectioning. Features in smears and imprints include those of neuroendocrine carcinomas, from bland to obviously malignant. In cytology, the appearance is usually similar to primary or recurrent lesions of the sella turcica. Positron emission tomography (PET) with radiolabeled octreotide, as well as *fluorodeoxyglucose (FDG)-PET*, aids in detecting and monitoring metastases of pituitary carcinomas.

Treatment
Since the tumors locally invade the cavernous sinus, and sellar floor, surgery is rarely curative. Intracranial metastatic deposits within the third or fourth ventricles are associated with increased morbidity and mortality. It is often possible to surgically debulk the tumor. Sometimes, gross total or subtotal resection of tumor tissues can be achieved. Repeated surgeries can be performed to remove secondary deposits that emerge. Recent advances in endoscopic techniques may offer advantages over craniotomy. Radiation therapy stops regrowth in subtotally resected pituitary carcinomas, and slows tumor growth. Usually, stereotactic radiosurgery is done via a single procedure, or fractionated radiation therapy is performed over five to six weeks. Radiation therapy modalities may include but are not limited to converging cobalt beams, modified linear accelerator, or proton beam therapy. Medications are similar to those used for pituitary adenomas, but in higher doses and combinations. These include dopamine agonists, somatostatins, somatostatin analogs, and less commonly, antiestrogens. Chemotherapy has shown varied results and will be limited to descriptive accounts and genomic profiling to best understand the balance of a preferred approach to treat a rare condition.

Prevention and Early Detection
Since pituitary carcinomas are not linked to any known lifestyle risk factors, there is no known way to prevent them currently. No imaging tests

or blood tests are recommended to screen for pituitary carcinomas when an individual has no predisposition. However, for family members at increased risk due to a genetic syndrome, regular blood testing of pituitary hormones is recommended. These tests increase the likelihood of finding the tumor early.

Prognosis

Overall prognosis of pituitary carcinomas is poor. Patients often die from complications of excessive hormones, instead of from the mass effect of metastases. Nearly 80% of patients die from pituitary carcinoma.

Before metastasis, multiple local recurrences are commonly seen. The time between onset and first recurrence varies, from several weeks to 30 years. There are varied latency periods between primary pituitary carcinoma diagnosis and metastasis, from weeks up to 40 years. Dissemination usually happens in the first 10 years after diagnosis. In early stages, metastases are rare. Once occurring, survival time is usually less than four years. Systemic metastases are more quickly fatal than CNS metastases. Corticotroph carcinomas have the shortest survival time. Prognosis for silent corticotroph carcinomas is like those that are hormonal. Some long-term survival after treatment has occurred.

Significant Point

Pituitary carcinomas are indistinguishable from pituitary adenomas simply via imaging studies. They are only defined by the presence of CNS or systemic metastases. Fortunately, their incidence is estimated at less than 0.5% of pituitary symptomatic tumors. Most of these tumors are hormonally active, and metastases occur through nearby lymphatic and vascular spaces, via hematogenous spread, or by invasion into the subarachnoid space. Their rarity and location usually require a multidisciplinary approach to treatment.

Pineoblastoma

A **pineoblastoma** is a well-differentiated malignant tumor arising in the pineal gland and is extremely rare. The World Health Organization classifies it as a grade 4 tumor. Pineoblastomas are typically localized to the pineal region at initial presentation. Pineoblastomas are the most aggressive pineal parenchymal tumors, occurring often in young children and young adults, and usually only spread within the central nervous system.

Epidemiology

Pineoblastomas are grade 4 tumors that make up 35% of all pineal parenchymal tumors, ranging between 24% and 61%. Their prevalence is 0.1% of all intracranial neoplasms. However, incidence is less than 1% of all primary brain tumors. Pineoblastomas can occur at any age, but most often in children. They usually develop during the first two decades of life, peaking at age 5.5 years and at 17.8 years. In adults, they occur between ages 20 and 40. Like other pineal parenchymal tumors, the male-to-female ratio is 0.7:1. There is no racial or ethnic predilection. Global statistics are nearly identical to those of the United States.

Etiology and Risk Factors

The actual cause of all pineal tumors is unknown, though research is ongoing. No specific genetic alterations have been found regarding pineocytomas. However, there have been some links associated with chromosomal abnormalities such as 22q11.2 deletion syndrome. There are also no identified risk factors.

Clinical Manifestations

Symptoms of pineoblastomas, due to hydrocephalus and increased intracranial pressure include headaches, dizziness, loss of upward gaze, tremor, ataxia, hearing changes, nausea and vomiting, papilledema, diplopia, and reduced visual acuity.

Pathology

Sheets of small, immature neuroepithelial cells are characteristic histologic findings in pineob lastomas. There is a high nuclear-to-cytoplasmic ratio, small amounts of cytoplasm, calcification, and hyperchromatic nuclei that sometimes have small nucleoli. The tumors usually spread aggressively, through CSF pathways. Pineoblastomas directly invade nearby brain structures: the **leptomeninges**, third ventricle, and **tectal plate**. Macroscopically, they are poorly demarcated and invasive. They have a soft texture, friability, and are pink to gray in color. There may be hemorrhage, often with necrosis. Microscopically, there are densely packed small blue cells with slightly irregular nuclear shapes. The nuclei can be angulated or oval. The cell borders are usually indistinct. With hematoxylin and eosin staining, a small number of rosettes may interrupt the diffuse growth pattern. Mitotic activity is usually high. Electron microscopy reveals large amounts of **euchromatin** and heterochromatin. The cytoplasm has polyribosomes, small numbers of rough endoplasmic reticulum, tiny mitochondria, and there may be intermediate filaments, lysosomes, and microtubules.

Diagnosis

Pineoblastomas appear as large, multi-lobulated masses, with frequent invasion of the splenium, tectum, and thalamus within the corpus callosum. Small cystic or necrotic areas may be present, with edema. In CT imaging, the tumors are usually hyperdense, with post-contrast enhancement. Calcifications may be present. Nearly all cases involve obstructive hydrocephalus. A T1-weighted MRI reveals the tumors to be hypointense to isointense, with heterogeneous contrast enhancement. In T2-weighted imaging, they are isointense to hyperintense.

Treatment

The treatment of choice for pineoblastoma is surgical resection. It is often performed with minimally invasive techniques that are very difficult but highly effective. Hydrocephalus is managed via a ventriculostomy or by shunt placement. High-dose chemotherapy may be given, along with surgery and radiation therapy.

Radiation therapy is used if the patient is over three years of age, due to the possibility of long-term cognitive damage in young patients.

Prevention and Early Detection

There is no known prevention regarding pineoblastomas. Early detection is rare prior to the onset of symptoms, but after treatment, monitoring should focus on early detection of recurrence. This allows for treatment of possible cognitive, endocrine, and neurological complications.

Prognosis

Pineoblastoma rarely results in extracranial drop metastasis. If this is the case, like most leptomeningeal involvement, this can lead to radiculopathy in the spine. Median overall survival is between four and nine years. Also, five-year overall survival rates are reported as being between 10% and 81%. Poor prognoses are given for disseminated disease, partial surgical resection, and younger patient age. Radiation therapy improves prognosis when safe for application. Because of better treatment modalities, five-year survival of patients with trilateral retinoblastoma syndrome has improved, from 6% to 44% of cases.

Significant Point

Pineoblastoma is more aggressive than other types of pineal gland tumors. It usually causes cerebrospinal fluid to build up in the brain. Fortunately, this tumor usually does not spread to other parts of the body. Pineoblastomas make up less than half of all pineal gland tumors, and usually occur in children and younger adults.

Clinical Case 3

1. In what age range does pineoblastoma most often clinically present?
2. How do pineoblastomas usually spread and progress?

3. Describe a characteristic appearance of pineoblastoma on head CT?

A 4-year-old girl with a known history of chromosome 22q11.2 deletion syndrome was brought to the emergency department due to vomiting that had worsened over several weeks. A head CT scan revealed a large pineal region calcified tumor, with hydrocephalus. An external ventricular drain was surgically inserted to alleviate the hydrocephalus. An MRI of the brain and spine confirmed a pineal tumor, with diffuse metastatic leptomeningeal spinal spread. Neuropathology assessment of the subtotal surgical resection revealed packed blue cells with oval and slightly angulated nuclei, and scant cytoplasm. In the pineal region, the neuropathic features indicated that it was a pineoblastoma. The patient was treated with craniospinal radiation with local boost and adjuvant chemotherapy. Despite these efforts, unfortunately, she died as a result of the tumor and its complications about 12 months later.

Answers:

1. **Pineoblastomas can occur at any age, but most often in children. They usually develop during the first two decades of life, peaking at age 5.5 years and at 17.8 years. In adults, they occur between ages 20 and 40.**
2. **Pineoblastomas usually spread aggressively, through cerebrospinal fluid pathways. They directly invade nearby brain structures such as the leptomeninges, third ventricle, and tectal plate.**
3. **In CT imaging, pineoblastomas are usually hyperdense, with post-contrast enhancement. Calcifications may be present. Nearly all cases involve obstructive hydrocephalus.**

Anaplastic Oligodendroglioma

An *oligodendroglioma* is a primary CNS tumor, beginning in the brain or spinal cord. Grade III oligodendrogliomas are malignant and fast growing. These are known as **anaplastic oligodendrogliomas**. They have focal or diffuse anaplastic features and usually occur in the supratentorial white matter. In most cases, anaplastic oligodendrogliomas are located in the frontal lobe. Another name for these tumors is *malignant oligodendrogliomas*.

Epidemiology

According to the *Central Brain Tumor Registry of the United States (CBTRUS)*, anaplastic oligodendroglioma has an annual prevalence of 0.11 cases out of every 100,000 people. Its incidence is 0.5% of all primary brain tumors and 2.5% of all gliomas. About 33% of all oligodendroglial tumors are anaplastic oligodendrogliomas; to this point, there are only two grades of oligodendrogliomas: grade 2 (low) and grade 3 (anaplastic). The median age at diagnosis is 49 years. Only about 6% occur in infants and children. These tumors are slightly more common in males than females. There is no racial or ethnic predilection for anaplastic oligodendrogliomas.

According to the World Health Organization, the reported prevalence rates of anaplastic oligodendroglioma ranges from 0.07 to 0.18 per 100,000, and the tumor comprises only 0.5–1.2% of all primary brain tumors. Only about 30% of oligodendroglial tumors have anaplastic features. As in the United States, anaplastic oligodendrogliomas are slightly more common in males, with no racial or ethnic predilection.

Etiology and Risk Factors

Anaplastic oligodendrogliomas are believed to originate from oligodendrocytes and usually occur sporadically, with no confirmed cause, and without familial inheritance. There are no proven risk factors. There are also no proven causes or risk factors for the *not otherwise specified anaplastic oligodendrogliomas*.

Clinical Manifestations

Anaplastic oligodendrogliomas often cause mental status changes, cognitive deficits, focal neurologic deficits, headache, or signs of increased intracranial pressure. Most patients may have seizures because of the location of lesion and its propensity to affect the cortical and subcortical areas.

Pathology

Anaplastic oligodendroglioma is usually located in the cerebral hemispheres, most often in the frontal lobe, followed by the temporal lobe. There have been rare cases of this tumor developing in the intramedullary parts of the spine. The histological features linked to high-grade malignancy include high cellularity, high mitotic activity, significant cytological atypia, necrosis with or without palisading, and pathological microvascular proliferation. Extracranial metastases are extremely rare. The detection of 1p/19q codeletion (codel) by FISH is mandatory for formal diagnosis.

Diagnosis

Accurate histologic diagnosis requires the presence of recognition of microvascular proliferation, which may or may not accompany brisk mitotic activity although there is usually a high mitotic index. There may be heterogeneous patterns with variable necrosis, calcification, cystic degeneration, and intratumoral hemorrhage. In CT and MRI, contrast enhancement is common. It can be homogeneous or patchy. Lack of contrast enhancement does not exclude anaplastic oligodendroglioma. Ring enhancement is less common than in malignant gliomas – especially glioblastomas without these molecular markers. It must be emphasized that irrespective of histologic appearances described above, the detection of 1p/19q codeletion (codel) by FISH is mandatory for formal diagnosis.

Macroscopically, anaplastic oligodendrogliomas resemble grade II oligodendrogliomas, except for areas of necrosis. Microscopically, they are cellular, diffusely infiltrating tumors with various morphologies. The majority of cells appear similar to oligodendroglial cells: They have round hyperchromatic nuclei, few cellular processes, and perinuclear halos. Local microcalcifications are usually present. There may be a high amount of cellular **pleomorphism** and

multinucleated giant cells. Rarely, there are sarcoma-like areas referred to as *oligosarcomas*. Branched capillaries are often seen, and pathological microvascular proliferation is usually prominent. An astrocytic component is also compatible with this diagnosis, and in rare occasions, mixed oligoastrocytoma is noted or so-called "collision tumors" of patches of separate and differentiated astrocytoma and oligodendroglioma coexist in mosaic. Differential diagnosis includes other clear cell tumor entities such as central neurocytoma distinguishable by unique immunohistochemistry and 1p19qcodel. It is important to distinguish these tumors from small cell astrocytic tumors, which are more aggressive.

Treatment

Treatments are usually varied for low-grade and high-grade oligodendrogliomas.

The first treatment option is maximum feasible surgical resection. Many patients with a low-grade oligodendroglioma remain in remission for years following surgery. For anaplastic oligodendrogliomas, surgery is focused on removing as much of the tumor as safely possible and sequencing radiotherapy and chemotherapy after surgery. Chemotherapy usually consists of PCV or modified PC therapy or potentially, temozolomide.

Prevention and Early Detection

There is no known prevention of anaplastic oligodendrogliomas. Early detection is the key to improving prognosis and life expectancy. Methods for early detection may involve medical history, physical examination, neurological examination, MRI, or if indicated CT.

Prognosis

Anaplastic oligodendrogliomas were historically believed to have a 5-year survival rate of 52% and a 10-year survival rate of 39%. Recent data reveals that the 5-year survival rate is now 74%, most likely due to more refined molecular classification of oligodendroglioma and identifying "look-alikes" with poorer prognosis. Local tumor progression is the usual cause of death. A better prognosis is provided via previous resection for a lower-grade tumor.

Significant Point

Anaplastic oligodendrogliomas rarely spread outside of the central nervous system. However, they can become more aggressive over time, and grow quickly. Anaplastic oligodendrogliomas are usually treated with a combination of radiation therapy and chemotherapy. Recurrence may be treated with surgery, chemotherapy, or possibility for clinical research study.

Anaplastic Ependymoma

Anaplastic ependymoma is a glioma made up of quickly proliferative small cells with polymorphic shapes. These cells have a greater tendency to spread via the cerebrospinal fluid, in comparison with grade II ependymomas. There are two grades of ependymoma, low (grade 2) and anaplastic (grade 3). Molecular classification has been updated to include supratentorial ependymomas with C11orf95-RELA fusion or YAP1 fusion, infratentorial ependymomas with or without a hypermethylated phenotype (CIMP), and spinal cord ependymomas. Myxopapillary ependymomas and subependymomas have a different and more indolent biology than ependymomas with typical WHO grade II or III histology.

Epidemiology

Approximately 800 cases of ependymomas are diagnosed every year within the United States with an incidence of roughly three per million population, and about 25% of these tumors show features of anaplasia with a high mitotic rate, microvascular proliferation, cellular pleomorphism, and intratumoral necrosis. Therefore, fewer than 250 cases of anaplastic ependymomas occur annually in the United States. This makes the incidence extremely small over the population. Anaplastic ependymomas occur in patients of all ages, but occur most often in children between birth and four years of age. However, adults over age 40 have nearly twice the risk of death compared with children. Anaplastic ependymomas occur nearly evenly between males and females. These tumors occur less often in African American children, yet they have a 78% increased risk of death from the tumors compared with Caucasian children, who have the highest rates of occurrence. Globally, the incidence of anaplastic ependymoma is also the highest in children under four years of age, and the prevalence is about the same as in the United States. Patient ages and gender distribution are also nearly identical. Tumors are most prevalent in Caucasians throughout the world.

Etiology and Risk Factors

Anaplastic ependymomas are usually not related to genetic mutations or inherited pathogenic conditions. They are however linked to **somatic mutations** of specific genes in certain cells of the body, resulting in the cells growing quickly. Rarely, these tumors are related to **neurofibromatosis type 2**, which increases risks for CNS tumors.

Clinical Manifestations

Signs and symptoms of anaplastic ependymomas include cognitive changes, headaches, hydrocephalus, lethargy, nausea, vomiting, nystagmus, and seizures. Clinical outcome is mostly based on the molecular group and extent of resection.

Pathology

Vital brain structures are often affected, so total resection is difficult, only possible in 30–40% of cases. The tumors have round nuclei in a fibrillary matrix. Perivascular pseudorosettes are common. The tumors often express *glial fibrillary acidic protein (GFAP)*, the S100 protein, and *vimentin*. There is a high nuclear-to-cytoplasmic ratio, and a high mitotic count. In about 25% of cases, there are ependymal rosettes present. Anaplastic ependymoma can invade adjacent CNS parenchyma significantly.

Diagnosis

Based on the signs and symptoms, an MRI or CT scan may be ordered to assess the location of the tumor. Diagnosis is usually confirmed via biopsy, if there is a high cell density, increased mitotic count, large microvascular proliferation, and necrosis. Ultrastructural examination shows cilia and microvilli. The tumors are usually intracranial, metastasizing through the CSF (see Figure 3.9). They occur in all ages, though most posterior fossa tumors occur in children. Clear cell, papillary, or tanycytic morphologies may be present.

Treatment

Treatment usually begins with surgery to remove as much of the anaplastic ependymoma as possible. Radiation therapy follows because it can reduce chances of recurrence. Chemotherapy may be used if there is recurrence. Genetic study of the tumor may provide information about prognosis and treatment options for the future. Additional treatments include steroids, antiseizure medications, physical or occupational therapy, and chemotherapy with stem-cell transplantation.

Prevention and Early Detection

There is no known prevention for anaplastic ependymomas. There are also no established methods for the early detection of these tumors, unfortunately.

Prognosis

The prognosis for anaplastic ependymomas is poorer than for other ependymomas, because of their fast growth. Prognosis is based on the extent of possible surgical resection and molecular subtyping as well as location of lesion. Younger patients have a worsened prognosis. Also, delays in radiation therapy and a lateral posterior fossa location make prognosis less positive.

Significant Point

Anaplastic ependymomas are grade III tumors that grow quickly, and usually occur in the brain. Less often, they develop in the spine. About 25% of all ependymomas have a high mitotic rate, microvascular proliferation, cellular pleomorphism, and intratumoral necrosis. These features signify them as anaplastic ependymomas.

Anaplastic Astrocytoma

Anaplastic astrocytoma can develop secondarily from a low-grade astrocytoma slowly over time, but it can also develop rapidly. The histologic and genomic profiling of astrocytomas make the grading type less likely fit the

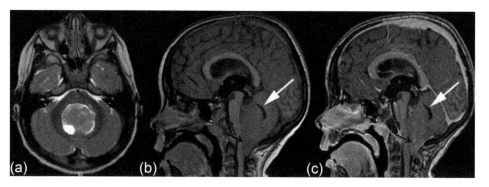

Figure 3.9 Anaplastic ependymoma in the fourth ventricle. (a) Axial T2-weighted MRI; (b) sagittal pre-contrast T1-weighted MRI; (c) Sagittal post-contrast T1-weighted MRI. *Source*: Poretti et al. (2011).

narrowing window of diagnostic criteria. Untreated tumor is usually fatal. Anaplastic astrocytomas usually occur sporadically, but can be linked to a genetic abnormality. The symptoms caused by this tumor are quite varied based on its actual location. Anaplastic astrocytoma is sometimes referred to as a malignant or high-grade glioma because under the umbrella of gliomas, malignant processes include grade 3 astrocytoma, grade 4 astrocytoma, grade 3 oligodendroglioma, and grade 3 ependymoma although independently, the biology of each of these is different.

Epidemiology

Anaplastic astrocytoma makes up 1–2% of all primary brain tumors and 7.5% of all gliomas. The overall survival rates are 24% at 5 years and 15% at 10 years. The prevalence of anaplastic astrocytoma in the United States is about 0.48 people per 100,000. The overall incidence is described as an age-adjusted rate of 3.5 per million person/years. There are only about 1,600 new cases diagnosed annually in the United States. Anaplastic astrocytoma is most often diagnosed at around 40 years of age, within a common range of 30–50 years. These tumors only affect males slightly more often than females. There is no predilection for any specific racial or ethnic groups.

Globally, the prevalence of anaplastic astrocytoma is about 0.44 people per 100,000. Overall incidence is described as an age-adjusted rate of 3.3 per million person/years. There are no accurate statistics about the number of new cases diagnosed annually. Anaplastic astrocytoma is, like in the United States, usually diagnosed at around 40 years of age. Males are slightly more affected in all countries, with no specific predilection for any races or ethnicities.

Etiology and Risk Factors

Anaplastic astrocytomas occur sporadically. Less than 5% of people with malignant astrocytomas have suspected hereditary predisposition, such as hereditary non-polyposis colorectal cancer, Li-Fraumeni syndrome, tuberous sclerosis, and **neurofibromatosis type 1**. Risk factors may include environmental factors and genetic disorders. Other risk factors may be immune system abnormalities and exposure to ultraviolet rays. Those individuals that deal and work in rubber manufacturing industries and oil refining have higher incidence of anaplastic astrocytomas.

Clinical Manifestations

The initial symptoms include depression, focal neurological deficits, seizures, and headache. Symptom onset and diagnosis are often 1.5–2 years apart. They may include personality and visual changes, walking difficulties, paralysis, and vomiting. The patient often has thinking, concentration, and memory abnormalities. If the tumor is in the temporal lobe, there are problems with speech and memory. When the tumor is located in the frontal lobe, there are usually gradual changes in mood and personality. A parietal lobe tumor causes abnormalities of motor skills, writing, and sensations. An occipital lobe tumor causes problems with vision and visual hallucinations. A cerebellar tumor results in coordination and balance problems.

Pathology

Anaplastic astrocytomas can range from diffuse to grossly well circumscribed, large, and have a soft yellow necrotic center with punctate hemorrhagic points. There may be a **pseudopalisading** appearance around the necrosis. Microscopically, they reveal increased cellularity, necrosis, pleomorphic astrocytes, and mitosis; as opposed to glioblastoma, necrosis and vascular proliferation are not seen. Molecular histology shows high vascularization and extensive heterogenic infiltration. The tumors may grow large enough to extend from the meningeal surface, pushing through the ventricular wall.

Diagnosis

Anaplastic astrocytomas may be detected via MRI and CT scan. An MRI usually exhibits lesions that have homogeneous enhancement. *Diffusion-weighted imaging* describes areas of increased cellularity in low-grade tumors, and may be useful in establishing early anaplastic changes. Maximum feasible surgical resection confirms diagnosis.

Treatment

To surgically remove as much of the tumor as possible is the initial treatment, and then follows radiation therapy. Recent studies show that irradiation with or without concurrent or adjuvant chemotherapy may be used upon initial diagnosis. Temozolomide or combination PCV chemotherapy may be helpful, but its role as an adjuvant to radiation therapy has not been fully proven. Quality of life after treatment is in part driven by the location of the tumor. The high molecular variability of anaplastic astrocytomas is related to poorer treatment outcomes than low-grade gliomas. Tumor location may make it more difficult to effectively deliver treatment. Some patients may develop paralysis, foot drop, speech difficulty, cognitive defect, and altered sensory perception. Many new therapies are being reviewed for anaplastic astrocytomas. These include most of the research relevant for glioblastoma.

Prevention and Early Detection

There is no known prevention for anaplastic astrocytomas. Unfortunately, no accurate methods of early detection have been developed.

Significant Point

Anaplastic astrocytomas can be fast-growing tumors that are treatable but usually not curable. As they continue to grow and become more aggressive, they can progress and advance into glioblastomas. Anaplastic astrocytomas often develop in the cerebral hemispheres, but can occur in nearly any area of the CNS. They are most common in adults, but also occur in children.

Prognosis

Prognosis across different ages is varied, especially during the first three years after diagnosis. Survival rates are 42% at two years and 24% at five years. The elderly population experiences relatively and progressively worse outcomes. Prognosis is best for patients receiving radiation therapy and surgery.

Clinical Case 4

1. What is the prevalence and incidence of anaplastic astrocytomas?
2. Are there any risk factors for developing an anaplastic astrocytoma?
3. What are some differences between glioblastoma and anaplastic astrocytoma?

A 33-year-old woman began experiencing seizures over several months. Her husband took her to the emergency department, where she was given antiseizure medications and released. Soon, the seizures began causing temporary right-sided paralysis, so an MRI of the brain was performed. It revealed a tumor in the left side of brain, located along the motor strip, in the areas that primarily control body movements. The patient underwent transcranial magnetic stimulation (TMS) to identify the motor control areas, especially in the left hemisphere around the tumor. It determined that areas located along the anterior and posterior tumor margins controlled her right leg function. The tumor was surgically removed, after which there was temporary foot drop, which resolved over several weeks. It was found that the tumor had been a grade III anaplastic astrocytoma. With continued physical therapy, and a six-week session of chemotherapy and radiation, the patient has remained seizure-free, and there has been no recurrence to date.

Answers:

1. **The prevalence of anaplastic astrocytoma in the United States is about 0.48 people per 100,000. The overall incidence**

is described as an age-adjusted rate of 3.5 per million person/years. There are only about 1,600 new cases diagnosed annually in the United States. Globally, the prevalence of these tumors is about 0.44 people per 100,000. Overall incidence is described as an age-adjusted rate of 3.3 per million person/years. There are no accurate statistics about the number of new cases diagnosed annually.

2. **Anaplastic astrocytomas have been linked to previous exposure to high doses of radiation therapy, and vinyl chloride. Risk factors include environmental factors, genetic disorders, immune system abnormalities, exposure to ultraviolet rays, and jobs in the rubber manufacturing and oil refining industries.**

3. **Anaplastic astrocytomas are noted to have increased cellularity, pleomorphic astrocytes with pyknotic nuclei, and active mitosis. Glioblastomas by definition display endothelial proliferation and/or necrosis, many times characterized by a pseudopalisading appearance around the necrosis.**

Embryonal Carcinoma

Embryonal carcinoma is an aggressive, *nongerminomatous* malignant germ cell tumor. There are large epithelioid cells, similar to embryonic **germ disk**, and geographical necrosis. Embryonal carcinoma may develop as part of a mixed germ cell tumor, along with other germ cell tumors. The major germ cell tumors include embryonal carcinoma, germinoma, yolk sac tumor, choriocarcinoma, and teratoma.

Epidemiology

Intracranial embryonal carcinomas occur as 2.2% of all primary pediatric CNS tumors. Most of these tumors in children are malignant. However, embryonal carcinoma is very rare in the CNS, usually occurring in the ovaries and testes. Incidence of embryonal carcinomas in the CNS is not well understood. Because of their

rarity, prevalence, and incidence, statistics are unknown in the United States or globally. In most cases, CNS embryonal carcinomas occur in infants and young children. Patients have ranged in age from newborns to 16 year olds, but the tumors are up to 10 times more likely to be diagnosed in children less than nine years of age. Embryonal tumors with multilayered rosettes are most common in children between two and three years of age. The development of embryonal carcinomas of the CNS occurs nearly equally in males and females, and there is no known racial or ethnic predilection.

Etiology and Risk Factors

Embryonal carcinomas of the CNS may begin in embryonic cells that remain in the brain after birth. Risk factors for embryonal carcinomas are unclear, but they may be linked to genetic such as **Fanconi anemia**, Gorlin syndrome, Li-Fraumeni syndrome, **Rubinstein-Taybi syndrome**, and Turcot syndrome.

Clinical Manifestations

Clinical manifestations of embryonal carcinomas include oculomotor difficulties or symptoms of increased intracranial pressure. No respond to light in the pupils, nystagmus, eyelid retraction, and vertical gaze paresis. There may be precocious puberty, and hemiparesis developed in some cases.

Pathology

Embryonal carcinomas are solid, with friable gray to white tissues that may have necrosis and focal hemorrhage. They are different from other germ cell tumors because of their cytoplasmic immunoreactivity for *cluster of differentiation 30 (CD30)*. They are strongly and uniformly reactive for cytokeratins. Embryonal carcinomas are usually negative for human placental lactogen, beta-hCG, and alpha-fetoprotein.

Diagnosis

Diagnostic methods include angiography, arteriography, CT scan with or without contrast, and MRI. Usually, imaging shows displacement of the deep venous system and origins of feeding tumor vessels. If located in the pineal region, there may be a heterogenous mass with scattered calcification, which enhances with contrast. Any suprasellar masses may be isodense and enhance homogenously with contrast. It is crucial to distinguish embryonal carcinomas, via biopsy, from other intracranial tumors. It is believed that embryonal carcinomas are more common than initially documented, and that current treatments for them may be insufficiently effective.

Treatment

Treatments for intracranial embryonal carcinomas include partial or total surgical resection, chemotherapy, and radiation therapy. Chemotherapies include cisplatin, citrovorum, and methotrexate.

Prevention and Early Detection

There is no known prevention for embryonal carcinomas. These tumors are usually not detected early, and there is no proven method for early detection.

Prognosis

Prognosis for intracranial embryonal carcinomas is varied, but generally is not good. Patients have survived for over two years following treatment, but the majority of children survive less than one year.

Significant Point

Embryonal carcinomas of CNS mostly occur in children, and are rarely seen in adults. Unfortunately, they are aggressive tumors that usually metastasize early in their development, with about 60% of patients already having metastasis upon initial presentation. These tumors are often associated with other cell types in the metastatic sites.

Choriocarcinoma

Choriocarcinoma is an aggressive, non-germinomatous and highly malignant germ cell tumor. It develops from the chorionic portion of the products of conception. This tumor is made up of intermediate trophoblasts and is a part of the spectrum known as *gestational trophoblastic disease*. Choriocarcinoma is rapidly invasive and metastasizes widely, but once identified responds well to chemotherapy.

Epidemiology

Choriocarcinoma in the brain is very rare that arises in 1 in 20,000–30,000 pregnancies in the United States. However, prevalence and incidence statistics globally are not fully understood. Documented cases in children have occurred between the ages of one month and eight years. However, they may be observed more often in young adults. They are most common in females of childbearing age. There appears to be no racial or ethnic predilection.

Etiology and Risk Factors

Choriocarcinomas in the brain originate from retained primordial germ cells that undergo abnormal migration during embryogenesis. There are no known risk factors.

Clinical Manifestations

Signs and symptoms of choriocarcinoma of the brain are varied, based on tumor location. Sometimes, symptoms include dizziness and headache that are related to increased intracranial pressure.

Pathology

Hemorrhage and necrosis are commonly seen in choriocarcinomas. There is an elevation of human chorionic gonadotropin (hCG) in the CSF and blood. Choriocarcinomas are solid tumors and may occur as components of mixed germ cell tumors. Neoplastic **syncytiotrophoblast** surrounds the cytotrophoblastic components, which consist of masses of large, mononucleated cells with vesicular nuclei. The cytoplasm is clear or acidophilic. Characteristics include pools of blood, **ectatic** vascular channels, and extreme hemorrhagic necrosis. The syncytiotrophoblasts have diffuse cytoplasmic immunoreactivity for beta-hCG, along with human placental lactogen.

Diagnosis

Imaging studies include X-rays MRI, and CT scan. Microscopic diagnosis requires cytotrophoblasts and syncytiotrophoblasts to be present. They usually contain multiple hyperchromatic or vesicular nuclei. The nuclei often form **knot-like clusters**, in significant amounts of purple or basophilic cytoplasm.

Treatment

Treatments for choriocarcinoma of the brain include surgery, radiation, and chemotherapy. Choriocarcinoma respond to chemotherapy very well, as many as 95% of patients. For intermediate to high-risk patients, EMACO therapy may be prescribed, which includes etoposide, methotrexate, actinomycin, cyclosporine, and vincristine (Oncovin).

Prevention and Early Detection

There is no known prevention for choriocarcinoma. Early consideration of an oncotic aneurysm that may be secondary to choriocarcinoma in a patient with multiple intracranial hemorrhages may result in early use of proper chemotherapy and a better prognosis.

Prognosis

Children with choriocarcinomas of the brain have a better prognosis in comparison with adults who develop these tumors. When there is no metastasis, the recovery rate is excellent; however, the tumor is usually fatal once metastasis has occurred.

Teratoma

A **teratoma** is a germ cell tumor consisting of somatic tissue, from the ectoderm, endoderm, and mesoderm. They are further classified as the following:

- *Immature* – containing embryonic, fetal, or immature only, or along with mature tissues
- *Mature* – containing only adult-type tissues, such as adipose tissue, bone, cartilage, gastrointestinal (GI) epithelium, mature skin or

---

Significant Point

Choriocarcinoma of the brain is difficult to treat, and patients are unlikely to fully recover. It is an extremely vascular tumor. In the brain, this tumor is clinically referred to as "primary intracranial choriocarcinoma." They are rare, and may be found in the pineal or suprasellar regions. There is usually increased cerebrospinal fluid and plasma beta-human chorionic gonadotropin, which aid in diagnosis.

---

skin appendages, minor salivary glands, neural tissue, respiratory epithelium, and smooth muscle
- *Malignant transformative* – a rare form, containing a component resulting from malignant transformation of somatic tissue, which is usually a carcinoma or sarcoma; embryonal tumors with features of primitive neuroectodermal tumors can also form in the CNS

Epidemiology

Teratomas are basically rare, yet are the most common fetal intracranial neoplasms. Prevalence, both in the United States and globally, is approximately 1 of every 100,000 births. Incidence is very low, with statistics that are difficult to prove. These tumors make up 26–50% of all fetal brain tumors, occurring in a wide range of ages in children. The female-to-male ratio is unclear, but is believed to be nearly identical. There appears to be no racial or ethnic predilection.

Etiology and Risk Factors

The causes of teratomas are based on abnormal development of *pluripotent cells*, such as germ cells and embryonal cells. Teratomas of embryonic origin are congenital, but teratomas of germ cell origin may or may not be congenital. Teratomas in the brain are usually derived from embryonic cells. Risk factors for teratomas are not known.

Clinical Manifestations

The signs and symptoms of teratomas in the brain are based on intra-axial or extra-axial locations. Intra-axial teratomas usually manifest before birth or in the newborn period. They are large head circumference that causing difficulty during delivery. They usually develop in the pineal gland or suprasellar regions. The tumor may cause hydrocephalus, optic chiasm compression, papilledema, headache, and vomiting.

Pathology

The ectodermal components contain nervous tissue, choroid plexus, and skin appendages. Common endodermal components are glands that are often dilated as cysts, and lined with epithelia that are like those of the enteric or respiratory areas. Sometimes, gastrointestinal-like structures with muscular coats or bronchus-like structures with cartilaginous rings, as well as mucosa, are found. Common mesodermal components include adipose tissue, bone, and both smooth and striated muscle.

Mature teratomas consist of differentiated adult-type tissues, with little or no mitotic activity. Immature teratomas have incompletely differentiated elements that resemble fetal tissues. Islands of primitive neuroectodermal elements may form tubules and rosettes that are neuroepithelial and multilayered. The rosettes may have a centralized lumen or **canalicular** structures

that resemble a developing neural tube. The primitive neuroepithelium has small cells and a small amount of cytoplasm, hyperchromatic oval or carrot-shaped nuclei, plus mitoses and apoptosis. Intracranial germ cell tumors may involve different somatic-type cancers. These are mostly undifferentiated sarcomas. Yolk sac tumor components may be relatives of enteric-type adenocarcinomas occurring in intracranial germ cell tumors.

Diagnosis

Careful evaluation is essential for the malignant of teratomas in the brain. Teratomas may be identified with increased levels of serum **alpha-fetoprotein** or serum **carcinoembryonic antigen**. Imaging reveals mixed tissue densities and intensity (see Figure 3.10). If fat is present, it helps to narrow the differential diagnoses. CT scans are performed without enhancement. Intermediate components are made of soft tissue, and hypointense components are due to calcification and blood products. Enhanced T1-weighted imaging provides enhancement of solid soft tissues. T2-weighted imaging reveals mixed signals from different components.

Treatment

The treatment for teratomas starts with surgical resection. For malignant teratomas, chemotherapy is usually given after surgery. When

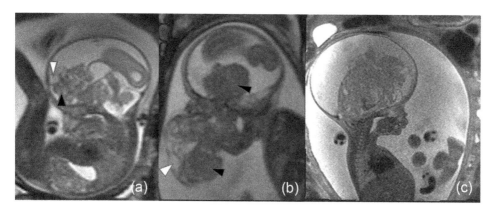

Figure 3.10 Teratomas within the brain. (a) Heterogeneous tumor with cystic (white arrowhead) and solid (black arrowhead) components; (b) Intracranial component (upper black arrowhead), cystic components (white arrowhead), and solid components (lower black arrowhead); (c) Large teratoma causing distortion and enlargement of the head. *Source*: Feygin et al. (2020).

teratomas in the brain are surgically inaccessible locations or difficult to remove the tumor, chemotherapy is the best option for the treatment.

Prevention and Early Detection
There is no known prevention for teratomas. Recurrences and complications may be prevented by early detection and treatment.

Prognosis
Prognosis of teratoma is determined by the tumor location and its size. For intra-axial tumors, a **stillbirth** is unfortunately relatively expected. Smaller extra-axial tumors have a good prognosis if they can be successfully resected.

Significant Point

Teratomas of the brain are complex tumors composed of multiple germ layers in various stages of maturation. This is why they may consist of tissue foreign to the area in which they arise. Because of their relatively strange appearance, mixing different types of tissues, they have been referred to as "monster tumors." In fact, the word *teras* means "monster," and is combined with *onkoma*, which means "swelling" or "tumor."

Metastatic Tumors

Metastatic tumors are commonly seen in the central nervous system. They originate from outside of the brain and spinal cord, and are spread via blood circulation to the CNS. Less frequently, they directly invade the CNS from nearby body structures. The outlook for each patient is based on the extent of metastasis and the aggressiveness of tumor growth.

Epidemiology
The exact prevalence of **metastatic brain tumors** is not fully understood, but is estimated at 200,000–300,000 people in the United States every year. The incidence rates for metastatic tumors to the brain has been underdiagnosed or underreported. Central nervous system metastases are generally seen in 25% of people who die of cancer. Leptomeningeal metastases occur in 4–15% of cases. With advanced cancer, 8–9% of cases involve dural metastases. Brain metastatic tumors are common in adults between ages 50 and 70, but in children make up only 2% of all CNS tumors. It appears to be no significant differences in distribution between females and males, and no racial or ethnic predilection.

Global cases of metastatic brain tumors are generally in the same proportions as those in the United States. For example, in Sweden alone, between 1987 and 2006, there were 14 cases out of every 100,000 people. This was two times the levels seen in earlier years, probably because of the development of better imaging techniques. Spinal epidural metastases actually occur in 5–10% of cases, which is much more common than spinal leptomeningeal or intramedullary metastases. Lung cancer, colorectal cancer, and melanoma are most commonly metastases to brain. Figure 3.11 illustrates primary tumors and their metastases in males, and Figure 3.12 shows the same information in females.

Etiology and Risk Factors
Metastatic brain tumors are commonly caused by lung cancer. For men, the second most common cause is colorectal cancer, and the third is melanoma. For women, the second most common cause involves breast cancers. The third most common cause is colorectal cancer. In children, the most common sources of CNS metastases are leukemias and lymphomas. **Ewing sarcoma**, osteosarcoma, germ cell tumors, **neuroblastoma**, and **rhabdomyosarcoma**. Primary head and neck neoplasms may extend intracranially via direct invasion. While actual risk factors for CNS metastases remain unknown, possible links exist to smoking, alcoholism, and chronic pancreatitis if patients have insulin-dependent diabetes.

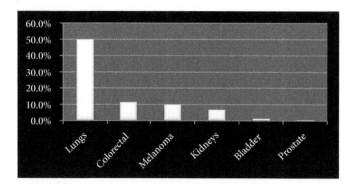

Figure 3.11 Primary tumors and resulting brain metastases in males.

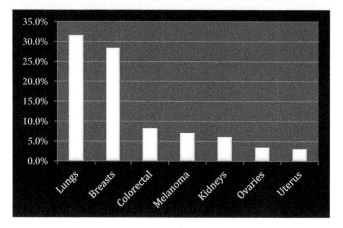

Figure 3.12 Primary tumors and resulting brain metastases in females.

Clinical Manifestations

Metastases to the brain may cause increased intracranial pressure. Symptoms may progress very slowly, including headache, nausea, visual changes, ataxia and other manifestation such as motor dysfunction, paresis, sensory abnormalities, altered mental status, and confusion. Sometimes, intracranial metastases may cause seizures, hemorrhages, or stroke.

Pathology

About 80% of brain metastases are observed in the central hemispheres. About 15% develop in the cerebellum and another 5% occur in the brainstem (see Figure 3.13). Less than half of all brain metastases are solitary lesions. Intracranial metastases may also occur in dura mater and leptomeninges. Sometimes, location of metastatic tumors may be in the walls of the ventricles, choroid plexus, or pituitary gland. Dural metastases are common with cancers of the breasts, lungs, and prostate, as well as in hematologic malignancies. Leptomeningeal metastases occur more commonly with breast and lung cancers, and melanoma. Spinal epidural metastases are commonly linked to cancers of the breasts, kidneys, lungs, prostate, and with non-Hodgkin lymphoma or multiple myeloma. Small cell lung carcinoma is regularly a component of intramedullary spinal cord metastases. Within the CNS, parenchymal metastases are rounded, with gray, white masses, and varied amounts of central necrosis and peritumoral edema. Cystic lesions are sometimes present. Lesions often impair CSF flow. Melanoma metastases have a large amount of melanin, so it

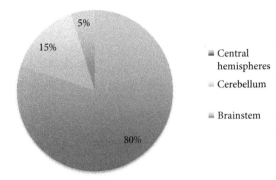

Figure 3.13 Locations of metastasis within the brain.

appears brown to black in color. Leptomeningeal metastasis of a non-Hodgkin lymphoma will have multiple nodules. Dural metastases may form localized nodules or plaques, and lesions with a diffuse appearance.

Diagnosis

Diagnostic examination reveals malignant cells in the first CSF sample in approximately half of all cases. Intraparenchymal metastases, via MRI, are usually circumscribed, with slight T1-hypointensity and T2-hyperintensity. Ring-like or diffuse contrast enhancement may exist, with surrounding parenchymal edema. Hemorrhagic metastases and metastatic melanomas containing melanin may show hyperintensity in non-contrast CT or MRI imaging. With leptomeningeal metastasis, MRI may reveal diffuse or focal leptomeningeal thickening with contrast enhancement. Tumor nodules may be dispersed through the subarachnoid space. Enlargement and enhancement of the cranial nerves, with communicating hydrocephalus, may be seen. An MRI can reveal dural metastases as nodular masses, or thickened dura mater along bone structures. Metastases in the vertebral bodies are confluent, diffuse, or discrete areas of low signal intensity. A CT scan may help detect any bone involvement.

Immunohistochemical characteristics of secondary CNS tumors are usually similar to tumors from which they originate. So, immunohistochemical analysis often helps in distinguishing primary from secondary CNS tumors.

It is good for the assessment of the natures and origins of metastatic neoplasms – especially unknown primary tumors.

Treatment

Systemic chemotherapy is regularly used for patients with CNS metastases. Treatment is often mostly palliative, to reduce symptoms and prolong life. In younger, healthier patients, aggressive treatments include maximal neurosurgical resection, craniotomy, chemotherapy, and **radiosurgical therapy**. Symptomatic care is given, including corticosteroids and anticonvulsants. Radiation therapy may include whole-brain irradiation, stereotactic, or fractionated radiotherapy. Targeted therapies, checkpoint inhibitors, immunotherapies, and various other treatment strategies have made CNS involvement from susceptible primary sources more successful.

Prevention and Early Detection

Surgery for treatment of the underlying primary tumor is one method to prevent a cancer from spreading to the brain. Other treatments that are used for various primary tumors can also be successful in preventing metastasis to the brain, but this is quite variable and contingent on an evolving molecular landscape. While early detection is an essential component of adequate treatment, this is unfortunately not always possible.

Significant Point

Intracranial metastatic tumors, beginning from non-CNS primary neoplasms, are being discovered more commonly today because of better diagnostic methods and ironically, because patients are living longer to allow for the natural history of the disease to advance in certain instances. Primary cancers that most often metastasize to the brain include lung cancer, breast cancer, renal cancer, and melanoma.

Prognosis

Prognosis for CNS metastases is based on age and the extension of metastases. Other factors include tumor type, and the molecular drivers that are involved. Prognosis may be affected by any peritumoral brain edema. Recent improvements in overall survival may be related to better focal and systemic therapies, plus earlier detection of CNS metastases.

Clinical Case 5

1. How prevalent are metastatic brain tumors?
2. What are the most common causes of metastases to the brain, in adults?
3. Where in the brain are metastatic tumors mostly found?

A 53-year-old man was evaluated because of headache, impaired vision, right-sided motor dysfunction, and intermittent confusion that had lasted for one week. He had previously been an alcoholic, had chronic pancreatitis with insulin-dependent diabetes, and smoked cigarettes for many years before quitting. A brain CT scan revealed a partially cystic lesion with significant contrast agent uptake, edema in the left temporoparietal lobe, and a small lesion in the right parietal lobe. Cerebrospinal fluid circulation was impaired. An acute craniotomy and neurosurgical resection of the left parieto-occipital lesion was performed. Histopathological examination revealed metastases of a solid carcinoma that was believed to be a non-small-cell carcinoma of the lung. A whole-body CT scan revealed tumorous lesions in both lungs, as well as metastases to the right adrenal gland and abdominal lymph nodes. The patient was treated with radiation therapy, stereotactic radiosurgery, and eight cycles of cisplatin with etoposide. The patient was stabilized for a while, but 11 months later, an MRI revealed two new intracerebral metastases, in the cerebellum and parietal lobe. Both were treated with radiosurgery. Confusion, seizures, and somnolence developed even though the symptoms were aggressively treated, and the patient died 14 months later.

Answers:

1. Metastatic tumors are the most common intracranial tumors. The exact prevalence is not fully understood, but is estimated at 200,000–300,000 people in the United States every year. Central nervous system metastases are generally seen in 25% of people who die of cancer, according to autopsy documentation. Global cases are generally in the same proportions.
2. Metastatic brain tumors are commonly caused by lung cancer. For men, the second most common cause is colorectal cancer, and the third is melanoma. For women, the second most common cause is breast cancer, and the third is colorectal cancer.
3. About 80% of brain metastases occur in the central hemispheres. About 15% develop in the cerebellum and another 5% occur in the brainstem. Additional locations include the dura mater and leptomeninges. Metastatic tumors may seed in the walls of the brain ventricles, pituitary gland, or choroid plexus.

Key Terms

Abducens nerve
Acrochordon
Acromegaly
Anaplastic astrocytoma
Anaplastic ependymoma
Anaplastic oligodendroglioma
Angiosarcomas

Astrocytomas
Bitemporal hemianopsia
Canalicular
Cerebellopontine
Choriocarcinoma
Clival
Cushing's disease

Cyberknife
Cytokines
Diffusion-weighted imaging
Drop metastases
Ectatic
Elephantiasis neuromatosa
Embryonal carcinoma
Endonasal
Euchromatin
Fanconi anemia
Gadolinium contrast
Gamma knife radiosurgery
Germ disk
Hemangioma
Leptomeninges
Li-Fraumeni syndrome
Meckel's cave
Meningioma
Metastatic brain tumors
Myxoid foci
Neurasthenia
Neurofibroma
Neurofibromatosis type 1
Neurofibromatosis type 2

Neurofibrosarcomas
Pineoblastoma
Pituitary adenoma
Pituitary apoplexy
Pituitary carcinoma
Pleomorphism
Prolactinomas
Proton therapy
Pseudopalisading
Radicular pain
Rosenthal fibers
Rubinstein-Taybi syndrome
Schwannoma
Somatic mutations
Somatic tissue
Spectroscopy
Stereotactic radiosurgery
Supratentorial
Syncytiotrophoblast
Tectal plate
Teratoma
Transsphenoidal
Tuberous sclerosis
Turcot syndrome

Bibliography

1 Adesina, A.M., Tihan, T., Fuller, C.E., and Young Poussaint, T. (2016). *Atlas of Pediatric Brain Tumors*, 2nd Edition. New York: Springer.

2 African Health Sciences Journal, Makerere Medical School. (2014). *Demographic profile of patients diagnosed with intracranial meningiomas in two academic hospitals in Johannesburg, South Africa: a 12-month prospective study.* V.14(4); PMC4370075. 959–945. https://www.ncbi.nlm.nih.gov/pmc/articles/PMC4370075 Accessed 2021.

3 Ahluwalia, M., Metellus, P., and Soffietti, R. (2020). *Central Nervous System Metastases*. New York: Springer.

4 Ali-Osman, F. (2005). *Brain Tumors (Contemporary Cancer Research)*. Totowa: Humana Press.

5 American Brain Tumor Association. (2020). *Meningioma*. https://www.abta.org/tumor_types/meningioma Accessed 2021.

6 American Cancer Society. (2021). *About Pituitary Tumors*. https://www.cancer.org/cancer/pituitary-tumors/about.html Accessed 2021.

7 Baehring, J.M. and Piepmeier, J.M. (2006). *Brain Tumors: Practical Guide to Diagnosis and Treatment*. Boca Raton: CRC Press.

8 Baskaya, M.K., Pyle, G.M., and Roche, J.P. (2019). *Vestibular Schwannoma Surgery*. New York: Springer.

9 Burrows, G. (2017). *Glioblastoma – A Guide for Patients and Loved Ones: Your Guide to Glioblastoma and Anaplastic Astrocytoma Brain Tumors*. Holywood (Ireland): NGO.Media.

10 Cancer Journal (American Cancer Society). (2007). *Pilocytic astrocytoma, T1-weighted axial MRI; T1-weighted sagittal MRI – Frequent recurrence and progression in pilocytic astrocytoma in adults.* https://acsjournals. onlinelibrary.wiley.com/doi/full/10.1002/ cncr.23148. Figure 2. Accessed 2021.

11 Central Brain Tumor Registry of the United States. (2010). *Average annual age-adjusted incidence rates for brain and central nervous system tumors by major histology groupings, histology and gender, CBTRUS statistical report: NPCR and SEER, 2006–2010.* https://academic. oup.com/view-large/18665155 Accessed 2021.

12 Chaichana, K. and Quinones-Hinojosa, A. (2019). *Comprehensive Overview of Modern Surgical Approaches to Intrinsic Brain Tumors.* Cambridge: Academic Press.

13 Chougule, M. (2020). *Neuropathology of Brain Tumors with Radiologic Correlates.* New York: Springer.

14. Colen, R.R. (2016). *Imaging of Brain Tumors, an Issue of Magnetic Resonance Imaging Clinics of North America (Volume 24-4, the Clinics: Radiology).* Amsterdam: Elsevier.

15 DeMonte, F., McDermott, M.W., and Al-Mefty, O. (2011). *Al-Mefty's Meningiomas*, 2nd Edition. Stuttgart: Thieme.

16 DeMonte, F., Gilbert, M.R., Mahajan, A., McCutcheon, I.E., Buzdar, A.M., and Freedman, R.S. (2007). *Tumors of the Brain and Spine (MD Anderson Cancer Care Series).* New York: Springer.

17 Dolgushin, M., Kornienko, V., and Pronin, I. (2018). *Brain Metastases: Advanced Neuroimaging.* New York: Springer.

18 Gajjar, A., Reaman, G.H., Racadio, J.M., and Smith, F.O. (2018). *Brain Tumors in Children.* New York: Springer.

19 German Pituitary Tumor Registry. (2007). *Pathohistological Classification of Pituitary Tumors: 10 Years of Experience with the German Pituitary Tumor Registry (In European Journal of Endocrinology).* Bioscientifica Ltd. Volume 156: Issue 2. 203–216. https://eje. bioscientifica.com/view/journals/ eje/156/2/1560203.xml

20 Goldman, S. and Turner, C.D. (2009). *Late Effects of Treatment for Brain Tumors (Cancer Treatment and Research, 150).* New York: Springer.

21 Hattingen, E. and Pilatus, U. (2016). *Brain Tumor Imaging (Medical Radiology).* New York: Springer.

22 Hayat, M.A. (2012). *Tumors of the Central Nervous System, Volume 8: Astrocytoma, Medulloblastoma, Retinoblastoma, Chordoma, Craniopharyngioma, Oligodendroglioma, and Ependymoma.* New York: Springer.

23 Internet Archive Book Images. (1904). *An individual with acromegaly.* https://www. flickr.com/photos/ internetarchivebookimages/14591960390. https://archive.org/stream/ sajoussanalytica01sajouoft/ sajoussanalytica01sajouoft#page/n304/ mode/1up. Accessed 2021.

24 Jain, R. (2015). *Brain Tumor Imaging.* Stuttgart: Thieme.

25 Journal of Magnetic Resonance Imaging. (2012). *Anaplastic ependymoma in the fourth ventricle, 3 views.* 35 (1): 32–47. https:// onlinelibrary.wiley.com/doi/full/10.1002/ jmri.22722. Figure 8.

26 Journal of Medical Imaging and Radiation Oncology. (2004). *CT scan showing a meningioma.* https://onlinelibrary.wiley.com/ cms/asset/61c6f66a-1338-48d1-846f-957589bbf3b9/jmiro_1278_f2.gif. https:// onlinelibrary.wiley.com/doi/ full/10.1111/j.1440-1673.2004.01278.x

27 Journal of Neuroscience, The. (2012). *Rosenthal fibers, amongst the astrocytes surrounding a blood vessel, and surrounded by intermediate filaments – Alexander Disease.* https://www.jneurosci.org/content/32/15/ 5017/tab-figures-data. 32(15); p. 5017–5023. https://doi.org/10.1523/jneurosci.5384-11.2012 Accessed 2021.

28 Kaye, A.H. and Laws, E.R., Jr. (2011). *Brain Tumors: An Encyclopedic Approach, Expert Consult, and 3rd Edition.* Philadelphia: Saunders.

29 Kesharwani, P. and Gupta, U. (2018). *Nanotechnology-Based Targeted Drug Delivery Systems for Brain Tumors*. Cambridge: Academic Press.

30 Kobayashi, T. and Lunsford, L.D. (2009). *Pineal Region Tumors: Diagnosis and Treatment Options (Progress in Neurological Surgery, Vol. 23)*. Basel: Karger Publishers.

31 Mattassi, R., Loose, D.A., and Vaghi, M. (2015). *Hemangiomas and Vascular Malformations: An Atlas of Diagnosis and Treatment*, 2nd Edition. New York: Springer.

32 Moliterno Gunel, J., Piepmeier, J.M., and Baehring, M.J. (2017). *Malignant Brain Tumors: State-of-the-Art Treatment*. New York: Springer.

33 Nachtigall, L.B. (2018). *Pituitary Tumors: A Clinical Casebook*. New York: Springer.

34 National Center for Biotechnology Information. (2015). *The Incidence of Meningioma, a Non-Malignant Brain Tumor, is Increasing in the U.S.* https://www.saferemr.com/2015/04/the-incidence-of-meningioma-non.html Accessed 2021.

35 National Library of Medicine, National Center for Biotechnology Information, World Health Organization. (2005). *Cerebral cavernous malformations*. 11;125(15):2008–2010. https://pubmed.ncbi.nlm.nih.gov/16100539 Accessed 2021.

36 Newton, H.B. and Maschio, M. (2015). *Epilepsy and Brain Tumors*. Cambridge: Academic Press.

37 Newton, H.B. (2018). *Handbook of Brain Tumor Chemotherapy, Molecular Therapeutics, and Immunotherapy*, 2nd Edition. Cambridge: Academic Press.

38 Nogales, F.F. and Jimenez, R.E. (2017). *Pathology and Biology of Human Germ Cell Tumors*. New York: Springer.

39 Obstetrics & Gynaecology. (2020). Prenatal diagnosis. *Teratomas within the Brain, 3 Views* 40 (10): 1203–1219. https://obgyn.onlinelibrary.wiley.com/doi/10.1002/pd.5722. Figure 1.

40 Ozsunar, Y. and Senol, U. (2020). *Atlas of Clinical Cases on Brain Tumor Imaging*. New York: Springer.

41 Paleologos, N.A. and Newton, H.B. (2019). *Oligodendroglioma: Clinical Presentation, Pathology, Molecular Biology, Imaging, and Treatment*. Cambridge: Academic Press.

42 Pope, W.B. (2020). *Glioma Imaging: Physiologic, Metabolic, and Molecular Approaches*. New York: Springer.

43 Quinones-Hinojosa, A. (2013). *Controversies in Neuro-Oncology (Best Evidence Medicine for Brain Tumor Surgery)*. Stuttgart: Thieme.

44 Singh, S.K. and Venugopal, C. (2018). *Brain Tumor Stem Cells: Methods and Protocols (Molecular Biology, 1869)*. Totowa: Humana Press.

45 Taylor, L.P., Porter Umphrey, A.B., and Richard, D. (2012). *Navigating Life with a Brain Tumors (Brain and Life Books)*. Oxford: Oxford University Press.

46 Walker, D.A., Perilongo, G., Taylor, R.E., and Pollack, I.F. (2020). *Brain and Spinal Tumors of Childhood*, 2nd Edition. Boca Raton: CRC Press.

47 Weis, S., Sonnberger, M., Dunzinger, A., Voglmayr, E., Aichholzer, M., Kleiser, R., and Strasser, P. (2020). *Imaging Brain Diseases: A Neuroradiology, Nuclear Medicine, Neurosurgery, Neuropathology, and Molecular Biology-based Approach*. New York: Springer.

48 Weiss, L., Gilbert, H.A., and Posner, J.B. (2011). *Brain Metastasis*. New York: Springer.

49 Wiley Online Library. (2020). Thoracic cancer. *MRI of a Cavernous Hemangioma, Seen in T1-weighted Imaging and T2-weighted Imaging* 11 (7): 2056–2058. https://onlinelibrary.wiley.com/doi/full/10.1111/1759-7714.13494. Figure 2.

50 World Health Organization. (2007). The 2007 WHO classification of tumours of the central nervous system. *National Center for Biotechnology Information, U.S. National Library of Medicine. Acta Neuropathol* 114 (2): 97–109. https://www.ncbi.nlm.nih.gov/pmc/articles/PMC1929165

4

Endocrine Tumors

OUTLINE

Thyroid Adenoma

Thyroid adenoma is a benign, encapsulated tumor that is noninvasive. It is the most common thyroid neoplasm. Adenomas of the thyroid may be inactive (non-functioning). An active (functioning) or *toxic adenoma* results in excessive thyroid hormone production from a single nodule within the thyroid gland. Palpable nodules of the thyroid are discovered in 5% of adults who live in areas where dietary iodine is sufficient. About 75% of these nodules are solitary when palpated, and are adenomas.

Epidemiology

Thyroid adenomas are usually solitary thyroid nodules. They are estimated to occur in 1–3% of the adult population. Thyroid nodules are detected by palpation in 6% of women and 2% of men. The majority of these represent, benign adenomatoid nodules or cysts, 5–10% of thyroid nodules are malignant. Follicular adenomas occur more often in areas of iodine deficiency. Females are affected slightly more often than males. However, the *follicular adenoma with papillary hyperplasia* variant occurs mostly in children and young adults. There is no proven

Global Epidemiology of Cancer: Diagnosis and Treatment, First Edition. Jahangir Moini,
Nicholas G. Avgeropoulos, and Craig Badolato.
© 2022 John Wiley & Sons Ltd. Published 2022 by John Wiley & Sons Ltd.

racial predilection for thyroid adenomas. As in the United States, thyroid adenomas affect between 1% and 3% of the global population. Global incidence is not well documented. The ages of people affected throughout the world peak at 45 years, with females being slightly more affected. There appears to be no racial predilection for thyroid adenomas.

Etiology and Risk Factors

The majority of follicular adenomas occur sporadically. The risk factors are iodine deficiency, exposure to radiation, and multinodular **goiter**. Exposure to radiation during childhood and adolescence increases the risk of follicular adenoma. This tumor has a longer latency period than papillary adenoma. Follicular adenomas develop 10–15 years after radiation exposure, and sometimes, the risks continue for 50 years. Follicular adenomas due to radiation exposure usually occur as single neoplasms. Palpable nodules are 2–3 times more common when iodine deficiency exists. The formation of thyroid nodules may be related to excessive DNA damage, **oxidative stress**, and increases in mutagenesis in the thyroid gland.

Clinical Manifestations

Adenoma of thyroid is a painless nodule, accidentally discovered during thyroid palpation, or seen in an imaging study. The submandibular region is a common location. The majority of adenomas are asymptomatic, but if large, there may be local symptoms such as difficulty swallowing. If hemorrhage occurs in the tumor, either spontaneously or after fine-needle aspiration or excessive palpitation, there may be acute pain and enlargement of the tumor. During ultrasound, an adenoma usually appears as a well-differentiated and solid homogeneous mass. It will be hypoechoic or isoechoic. Although the patients may have normal thyroid function, if a patient has a hyperfunctioning adenoma, hyperthyroidism may occur.

Pathology

Most follicular adenomas are encapsulated with solitary round nodules. The capsule can be thick or thin. Most tumors are 1–3 cm in size; however, they may grow much larger. Cut surfaces show homogeneous gray–white, brown-fleshy, or tan colors. In most cases, tumors that are gray–white have more cellularity, plus a trabecular, irregular, or solid growth pattern. The brown–tan tumors have follicles that are well developed and contain large amounts of colloid. There may be secondary hemorrhage and cystic degeneration, as well as fibrous qualities.

Diagnosis

Accurate diagnosis of follicular adenoma can be obtained by fine-needle aspiration biopsy. Imaging studies include ultrasound, **scintigraphy**, MRI, and CT. The nodules are often hypoechoic. The lesions can be of different shapes, have irregular T1-weighted signals, and increased intensity with T2-weighted imaging. The differential diagnoses for follicular adenomas include multinodular goiter and follicular carcinoma.

Treatment

Observation over time, with regular checkups is important and surgery may indicate if there are changes in nodule size and symptoms. Total surgical thyroidectomy is the goal. Prior to surgery, ultrasonography and fine-needle aspiration biopsy are indicated.

Prevention and Early Detection

There is no known method of prevention for thyroid adenomas. Though early detection can help prevent the development of future thyroid cancer, there are no effective methods of early detection, and most adenomas are discovered incidentally during other procedures.

Prognosis

Once a follicular adenoma is totally removed, there is no additional risk of recurrence. Therefore, the prognosis is generally excellent. The only potentially poor prognostic factors involve unexplained voice changes, age less than 18 years, palpable cervical lymphadenopathy, rapid enlargement of the mass, and stridor.

Clinical Case

1. How common are thyroid adenomas?
2. What are the facts about follicular thyroid adenoma in regard to radiation exposure?
3. What is the outlook for follicular thyroid adenomas?

A 47-year-old woman went to her physician for assessment of left submandibular swelling and slight pain below it. The swelling and gradual growth had been noticed a few months before. Physical examination revealed a bulky mass under the left mandible, near the submandibular gland. Diagnostic ultrasound revealed a normal thyroid and morphology, but with the parenchyma having an irregular structural pattern, fibrous qualities, and two nodules on the right lobe – one 6 mm in size and the other, 12 mm. An MRI was ordered, which indicated an oval formation with an irregular T1-weighted signal due to a slightly hyperintense centralized area, which increased in intensity with T2-weighted imaging. A follicular thyroid adenoma was diagnosed, and surgical resection occurred. The tumor was capsulated and superficial, and the patient recovered soon after surgery.

Answers:

1. **Thyroid adenoma is the most common thyroid neoplasm. They are estimated to occur in 1–3% of the adult population. Follicular adenomas occur more often in areas of iodine deficiency.**
2. **Exposure to radiation during childhood and adolescence increases the risk of follicular adenoma. They develop 10–15 years after radiation exposure, and sometimes, the risks continue for 50 years. Follicular adenomas due to radiation exposure usually occur as single neoplasms.**
3. **Once a follicular adenoma is totally removed, there is no additional risk of recurrence, so the prognosis is generally excellent. The only potentially poor prognostic factors involve unexplained voice changes, age less than 18 years, palpable cervical lymphadenopathy, rapid enlargement of the mass, and stridor.**

Thyroid Cancers

According to the American Cancer Society, estimates of cases of thyroid cancer in the United States for 2021 are 32,130 in women and 12,150 in men, totaling 44,280. Thyroid cancer is most common between the ages of 20 and 50. Women are generally three times more likely to develop thyroid cancer than men. In the United States, Caucasians have the highest rates of thyroid cancer, while African Americans have the lowest rates. Globally, thyroid cancer affects about 0.4 of every 100,000 women and 0.3 of every 100,000 men. Incidence of thyroid cancer has doubled globally since 1990. Interestingly, the figures for thyroid cancer occurring throughout the world have some gender differences. For women, most cases occur in the countries of Ecuador, Columbia, and Israel. For men, most cases occur in Latvia, Hungary, the Republic of Moldova, and in Israel. Generally, Caucasians throughout the world have the highest rates of thyroid cancer.

Papillary Carcinoma

Papillary carcinoma of the thyroid is a malignant epithelial tumor. It has follicular cell differentiation and distinct nuclei. This carcinoma is usually invasive. It is also referred to as *papillary thyroid adenocarcinoma*.

Epidemiology

The prevalence of papillary carcinoma of the thyroid has increased since 1975, from 4.8 to

14.9 cases per 100,000 individuals. In the United States, it makes up about 45,000 new diagnoses every year. Incidence rates tripled over the past 30 years. Most cases are diagnosed between ages 40 and 50, within a total range of 20–55 years. Papillary carcinoma is also the predominant type of thyroid cancer in children, and in patients of all ages with thyroid cancer who had previous head or neck radiation. Females have a 2.5 : 1 higher incidence compared with males. There is an increasing number of cases of papillary carcinoma over the past 20 years due to better recognition of thyroid nodules in imaging studies. There is no racial or ethnic predilection for these tumors.

Globally, the prevalence and incidence statistics for most countries are not well documented. The age range is the same, between 20 and 55 years. As in the United States, women are 2.5 times more likely to develop papillary thyroid carcinoma. It appears that there is a slight Caucasian predilection for papilloma thyroid carcinoma throughout the world. Fortunately, death rates have remained nearly stable or even slightly decreased in most countries. Percentages of papillary carcinoma out of all thyroid cancers are approximately 90% in Japan, 80% in Korea, and 80% in the United States (see Figure 4.1).

Etiology and Risk Factors

Exposure to ionizing radiation is the main cause of papillary thyroid carcinoma. Risk factors may include genetic factors, alcohol consumption, diabetes mellitus, dietary nitrites, excessive dietary iodine, obesity, and smoking.

Clinical Manifestations

Papillary carcinoma often is detected as a painless mass, with enlargement of the cervical lymph nodes. However, some patients may complain about neck pain, hoarseness, and dysphagia. Patients have also nodal metastases in the lateral neck.

Pathology

Papillary carcinoma may appear in one or both lobes. It is poorly defined with a firm texture and a granular white cut surface. Size of the tumor is between 2 and 3 cm in diameter, with calcifications. The cytoplasm is eosinophilic. **Psammoma bodies** are classic features, and are round, calcified, and hard masses (see Figure 4.2). There is a great amount of fibrous stroma, particularly at the advancing edge of the tumor. Often, there are multinucleated giant cells of a non-neoplastic histiocytic nature scattered throughout, which are easily found in cytology studies. Secondary cystic changes often occur, with most cysts being lined with papillary formations that aid in diagnosis.

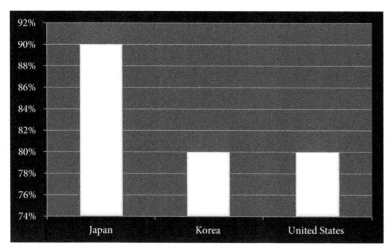

Figure 4.1 Percentages of papillary carcinoma (out of all thyroid cancers) in several countries.

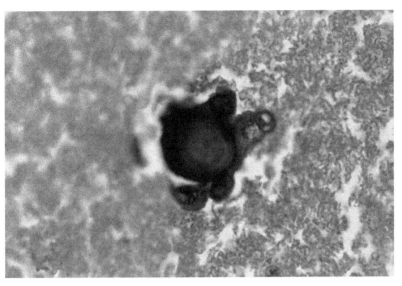

Figure 4.2 Psammoma bodies in a papillary carcinoma of the thyroid. *Source*: Ellison et al. (1998).

Diagnosis

Ultrasonography is a very helpful method that reveals hypoechoic or isoechoic solid nodules. Thyroid scans using iodine-123 (^{123}I) result in most papillary carcinomas appearing hypofunctional. However, in rare cases, they may appear hyperfunctionality. Ultrasound guides fine-needle aspiration biopsy of abnormal nodes. In some cases, CT and MRI can determine how much extrathyroidal extension is present. Cystic changes may be present, which indicate papillary carcinoma. However, biopsy is still needed. Immunostains are able to differentiate between papillary carcinoma and benign lesions. For recurrence, measurement of serum thyroglobulin provides 96% sensitivity for detection. The staging for differentiated thyroid carcinoma, which includes the papillary subtype, is as follows:

- Stage I – patient age below 55 years – any T, any N, M0 – the cancer is any size and may or may not have spread to nearby lymph nodes, with no distant metastasis; OR: the patient is age 55 or older – T1, N0 or NX, M0 – the cancer is no larger than 2 cm across and is only in the thyroid gland, has not spread to nearby lymph nodes, with no distant metastasis, OR: the patient is age 55 or older – T2, N0 or NX, M0 – the cancer is between 2 and 4 cm across and is only in the thyroid, has not spread to nearby lymph nodes, with no distant metastasis

- Stage II – patient age below 55 years – any T, any N, M1 – the cancer is any size and may or may not have spread to nearby lymph nodes, but has spread to other parts of the body; OR: the patient is age 55 or older – T1, N1, M0 – the cancer is no larger than 2 cm across and is only in the thyroid, has spread to nearby lymph nodes, with no distant metastasis; OR: the patient is age 55 or older – T2, N1, M0 – the cancer is between 2 and 4 cm across and is only in the thyroid, has spread to nearby lymph nodes, with no distant metastasis; OR: the patient is age 55 or older – T3a or T3b, any N, M0 – the cancer is larger than 4 cm across but is only in the thyroid or has grown into the strap muscles around the thyroid, may or may not have spread to nearby lymph nodes, with no distant metastasis

- Stage III – the patient is age 55 or older – T4a, any N, M0 – the cancer is any size and has grown beyond the thyroid into the larynx, trachea, esophagus, or laryngeal nerve, may or may not have spread to nearby lymph nodes, with no distant metastasis

- Stage IVA – the patient is age 55 or older – T4b, any N, M0 – the cancer is any size and has grown beyond the thyroid back toward the spine or into nearby large blood vessels, may or may not have spread to nearby lymph nodes, with no distant metastasis
- Stage IVB – the patient is age 55 or older – any T, any N, M1 – the cancer is any size and may or may not have spread to nearby lymph nodes, and has spread to other parts of the body

Note that there are also three more abbreviations used for classification, which include:

- TX – the primary tumor cannot be evaluated due to insufficient information
- T0 – there is no evidence of a primary tumor
- NX – the regional lymph nodes cannot be evaluated due to insufficient information

Treatment

Total surgical resection via thyroidectomy with or without isthmectomy is the treatment of choice for papillary thyroid carcinomas. This includes dissection of any involved cervical lymph nodes. After total surgical resection, the patient must receive lifelong hormone replacement therapy. In some cases, recurrence may occur during the first 10 years. However, recurrence can happen after more than 20 years. Thyroid lobectomy may be sufficient for small tumors. For minimal tumors, less than 1 cm, unilateral lobectomy is sufficient. When a residual tumor cannot be removed, radiation therapy is needed. Chemotherapy options include cisplatin and doxorubicin. Antineoplastic agents are used to inhibit cell growth and proliferation in the case of metastases.

Prevention and Early Detection

Since the actual cause of papillary thyroid carcinoma is unknown, it cannot be fully prevented. Reducing radiation exposure during childhood

may be preventive. Other preventive measures may include genetic testing, limiting alcohol consumption, treating diabetes mellitus, reducing dietary nitrites, having adequate dietary iodine, treating obesity, and avoiding smoking. For high-risk patients, surgical removal of the thyroid may prevent papillary thyroid carcinoma from developing. Better diagnostic methods are resulting in earlier detection of papillary thyroid carcinoma.

Prognosis

Prognosis is based on the extent of the disease. Prognosis is further based on patient age at diagnosis, tumor size, staging, and distant metastases. There is increased mortality for patients between 40 and 45 years of age, as well as for tumors that are larger than 3–4 cm in diameter. Overall mortality rates are 1–7%.

The five-year survival rate for papillary carcinoma is 97.9% in the United States. The global survival rate is 96%. Extrathyroidal tumor extension worsens prognosis, with extensive extension being worse than only minimal extension. Prognosis is very poor for bones and visceral metastases. Other factors that worsen prognosis include tumor cell type, incomplete surgical excision, and male gender. Total surgical resection is very important regarding prognosis. Recurrence within 10 years after initial surgery is usually related to increased mortality.

Significant Point

Papillary thyroid carcinoma is the most common type of thyroid cancer. It ranges from being mild and easy to cure to being more aggressive and difficult to cure. This cancer usually starts within the thyroid gland as a growth or nodule that grows out of normal thyroid tissue. It is one of the few cancers that has been becoming more common throughout the world, for unknown reasons.

Clinical Case

1. Are papillary carcinomas increasing or decreasing in prevalence and incidence?
2. What are the classic features of papillary thyroid carcinomas?
3. After the thyroid gland is totally resected, what must the patient receive?

A 28-year-old woman was hospitalized because of a palpable lump on the right side of the thyroid isthmus. There was no thyroid disease in the patient's family, but she did have a congenital heart disease. Ultrasound revealed the mass to be 2 cm in diameter with an unclear border, with many dot-like calcifications and blood flow signals. A CT scan revealed multiple nodular shadows of lower density, some of which were calcified. There was a larger shadow in the isthmus. The diagnosis was of papillary thyroid carcinoma. Echocardiography revealed her heart disease to be a ventricular septal defect, left to right shunt, and mild pulmonary hypertension. A right thyroidectomy plus isthmectomy with right central node dissection was performed. Intraoperative frozen section revealed multifocal papillary thyroid carcinoma in the right thyroid lobe, since many psammoma bodies were present. Therefore, left thyroidectomy and left central node dissection were also performed. After three days, the patient was discharged, with no symptoms of hypoparathyroidism, and started on lifelong hormone replacement therapy.

Answers:

1. **The prevalence of papillary carcinoma of the thyroid has increased since 1975, from 4.8 to 14.9 cases per 100,000 individuals. Incidence rates tripled over the past 30 years. There is an increasing number of cases, over the past 20 years, due to better recognition of thyroid nodules in imaging studies. Fortunately, death rates have remained**
nearly stable or even slightly decreased in most countries.
2. **Psammoma bodies are classic features of papillary thyroid carcinomas, and are round, calcified, and hard masses.**
3. **After total surgical resection of the thyroid, the patient must receive lifelong hormone replacement therapy.**

Follicular Carcinoma

Follicular carcinoma is the second most common type of thyroid carcinoma. It is encapsulated and has invasive growth. These tumors are also called *follicular thyroid adenocarcinomas*.

Epidemiology

The annual prevalence of follicular thyroid carcinomas in the United States, in 2009, was 12 cases per 1 million women, and 5.5 cases per 1 million men. This form makes up 10–15% of all thyroid cancers. Follicular carcinomas are very rare in children. Highest annual cases were in patients between the ages of 70 and 79 years. Women over 50 years of age develop follicular thyroid carcinomas more than two times as often as men. There is no clear racial or ethnic predilection.

Because follicular thyroid carcinomas are rare, global statistics on the prevalence and incidence of this carcinoma are not well documented. In patients under 19 years of age, the female-to-male ratio is 4 : 1, as it is in patients older than 45 years. For some reason, in patients between 20 and 45 years of age, the ratio is lower, at 3: 1. In older adults only, follicular thyroid carcinoma is more common than papillary thyroid carcinoma. Overall, this form of thyroid cancer is two to three times more prevalent in women throughout the world compared with men. There is a slightly Caucasian predilection for this cancer. The European Network of Cancer Registries has reported the highest rates of follicular thyroid carcinomas in Lithuania, Italy, Austria, Croatia, and Luxembourg.

Etiology and Risk Factors

The actual causes of follicular thyroid carcinoma are unknown, but inadequate dietary iodine is a significant risk factor. Since iodine supplementation was started in some parts of the world, the number of follicular carcinomas, compared with papillary carcinomas, has decreased. There is a link between ionizing radiation and increased risk of follicular carcinoma, but this is much lower than of papillary carcinoma. Genetic factors are considerable risk factors for follicular thyroid carcinomas.

Since inherited tumor syndromes are linked to follicular-origin tumors and malignancies, the tumors seen in these syndromes are often follicular carcinomas. Cowden's syndrome is an example associated with these tumors as well as with the follicular variant of papillary thyroid carcinomas. It is caused by several germline gene mutations. In 66% of Cowden's syndrome cases, thyroid lesions are present. Patient ages are younger, and there are usually multiple well-defined thyroid nodules, which are often encapsulated. Follicular carcinomas may develop along with **Werner's syndrome**, which is caused by a WRN gene mutation. Follicular carcinoma is seen in about 3% of Werner's syndrome patients. In the United States, family history of thyroid carcinoma is present in 3.8% of follicular carcinoma cases.

Clinical Manifestations

Follicular thyroid carcinoma is often a painless tumor, from less than 1 cm in diameter up to several centimeters. Large tumors cause dyspnea or dysphagia, and throat or neck soreness and pain. There may be unintended weight loss and night sweats. Cervical lymph node enlargement at diagnosis is not common. Sometimes, the first symptom is metastasis that can be signified by a lung nodule or a bone fracture. If a metastasis is diagnosed as being from the thyroid, a neck examination will usually reveal a thyroid mass. In certain cases, findings of bone metastases prompt a reexamination of an earlier resected thyroid mass that was believed to be an adenoma. Rare cases of functional follicular thyroid carcinoma also relate to hyperthyroidism.

Pathology

Follicular thyroid carcinomas are solid and encapsulated. Some have cystic features. Hemorrhage may be seen in biopsied lesions. In extremely invasive tumors, there is prominent extension into the thyroid or extrathyroidal tissue. Structurally, these tumors are similar to follicular adenomas. Most pathologists diagnose them based on total thickness penetration of the tumor capsule. Invasion is not related to capsule rupture from surgical manipulation, **pseudoinvasion** caused by biopsy trauma. Most invasive follicular carcinomas are large in size. If there is a solid or trabecular growth pattern, the tumor must be distinguished from poorly differentiated thyroid carcinoma. Clear-cell cytoplasm is most common with oval or round nuclei, and small nucleoli. Cytoplasmic clearing occurs because of lipid, thyroglobulin, glycogen, and mucin accumulation. It is important to exclude metastatic clear-cell carcinoma that arises from the kidney, parathyroid tumors, and medullary thyroid carcinoma (MTC). The clear-cell variant may be more aggressive than the classic form of follicular carcinoma, but this is not proven.

Diagnosis

Benign and malignant follicular-patterned tumors cannot be distinguished via fine-needle aspiration, but this procedure does assist in the assessment of morphology. Cytological diagnosis of a follicular neoplasm demonstrates that thyroid cytology is limited, since follicular carcinoma diagnosis is based on demonstrating capsular invasion, vascular invasion, or both. Imaging studies include X-rays and CT scans. Follicular thyroid carcinomas, like the papillary subtype, are differentiated tumors, so the identical staging system is used for both.

Treatment

Surgery is the treatment of choice for follicular thyroid carcinoma. Hemithyroidectomy is commonly done first to distinguish between follicular carcinoma and follicular adenoma. Once carcinoma is confirmed, thyroidectomy is performed. After radioactive iodine treatment, the patient is placed on a two-week low-iodine diet. Iodine-131 is used for ablation of thyroid tissue. For cases in which nodules are small, minimally invasive thyroidectomy has been used. Patients then have to receive lifelong hormonal replacement therapy.

Prevention and Early Detection

There is no actual prevention for follicular thyroid carcinoma and the same risk reduction strategies exist as for papillary thyroid carcinoma. There are also no specific methods for its early detection. However, genetic testing may be considered.

Prognosis

Prognosis for follicular carcinomas is excellent with capsular invasion, but not vascular invasion. Tumors invading even only one to two vessels may show hematogenous metastasis. Prognosis is worsened with larger numbers of vessels being invaded. Distant metastases most often occur in the lungs, bones, brain, and liver. Prolonged survival is possible when the tumor responds to radioactive iodine.

Clinical Case

1. How does patient age affect development of follicular thyroid carcinoma?
2. What inherited tumor syndrome may be related to follicular carcinomas?
3. What is the prognosis for follicular thyroid carcinomas?

A 70-year-old man presented with a severely sore throat, neck pain, and difficulty swallowing. He had lost 10 pounds over the past few months without changing his diet or exercise, and was having night sweats. Physical examination revealed a hard and fixed left-sided neck mass. Laboratory tests revealed normal bloodwork. Intravenous dexamethasone improved his throat pain. A chest X-ray showed focal tracheal deviation toward the right side. A neck CT revealed a large left thyroid mass with pathological cervical lymphadenopathy, which extended to the intrathoracic region, and had cystic as well as solid features. A fine-needle aspiration was performed, showing follicular cell morphology. The patient was scheduled for surgical resection. Thyroidectomy confirmed follicular thyroid cancer. The patient was treated with thyroid hormone therapy and radioiodine, and monitored for any recurrence.

Answers:

1. **Follicular carcinomas of the thyroid are very rare in children. Highest annual cases in the United States are in patients between the ages of 70 and 79 years. Women over 50 years of age develop them more than two times as often as men. Globally, in patients under 19 years of age, the female-to-male ratio is 4 : 1, as it is in patients older than 45 years. For some reason, in patients between 20 and 45, the ratio is only 3:1. In older adults only, this type of carcinoma is more common than papillary thyroid carcinoma.**
2. **Related inherited tumor syndromes include Cowden's syndrome and Werner's syndrome.**
3. **The prognosis for follicular thyroid carcinomas is excellent with capsular invasion, but not vascular invasion. Prognosis is worsened, with larger numbers of vessels being invaded.**

Medullary Carcinoma

Medullary thyroid carcinoma (MTC) is made up of cells that demonstrate C-cell (parafollicular cell) differentiation. It is a malignant thyroid tumor and is the third most common of all thyroid tumors. Other names for **medullary carcinoma** include: *C-cell carcinoma* and *parafollicular cell carcinoma*. Medullary carcinomas of the thyroid were first identified in 1959.

Epidemiology

MTC makes up less than 2.5% of all malignant thyroid tumors. Approximately 1,000 patients are diagnosed each year with MTCs in the United States. MTCs usually occur in patients over age 45. Overall, there is a slight female prevalence, but no apparent racial or ethnic predilection. The sporadic form occurs during the fifth or sixth decades, while the hereditary cases occur in younger people. Almost 30% of MTCs are inherited.

Because of its rarity, the global prevalence and incidence of MTC are not well documented. Most cases occur between the ages of 40 and 50. The female-to-male ratio only shows a slight predominance in women. There is no racial or ethnic predilection, and no clear statistics as to which countries have more cases than others.

Etiology and Risk Factors

The cause of MTC is not known, and there is no relationship to external ionizing irradiation of the head and neck. Often, the tumor develops along with **Hashimoto's thyroiditis**, but this is not fully understood. However, there is a link between MTC and multiple endocrine neoplasia 2 (MEN2). If a patient has this inherited cancer syndrome, offspring have a 50% chance of having inherited it as well. In rare cases, chronic hypercalcemia appears to increase risks for MTC. Otherwise, there are no other risk factors identified.

Clinical Manifestations

The majority of MTCs are painless. Extensive localized tumor growth causes upper airway obstruction plus dysphagia. With metastases, some patients experience flushing and severe diarrhea because of high circulating calcitonin levels and other products that result from the tumor.

Pathology

MTCs are usually single, circumscribed, and unencapsulated tumors with a gray–tan–yellow color. The size usually is 2–3 cm in diameter. Differently, the inherited tumors are usually multicentric and bilateral. For members of families with tumor syndromes, a full examination is required of the thyroid gland since gross tumors may not be visualized, and prophylactic thyroidectomies are often performed. Tumors less than 1 cm in diameter are identified incidentally from resected thyroid glands, or in patients with nodular thyroid disease after screening for calcitonin-level changes.

Cells are of various sizes, round, or spindle-shaped. The nuclei are round and have small nucleoli plus chromatin. The mitotic activity is low in most primary tumors. In fixed samples, cytoplasm is eosinophilic, with fine granules. Measurement of serum calcitonin is highly helpful. In MTC patients with palpable thyroid nodules, there may be cervical lymph node metastases. Nodal metastases often involve central compartment nodes. Hematogenous metastases are often to the lungs, bones, and liver.

Diagnosis

Early diagnosis of MTC is essential to improve the chances for a cure. Cervical ultrasonography helps confirm that a mass is within the thyroid, accurately define its size, classify it as cyst or solid, and determines whether additional nodules are present. Radionuclide scanning with radioiodine or technetium pertechnetate is helpful only in selected cases. For sporadic tumors, there must be screening of nodules for serum calcitonin. Many MTCs mimic other thyroid malignancies. The tumor usually has lobular, solid, or trabecular growth patterns. Cells are of various sizes, and may be **plasmacytoid**, spindle-shaped, polygonal, or round. The nuclei are round and contain small nucleoli. Small amounts of nuclear pseudoinclusions may be present. Diagnosis of MTCs involves biochemical or genetic screening studies after fine-needle aspiration. Patients with sporadic or inherited MTCS presenting with bone pain, diarrhea, and flushing usually have widespread metastases. The staging for MTC is as follows:

- Stage I – patient age is not a factor – T1, N0, M0 – the cancer is 2 cm or smaller and is only in the thyroid, has not spread to nearby lymph nodes, with no distant metastasis
- Stage II – patient age is not a factor – T2, N0, M0 – the cancer is 2–4 cm across and is only in the thyroid, has not spread to nearby lymph nodes, with no distant metastasis; OR: the cancer is larger than 4 cm across and only in the thyroid, or is of any size and growing outside of the thyroid yet not involving nearby structures, has not spread to nearby lymph nodes, with no distant metastasis
- Stage III – patient age is not a factor – T1 to T3, N1a, M0 – the cancer is of any size and may be growing outside of the thyroid but is not involving nearby structures, has spread to lymph nodes in the neck but not to other lymph nodes, with no distant metastasis
- Stage IVA – patient age is not a factor – T4a, any N, M0, the cancer is of any size and has grown beyond the thyroid into the larynx, trachea, esophagus, or laryngeal nerve, may or may not have spread to nearby lymph nodes, with no distant metastasis; OR: T1 to T3, N1b, M0 – the cancer is of any size and may be growing outside of the thyroid but is not involving nearby structures, has spread to the cervical or jugular lymph nodes of the neck, with no distant metastasis
- Stage IVB – patient age is not a factor – T4b, any N, M0 – the cancer is of any size and has grown back toward the spine or into nearby large blood vessels, may or may not have spread to nearby lymph nodes, with no distant metastasis
- Stage IVC – patient age is not a factor – any T, any N, M1 – the cancer is of any size and may have grown into nearby structures, may or may not have spread to nearby lymph nodes, and has spread to distant body sites such as the liver, lungs, bones, or brain

Treatment

Surgical resection and radiation therapy are the principal treatments for MTCs. Sometimes a total thyroidectomy is the best method to accomplish a cure if there are no distant metastases or extensive involvement of the lymph nodes. Recurrence is more likely if there are multiple positive lymph nodes or extracapsular invasion. Radiation therapy is recommended if there is a high risk of regional recurrence, even after total thyroidectomy. There is no role for radioactive iodine treatment in relation to MTCs. Protein kinase inhibitors such as vandetanib and cabozantinib have been successful in some patients.

Prevention and Early Detection

There is no known method of prevention for medullary thyroid cancer. Newly identified *rearranged-during-transfection point mutations* have helped to detect MTC earlier than in previous decades, and new treatment guidelines have resulted. Screening methods are based on serum calcitonin levels, and for metastatic or recurrent MTCs, neck ultrasonography, chest CT, liver MRI, bone scintigraphy, and axial skeleton MRI.

Prognosis

For MTC, 5-year survival rates are 77% and 10-year survival rates are 65% based on staging. Patient age is important along with staging to determine prognosis for MTCs. A poor prognosis is related to the presence of highly calcitonin after surgical resection. When the tumor is more aggressive, the prognosis is poor. Vascular invasion also worsens outlook.

Significant Point

MTC begins when the parafollicular C cells of the thyroid become cancerous and grow without control. It is the rarest type of thyroid cancer. In most cases, it is treated by removal of the thyroid gland, with or without adjuvant radiation therapy or chemotherapy. About 25% of cases are familial.

Clinical Case

1. How common are MTCs in comparison with other forms of thyroid cancer?
2. What are the best surgical options for MTCs?
3. What are the new methods used for early detection?

A 45-year-old woman recently noticed a lump on her neck and went to see her physician. She has no family history of thyroid or any other cancer, but her mother died of complications of pheochromocytoma after having had a routine hysterectomy. Physical examination revealed an asymmetric thyroid gland, with a 1.5 cm nodule on the right side. Fine-needle aspiration reveals C-cell hyperplasia. A thyroidectomy is performed, and medullary carcinoma is confirmed. The patient recovers soon after surgery. Her physician recommends ongoing surveillance for the inherited cancer syndrome called multiple endocrine neoplasias 2 (MEN2), because her children have a 50% chance of having inherited it. The diagnosis of MTC can be an indicator of MEN2, and since the patient developed her cancer at only age 40, her younger age is an indicator of having an inherited cancer syndrome. Also, her mother's history of pheochromocytoma is highly suggestive of MEN2.

Answers:

1. **Medullary thyroid carcinoma makes up less than 2.5% of all malignant thyroid tumors. About 1,000 patients are diagnosed each year in the United States. Global prevalence and incidence are not well documented.**
2. **Surgical resection and radiation therapy are the principal treatments for MTCs. Sometimes a total thyroidectomy is the best method to accomplish a cure if there are no distant metastases or extensive involvement of the lymph nodes.**
3. **Newly identified rearranged-during-transfection point mutations have helped to detect MTC earlier than in previous decades, and new treatment guidelines have resulted. Screening methods are based on serum calcitonin levels, and for metastatic or recurrent MTCs, neck ultrasonography, chest CT, liver MRI, bone scintigraphy, and axial skeleton MRI.**

Anaplastic Thyroid Carcinoma

Anaplastic thyroid carcinoma (ATC) is very aggressive and malignant. It is made up of undifferentiated follicular thyroid cells, which do not look like normal thyroid cells. Nearly every **anaplastic carcinoma** of the thyroid is a grade IV tumor.

Epidemiology

Anaplastic carcinoma of the thyroid is also very rare, affecting less than 2% of thyroid cancer patients, but is responsible for 20–50% of deaths. ATC affects one to two out of every one million people annually in the United States. The majority of patients are over age 65, and 90% of cases occur above the age of 50. There is a female-to-male predilection of 2 : 1. There appears to be no racial predilection for ATCs. Globally, statistics on prevalence and incidence are poorly documented. The mean age at diagnosis is 55–65 years. Women make up 55–77% of all patients. There appears to be no racial or ethnic predominance.

Etiology and Risk Factors

The etiology of ATCs is unclear. Epigenetic and microRNA changes may be related. The ATCs may develop via progressive increases in genetic alteration in preexisting differentiated carcinoma. Risk factors include inherited cancer syndromes, including Cowden's syndrome, Carney complex, Werner's syndrome, and familial adenomatous polyposis.

Clinical Manifestations

Patient may present with firm neck mass that is fixed in one location. The tumor is widely infiltrative. Hoarseness, breathing problems, dysphagia, and pain are common symptoms as well as dyspnea and vocal cord paralysis. Approximately 35% of patients initially present with distant metastasis to the lungs and bones.

Pathology

ATC is the primary malignancy of the gland and often spreads to regional lymph nodes as well as distant locations. The tumor is often large, multicolored, with necrosis, and an infiltrative growth pattern. Vascular invasion is common, and involves penetration of the vessel walls by spindle cells, protruding into the lumina. The cells usually include epithelioid and spindle cells, plus giant cells that resemble osteoclasts, and tumor diathesis. Clusters of tumor cells are often infiltrated by neutrophils.

Diagnosis

There is cellularity via fine-needle aspiration, and it depends on which area of the tumor is biopsied. Malignant cells and obvious nuclear pleomorphism signify high-grade malignancies. Immunohistochemistry helps to distinguish ATCs from other undifferentiated tumors by using lymphoid markers. If there are high levels of inflammatory cells and necrotic debris, a core biopsy is used after the fine-needle aspiration. Imaging studies often include CT. The staging for anaplastic (undifferentiated) thyroid carcinoma is as follows:

- Stage IVA – T1 to T3a, N0 or NX, M0 – the cancer is of any size but is only in the thyroid gland; has not spread to nearby lymph nodes, with no distant metastasis
- Stage IVB – T1 to T3a, N1, M0 – the cancer is of any size but is only in the thyroid, has spread to nearby lymph nodes, with no distant metastasis; OR: T3b, any N, M0 – the cancer is of any size and has grown into the strap muscles around the thyroid, may or may not have spread to nearby lymph nodes, with no distant metastasis; OR: the cancer is of any size and

has grown beyond the thyroid into the larynx, trachea, esophagus, laryngeal nerve, or back toward the spine or into nearby large blood vessels, may or may not have spread to nearby lymph nodes, with no distant metastasis
- Stage IVC – any T, any N, M1 – the cancer is of any size, may or may not have spread to nearby lymph nodes, but has spread to other parts of the body such as distant lymph nodes, internal organs, or bones

Treatment

Most cases of ATCs are unresectable at presentation because of invasion of cervical structures. Surgery is not curative and should aim to secure the patient's airway. Often, radiation therapy and chemotherapy are administered. The multiple kinase inhibitor *lenvatinib* is a common medication for many thyroid cancers. Thyroid-stimulating hormone suppression therapy may also be used.

Prevention and Early Detection

There is no known method of preventing ATC. There is also no way to diagnose the disease early. By the time symptoms are present, there is often evidence that the carcinoma has spread to distant body sites.

Prognosis

The one-year survival rate for ATCs is 10–20%. Mortality rates are 90%. A primary presentation with a large, infiltrative tumor suggests a poor prognosis. There is a better outlook when the tumor is found incidentally during another surgery.

Clinical Case

1. How often does ATC affect women?
2. During diagnosis, what signifies high-grade ATC malignancies?
3. What is the usual prognosis for ATCs?

A 70-year-old woman had previously undergone surgery for papillary thyroid carcinoma. Five years later, multiple pulmonary metastases were found. Radiation therapy was ineffective for treatment. Active surveillance continued along with thyroid-stimulating hormone suppression therapy, but the pulmonary tumors continued to grow. Lenvatinib therapy was started, which caused a number of adverse effects, but did cause the tumors to shrink. The patient's condition remained stable for almost five years, but then her white blood count suddenly increased to extremely high levels, and a CT scan showed worsening of the pulmonary metastases. Over time, the patient's condition deteriorated, with weight loss and an inability to walk. A CT scan revealed metastases to her liver, left adrenal gland, and kidneys. The patient died seven weeks later.

Answers:

1. **There is a female-to-male predilection for ATC of 2 : 1 in the United States. Globally, women make up 55–77% of all patients.**
2. **In anaplastic thyroid carcinoma, malignant cells and obvious nuclear pleomorphism signify high-grade malignancies.**
3. **The one-year survival rate for anaplastic thyroid carcinomas is 10–20%. Generally speaking, mortality rates are 90%. A primary presentation with a large, infiltrative tumor suggests a poor prognosis. There is a better outlook when the tumor is found incidentally during another surgery.**

Parathyroid Tumors

Parathyroid adenomas are benign tumors that may cause hyperparathyroidism. Parathyroid hormone causes calcium concentrations in the blood to increase (hypercalcemia). Parathyroid carcinoma is less common than parathyroid adenoma, and is a malignant tumor that may have progressed from a parathyroid adenoma. It usually results in severe hypercalcemia and high parathyroid hormone levels, and often causes kidney and bone abnormalities.

Adenoma

Adenoma of the parathyroid gland is a benign neoplasm and is the main cause of primary hyperparathyroidism. The lower parathyroid glands are more commonly affected by adenomas.

Epidemiology

Parathyroid adenomas are very rare causes of hyperparathyroidism, accounting for less than 1% of that disease. About 100,000 people in the United States develop primary hyperparathyroidism annually due to a parathyroid adenoma. In most cases (80–85%), there is only a single parathyroid adenoma. These tumors can occur at any age, but are most common in patients between 50 and 70 years. Women are affected three times more often than men. There is no clear racial or ethnic predilection. The only available global statistics appear to be identical to those of the United States.

Etiology and Risk Factors

The etiology of parathyroid adenomas is unknown. There has been a link to external ionizing radiation treatments of the head and neck during childhood. Parathyroid adenoma and primary hyperparathyroidism may coexist in people exposed to radiation. Survivors of atomic bombs in Japan have shown a four times higher rate of parathyroid adenomas.

Clinical Manifestations

Hyperparathyroidism may result in renal disease and severe metabolic bone disease, such as osteitis fibrosa cystica. However, most cases are asymptomatic. If symptoms occur, they may include fatigue, weakness, anxiety, and various amounts of cognitive impairment. With primary hyperparathyroidism, risks for bone fractures and nephrolithiasis are higher.

Pathology

Parathyroid adenomas occur more commonly in the inferior parathyroid glands. These noninvasive adenomas may also arise in other parts of the neck, the thyroid gland, the mediastinum, the thymus, and the retro-esophageal space. The size of tumors range between 1 and 10 cm. Parathyroid adenomas are oval shaped, with a thin surrounding capsule. Cross sections reveal a soft appearance and a pink–tan color. There may also be foci of calcification with marked fibrotic areas. Microadenomas are hard to identify. Spindle-shaped cells are sometimes present. The cytoplasm is slightly eosinophilic. The nuclei are usually round and located in the centers of the cells.

Diagnosis

Ultrasound, *scintigraphy*, MRI, arterial phase MRI, single-photon emission computerized tomography (SPECT), and four-dimensional parathyroid CT are helpful. When parathyroid adenomas are aspirated, there is varied cellularity. Usually, the samples have dissociated epithelial cells, along with small-cell aggregates having oval to round hyperchromatic nuclei.

Treatment

The treatment of choice for parathyroid adenoma is surgery to remove the tumor. Occasionally, hemithyroidectomy is required, and parathyroidectomy is common. Preoperatively, the extent of possible removal of adenoma is determined by localization studies. After excision of the affected gland, a decrease of PTH is expected.

Prevention and Early Detection

There is no known method of prevention for parathyroid adenomas. They are often detected incidentally. The only methods of early detection may be to look for germline mutations that may be implicated in familial cases of isolated hyperparathyroidism.

Prognosis

Prognoses for parathyroid adenomas are excellent. Recurring or persisting hyperparathyroidism occurs in a subgroup of cases. This may be due to the inability to find a normally positioned parathyroid gland.

Clinical Case

1. How often do parathyroid adenomas cause primary hyperparathyroidism?
2. What are some severe results of hyperparathyroidism?
3. Are there any methods for early detection of parathyroid adenomas?

A 51-year-old woman underwent parathyroid surgery, but then had persistent hypercalcemia. When imaging could not localize any abnormal parathyroid tissues, the patient underwent bilateral neck exploration with total left parathyroidectomy and right superior parathyroidectomy. Her PTH levels remained elevated. Single-photon emission computerized tomography (SPECT) showed sestamibi uptake in the lower right mid-chest area, and a 1 cm soft tissue nodule was found, consistent with a solitary parathyroid gland in the anterior mediastinum. Arterial phase MRI of the chest confirmed a 7 mm nodule in the right lobe of the remaining thymus gland. A partial thymectomy was performed, with resection of intrathymic ectopic parathyroid gland via right thoracoscopy. The PTH levels decreased. Pathology revealed an intrathymic parathyroid adenoma with hypercellular parathyroid tissue. The thymus has been reported as the most common ectopic site for parathyroid adenomas. The patient recovered well.

Answers:

1. **Adenoma of the parathyroid gland is the main cause of primary hyperparathyroidism. Even so, the tumor accounts for less than 1% of that disease. About 100,000 people in the United States develop primary hyperparathyroidism annually due to parathyroid adenoma.**
2. **Hyperparathyroidism may result in renal disease and severe metabolic bone disease, such as osteitis fibrosa cystica.**

3. **The only methods of early detection may be to look for germline mutations that may be implicated in familial cases of isolated hyperparathyroidism.**

Carcinoma

Malignant tumors of the parathyroid glands are not common. They originate from parenchymal cells. Most cases occur sporadically, though there are documented cases of familial carcinomas.

Epidemiology

Parathyroid carcinoma makes up less than 1% of cases of primary hyperparathyroidism. It accounts for just 0.005% of all malignant tumors in the United States. According to the *Surveillance, Epidemiology, and End Results (SEER)* program, parathyroid carcinoma affects less than one person per million people in the United States. Even so, incidence has increased over the last 30 years, from 3.58 to 5.73 per 10 million. The increases could be due to better screening, improved methods of diagnosis, or an actual disease increase. Within a range of 15–89 years, the mean patient age is 57 years. The female-to-male ratio is nearly even, with a slight female predominance. There is no racial or ethnic predilection.

Global incidence is increasing, but parathyroid carcinoma also accounts for only 0.005% of all malignant tumors in Western Europe. In Japanese studies, 6% of primary hyperparathyroidism patients may result in parathyroid carcinomas. There is little other data available, but according to a study in the United Kingdom, there are about 400 cases reported globally every year. The peak age range is between 50 and 60 years, with a slight female predominance, but no racial or ethnic predilection.

Etiology and Risk Factors

The etiology of parathyroid carcinomas is not clear. However, there may be a genetic link. There have been a few cases reporting a connection with MEN1 and MEN2. Radiation exposure may be another factor. With renal failure, parathyroid carcinomas are often present. There appear to be no other risk factors for parathyroid carcinomas.

Clinical Manifestations

Signs and symptoms are linked to the overproduction of PTH. Calcium levels are high. Most patients may have nephrolithiasis. Some patients may exhibit signs of bone disease, including osteitis fibrosa cystica, osteoporosis, and bone fractures. Hypercalcemia may result in anorexia, fatigue, weakness, weight loss, nausea, vomiting, polydipsia, and polyuria. The presence of a carcinoma may be indicated by recurrent laryngeal nerve paralysis.

Pathology

Macroscopically, the tumors have wide variations in appearance. They are usually large, but have variable encapsulation. They weigh from 1.5 g to over 50 g. The tumors can be dense in their adherence to nearby soft tissues or the thyroid. Some of these tumors are not distinguishable from adenomas. Microscopically, there are round to oval nuclei with dense chromatin. The cells may closely resemble those of the adenomas. Identifiers of carcinoma include an increase in serum calcium and PTH, vascular or perineural invasion, and a palpable neck mass.

Diagnosis

Ultrasound and CT scans are useful to diagnose parathyroid carcinomas. Blood or urine tests include serum calcium, PTH, and blood phosphorus. A Sestamibi/SPECT scan uses the **sestamibi protein**, mixed with a radioactive material and injected IV. It is recommended if laboratory tests reveal elevated PTH levels, to evaluate possible spread of the carcinoma, and to assess recurrence. An MRI can also be used to assess tumor size, using a contrast agent, though this is not as accurate as the other methods. Surgical resection is the most common method of diagnosis, confirmed by pathology. A biopsy is usually not recommended as a separate procedure from surgery. There is no standard staging system for parathyroid carcinoma because it is very rare. Therefore, it is simply referred to as localized, metastatic, or recurrent.

Treatment

Calcimimetic agents are used to lower calcium levels to decrease hypercalcemia. Aggressive surgical excision is performed for parathyroid carcinoma. It may involve **en bloc resection**, tumor debulking, or metastasectomy. Parathyroidectomy can damage the vocal cords, so treatments may be required to improve speech problems that result. External or internal radiation therapy may be required. Systemic or regional chemotherapy may also be needed. Supportive care for hypercalcemia includes IV fluids, drugs to increase urine production, and drugs to stop the manufacture of PTH from the parathyroid glands.

Prevention and Early Detection

There is no known method of preventing parathyroid carcinoma. Early detection utilizes the same methods as for parathyroid adenoma – identifying related germline mutations, based on familial cases of isolated hyperparathyroidism.

Prognosis

Unfortunately, prognosis for parathyroid carcinomas is fair to poor. It may recur locally and metastasize to the neck structures. Recurrence often involves extreme hypercalcemia, plus various metabolic complications. Metastatic spread often appears late in the disease development. The estimated 5-year survival rate is 82%, and the 10-year survival rate is 60%. According to the *United States National Cancer Database*, negative prognoses are most prevalent in older patients, in males, and with larger tumor size. When the lymph nodes are affected, the prognosis is also worsened.

Significant Point

Parathyroid carcinoma is so rare that many physicians have never encountered it. It is most often signified by extremely high production of parathyroid hormone, accompanied by very high serum calcium levels. Since this type of cancer is associated with a genetic defect, it can occur in family members. These tumors can reappear decades after their first appearance. Therefore, long-term monitoring is required.

Clinical Case

1. What are the most common signs and symptoms of parathyroid carcinoma?
2. What type of surgical excision is indicated for parathyroid carcinoma?
3. Is the outlook good or bad for parathyroid carcinoma?

A 60-year-old woman had a previous history of primary hyperparathyroidism. She had undergone a left parathyroidectomy of one parathyroid gland. Two years later, hypercalcemia and persistent hyperparathyroidism were detected. The patient was hospitalized, with other complaints of osteoporosis, hypertension, constipation, irritability, and depression. Laboratory tests revealed increased serum parathyroid hormone, calcium, phosphorous, albumin, and magnesium. Ultrasonography revealed a thyroid nodule on the right lobe of 22 mm and 35 mm nodule on the posterior face of the left lobe. A CT scan revealed a heterogeneous mass of about 5 cm in diameter, posterior to the left inferior pole and extending to the mediastinum. The patient was referred for a formal cervical exploration with parathyroidectomy. The inferior left parathyroid gland was totally removed, along with the left thyroid lobe and all involved tissue. Within 10 minutes, her PTH levels decreased. Pathological examination revealed the mass to be a parathyroid carcinoma. The patient recovered, and at 12 months of follow-up is asymptomatic with no recurrence.

Answers:

1. **Most patients have nephrolithiasis. Some may have signs of bone disease, including osteitis fibrosa cystica, osteoporosis, and bone fractures. There may be anorexia, fatigue, weakness, weight loss, nausea, vomiting, polydipsia, polyuria, and recurrent laryngeal nerve paralysis.**

2. **Aggressive surgical excision is performed for parathyroid carcinoma. It may involve en bloc resection, tumor debulking, or metastasectomy.**
3. **Unfortunately, prognosis is poor. It may recur locally and metastasize to the neck structures. Recurrence often involves extreme hypercalcemia, plus various metabolic complications. Negative prognoses are most prevalent in older patients, in males, and with larger tumor size. When the lymph nodes are affected, the prognosis is also worsened.**

Thymus Tumors

The thymus has important functions primarily during the early phase of life. It is found in the inferior neck and extended into the superior thorax. The thymus is a primary lymphoid organ and differs from secondary lymphoid organs. Overall, thymus tumors are rare, and develop when cancer cells form on the outside surface of the organ. Thymus tumors are often asymptomatic at the time of diagnosis, and are often found when an unrelated medical test or examination is performed.

Thymoma

Thymoma is a tumor of the epithelial cells of the thymus. It is classified based on biologic or cytologic criteria. Benign or encapsulated thymomas are both biologically and cytologically benign. Malignant thymoma may be of two types. *Type I* is cytologically benign, but infiltrative as well as locally aggressive. Once a thymoma progresses to *Type II*, it is known as *thymic carcinoma*, and is biologically and cytologically malignant. Squamous cell carcinoma of the thymus is a common subtype.

Epidemiology

Thymomas are uncommon tumors, affecting only about 0.13 out of every 100,000 people in the United States. This means that there are approximately 390 cases per year. Thymomas develop at any age. The usual age at diagnosis is 30–40 years, though they have occurred in every age group, including children. Men and women appear to be equally affected by thymomas. Globally, most cases occur in Asians and Pacific Islanders (0.25 per 100,000), followed by African Americans (0.18), non-Hispanic Caucasians (0.10), and Hispanic-Americans (0.08). Thymomas are reported in about 0.15 per 100,000 people, and no actual incidence statistics are available.

Etiology and Risk Factors

Myasthenia gravis, pure red cell aplasia, and hypogammaglobulinemia may cause thymomas. Lymphocytic leukemia, autoimmune disorders, and drug exposures may also be related. Less common potential risk factors for thymomas include acute agranulocytosis, hemolytic anemia, pernicious anemia, myocarditis, pericarditis, **alopecia areata**, thyroiditis, Cushing's disease, ulcerative colitis, nephrotic syndrome, rheumatoid arthritis, scleroderma, and systemic lupus erythematosus.

Pathology

Thymomas are lobulated, well-circumscribed, firm masses of a gray–white color. They arise in the anterior superior mediastinum. They may also be seen in the thyroid or neck. Thymomas can reach 15–20 cm in diameter. There is often calcification and cystic necrosis. Macroscopically, thymomas are encapsulated and may infiltrate to the perithymic tissues. Microscopically, they are made up of epithelial tumor cells in a swirling pattern and immature T cells. The epithelial cells are elongated or spindled. The cells have oval to elongated nuclei, with only a few small reactive lymphoid cells interspersed.

Malignant thymoma type I has bland cytology, but is locally invasive. They contain significant cytoplasm and vesicular nuclei. Many small reactive lymphoid cells are interspersed. The identifying feature is capsule penetration and invasion of surrounding tissues. *Malignant thymoma Type II* is more accurately termed thymic carcinoma. They only make up about 5% of all thymomas. They appear fleshy, with obvious invasion, and often metastasize to the lungs and abdomen. The majority of these tumors resemble squamous cell carcinoma when viewed under a microscope.

Clinical Manifestations
About 30% of thymomas are asymptomatic, and about 40% have symptoms caused by impingement upon mediastinal structures. Between 35% of thymomas cause localized signs and symptoms, including dyspnea, coughing, chest pain and tightness, and **superior vena cava syndrome**. The remaining percentage is related to myasthenia gravis or other systemic diseases. Fatigue and difficulty swallowing have also been reported.

Diagnosis
Diagnosis of thymoma is made via histologic examination. About 33% of patients have thymomas discovered because of a related autoimmune disorder. The tumors are often found on a chest X-ray or CT scan that is performed for another reason. The tumor is sampled with a CT-guided needle biopsy. On CT scans, increased vascular enhancement or pleural deposits may indicate malignancy, and axial positron emission tomography (PET) as well as fused FDG-PET/CT may also be used. Other diagnostic tests include full blood cell count, protein electrophoresis, electrolytes, liver enzymes, and renal function. Laboratory testing may reveal abnormal amounts of hematocrit, hemoglobin, platelets, sodium, and white blood cells. The staging of thymic carcinomas is as follows:

- Stage I – T1a, N0, M0 – the cancer has not spread into the outer layer of the thymus, or it has grown into nearby fatty tissues, but not into the mediastinal pleura, has not spread to nearby lymph nodes, with no distant metastasis; OR: T1b, N0, M0 – the cancer has grown into nearby fatty tissues and the mediastinal pleura, has not spread to nearby lymph nodes, with no distant metastasis
- Stage II – T2, N0, M0 – the cancer has grown into nearby fatty tissues and into the pericardium, has not spread to nearby lymph nodes, with no distant metastasis

- Stage IIIA – T3, N0, M0 – the cancer is growing into nearby tissues or organs, including the lungs, vessels carry blood into or out of the lungs, superior vena cava, or the phrenic nerve; has not spread to nearby lymph nodes, with no distant metastasis
- Stage IIIB – T4, N0, M0 – the cancer is growing into nearby tissues or organs, including the trachea, esophagus, or main blood vessels pumping blood away from the heart; has not spread to nearby lymph nodes, with no distant metastasis
- Stage IVA – any T, N1, M0 – the cancer may or may not have grown into nearby tissues or organs, and has spread to nearby lymph nodes in the front chest cavity, with no distant metastasis; OR: any T, N0 or N1, M1a – the cancer may or may not have grown into nearby tissues or organs, may or may not have spread to nearby lymph nodes, but has spread to the pleura or the pericardium
- Stage IVB – any T, N2, M0, or M1a – the cancer may or may not have grown into nearby tissues or organs, has spread to the lymph nodes deep in the chest cavity or neck, and may or may not have spread to the pleura or pericardium; OR: any T, any N, M1b – the cancer may or may not have grown into nearby tissues or organs, may or may not have spread to nearby lymph nodes in the chest cavity or neck, but has spread to the inside of the lungs or to other distant organs

Treatment
Surgical resection of a thymoma often improves any coexisting neuromuscular disorder. When a thymoma is invasive and large in size, preoperative chemotherapy with or without radiation therapy may be used to shrink the tumor and improve surgical resectability. Also, medications can be administered to balance thyroid hormones in relation to Graves' disease, which sometimes result in the resolution of the tumor. If the thymoma is stage I through IIB, there is no need for additional therapy. Surgical removal is not believed to result in immune deficiency in adults. However, in children, immunity following surgery may be reduced, so vaccinations for various infectious agents such as yellow fever can be dangerous. This is likely

because of inadequate T-cell response to the live, attenuated vaccine, and can be fatal. An invasive thymoma may need radiation therapy and chemotherapy with cisplatin, cyclophosphamide, and doxorubicin. Recurrences have been seen in 10–30% of cases up to 10 years after surgery. For most cases, pleural recurrences can be resected. Surgical removal of pleural recurrences may be followed via intrathoracic hyperthermic perfused chemotherapy (ITH). In some cases, total surgical resection of the thymus is required.

Prevention and Early Detection

There is no known method of prevention for thymomas. There are no widely recommended screening tests. Early detection can occur via a chest X-ray or CT scan for another medical reason. If present, paraneoplastic syndromes can be highly important for early detection since they may be present while the tumor is still in its early stages.

Prognosis

Prognosis is based on the stage of the thymoma, and the ability to remove the tumor surgically. Thymic carcinomas have a worsened prognosis than thymomas, which usually grow slowly. Prognosis is good to excellent for stage I thymomas, and also for stage II thymic carcinomas. In one study, only 3% of thymomas recurred after surgery. For stage III thymomas, 83% of patients survived for 10 years or more after diagnosis. The 10-year survival rate for stage IV thymoma is about 47%. Overall, most patients live for at least five years after a thymoma is diagnosed, but less than half of patients with thymic carcinoma will live for five more years.

Significant Point

Thymomas are described based on their degree of spread. While most of them can spread beyond the thymus, many are noninvasive. When the pattern of spread is typical for cancer, these tumors are usually described as thymic carcinomas.

Clinical Case – Thymic Carcinoma

1. What are the most prominent causes of thymic carcinoma?
2. What is the macroscopic and microscopic appearance of thymic carcinomas?
3. Which chemotherapies are often used for thymic carcinomas?

A 43-year-old African American man complained of chest pain and dyspnea. A chest X-ray showed a mass near his heart of about 9 cm in diameter, close to the aorta and pulmonary artery. Laboratory tests revealed abnormal amounts of white blood cells, hemoglobin, hematocrit, sodium, and platelets. The tumor was large enough to be impinging the right side of the heart near the pulmonic valve. Squamous cell carcinoma of the thymus was diagnosed. The tumor was carefully resected, and adjuvant treatments included radiation therapy and chemotherapy. After one year of follow-up, the patient had no recurrence of the carcinoma and was doing well.

Answers:

1. **Myasthenia gravis, pure red cell aplasia, and hypogammaglobulinemia may cause thymomas. Lymphocytic leukemia, autoimmune disorders, and drug exposures may also be related.**
2. **Macroscopically, these tumors are encapsulated and may infiltrate to the perithymic tissues. Microscopically, they are made up of elongated or spindled epithelial cells in a swirling pattern, and immature T cells. The epithelial cells have oval to elongated nuclei, with only a few small reactive lymphoid cells interspersed.**
3. **Chemotherapies for thymic carcinomas include cisplatin, cyclophosphamide, and doxorubicin.**

Thymolipoma

Thymolipoma is a benign tumor, located in anterior mediastinum that originates from the thymus cells. It contains both thymic and adipose tissue. Thymolipomas have been reported since 1916. A subtype is known as *thymofibrolipoma*.

Epidemiology

Thymolipomas make up 5.5% of all thymic neoplasms, and affect about 0.12 of every 100,000 people in the United States. They are less common than mediastinal lipomas of non-thymic origin. The reported age range is between 3 and 56 years, with a mean age of 22 years, though more cases are discovered in the third and fourth decades of life. There is no difference in prevalence between males and females. There is no racial or ethnic predilection.

Globally, thymolipomas account for 2–9% of all thymic tumors. About half of all diagnosed patients also have an autoimmune disease. Only a few hundred cases of thymolipomas have ever been reported from countries outside of the United States. The same age range has been seen as in the United States, and there is no difference in occurrence between males and females. There is no racial or ethnic predilection as well.

Etiology and Risk Factors

Causes of thymolipomas are unknown, though it is believed they may be either true neoplasms of the thymus, or neoplasms made of mediastinal fat that engulf the thymus. Thymolipomas are only rarely associated with myasthenia gravis. They may be linked to Graves' disease, Hodgkin's lymphoma, chronic lymphocytic leukemia, aplastic anemia, or hypogammaglobulinemia. Thymolipomas may be related to an abnormal chromosome, such as 5q21-22 or 12q15. There are no known environmental risk factors.

Pathology

Thymolipomas are developed from mature adipose tissue mixed with islands of thymic tissue. They grow slowly, and gradually increase in size. The tumors are soft in consistency and form around the mediastinum and diaphragm, often mimicking cardiomegaly. There is usually a thin, fibrous capsule. The color is yellow, and focal, solid areas may be present. The polygonal, striated myoid cells have abundant eosinophilic cytoplasm.

Clinical Manifestations

The majority of thymolipomas are asymptomatic. When symptoms are present, they are related to the displacement of mediastinal structures. About 25% of patients have chest pain, coughing, and dyspnea – which may or may not be related to the tumor. Some patients experience sneezing and nasal congestion. Tachypnea and palpitations have also been documented.

Diagnosis

Most thymolipomas are diagnosed incidentally, by imaging of a respiratory tract infection. By the time of diagnosis, thymolipomas are usually large in size. Thymolipomas often appear as large anterior mediastinal masses. The mostly fatty density can be hard to identify on plain X-rays. CT scans reveal almost completely fatty tumors with some areas of inhomogeneous soft tissue density, representing thymic tissue. On MRI, they have fat and soft tissue signal characteristics. Differential diagnoses include cardiomegaly, mediastinal liposarcoma, thymoliposarcoma, focal thymic hyperplasia, and anterior mediastinal masses. Transthoracic biopsy is a diagnostic option for certain thymolipomas.

Treatment

Surgical resection of thymolipomas is curative, with thoracotomy being common. For patients with myasthenia gravis, extended thymectomy is the treatment of choice, and provides a better complete remission rate after resection. With this procedure, there have been no reports of recurrences, metastases, or deaths from these tumors.

Prevention and Early Detection

There is no known method of prevention for thymolipomas. Though early detection can help to find a thymolipoma before it becomes very large, this has no general effect upon outcome, since extended thymectomy is usually curative.

Prognosis

The prognosis for thymolipomas is excellent because of surgical resection being curative.

***

Significant Point

A thymolipoma is a rare, benign anterior mediastinal mass that originates from the thymus. It contains thymic and mature adipose tissue. They may be true thymic neoplasms, variants of thymomas, neoplasms of mediastinal fat that engulfs thymic tissue, or simply hyperplasia of mediastinal fat.

***

Clinical Case – Thymolipoma

1. What other conditions may be risk factors for thymolipomas?
2. Though often asymptomatic, what may symptoms of a thymolipoma be related to?
3. What subclassifications may be made for a thymolipoma?

A 44-year-old woman complained of shortness of breath, nasal congestion, and sneezing that had continued for several months. Bronchodilators were given, but then she developed a productive cough and became tired very easily. The dyspnea even bothered her while resting, and she experienced tachypnea and palpitations. Physical examination revealed decreased breath sounds on the right side. When her symptoms worsened, she was hospitalized. A chest X-ray revealed a large mass in the anterior mediastinum that extended to the right hemothorax, with collapse of the right inferior and middle lobes. A CT scan showed a large right subpulmonary fat-containing lesion with a transverse diameter of 23 cm. A transthoracic biopsy revealed that fatty tissue was present. A right thoracotomy was performed with the intention of either resecting the tumor or obtaining an open biopsy. The tumor was solid, well-circumscribed, and encapsulated. Because of its size, it was resected in two parts. Diagnosis was of a benign thymolipoma with no evidence of malignancy. After surgery, the patient's pulmonary function was immediately improved. After four years of follow-up, the patient is fully functioning with no recurrence.

Answers:

1. **Thymolipomas may be related to Graves' disease, Hodgkin's lymphoma, chronic lymphocytic leukemia, aplastic anemia, hypogammaglobulinemia, abnormal chromosomes, and rarely, to myasthenia gravis.**
2. **If symptoms of a thymolipoma are present, they may be related to displacement of mediastinal structures – chest pain, coughing, dyspnea, sneezing, nasal congestion, tachypnea, and palpitations.**
3. **Thymolipomas may be true thymic neoplasms, variants of thymomas, neoplasms of mediastinal fat that engulf thymic tissue, or simply hyperplasia of mediastinal fat.**

Thymoliposarcoma

Thymoliposarcoma is a very rare malignant tumor. They are often very large by the time they are diagnosed.

Epidemiology

There have only been five reports of thymoliposarcomas, so there is no available prevalence or incidence. The median age is 56 years. They are slightly more common in women. There is no racial or ethnic predilection. This information is for the United States and the rest of the world.

Etiology and Risk Factors

The cause of thymoliposarcomas is unclear. They may develop based on genetic mutations during fat cell development. Risk factors include **Gardner's syndrome**, Werner's syndrome, tuberous sclerosis, **Gorlin's syndrome**, retinoblastoma, and Li–Fraumeni syndrome. Other risk factors may include doses of ionizing radiation, and some chemical exposures.

Pathology

Thymoliposarcomas appear as soft, gray–yellow masses that are well-circumscribed and very elastic. They have been as large as 12.5 cm in diameter. Cut sections reveal multicolored gray–white–yellow fatty areas of varying size. Microscopically, there are lobules of thymic tissue with **Hassall's corpuscles** embedded in the fatty component. Vacuoles may be of various sizes. Large, atypical spindle and multinucleated stromal cells have hyperchromatic and pleomorphic nuclei. These are scattered in the adipose tissue and thymic cortex. There may also be broad, short, and coarse collagen fibers (see Figure 4.3). Small amounts of lipoblasts with indented hyperchromatic nuclei and multivacuolated lipid droplets may be within the fatty components.

Clinical Manifestations

Patients are mainly asymptomatic. Sometimes a large thymoliposarcoma may be symptomatic because of compression to surrounding tissues.

Therefore, patients may complain of dyspnea and chest pain.

Diagnosis

Chest X-rays and CT scans are done to diagnose thymoliposarcoma. CT will reveal a tumor of soft tissue density and prominent fat components. These tumors may be diagnosed incidentally during imaging studies. Differential diagnoses include thymolipoma, thymofibrolipoma, Hodgkin's lymphoma, inflammatory pseudotumors, and sclerosing mediastinitis. Staging of thymoliposarcomas is the same as for thymic carcinomas.

Treatment

Surgical resection is the treatment of choice. However, radiation therapy may be used after surgery. Radiation may be combined with chemotherapy, though the use of chemotherapy is still controversial. Targeted therapies may also be used.

Prevention and Early Detection

Prevention for thymoliposarcoma is unknown. Early detection is, of course, an optimal method of improving treatment and prognosis, but due to the lack of cases, no methods for early detection have been developed.

Prognosis

Though data is very limited, prognosis appears to be good since there has been only one documented

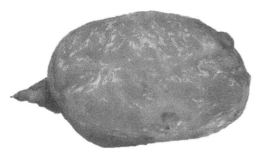 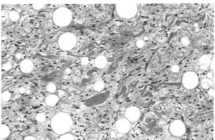

Figure 4.3 Spindle cell thymoliposarcoma. (a) Macroscopy of resected specimen; (b) histology of fat cells with variations of vacuole size, hyperchromatic stromal cells, and broad short coarse collagen fibers. *Source*: Courtesy: Dr. Margaret Burke, Harefield Hospital, Royal Brompton & Harefield NHS Trust, London, UK. den Bakker and Oosterhuis.

case of tumor recurrence, and this was 25 years after surgical resection of the primary tumor.

Adrenal Tumors

Adrenal tumors are common neoplasms and fortunately most of them are benign. Adrenal carcinomas are rare and observed mostly in adults between ages 30 and 40. They are also seen in children under five. Pheochromocytomas originate from the adrenal medulla. The most common sites of primary tumors related to adrenal metastasis are the lungs, liver, and stomach. The adrenal glands are the fourth most common metastatic site, for all cancers.

Adenoma of the Cortex

Adrenal cortical adenoma is a benign epithelial tumor. It arises from different layers of the adrenal cortex, and is also referred to as *adrenocortical adenoma*. This tumor may cause Cushing's syndrome, aldosteronism, and hirsutism. This type of tumor can affect one or all of the layers of the adrenal cortex. If only one layer of the adrenal cortex is involved, the tumor may release cortisol, aldosterone, or androgens.

Epidemiology

Adenomas of the adrenal cortex are common. They affect up to 10% of the global population. It is difficult to make an accurate diagnosis between hyperplastic nodules and actual adrenal cortical neoplasms. Because of this, *actual incidence* of adrenal cortical adenomas is unknown. There has been a recent increase in adenoma, which may be linked to the aging population, and to more use of CT for abdominal imaging. Incidence increases with age, but they may occur in all age groups. Adenomas also occur in both genders with nearly the same frequency, but in females usually have an onset in early adulthood (before age 20), while males usually develop the tumors before age 30. Adrenal cortical adenomas make up a large amount of *adrenal incidentalomas*, which are adrenal tumors that are discovered incidentally.

The global prevalence and incidence are not well documented. The adenomas are most prevalent in younger adults, with females developing them earlier. There is no obvious racial or ethnic predilection.

Etiology and Risk Factors

Adrenal cortical adenomas are sometimes linked to hereditary syndromes. While no environmental factors have been documented, aldosterone-producing adenomas appear to emerge from clusters of cells in the zona glomerulosa. They are called *aldosterone-producing cell clusters*. Mutations linked with autonomous aldosterone production are supportive of these tumors' formation. There are underlying molecular mechanisms resulting in excessive, autonomous aldosterone production. Its mutation is common with cortisol-producing adenomas and observable **Cushing's syndrome**, found in 35–65% of cases. Other mutations in known cancer genes have also been identified in adrenal cortical adenomas.

Clinical Manifestations

The aldosterone-producing adenomas usually cause hypertension and hypokalemia or normokalemia. Other symptoms are cramping, muscle weakness, headaches, palpitations, polydipsia, polyuria, and nocturia. Cortisol-producing adenomas cause Cushing's syndrome that is independent of adrenocorticotropic hormone (ACTH). Signs and symptoms include central obesity, weight gain, facial roundness, a buffalo hump on the posterior lower neck, easy bruising, hirsutism, poor wound healing, purple-red striae on the skin, hyperglycemia, proximal muscle weakness, hypertension, osteoporosis, and increased susceptibility to opportunistic infections (see Figure 4.4). Signs and symptoms resulting from the individual hormones being secreted by the tumor signify sex hormone-producing adenomas. In females, excessive androgen leads to amenorrhea, hirsutism, and virilization. In males, excessive estrogen causes impotence and gynecomastia.

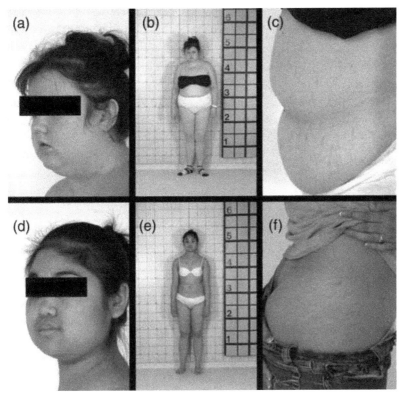

Figure 4.4 Manifestations of Cushing's syndrome. (a) Caucasian female face changes; (b) overall body shape; (c) fat distribution; (d) Asian female face changes; (e) overall body shape; (f) fat distribution. *Source*: Hsiao et al. (2007).

Pathology

A large majority of adrenal cortical adenomas are unilateral, since most multinodular processes are likely to be classified as hyperplasia. There is no precise localization to any particular areas of the adrenal glands. The tumors may be non-functioning, or related to various endocrinopathies, based on their hormonal secretions. The majorities of adrenal cortical adenomas are well-circumscribed, and are only present within the adrenal gland. They are usually solitary, 5–6 cm in diameter, and have a weight of less than 50–100 g. Larger adenomas usually have acute hemorrhage, then centralized organization and degeneration. These tumors may be encapsulated. There have been cases of adenomas that were black, which is usually linked to intracellular accumulation of **lipofuscin**, or melanin. Microscopically, adrenal cortical adenomas have lipid-rich cells, abundant intracytoplasmic lipid droplets that resemble the zona fasciculata, and various amounts of lipid-poor compacted cells that resemble the zona reticularis. Growth patterns involve cords, cell nests, cortical cell islands, and sinusoidal components.

Diagnosis

Measuring plasma aldosterone levels is the primary step in diagnosis. Evaluation of cortisol-producing adenomas requires baseline morning and evening measurements of free cortisol in the serum and saliva. A 24-hour urinary free cortisol test is also done. A dexamethasone suppression test can confirm autonomy. The hypercortisolism is identified as ACTH-independent by suppressed plasma ACTH levels. Diagnosis of sex-hormone-producing adenomas is based on the obvious signs and symptoms. Non-functioning adenomas are often found incidentally during radiological imaging, as *adrenal incidentalomas*. They are found more often because of the increased use of CT abdominal imaging. Other imaging studies include axial PET and MRI. Various diagnoses of these tumors have included examples that were rich in fluorodeoxyglucose (FDG).

Treatment

Surgical resection is required in most cases. Treatment is highly individualized based on the subtype. Non-functioning adrenocortical adenomas can be managed via long-term follow-up and monitoring. If there is severe atrophy of the adrenal cortex, with extensive suppression of the hypothalamic-pituitary-adrenal axis, the patient will need glucocorticoid supplementation. Hydrocortisone may be given intravenously if needed.

Prevention and Early Detection

There is no method of prevention for adrenocortical adenomas. They are not usually detected early in their development, though earlier detection may occur more often, incidentally, in children than in adults.

Prognosis

Overall prognosis is good. Prognosis for functional tumors is good as long as there is early diagnosis and treatment. The long-term outlook for non-functioning tumors is excellent.

Clinical Case

1. What do androgen-producing adenomas cause in women?
2. What imaging studies can be used for diagnosis?
3. What is the prognosis for adrenal cortical adenomas?

An 18-year-old woman was referred for assessment of an adrenal mass. Her past medical history included hirsutism and hypertension. So far, she has never had a menstrual period. She has experienced a hypertensive crisis with chest pain. An MRI showed that she did not have a stroke. Her heart enzymes were normal, as were the results of an electrocardiogram. A CT scan revealed a left adrenal mass of 10 cm in diameter. A hormonal study was undertaken, and the patient had definite shifts in androgens that were excessive for the female gender. However, her FSH, LH, prolactin, estrogen, and progesterone levels were normal. Once her blood pressure was controlled, the patient underwent a successful left adrenalectomy. It was a pure androgen-secreting adrenal cortical adenoma with no signs of malignancy. After surgery, her hormone levels normalized, as did her blood pressure. The male pattern hair growth stopped, and she began to develop more feminine body characteristics.

Answers:

1. **In females, excessive androgen leads to amenorrhea, hirsutism, and virilization.**
2. **Imaging studies include CT, PET, MRI, and fused PET/CT.**
3. **Overall prognosis for adrenal cortical adenomas is good. Prognosis for functional tumors is good as long as there is early diagnosis and treatment. The long-term outlook for non-functioning tumors is excellent.**

Carcinoma of the Cortex

Adrenal cortical carcinoma is uncommon but aggressive. It is derived from the cortical cells of the adrenal gland, and is also referred to as *adrenocortical carcinoma*. The left adrenal gland is affected in the majority of cases.

Epidemiology

Accurate data for the prevalence, incidence, and mortality of adrenal cortical carcinomas are lacking. They are rare and appear to occur in 0.5–2 of every 1 million people *globally*, except for in southern Brazil, where cases are higher.

Median patient age at diagnosis is in the fifth to sixth decade. Females are more likely to develop adrenal cortical carcinomas in a 2.5 : 1 ratio. There is no racial or ethnic predisposition.

Etiology and Risk Factors

The increased number of cases in southern Brazil have been linked to gene mutations. The mutations may occur during DNA replication. There are no other established risk factors, except for smoking, which is believed to be an associated risk factor.

Adrenal cortical carcinomas occur sporadically. There are several hereditary syndromes that account for rare familial cases such as Li–Fraumeni syndrome in children – especially southern Brazil. Hereditary syndromes linked to adrenal cortical carcinoma include Carney complex and Lynch syndrome.

Clinical Manifestations

Almost half of patients have excessive steroid hormones, and complain about abdominal fullness or pain. Signs and symptoms of excessive hormones reveal specific endocrinopathies. Therefore, signs and symptoms of Cushing's syndrome are present. Weight gain, severe hypertension, muscle atrophy, and diabetes occur.

In women, excessive androgen is linked to menstrual irregularities, hirsutism, and virilization. In men, it is often unrecognized because of only minimal symptoms. However, gynecomastia and testicular atrophy are seen. In rare cases, hypertension and hypokalemia are caused by mineralocorticoid excess. The suspicion of an adrenal cortical carcinoma is raised by androgen and estrogen production. Generally, adrenal cortical carcinomas are large, over 10–25 cm.

Pathology

Adrenal cortical carcinomas often involve one adrenal gland – usually the left gland. If both adrenal glands are involved, there may be other conditions present. In rare cases, they may result from ectopic adrenal tissue. They are often large, circumscribed, encapsulated, and solitary. They can reach a weight of 2 kg. Cut surfaces have a yellow–tan multicolored appearance. Necrosis

and hemorrhage are common. Microscopically, growth patterns are either broad trabecular, large-nested, or solid. Tumor encapsulation involves thick, fibrous capsules. There are often degenerative changes after hemorrhage. Adrenal cortical carcinomas usually displace and invade nearby organs, such as the liver, pancreas, kidneys, and inferior vena cava. Metastases are common to the lungs, bones, and brain.

Diagnosis

Imaging of the adrenal gland is accurate for distinguishing between carcinomas and adenomas. Carcinomas may be mimicked by benign tumors that have hemorrhage and revascularization. In most cases, imaging of a carcinoma shows tumor size larger than 4 cm, hemorrhage, and necrosis. Axial sections of MRI of the abdomen reveal a heterogeneous adrenal cortical carcinoma. Coronal sections with T1-weighting and opposite phasing show diffuse homogeneous signal dropout (see Figure 4.5). The use of FDG-PET may improve diagnostic accuracy. Differential diagnosis with adrenal cortical adenoma is often simple, though cases with intermediate factors are more difficult. Rarely, a tumor with an unclear border can be diagnosed as an adrenal cortical neoplasm of uncertain malignant potential. Immunostaining for Ki-67 may be helpful for adenomas having a Ki-67 proliferation index of less than 5%, and carcinomas with this index being higher than 5%. Also, overexpression of *insulin-like growth factor 2 (IGF2)* is supportive of a carcinoma diagnosis. Reticulin staining reveals a loss of nested structure and is diagnostic. This has been used for diagnosis along with the presence of necrosis, mitotic rates, and vascular invasion. However, accurate classification of these neoplasms is still challenging, and up to 9% of cases are misdiagnosed.

The staging for adrenal cortical carcinoma is as follows:

- Stage I – T1, N0, M0 – the tumor is 5 cm or less in size, has not grown into tissues outside of the adrenal gland, has not spread to nearby lymph nodes, with no distant metastasis

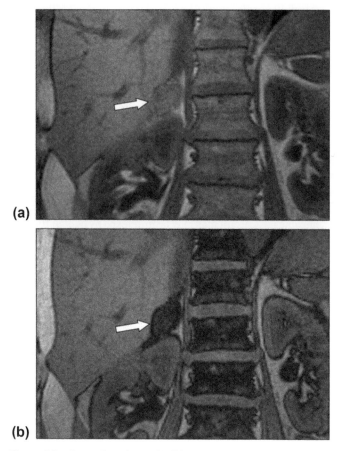

Figure 4.5 Coronal sections with T1-weighting of an adrenal cortical adenoma with (a) in-phase; (b) opposed phase, showing diffuse homogeneous signal dropout. The arrows indicate the adenoma. *Source*: Siddiqi et al. (2009).

- Stage II – T2, N0, M0 – the tumor is greater than 5 cm in size, has not grown into tissues outside the adrenal gland, has not spread to nearby lymph nodes, with no distant metastasis
- Stage III – T1, N1, M0 – the tumor is 5 cm or less in size, has not grown into tissues outside the adrenal gland, has spread to nearby lymph nodes, with no distant metastasis; OR: T2, N1, M0 – the tumor is larger than 5 cm in size, has not grown into tissues outside the adrenal gland, has spread to nearby lymph nodes, with no distant metastasis; OR: T3, any N, M0 – the tumor is growing in the fat surrounding the adrenal gland, can be of any size, may or may not have spread to nearby lymph nodes, with no distant metastasis; OR: the tumor is growing into nearby organs such as the kidney, pancreas, spleen, liver, renal vein, or vena cava, can be of any size, may or may not have spread to nearby lymph nodes, with no distant metastasis

- Stage IV – any T, any N, M1 – the cancer has spread to distant sites such as the liver or lungs, can be of any size, and may or may not have spread to nearby tissues or lymph nodes

Treatment

Total surgical resection is the goal of treatment for adrenal cortical carcinomas. Unfortunately, many patients are not candidates for surgery due to adhesions to various organs. Therefore, radiation therapy and radiofrequency ablation may be used palliatively. Also, open adrenalectomy and laparoscopic minimally invasive techniques have been successful. Standard cytotoxic drugs can be used. There are two common multiple chemo-therapy regimens: cisplatin+doxorubicin+etoposide+mitotane, and streptozotocin+mitotane.

Prevention and Early Detection

There is no known method of prevention for adrenal cortical carcinomas. Early detection is not common, but these tumors have been found earlier in children than in adults, since they are more likely to secrete hormones that cause the signs and symptoms. A child with an adrenal cortical carcinoma may develop early signs of puberty as a result, aging in tumor detection.

Prognosis

The five-year survival rate is about 42% for adrenal cortical carcinoma. After total surgical resection of the carcinoma, if hypercortisolism manifests, the prognosis is worsened. The outlook for metastases of adrenal cortical carcinoma is poor.

Significant Point

Adrenal cortical carcinoma is rare, and may be functioning, making more hormones than normal, or non-functioning, in which excessive hormones are not made. The majority of these tumors are functioning. Genetic conditions that predispose individuals to these tumors include: Li–Fraumeni syndrome, Lynch syndrome, Beckwith–Wiedemann syndrome, and Carney complex.

Clinical Case

1. What hereditary syndromes are linked to adrenal cortical carcinoma?
2. What are the common pathological features of adrenal cortical carcinomas?
3. What are the two common multiple chemotherapy regimens?

A 48-year-old woman was hospitalized after experiencing blurred vision, fatigue, muscle weakness, weight gain, swelling of the abdomen, hair loss, abdominal striae, and indurated swelling on the back of the neck. There were elevations of her morning cortisol level, 24-hour urine-free cortisol level, and very low ACTH levels. A diagnosis of Cushing's syndrome was confirmed. A CT scan revealed a 9 cm left adrenal mass. A left adrenalectomy was performed, and a high-grade carcinoma was diagnosed. Soon, the patient was started on adjuvant chemotherapy with mitotane. She received replacement doses of hydrocortisone and fludrocortisone, with close monitoring. Four years later, an FDG-PET scan revealed a recurrence in the same body area. Extensive surgery was performed along with intraperitoneal chemotherapy, using cisplatin. There was a small metastasis to her left lung, which was successfully removed. The patient was continued on mitotane therapy, without any further recurrence.

Answers:

1. **Several hereditary syndromes account for rare familial cases of adrenal cortical carcinomas. These include Li–Fraumeni syndrome (in children – especially in southern Brazil), Carney complex, and Lynch syndrome.**
2. **Adrenal cortical carcinomas often involve one adrenal gland – usually the left gland. They are often large, circumscribed, encapsulated, and solitary. Necrosis and hemorrhage are common. There are often degenerative changes after hemorrhage. Adrenal cortical carcinomas usually displace and invade nearby organs, such as the liver, pancreas, kidneys, and inferior vena cava. Metastases are common to the lungs, bones, and brain.**
3. **For adrenal cortical carcinomas, the two common multiple chemotherapy regimens are cisplatin + doxorubicin + etoposide + mitotane, and streptozotocin + mitotane.**

Pheochromocytoma

Pheochromocytoma is a tumor of the chromaffin cells. It arises in the adrenal medulla. Other names for pheochromocytoma include: *benign pheochromocytoma, malignant pheochromocytoma, chromaffinoma,* and *paraganglioma.* Pheochromocytomas are intra-adrenal sympathetic paragangliomas.

Epidemiology
The estimated prevalence of pheochromocytomas in hypertensive adults is believed to range from 0.1% to 0.6% of the population. Incidence in the general population is believed to be about 0.05%, based on autopsy studies. However, there are other studies that state pheochromocytomas occur in 1 of every 4,500 people with an annual incidence of 5.5 cases per 1 million people. About 35% are familial and 3–50% are malignant. Up to 61% of cases are found incidentally. Pheochromocytomas can occur at any age but are usually diagnosed between the ages of 30 and 50 years. However, up to 20% of cases are diagnosed in children, with 70% of these being diagnosed below the age of 10 years. The youngest patient ever diagnosed was only 2.7 years. There is a nearly even male-to-female ratio. The tumors occur in people of all races but are diagnosed least often in the African American population.

There are wide geographical variations in prevalence and incidence. This may be linked to founder mutations causing various hereditary tumor prevalence rates, and to case reporting variances. The primary age range worldwide is between 30 and 50 years, though children are also diagnosed. The male-to-female ratio is also nearly even, and the tumors occur in all racial and ethnic groups.

Etiology and Risk Factors
The most common cause of pheochromocytomas is genetic. More than 30% develop along with germline mutations in hereditary susceptibility genes, meaning that these tumors are among the most strongly hereditary of all tumors. Therefore, genetic testing is considered for the most common germline mutations in all patients, even without a family history. They are autosomal dominant inheritance.

Clinical Manifestations
Signs and symptoms of pheochromocytoma are related to excessive catecholamine production. The majority of patients develop hypertension with sudden onset. Headache, palpitations, tachycardia, abdominal pain, and sweating are other clinical manifestations. Uncommon signs and symptoms are tremors, anxiety, and panic attacks.

Pathology
Macroscopically, pheochromocytomas are circumscribed, and unencapsulated. As they increase in size, the capsule of the gland is expanded, compressing or destroying the cortex. The cut surface is pink–gray–tan, yet may have a slight yellow coloring after being exposed to air, or during fixation with formalin. Central degenerative changes, hemorrhage, cystic changes, and fibrosis may be present. Size of the tumor is usually 3–5 cm. Microscopically, pheochromocytomas can extend to the adrenal capsule. They have an alveolar pattern, with nests of polygonal cells that are separated by peripheral capillaries. There may be extreme hemosiderin deposition, hemorrhage, and sclerosis. Pheochromocytoma cells can be very similar to normal chromaffin cells, or larger or smaller. Larger cells usually have prominent nucleoli and vesicular nuclei. The cytoplasmic staining is often granular and basophilic, or amphiphilic. It can be greatly affected by how fixation is performed.

Diagnosis
Blood tests reveal an increase in catecholamines and their metabolites, confirming a pheochromocytoma. Tests vary, but it is recommended that initial testing should include measurements of urinary fractionated or plasma-free **metanephrines**. Specific genetic disorders can be indicated by the catecholamine metabolite profile. Pheochromocytomas may linked to

multiple endocrine neoplasia type 2 (MEN2) or neurofibromatosis type 1 (NF1), usually involving production of epinephrine. Oppositely, von Hippel–Lindau syndrome is suggested by isolated increases in norepinephrine and **normetanephrine**. There is no standard staging system for pheochromocytoma, so the tumor is described as localized, regional, or metastatic.

Imaging studies may be needed when there is clear biochemistry indicating a pheochromocytoma. Anatomical imaging is done first, either CT or MRI (see Figure 4.6). An MRI usually shows an enhancing mass, with high T2-weighted signal intensity. Functional imaging via *scintigraphy* is very helpful and specific. Newer techniques are also used, such as single-photon positron emission CT (SPECT). They are highly sensitive techniques, but not widely available.

Treatment

Total surgical resection is the treatment of choice for pheochromocytoma. The preferred technique, though requiring a high level of specialization, is mini posterior retroperitoneal scope adrenalectomy (Mini-PRSA). A scope is used, and three small incisions are made into the lower back of the patient. Prior to surgery, the patient may be given alpha adrenoceptor blocker *phenoxybenzamine*, or a short-acting alpha antagonist such as *doxazosin, prazosin,* or *terazosin*. These allow surgery to proceed while minimizing likelihood of severe intraoperative hypertension. A combined alpha/beta blocker, such as *labetalol*, may also be given to slow the heart rate. After surgery, there may be profound hypotension, so the patient (preoperatively) may require intravenous saline solution.

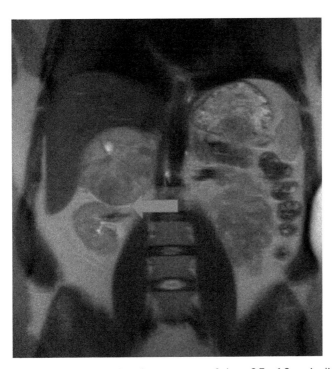

Figure 4.6 MRI of a pheochromocytoma of about 9.7 × 6.9 cm in diameter with good demarcation to the surrounding tissue (above arrow). The inferior vena cava and kidney are slightly compressed (arrow). *Source*: Harsch and Helfritzsch.

Prevention and Early Detection

There are no known methods of prevention of pheochromocytoma. Though early detection is difficult, screening is indicated in asymptomatic patients with an inherited disorder linked to an increased risk, such as multiple endocrine neoplasia 2A and 2B, von Hippel–Lindau disease, and neurofibromatosis type 1.

Prognosis

Prognosis for pheochromocytoma depends on surgical resectability and the tumor's genetic profile. The overall five-year survival rate, with metastases, is 34–60%. Survival times are usually less than five years if metastasis affects the liver or lungs, but can be longer if the bones are involved.

Significant Point

A pheochromocytoma is a tumor that increases blood pressure by secreting catecholamines. Most are benign, and often are caused by genetic diseases, including multiple endocrine neoplasia (MEN), von Hippel–Lindau disease, and neurofibromatosis. The tumors are surgically removed once the patient's blood pressure is under control by medications.

Clinical Case

1. What is the most common cause of pheochromocytoma?
2. Which genetic disorders are linked to pheochromocytomas?
3. What is the prognosis for pheochromocytoma?

A 50-year-old woman had experienced hypertension, palpitations, headache, sweating, abdominal pain, nausea, and vomiting. Her physician performed a urinalysis, which revealed catecholamines and their metabolites to be present. A CT scan confirmed the presence of a pheochromocytoma of the right adrenal medulla. Surgical resection was scheduled, and a mini posterior retroperitoneal scope adrenalectomy (Mini-PRSA) was performed. A scope was used for the operation, with three small incisions made into the patient's lower back. Soon after surgery, the patient's condition was almost totally resolved, and she recovered very quickly.

Answers:

1. **More than 30% of pheochromocytomas develop with germline mutations in hereditary susceptibility genes, meaning that these tumors are among the most strongly hereditary of all tumors.**
2. **Pheochromocytomas may be linked to MEN2 or NF1, usually involving the production of epinephrine, and with von Hippel–Lindau syndrome, suggested by increases in norepinephrine and normetanephrine.**
3. **Prognosis for pheochromocytoma depends on surgical resectability and the tumor's genetic profile. The overall five-year survival rate, with metastases, is 34–60%. Survival times are usually less than five years if metastasis affects the liver or lungs, but can be longer if the bones are involved.**

Neuroblastoma

Neuroblastoma of the adrenal gland is a highly malignant tumor composed of primitive ectodermal cells derived from the neural plate during embryonic life. The tumor may originate in any part of the sympathetic nervous system, but is most common in the adrenal medulla. It is a rare, and aggressive cancer. Neuroblastomas metastasize early and widely to lymph nodes, liver, lungs, and bone.

Epidemiology

Neuroblastoma of the adrenal gland is most common in infants and young children. It is also seen in older children and teenagers. Rarely, it occurs in adults. There is no specific gender, racial, or ethnic predilection. The same statistics are true in the United States and throughout the world.

Etiology and Risk Factors

The cause of neuroblastoma of the adrenal gland may be due to genetic mutations, since several genetic abnormalities have been found. Risk factors include genetic disorders such as **Beckwith–Wiedemann syndrome** and **DiGeorge syndrome**, and a positive family history. Other risk factors include **Hirschsprung disease**, hypoventilation syndrome, chemical exposures, excessive alcohol use, smoking, and use of certain drugs or medications during pregnancy. Hormone supplements, fertility drugs, and hair dyes used by pregnant women are also considered as the risk factors.

Clinical Manifestations

Signs and symptoms may include an abdominal mass, respiratory distress, and anemia. Hormonally active adrenal lesions may cause irritability, flushing, sweating, weight loss, hypertension, tachycardia, and unexplained fever. The cancer can metastasize to other parts of the body, causing other manifestations. Additional manifestations include fatigue because of anemia, pedal edema, night sweats, and generalized weakness. Paraneoplastic syndrome can develop, which includes permanent neurologic symptoms.

Pathology

The neuroblastic cells of a neuroblastoma of the adrenal gland are separated by thin, fibrovascular stromal septa, with no Schwannian proliferation. There are three subtypes: undifferentiated, poorly differentiated, and differentiated. The undifferentiated subtype is the least common. Fewer than 5% of the neuroblastic cells have cytomorphological differentiation toward mature neurons. The neuroblasts, in both the poorly differentiated and undifferentiated subtypes, have a nuclear morphology described as "salt-and-pepper."

Diagnosis

Initially, personal and family histories are evaluated, and there is a complete physical examination. Blood tests include CBC, serum calcium and albumin, and liver function tests. Since the proliferating cells have a regularly primitive small round blue cell appearance, with no clearly identifiable neuropil formation, diagnosis requires immunohistochemistry, with or without molecular testing. Imaging includes plain abdominal X-rays, ultrasound, CT, MRI, and PET, which can reveal calcification. Tissue biopsy may be required, using hematoxylin and eosin (H&E) staining, immunohistochemical stains, and molecular testing. Rarely, electron microscopic studies are required. Staging is determined by two different systems – the International Neuroblastoma Risk Group Staging System (INRGSS), which is based on imaging tests – and the International Neuroblastoma Staging System (INSS), which uses results from surgical resection. The staging for neuroblastoma, using the INRGSS criteria, is as follows:

- Stage L1 – the tumor has not spread, has not grown into vital structures, and is confined to one area of the body
- Stage L2 – the tumor has not spread very far, but has at least one image-defined risk factor (IDRF)
- Stage M – the tumor has metastasized to a distant part of the body – except for a tumor classified as stage MS
- Stage MS – there is metastatic disease in a child younger than 18 months, with cancer spread only to the skin, liver, and/or bone marrow; no more than 10% of the marrow cells are cancerous; a **metaiodobenzylguanidine** (MIBG) scan does not show that the cancer has spread to the bones and/or bone marrow

The staging for neuroblastoma, using the INSS system, is as follows:

- Stage I – the cancer has not spread, is on one side of the body, all visible tumor has been completely resected, and lymph nodes outside the tumor are free of cancer
- Stage IIA – the cancer has not spread, is on one side of the body, but not all of the visible tumor could be resected, and lymph nodes outside the tumor are free of cancer
- Stage IIB – the cancer is on one side of the body, may or may not have been completely resected, nearby lymph nodes contain neuroblastoma cells, but the cancer has not spread to lymph nodes on the other side of the body or to other areas
- Stage III – the cancer has not spread to distant sites, but one of the following exists: the cancer cannot be completely resected and it has crossed the spine to the other side of the body, and may or may not have spread to nearby lymph nodes; the cancer has not spread and is on one side of the body, but has spread to relatively nearby lymph nodes on the other side of the body; the cancer is in the middle of the body and is growing toward both sides, and cannot be completely resected
- Stage IV – the cancer has spread to distant sites such as the distant lymph nodes, bones, liver, skin, bone marrow, or other organs; the child still does not meet the criteria for stage IVS
- Stage IVS – "special neuroblastoma" – the child is younger than one year of age, the cancer is on one side of the body, it may have spread to lymph nodes on the same side, but not to nodes on the other side; it has spread to the liver, skin, and/or bone marrow, but no more than 10% of the marrow cells are cancerous; imaging tests such as the MIBG scan do not show cancer in the bones or bone marrow

Neuroblastoma can also be described as "recurrent" if it has returned after treatment, either to the original site or to another part of the body.

Treatment

Before metastasis, treatment options for neuroblastoma of the adrenal gland include radical surgery, radiation therapy, chemotherapy, and targeted drug therapy. Treatments are based on risks and the stage of malignancy. For most patients, surgical resection is performed, with clear margins, especially when the tumor is only within the adrenal gland. For low-risk patients, surgery may be all that is needed. Postoperative care requires maintaining minimum activity levels until the surgical wound heals. For intermediate-risk patients, chemotherapy may also be required. For high-risk patients, chemotherapy, radiation therapy, stem cell transplantation, biological therapy, and immunotherapy may be required.

Prevention and Early Detection

There is no known method to prevent neuroblastoma of the adrenal gland. However, stopping smoking, eating a healthy diet, exercising regularly, maintaining a healthy weight, avoiding toxin exposures, and avoiding unnecessary medications during pregnancy factors are important for prevention. There are no standardized screening methods for early detection. If detected in the early stages, prognosis will be better.

Prognosis

Prognosis is based on tumor size, localization, and metastasis. Generally, prognosis is highly individualized on each patient's health status. It is often poor due to the aggressiveness of these tumors.

Clinical Case

1. What are the risk factors for neuroblastoma of the adrenal gland?
2. What are the three subtypes of neuroblastomas?
3. Since this patient's neuroblastoma has already metastasized, what are his treatment options.

A 17-year-old boy with scoliosis was having X-rays taken of his spine. Calcifications in the right upper quadrant were found. An abdominopelvic CT scan revealed a 4 cm lobular mass in the right adrenal gland, with calcifications. A right adrenalectomy was performed. The resected tumor was encapsulated. When the surrounding soft tissues were dissected, several lymph nodes were found to be enlarged. They were positive for metastasis. The final diagnosis was of a poorly differentiated neuroblastoma. A bone marrow biopsy indicated there was metastasis as well, and the patient was started on chemotherapy.

Answers:

1. **Risk factors include Beckwith–Wiedemann syndrome, DiGeorge syndrome, positive family history, Hirschsprung disease, hypoventilation syndrome, chemical exposures, excessive alcohol use, smoking, and use of certain drugs or medications during pregnancy. Additionally, hormone supplements, fertility drugs, and hair dyes used by pregnant women are considered to be risk factors.**

2. **The three subtypes of neuroblastomas are: undifferentiated, poorly differentiated, and differentiated. The undifferentiated subtype is the least common.**

3. **Since this patient is considered "high-risk," treatment options include chemotherapy, radiation therapy, stem cell transplantation, biological therapy, and immunotherapy.**

Multiple Endocrine Neoplasia

Multiple endocrine neoplasia (MEN) syndrome types 1 and 2 are hereditarily linked cancer syndromes. Various benign and malignant tumors develop. Both types are associated with the parathyroid glands. The difference is that MEN1 is mainly associated with parathyroid *tumors* while MEN2 is mainly associated with parathyroid *disorders*. Both types are also related to tumors in other body sites, often within the gastrointestinal tract. Patients with MEN 1 usually have parathyroid proliferative disorder, and almost 90% are diagnosed with parathyroid hyperplasia. Parathyroid adenoma and carcinoma can be part of MEN1 and MEN2. Therefore, chances for MEN syndromes must be considered when parathyroid adenoma or carcinoma is being evaluated. MEN1 is an autosomal dominant disease. It involves multifocal neoplastic endocrine lesions of the anterior pituitary, parathyroid glands, and pancreatic islet cells. Sometimes, different types of non-endocrine lesions occur in the central nervous system, skin, and soft tissues.

MEN2 is also an autosomal dominant tumor syndrome. There are subtypes known as MEN2A **(Sipple syndrome)** and MEN2B. However, "MEN2B" is also known as "MEN3," so its information is listed under a separate heading. Classic MEN2A involves MTC, usually along with pheochromocytoma, with or without parathyroid neoplasia that causes hyperparathyroidism.

MEN3 also known as MEN2B is rare, and is also an autosomal dominant disorder. This involves oral mucosal neuromas, a **Marfanoid body habitus**, intestinal ganglioneuromatosis, and myelinated corneal nerve fibers. It is believed that the U.S. President Abraham Lincoln had MEN3, based on his appearance alone, as well as his Marfanoid body shape. Experts believe that because of photographs taken shortly before his death, Lincoln had MEN3, with an aggressive thyroid tumor, due to the "hooding" of his eyelids, an asymmetric jaw, and lip enlargement. MEN4 is another autosomal dominant tumor syndrome. The tumor mostly is seen in the pituitary, parathyroid glands, and pancreas.

Epidemiology

The global prevalence, for various populations, is between 1 in every 30,000. Approximately 10% of patients have MEN1 germline mutations that develop on their own, without any family history. All age groups, with equal gender distribution, are affected by parathyroid involvement, which is present in 92% of MEN1 patients. The proportion for developing hyperparathyroidism increases with patient age. Males and females are equally affected. There are no geographical, ethnic, or racial differences. Pituitary tumors occur in about 35% of patients with MEN1. The mean patient age of patients with sporadic pituitary tumors is 40 years. The youngest reported patient age was five years. Females are affected more than males – especially younger females. Lactotroph adenomas are most common (30%), followed by non-functioning adenomas (15%) of cases, somatotroph adenomas (9%), corticotroph adenomas (4%), and thyrotroph adenomas (about 1%) – see Figure 4.7. Gonadotroph carcinomas are extremely rare.

Incidence of MEN1-related duodenal and *pancreatic neuroendocrine tumors* peaks between 40 and 60 years, though patients of any age may be affected. The gender distribution is even. MEN1-related Zollinger–Ellison syndrome (ZES) makes up 25% of all ZES cases. For MEN2, actual yearly incidence rates are unknown, but are estimated at 1 case per 1,974,000 people, globally. Prevalence is believed to be about 1 in 30,000. The total age range of patients is not well documented. The female-to-male ratio is nearly equal. There appears to be no racial predilection. For MEN3, actual yearly incidence rates are unknown, but are estimated at 1 case per 39,000,000 people, globally. MEN3 has been estimated to occur in only 4 cases per 100 million people, annually. There is no racial predilection. Incidence and prevalence of MEN4 is extremely low. Global statistics are not well documented. For unknown reasons, most patients with a MEN4 gene mutation have been women. Hyperparathyroidism occurs at an average patient age of 56 years. There appears to be no racial predilection.

Etiology and Risk Factors

MEN1 is caused by germline mutations of genes. Overall, there are no significant correlations between **genotype** and **phenotype**. There are no risk factors except for genetics. Activating germline mutations causes MEN2. About 30% of MTCs are related to germline mutations. Each organ has a different threshold level for transforming to neoplasia. The highest threshold is in the parathyroid glands, while the lowest is in the C cells of the thyroid, which are the precursor cells of MTC. Like MEN2, about 30% of MTCs are related to germline RET mutations manifesting as MEN3. Non-syndrome-related gene mutations occur in more than 90% of cases of MEN3. MEN4 is caused by germline mutations, creating a phenotype that is similar to that of MEN1.

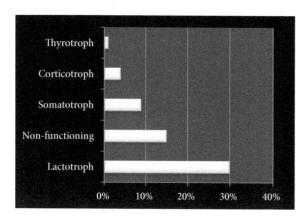

Figure 4.7 The most commonly occurring types of pituitary adenomas as part of MEN1.

Clinical Manifestations

With MEN1, primary hyperparathyroidism is clinically present by the age of 20 years. This is the first manifestation in patients, who usually present with multiglandular parathyroid disease instead of a solitary adenoma. For pituitary tumors, clinical manifestations may be related to the types of hormones secreted. For example, in hyperprolactinemia, signs and symptoms include nausea, vomiting, weakness, changes in menstruation, sexual dysfunction, and weight loss or gain. Pituitary tumors may also cause symptoms that are related to tumor growth and pressure upon other structures. They can cause headache and vision loss. The clinical manifestations of duodenal tumors are seen in patients with MEN1, and Zollinger–Ellison syndrome is present in 60% of cases. This is followed by hyperinsulinemia and hypoglycemia. Life-threatening events are possible with MEN2, including myocardial infarction and stroke. The most commonly seen MEN4-related tumors include: neuroendocrine neoplasms of the parathyroid, pituitary, and pancreas, followed by the cervix, bronchus, and stomach. The most common manifestation of MEN4 is primary hyperparathyroidism and in some cases, pituitary adenomas.

Pathology

Multiple abnormal parathyroid glands can easily diagnose parathyroid hyperplasia. Macroscopically, they are usually more than 6–8 mm in diameter, and their weight is 40–60 mg. In histology, they have multinodular proliferations that are mostly made up of chief cells, containing clear cells, oncocytic cells, or both. Microscopically in angiofibromas, there are concentric layers of collagen around vessels, and even hair follicles. In patients with MEN1 and Zollinger–Ellison syndrome, excessive **gastrin** is caused by multicentric neuroendocrine tumors – usually in the mucosa and submucosa of the upper part of the duodenum. Sometimes, this occurs at the edge of an ulcer. They are usually less than 1 cm in size, making them hard to find. Liver metastases only occur in 3–4% of MEN1 patients, late in the disease course. They are grade 1, well-differentiated tumors, with a trabecular pattern. Diffuse microadenomatosis, related to one or more macrotumors of over 0.5 cm, is a unique feature of the pancreas when MEN1 is present.

Severe obstructive pancreatitis may occur, caused by duct stenosis from macrotumors. Many tumors are multihormonal, and usually, one hormone dominates. Glucagon is most often secreted, followed by insulin and somatostatin. The glucagon-positive tumors can be cystic. Gastrin is hardly ever secreted. Adrenal cortical lesions occur in patients with MEN1, as cortical adenomas. Tumors are often bilateral, 3 cm or less in size, and non-functional. Adrenal cortical carcinomas are rare, and also occur bilaterally. Skin lesions are present in 40–80% of MEN1 patients, including collagenomas and facial angiofibromas. Primary malignant melanomas in MEN1 patients may also occur. Most patients with MEN2 develop MTC, with frequency related to age and the specific mutation. The identifying pathological factor of inherited forms of MTC is C-cell hyperplasia-to-neoplasia progression. Primary C-cell hyperplasia is considered when there are more than 6–8 C cells per low-power field. The identifying pathological factor of MEN2-related pheochromocytoma is the adrenal medullary hyperplasia-to-neoplasia progression sequence. This leads to bilateral and multifocal pheochromocytomas. Medullary thyroid carcinomas occurring in MEN3 patients are linked to early onset – even during the first year of life. The syndrome involves development of pheochromocytomas in 50% of patients. The tumors are often bilateral and can be extra-adrenal. All patients develop medullary thyroid cancer that is aggressive and may secrete calcitonin. The pathology of MEN4 is most like that of MEN1.

Diagnosis

The diagnosis of MEN1 must be considered when an individual has newly diagnosed MEN1-associated lesions, if patient meets criteria that are considered to be related to inherited cancers. These include age that is usually over 50 years, multifocal or recurrent neoplasia, positive family history, and two or more endocrine organs or systems affected. Diagnosis requires proof of invasion into nearby organs, vessels, or the perineural space, with or without the presence of metastases. Contrast-enhanced CT through the abdomen may show multiple well-circumscribed lesions in various structures, such as the duodenum and pancreas.

The diagnosis of MEN2 is made based on the determination of a germline DNA variant in the RET gene. Analysis of the mutation should be done for any patient, regardless of age, diagnosed with MTC, with or without lack of disease features or family history. A diagnosis of adrenal medullary hyperplasia is made when the adrenal medulla is larger than 33% of the gland's thickness. CT with contrast is able to show adrenal tumors with extreme clarity. Screening for parathyroid neoplasia and MEN2 requires annual blood tests to measure calcium and intact parathyroid hormone levels. This usually begins at the time of diagnosis. If one or more adenomas are diagnosed, surgery is required. There is often difficulty in recognizing the MEN3 phenotype in younger patients. Calcitonin and carcinoembryonic antigen (CEA) are strong tumor markers for MTC. No screening for hyperparathyroidism is necessary with MEN3 since this type does not involve the parathyroid. There are no specific diagnostic guidelines for MEN4. There are no formal staging criteria for any of the various types of MENs except for the actual types of tumors that are present.

Treatment

Resection is required for MEN1 pituitary adenomas. Prophylactic partial thymectomy is also considered in this procedure. It is important to diagnostically differentiate the parathyroid glands from other structures that could be mistaken for a parathyroid gland during surgery. Parathyroidectomy is also performed.

Lateral neck lymph node compartments are dissected only if they are clinically or radiologically suspicious for metastasis. Targeted therapies are used, for MEN2-related MTC. Cabozantinib and vandetanib have been approved to treat locally advanced and metastatic MTC. Without treatment, the patient with MEN3 usually dies prematurely. The primary preventive measure for MTC is prophylactic thyroidectomy. Genetic screening for MEN4 has enabled earlier diagnoses, and has become routine for affected patients and their families. Prophylactic thymectomy may be done. Subtotal or total parathyroidectomy may also be needed.

Prevention and Early Detection

There is no known prevention for any form of MEN, though genetic counseling may help families with the disease to plan for their futures. Regular screening allows for early detection and treatment of endocrine tumors.

Prognosis

The most important prognostic factors for patients with MEN1 are tumor size and histological grade. Patients with MEN1 are at a higher risk of premature death, because of its complications. Primary causes of death are thymic tumors and the aggressiveness of adrenal tumors. Patients with smaller neuroendocrine tumors of the duodenum have a 15-year survival rate of almost 100%. There are also high-risk MEN1 mutations. For gastric lesions related to MEN1, tumors less than 1 cm in diameter usually have a good prognosis after surgery. Larger tumors can metastasize, requiring surgery, but related deaths are rare. Worsened survival is closely related to older patient age at diagnosis, lymph node disease, larger tumor size, and distant metastases. The average survival rate, combining all patients with MEN2, is 97% over 10 years, after surgery has been performed. Patients with pheochromocytoma have a high risk of hypertensive crisis, stroke, or myocardial infarction. The average survival rate for MEN3, combining patients in all stages of disease, is 76%. Overall survival is affected by early onset and late diagnosis of MTC. Without treatment, the prognosis is poor. The prognosis of MEN4 is based on the tumors that are already present, or develop in the future. There is no current way to accurately predict exactly which tumors will develop.

Significant Point

Multiple endocrine neoplasia type 1 (MEN1) involves tumors that are usually in the parathyroid gland, islet cells of the pancreas, and pituitary gland – most are benign. MEN2, however, is associated with more aggressive medullary thyroid cancer during childhood, and with benign neuromas of the mucous membranes.

Clinical Case

1. How common are pituitary tumors in relation to MEN1, and when do they occur?
2. What are the clinical manifestations of MEN1?
3. What is the prognosis for MEN1?

A 31-year-old man went to the local emergency department because of several weeks of burning epigastric abdominal pain, nausea, vomiting, and diarrhea. He had previously had a pituitary prolactinoma, which was surgically resected. The patient had also experienced hypercalcemia and hyperparathyroidism. Family history was positive for pituitary and thymic tumors. A CT scan showed duodenal inflammation and 2 hyperenhancing pancreatic masses. Gastrinoma with resultant peptic ulcer disease was suspected. These findings, along with the patient's history, suggested MEN1 syndrome. On contrast-enhanced CT, bilateral hypoattenuating adrenal nodules were also identified. Esophagogastroduodenoscopy showed multiple non-bleeding duodenal ulcers. Endoscopic ultrasound confirmed the pancreatic mass and biopsy revealed a well-differentiated neuroendocrine tumor, compatible with a gastrinoma. His burning epigastric pain was well controlled by proton pump inhibitors. In a short period of time, the patient underwent distal pancreatectomy with lymph node resection. The largest tumor was classified as a grade 2 neuroendocrine tumor of at least 6.6 cm in diameter, and one metastatic inferior pancreatoduodenal lymph node was identified. The adrenal lesions were diagnosed as benign adenomas. Scintigraphy revealed a parathyroid adenoma, and a subtotal parathyroidectomy was performed, with three of the parathyroid glands removed. Since there was regional nodal metastasis from the gastrinoma, the patient is being treated every month with lanreotide infusions and has follow-up imaging studies. He is on daily cabergoline therapy for his residual prolactinoma, followed by periodic MRI and prolactin-level monitoring. Since the adrenal adenomas are non-functioning, no follow-up for them is required.

Answers:

1. **Pituitary tumors occur in about 35% of patients with multiple endocrine neoplasias 1 (MEN1). The mean patient age of patients with sporadic pituitary tumors is 40 years. The youngest reported age was 5 years.**
2. **With MEN1, primary hyperparathyroidism is clinically present by the age of 20 years. This is the first manifestation in patients, who usually present with multiglandular parathyroid disease instead of a solitary adenoma. For pituitary tumors, clinical manifestations may be related to the types of hormones secreted. In hyperprolactinemia, signs and symptoms include nausea, vomiting, weakness, changes in menstruation, sexual dysfunction, and weight loss or gain. Pituitary tumors may also cause symptoms related to tumor growth and pressure upon other structures. They can cause headache and vision**

loss. Manifestations of duodenal tumors are seen, and Zollinger–Ellison syndrome is present in 60% of cases, followed by hyperinsulinemia and hypoglycemia.

3. The most important prognostic factors for patients with MEN1 are tumor size and histological grade. Patients with MEN1 are at a higher risk of premature death, because of its complications. Patients with smaller neuroendocrine tumors of the duodenum have a 15-year survival rate of almost 100%. For gastric lesions related to MEN1, tumors less than 1 cm in diameter usually have a good prognosis after surgery. Larger tumors can metastasize, requiring surgery, but related deaths are rare. Worsened survival is closely related to older patient age at diagnosis, lymph node disease, larger tumor size, and distant metastases.

Key Terms

Adenoma
Adrenal cortical carcinoma
Alopecia areata
Anaplastic carcinoma
Beckwith–Wiedemann syndrome
Calcimimetic
Cushing's syndrome
DiGeorge syndrome
En bloc resection
Follicular carcinoma
Gardner's syndrome
Gastrin
Genotype
Goiter
Gorlin's syndrome
Hashimoto's thyroiditis
Hassall's corpuscles
Hirschsprung disease
Lipofuscin
Marfanoid body habitus

Medullary carcinoma
Metaiodobenzylguanidine
Metanephrines
Normetanephrine
Osteitis fibrosa cystica
Oxidative stress
Papillary carcinoma
Phenotype
Pheochromocytoma
Plasmacytoid
Psammoma bodies
Pseudoinvasion
Scintigraphy
Sestamibi protein
Sipple syndrome
Superior vena cava syndrome
Thymolipoma
Thymoliposarcoma
Thymoma
Werner's syndrome

Bibliography

1 Ali, S.Z. and Cibas, E.S. (2018). *The Bethesda System for Reporting Thyroid Cytopathology: Definitions, Criteria, and Explanatory Notes*, 2nd Edition. New York: Springer.

2 American Cancer Society. (2021). *Key Statistics for Thyroid Cancer*. https://www.cancer.org/cancer/thyroid-cancer/about/key-statistics.html Accessed 2021.

3 American College of Surgeons, United States National Cancer Database. (2017). *Helpful Tool Allows Physicians to More Accurately Predict Parathyroid Cancer Recurrence*. https://www.facs.org/media/press-releases/2017/parathyroid042817

4 Anastasiadis, K. and Ratnatunga, C. (2007). *The Thymus Gland: Diagnosis and Surgical Management*. New York: Springer.

5 Angelos, P., and Grogan, R.H. (2018). *Difficult Decisions in Endocrine Surgery: An Evidence-Based Approach*. New York: Springer.

6 Arnold, A. (2012). *Endocrine Neoplasms (Cancer Treatment and Research Book 89)*. New York: Springer.

7 Bhansali, A., Aggarwal, A., Parthan, G., and Gogate, Y. (2016). *Clinical Rounds in Endocrinology: Volume II – Pediatric Endocrinology*. New York: Springer.

8 Bodey, B., Siegel, S.E., and Kaiser, H.E. (2006). *Immunological Aspects of Neoplasia – the Role of the Thymus (Cancer Growth and Progression Book 17)*. New York: Springer.

9 Cancer Cytopathology. (2000). *Psammoma bodies in fine-needle aspirates of the thyroid – Predictive value for papillary carcinoma.* 84 (3): https://acsjournals.onlinelibrary.wiley.com/doi/10.1002/(SICI)1097-0142(19980625)84:3%3C169::AID-CNCR9%3E3.0.CO;2-J. Figure 1. Accessed 2021.

10 Chung, D.C. and Haber, D.A. (2010). *Principles of Clinical Cancer Genetics: A Handbook from the Massachusetts General Hospital*. New York: Springer.

11 Clinical Case Reports. (2019). *MRI of a pheochromocytoma with good demarcation to the surrounding tissue.* https://onlinelibrary.wiley.com/doi/full/10.1002/ccr3.2464. Figure 1. Accessed 2021.

12 Clinical Endocrinology. (2007). *Manifestations of Cushing's syndrome.* https://onlinelibrary.wiley.com/doi/abs/10.1111/j.1365-2265.2007.02793.x. Figure 1. Accessed 2021.

13 Cloyd, J.M. and Pawlik, T.M. (2021). *Neuroendocrine Tumors: Surgical Evaluation and Management*. New York: Springer.

14 Cooper, D.S. and Durante, C. (2016). *Thyroid Cancer: A Case-Based Approach*. New York: Springer.

15 Duick, D.S., Levine, R.A., and Lupo, M.A. (2018). *Thyroid and Parathyroid Ultrasound and Ultrasound-Guided FNA*, 4th Edition. New York: Springer.

16 Gasparri, G., Camandona, M., and Palestini, N. (2016). *Primary, Secondary and Tertiary Hyperparathyroidism – Diagnostic and Therapeutic Updates (Updates in Surgery)*. New York: Springer.

17 Hammer, G.D. and Else, T. (2010). *Adrenocortical Carcinoma: Basic Science and Clinical Concepts*. New York: Springer.

18 Histopathology. (2009). *Spindle cell thymoliposarcoma, macroscopy of resected specimen and histology of fat cells.* 54: 69–89. https://onlinelibrary.wiley.com/doi/pdf/10.1111/j.1365-2559.2008.03177.x. Accessed 2021.

19 Hubbard, J., Inabnet, W.B., and Lo, C.Y. (2009). *Endocrine Surgery: Principles and Practice*. New York: Springer.

20 Jain, D., Bishop, J.A., and Wick, M.R. (2020). *Atlas of Thymic Pathology*. New York: Springer.

21 Journal of Magnetic Resonance Imaging. (2009). *Coronal sections with T1-weighting of an adrenal cortical adenoma, in-phase and opposed phase.* https://onlinelibrary.wiley.com/doi/full/10.1002/jmri.21430. Figure 2. Accessed 2021.

22 Kearns, A.E. and Wermers, R.A. (2016). *Hyperparathyroidism: A Clinical Casebook*. New York: Springer.

23 Kebebew, E. (2017). *Management of Adrenal Masses in Children and Adults*. New York: Springer.

24 Landsberg, L. (2018). *Pheochromocytomas, Paragangliomas and Disorders of the Sympathoadrenal System – Clinical Features, Diagnosis and Management (Contemporary Endocrinology)*. Totowa: Humana Press.

25 Licata, A.A. and Lerma, E.V. (2012). *Diseases of the Parathyroid Glands*. New York: Springer.

26 Lin, F., Liu, H., and Zhang, J. (2018). *Handbook of Practical Fine Needle Aspiration and Small Tissue Biopsies*. New York: Springer.

27 Luster, M., Duntas, L.H., and Wartofsky, L. (2019). *The Thyroid and its Diseases: A Comprehensive Guide for the Clinician*. New York: Springer.

28 Mancino, A.T. and Kim, L.T. (2017). *Management of Differentiated Thyroid Cancer*. New York: Springer.

29 Manger, W.M. and Gifford, R.W., Jr. (2012). *Pheochromocytoma*. New York: Springer.

30 Metcalf, D. and Burnet, M. (2012). *The Thymus: Its Role in Immune Responses, Leukaemia Development and Carcinogenesis*

(Recent Results in Cancer Research Book 5). New York: Springer.

31 Nelkin, B.D. (2013). *Genetic Mechanisms in Multiple Endocrine Neoplasia Type 2 (Medical Intelligence Unit)*. New York: Springer.

32 Nikiforov, Y.E., Biddinger, P.W., and Thompson, L.D.R. (2019). *Diagnostic Pathology and Molecular Genetics of the Thyroid: A Comprehensive Guide for Practicing Thyroid Pathology*, 3rd Edition. Philadelphia: Lippincott, Williams, & Wilkins.

33 Ozyigit, G., Selek, U., and Topkan, E. (2016). *Principles and Practice of Radiotherapy Techniques in Thoracic Malignancies*. New York: Springer.

34 Parathyroid UK. (2008) *Parathyroid cancer*. https://parathyroiduk.org/ hyperparathyroidism/parathyroid-cancer Accessed 2021.

35 Pathak, K.A., Nason, R.W., and Pasieka, J.L. (2015). *Management of Thyroid Cancer: Special Considerations (Head and Neck Cancer Clinics Book 2)*. New York: Springer.

36 Raue, F. (2015). *Medullary Thyroid Carcinoma: Biology – Management – Treatment (Recent Results in Cancer Research)*. New York: Springer.

37 Sarnacki, S. and Pio, L. (2020). *Neuroblastoma: Clinical and Surgical Management*. New York: Springer.

38 Shifrin, A.L., Neistadt, L.D., and Thind, P.K. (2020). *Atlas of Parathyroid Imaging and Pathology*. New York: Springer.

39 Solcia, E., Kloppel, G., and Sobin, L.H. (2012). *Histological Typing of Endocrine Tumours (World Health Organization International Histological Classification of Tumours)*, 2nd Edition. New York: Springer.

40 Stratakis, C.A. (2013). *Endocrine Tumor Syndromes and Their Genetics (Frontiers of Hormone Research Book 41)*. Basel: S. Karger.

41 Sturgeon, C. (2009). *Endocrine Neoplasia (Cancer Treatment and Research Book 153)*. New York: Springer.

42 Surveillance, Epidemiology, and End Results (SEER) Program. (2017). Current Understanding and Management of Parathyroid Carcinoma. *Journal of Cancer Treatment and Research* 5 (3). 51–61. https:// www.cancer.org/cancer/thyroid-cancer/ about/key-statistics.html. Accessed 2021.

43 Van Nostrand, D., Wartofsky, L., Bloom, G., Wu, D., and Dellar, S. (2019). *Thyroid Cancer: A Guide for Patients*, 3rd Edition. Harrisburg: Keystone Press.

44 Wang, T.S. and Evans, D.B. (2016). *Medullary Thyroid Cancer*. New York: Springer.

5

Respiratory Tumors

Nasopharyngeal Tumors

Nasopharyngeal tumors are growths within the nasopharynx, the upper portion of the throat, behind the nasal cavity. The nasopharynx is a passageway for air, from the nose to the throat and lungs. Tumors of the nasopharynx may be benign angiofibromas, benign hemangiomas, or malignant carcinomas. Benign tumors can also develop in the nasopharynx, but less often. They are more common in children and younger adults. When a nasopharyngeal tumor is malignant, it has the potential to spread to nearby tissues as well as the rest of the body.

Nasopharyngeal Angiofibroma

Nasopharyngeal angiofibromas are growths that are filled with blood vessels, making them likely to bleed. These tumors are most common in teenage boys, and grow at the posterior aspect of the nose. Boys with light skin and red hair are most affected. During puberty, the growth of these tumors is usually fast, but then they indicate a slow down in growth rate or stop growing completely after adolescence. These tumors usually cause nasal obstruction and nosebleeds, but sometimes cause nasal discharge and sinusitis. If these tumors are more extensive, they can grow into the paranasal sinuses, eye orbits, or brain, resulting in headaches and vision changes. Diagnosis is usually via nasal endoscopy, followed by an MRI or CT scan. Biopsy usually causes significant bleeding, so surgery is usually scheduled based on imaging studies instead of biopsy. Prior to surgery, embolization may be performed to block the blood vessels that supply the tumor. This will reduce bleeding during surgical resection. Surgical options include open surgery, stereotactic radiosurgery, and the *Expanded Endonasal Approach*, which is minimally invasive, and involves tumor removal

Global Epidemiology of Cancer: Diagnosis and Treatment, First Edition. Jahangir Moini,
Nicholas G. Avgeropoulos, and Craig Badolato.
© 2022 John Wiley & Sons Ltd. Published 2022 by John Wiley & Sons Ltd.

through the nasal passages without any incisions being made.

Nasopharyngeal Hemangioma

Nasopharyngeal hemangiomas are benign vascular tumors that are extremely rare. There have only been a few reported cases. They develop from unknown causes, and usually cause nosebleeds, nasal obstruction, discharge, facial pain, alterations of the sense of smell, and headaches. There is one theory that hemangiomas of the nasopharynx may be related to a malformation during fetal development. These tumors can occur in any age, in males and females. Hemangiomas grow quickly. Like angiofibromas, their extreme vascularity makes them likely to bleed. These tumors are diagnosed via nasal endoscopy, followed by MRI or CT scan, and biopsy. Treatment techniques include cryotherapy, sclerosing solutions, endoscopic surgery, corticosteroids, and *yttrium aluminum garnet (YAG) laser surgery*. With incomplete surgical removal, there have been cases of recurrences. Endoscopic surgery is the treatment with the best success at complete tumor removal and prevention of recurrence.

Nasopharyngeal Carcinoma

Nasopharyngeal carcinoma is usually of the squamous cell subtype. It begins in the nasopharynx – the upper area of the throat, behind the nose and near the base of the skull. The three forms of nasopharyngeal carcinoma are *non-keratinizing undifferentiated, non-keratinizing differentiated*, and *keratinizing squamous cell* carcinomas.

Epidemiology

Nasopharyngeal carcinoma affects less than 1 person of every 100,000 in the United States annually. Incidence statistics are not well documented. Nasopharyngeal carcinoma occurs in people of all ages, including teenagers, though risks slowly increase with aging. About 50% of diagnosed patients are under age 55. Men are two times more likely than women to develop nasopharyngeal carcinoma. Chinese immigrants to the United States have high rates of nasopharyngeal carcinoma, especially when they come from the southern part of China or have Southeast Asian ancestry. Cases of nasopharyngeal carcinoma in Chinese-Americans slowly decrease over the generations to rates seen in Americans that did not come from China. This may be environmentally related. The most common subtype of nasopharyngeal carcinoma in the United States is non-keratinizing undifferentiated carcinoma.

Globally, there are up to 21 cases of nasopharyngeal carcinoma per 100,000 people every year. There are over 129,000 new cases per year throughout the world. Most diagnosed patients are under age 55. This cancer is more common in men than in women (18th most common cancer in men and 22nd most common cancer in women). Nasopharyngeal carcinoma is most common in countries of the South China Sea and in Asia. The countries with the highest rates of nasopharyngeal carcinoma include: Brunei (9.9 cases out of every 100,000 people), Maldives (6.7 cases), Singapore (6.7), Indonesia (6.6), Malaysia (6.3), Vietnam (5.7), Timor-Leste (5.1), Laos (4.3), Myanmar (3.7), Algeria (3.2), Kenya (3.2), and the Philippines (3.2) – see Figure 5.1.

Etiology and Risk Factors

The exact causes of nasopharyngeal carcinoma are not known, though there are dietary, infectious, and family history factors. There is a genetic predisposition to nasopharyngeal carcinoma. Risk factors include dietary exposure to salted fish and nitrites, along with the Epstein–Barr virus. Smoking, alcohol, and certain workplace chemicals may also increase risks.

Clinical Manifestations

Often, palpable lymph node metastases in the neck are an early indication of nasopharyngeal cancer. Hearing loss may also be present, often caused by obstruction of the nasal or eustachian tubes, which results in middle ear effusion. Additional manifestations include dizziness, ear

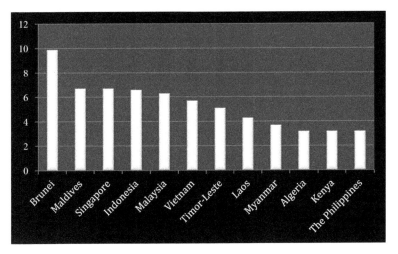

Figure 5.1 Countries with the highest rates of nasopharyngeal carcinoma, out of every 100,000 people.

pain, headaches, serious nosebleeds, rhinorrhea that is purulent and bloody, cervical lymphadenopathy, and cranial nerve palsies. These palsies usually affect the third, fourth, and sixth cranial nerves, since these are located within the cavernous sinus, near to the foramen lacerum. This is the most common route in which these tumors spread intracranially. Since the nasopharynx lymphatics connect across the midline, bilateral metastases often occur.

Pathology

Though squamous cell carcinoma is the most common variant of nasopharyngeal carcinoma, other variants include adenoid cystic and mucoepidermoid carcinomas, adenocarcinomas, malignant mixed tumors, fibrosarcomas, lymphomas, chondrosarcomas, osteosarcomas, and melanomas. The three primary subtypes of nasopharyngeal carcinoma include the following:

- *Non-keratinizing undifferentiated carcinoma* – the most common subtype in the United States
- *Non-keratinizing differentiated carcinoma*
- *Keratinizing squamous cell carcinoma*

Diagnosis

For diagnosis, a nasopharyngeal mirror or endoscope is required, and any lesions that are found must be biopsied. A needle biopsy is often preferred, and open cervical node biopsy should not be the first procedure performed. Electronic nasopharyngeal biopsy is an effective diagnostic option. Imaging studies include the following:

- Gadolinium-enhanced MRI with fat suppression – special attention is paid to the nasopharynx and base of the skull, since this area is involved in about 25% of cases
- CT scan – accurately evaluates changes to the bones of the skull base better than MRI
- PET scan – evaluates disease that extend to the cervical lymph nodes

The staging of nasopharyngeal carcinoma is as follows:

- Stage I – tumor confined to the nasopharynx, or extends to the oropharynx and/or nasal cavity, with no parapharyngeal involvement (T1); no regional lymph node metastasis (N0); and no distant metastasis (M0)
- Stage II – T1; with N1 (unilateral cervical or bilateral retropharyngeal nodes are 6 cm in diameter or less); with M0, OR: T2 (tumor extends to the parapharyngeal space and/or adjacent soft tissue); with N0 or N1; with M0
- Stage III – T1 or T2; with N2 (bilateral cervical nodes are 6 cm in diameter or less); with

M0, OR: T3 (tumor infiltrates bony structures at the skull base, cervical vertebrae, pterygoid, and/or paranasal sinuses); with N0 to N2; with M0

- Stage IVA – T4 (tumor with intracranial extension, or involvement of cranial nerves, hypopharynx, orbit, parotid, and/or extensive soft tissue infiltration); with N0 to N2; with M0, OR: any "T" level, with N3 (unilateral or bilateral node is larger than 6 cm, and/or extension below the cricoid cartilage); with M0
- Stage IVB – any "T" level; with any "N" level; with M1 (distant metastasis is present)

Treatment

Nasopharyngeal cancers are often not surgically resectable due to their location and the amount of tissues involved. They are usually treated with chemotherapy and radiation therapy, and adjuvant chemotherapy often follows. Surgery is often reserved for lymph nodes that do not regress after radiation therapy, or for lymph node recurrence after all treatments are completed. Radiation therapy doses and field margins are chosen on an individual patient basis, based on the size and location of the primary tumor and lymph nodes. Externa-beam radiation therapy (EBRT) is most often used as a single method of treatment. There may be a 30–40% incidence of hypothyroidism if EBRT is delivered to the entire thyroid or pituitary glands. Thyroid function testing should be part of treatment. For some tumors, intracavitary or interstitial implants are used, or stereotactic radiosurgery is performed. Intensity-modulated radiation therapy (IMRT) is also often successful and causes less incidence of xerostomia.

If a tumor recurs, another course of radiation may be given – often using brachytherapy, which is a radioactive implant placement. However, radionecrosis of the base of the skull is a risk factor. For individually selected patients, skull base resection is performed instead of radiation therapy. The resection usually involves removing a section of the maxilla bone for access. However, for some patients, resection may be performed endoscopically, though this is a newer method with not a large degree of information. Under clinical study, dose escalation with new radiation therapy techniques is being reviewed, such as *stereotactic radiation therapy boost.*

Prevention and Early Detection

There is no known method of preventing nasopharyngeal cancer. It is suspected that avoiding tobacco use and limiting alcohol use could be preventive. There is no routine screening method for early detection. Regular medical check-ups and dental visits are recommended. In countries with high rates of nasopharyngeal cancer, there are routine screening programs available. Finding the Epstein–Barr virus to be present may be an early determining factor. Sometimes, this carcinoma is detected early because of symptoms such as a feeling of fullness in the ear, but most patients have no symptoms until the disease has advanced.

Prognosis

Early-stage nasopharyngeal carcinoma usually has a good prognosis, with five-year survival between 60% and 75%. However, patients with stage IV disease have a poor prognosis, with five-year survival being less than 40%. The five-year survival rate for localized disease is 85%; for regional disease, it is 71%; and for distant disease, it is 49%.

Significant Point

While the treatment for nasopharyngeal carcinomas is the same for all subtypes, the non-keratinizing subtypes usually respond better. Many of these tumors also contain large amounts of lymphocytes and other immune system cells. Undifferentiated nasopharyngeal carcinomas are often described as *lymphoepitheliomas.*

Clinical Case

1. What are the statistics on people from a Chinese background having nasopharyngeal carcinoma?
2. What are the three primary subtypes of nasopharyngeal carcinoma?
3. What is the prognosis for nasopharyngeal carcinoma?

A 54-year-old Chinese man started experiencing headaches that were focused more on the left side of his head. He went to his physician for evaluation, and also complained of occasional dizziness. A PET-CT revealed a high metabolic mass in the left side of the nasopharynx, multiple mild hypermetabolic lymph nodes in the bilateral neck, and a hypermetabolic nodule in the right middle lung lobe. An electronic nasopharyngeal biopsy revealed a non-keratinizing undifferentiated nasopharyngeal carcinoma. A resection of the nodule in the right middle lung lobe was performed and later diagnosed as a lung metastasis of the nasopharyngeal carcinoma. The patient was given chemotherapy with docetaxel, cisplatin, and nimotuzumab. Radical IMRT radiation therapy was given adjunctively. He was also placed on capecitabine as a maintenance treatment over one year. While still present, the nasopharyngeal carcinoma had become smaller and the lymph nodes in the neck had resolved. The patient continues to be monitored.

Answers:

1. **Chinese immigrants to the United States have high rates of nasopharyngeal carcinoma, especially when they come from the southern part of China or have Southeast Asian ancestry. Cases of nasopharyngeal carcinoma in Chinese-Americans slowly decrease over the generations to rates seen in Americans that did not come from China. This may be environmentally related.**
2. **The three primary subtypes of nasopharyngeal carcinoma include: non-keratinizing undifferentiated carcinoma (the most common subtype in the United States), non-keratinizing differentiated carcinoma, and keratinizing squamous cell carcinoma.**
3. **Early-stage nasopharyngeal carcinoma usually has a good prognosis, with the five-year survival rate between 60% and 75%. However, patients with stage IV disease have a poor prognosis, with the five-year survival rate being less than 40%. The five-year survival rate for localized disease is 85%; for regional disease it is 71; and for distant disease it is 49%.**

Laryngeal Cancer

Laryngeal cancer affects the larynx, and in most cases, about 90% is diagnosed as squamous cell carcinoma. Fortunately, this type of cancer is often diagnosed relatively early if it affects the vocal cords, because this causes hoarseness of the voice. Unfortunately, the supraglottic tumors and subglottic tumors are often diagnosed only once they have become advanced, since they take a much longer time to cause symptoms.

Epidemiology

Laryngeal cancer is diagnosed in about 13,000 people per year in the United States, though changes in smoking habits are causing the number of cases to decrease – especially in men. There are about 3,700 deaths every year in the United States. The current incidence is estimated to be 2.76 cases out of every 100,000 people. The disease affects people between 55 and 74 more often than all other age groups, though it has occurred in all ages of adults. Laryngeal cancer is about four times more common in men than in women. It is also more common in people from a lower socioeconomic status. The disease affects African American men the most (7.3 cases out of 100,000), followed by Caucasian men (5.1), and Hispanic men (4.2). For women, the statistics are different. African American women are affected the most (1.4 cases out of 100,000), followed by Caucasian women (1.1) and American Indian/Alaskan Native women (0.9) – see Figure 5.2.

According to the Global Health Data Exchange, the current worldwide prevalence of laryngeal cancer is 14.33 cases per year out of every 100,000 people. Incidence is estimated at 2.76 cases per year per 100,000. There are about 1.66 deaths per year per 100,000 people. Global prevalence has increased by 24% over the past 30 years, and global incidence has increased 12% over the same period. Fortunately, global mortality has declined by about 5%. The disease is more common after age 65, and males are affected five times more than females. Incidence and mortality are higher in Europe and lower in Africa. The ratio between deaths and incidence is highest in Africa. The incidence in Europe gradually declined over the past 30 years, but it increased in Southeast Asia and the Western Pacific countries.

Etiology and Risk Factors

The most common cause of laryngeal cancer is smoking, with more than 95% of patients being current or former smokers. However, risks are increased by 30 times when a person has smoked for 15 or more years of at least one pack of cigarettes per day. Moderate to heavy alcohol use also increases the risk of laryngeal cancer, but not as much as smoking does. Those that both smoke and drink alcohol have the highest risk for developing this cancer. Other possible risk factors for laryngeal cancer include poor nutrition, the human papillomavirus infection, Fanconi anemia, **dyskeratosis congenita**, wood dust, paint fumes, exposure to chemicals from workplaces, and asbestos. The male gender, older age, and the African American race are also risk factors. Gastroesophageal reflux disease is being studied as to its relationship with laryngeal cancer.

Clinical Manifestations

Upon diagnosis, 60% of cases are localized and 25% are localized with regional lymph node metastasis. Only 15% of cases present with advanced cancer, distant metastases, or both. Because of the small amount of lymphatic drainage of the glottis, lymph node metastases are more common with the supraglottic and

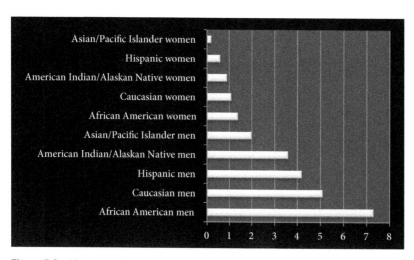

Figure 5.2 New annual cases of laryngeal cancer in the United States, per 100,000 people, separated by gender.

subglottic tumors than with the glottic (true vocal cord) tumors. The most common sites of distant metastases are the lungs and liver. Hoarseness of the voice is commonly seen early with glottic cancers. With supraglottic cancers, there is often dysphagia, and with subglottic cancers, there may be airway obstruction, a neck mass, otalgia, and a muffled sound to the voice (known as "hot potato voice"). A direct laryngoscopy is required for these symptoms immediately.

Pathology

Squamous cell carcinoma is by far the most common type of laryngeal cancer. The most common site of pathological origin is the glottis, followed by the supraglottic larynx. Only 1% of primary laryngeal cancers begin in the subglottic larynx. Verrucous carcinoma is a rare subtype of squamous cell carcinoma that usually forms in the glottic area – meaning it has a better survival rate than the standard form of squamous cell carcinoma.

Diagnosis

A specialist for any patient who has had hoarseness of the voice for over 2–3 weeks must examine the larynx. A flexible fiberoptic scope is preferred, though a mirror can be used. Any present lesions usually require operative endoscopy and biopsy. There must be evaluation of the upper airway and GI tract for concurrent cancers. Up to 10% of cases of laryngeal cancer also have a concurrent second primary tumor. Imaging with CT, MRI, and sometimes PET is done.

Laryngeal staging is done with standard TNM features as well as separate "N" categories for cancers that are related or unrelated to the human papillomavirus. Clinical staging (cTNM) requires results of physical examination and pre-surgical tests. Pathologic staging (pTNM) is based on pathology of the primary tumor and the amount of positive lymph nodes found during surgery. Extranodal extension is part of the "N" category, based on evidence of gross extension during physical examination and confirmed by imaging. Extranodal extension is histological proof of a lymph node tumor extending through the capsule into the surrounding connective tissue, even though there may or may not be a stromal reaction. Staging of laryngeal cancer is summarized as follows:

- Stage 0 – T, N0, M0 – the tumor is in the top cell layer lining the larynx only, has not spread to lymph nodes or had distant metastasis
- Stage I – T1, N0, M0 – the tumor has reached only one part of the supraglottis and the vocal cords move normally; no spread to lymph nodes or distant sites
- Stage II – T2, N0, M0 – the tumor has grown into several parts of the supraglottis or glottis, but the vocal cords move normally; no spread to lymph nodes or distant sites
- Stage III – T3, N0, M0 – the tumor is only in the larynx but has caused a vocal cord to stop moving, OR is growing into the postcricoid area, paraglottic space, pre-epiglottic tissues, or inner part of the thyroid cartilage; no spread to lymph nodes or distant sites, OR: T1 to T3, N1, M0 – the tumor may have reached structures outside the larynx and might have affected a vocal cord; it has spread to one lymph node on the same side of the neck as the tumor, which is no larger than 3 cm across; no distant metastasis
- Stage IVa – T4a, N0 or N1, M0 – the tumor has grown through the thyroid cartilage or into tissues beyond the larynx (moderately advanced local disease); has not spread to one lymph node on the same side and the tumor is not larger than 3 cm across; no distant metastasis, OR: T1 to T4a, N2, M0 – the tumor may have grown outside the larynx and may have affected a vocal cord; it has reached one lymph node on the same side, and is 3–6 cm across, OR: has spread to several nodes on the same side that are not larger than 6 cm across, OR: has spread to one or more nodes on the other side of the neck that are not larger than 6 cm across; no distant metastasis

- Stage IVb – T4b, any "N," M0 – the tumor has reached the prevertebral space, surrounds a carotid artery, or is growing down between the lungs (very advanced local disease); it may have spread to lymph nodes; no distant metastasis, OR: any T, N3, M0, the tumor may or may not have infiltrated structures outside the larynx, and may or may not have affected a vocal cord; it has spread to one or more lymph nodes larger than 6 cm across, OR: it has spread to a lymph node and then grown outside of the node, but not spread to distant sites
- Stage IVc: Any T, Any N, M1 – the tumor may or may not have grown into structures outside of the larynx, and may or may not have affected a vocal cord; the cancer may or may not have spread to nearby lymph nodes, and has spread to distant sites

Treatment

Treatment of early-stage *glottic carcinoma* is laser excision, radiation therapy, and sometimes, open laryngeal surgery. Normality of the voice and vocal cord function, as well as similar cure rates, is usually preserved by endoscopic laser resection and radiation therapy. The choice of surgery or radiation is usually based on where the lesion is located in the glottis, preferences of the physicians, and the patient's choice. Advanced glottic carcinoma is defined as the lack of vocal cord mobility or extension into the tongue. The majority of patients receive chemotherapy as well as radiation therapy. If there is extension outside of the larynx, or cartilage invasion, a laryngectomy will be the treatment chosen. This is usually total, but for some individuals, endoscopic laser resection or open partial laryngectomy can be used. For salvage, a total laryngectomy is often used, but endoscopic resection or open partial laryngectomy is sometimes possible.

For early *supraglottic carcinoma*, radiation therapy or partial laryngectomy can be effective. Laser resection is highly successful for early supraglottic squamous cell carcinomas, and reduces functional changes following surgery. If advanced but not affecting the true vocal cords, a supraglottic partial laryngectomy can preserve the voice and glottic sphincter. If the true vocal cords are affected, a total laryngectomy is indicated. Most advanced stage supraglottic carcinomas are first treated with chemotherapy and radiation therapy. For early *subglottic carcinoma*, radiation therapy is needed, since this cancer is not usually treatable via endoscopic resection. When the lesion is more advanced or has metastasized, chemoradiation is used, unless there is extension outside of the larynx, or there is extensive invasion of the cartilage. In these cases, a total laryngectomy is performed.

Prevention and Early Detection

The prevention of laryngeal cancer begins with avoiding smoking and limiting alcohol intake. Avoiding workplace chemicals, following a healthy eating pattern, and avoiding the human papillomavirus infection are also methods of prevention. There is no simple screening test for laryngeal cancer. Early detection is via voice changes, which should be discussed soon with a physician.

Prognosis

Fortunately, early-stage glottic carcinoma has a five-year survival rate of 90%. Overall, the five-year survival rate for all forms of laryngeal cancer is 60%. If there is regional nodal disease, the five-year survival rate is 43%, and there is only a 30% rate with distant metastasis.

Significant Point

Tobacco use is the major predisposing factor for laryngeal cancer. The vast majority of laryngeal cancers are squamous cell carcinomas that arise from the covering of the vocal cords. Generally, laryngeal cancers are not difficult to diagnose. Precise and direct visualization of the cancer is required since most treatment decisions are based on the size and extent of the carcinoma.

Clinical Case

1. What is the most common cause of laryngeal cancer?
2. How does diagnosis for laryngeal cancer begin?
3. Are there any methods of preventing laryngeal cancer?

A 65-year-old man who had smoked two packs of cigarettes per day for 40 years goes to see his physician because of a sore throat and persistent hoarseness. The man also admits to drinking three to four alcoholic beverages per night, also for about 40 years. After examination and visualization, the patient is diagnosed with laryngeal cancer, specifically of the glottis. He is hospitalized, and a total laryngectomy is performed. During the surgery, the entire larynx, strap muscles, paratracheal lymphatics, and the ipsilateral thyroid lobe were removed. The patient is started on chemotherapy and radiation therapy, and is advised that he will also receive rehabilitation therapy to be able to speak again, which will be quite different from how he sounded before, but still functional.

Answers:

1. **The most common cause of laryngeal cancer is smoking, with more than 95% of patients being current or former smokers. Risks are increased by 30 times when a person has smoked for 15 or more years of at least on pack of cigarettes per day. Moderate to heavy alcohol use also increases the risk of laryngeal cancer. Those that both smoke and drink alcohol have the highest risk for developing this cancer.**
2. **A specialist must examine the larynx if there has been hoarseness of the voice for over 2–3 weeks. A flexible fiberoptic scope is preferred, though a mirror can be used. Lesions usually require operative endoscopy and biopsy.**
3. **Prevention of laryngeal cancer begins with avoiding smoking and limiting alcohol intake. Avoiding workplace chemicals, following a healthy eating pattern, and avoiding the human papillomavirus infection are also suggested.**

Lung Cancer

Lung cancer, specifically *lung carcinoma*, is the leading cause of cancer-related deaths throughout the entire world. It is also called *bronchogenic carcinoma*. Cigarette smoking causes most cases. Lung cancer can affect any part of the two left lung lobes or the three right lung lobes. The majority of lung cancers are adenocarcinomas, which form in the alveoli and other mucus-secreting glands. Most lung nodules, also known as pulmonary nodules, are benign and asymptomatic growths. However, some lung nodules are cancerous tumors that will grow over time. The classifications of lung cancer include non-small cell lung cancer, which is the most common form, small cell lung cancer, and also cancers that begin in the bronchi, bronchioles, or alveoli.

Epidemiology

Approximately 229,000 new cases of lung cancer are diagnosed annually in the United States. According to the American Lung Association, there are approximately 57.8 cases in men out of every 100,000 and about 45.9 cases in women out of every 100,000. Fortunately, incidence in men has been declining over the past 20 years, and has also started to decline in women. The number of deaths caused by lung cancer peaked in 2005 at 159,292. Lung cancer is mostly a disease of the elderly, with 86% of cases being in people aged 60 or older. More than 116,000 men are diagnosed annually, and more than 112,000 women. African American men and women are more likely to develop and die from lung cancer than people from any other racial or ethnic group. Age-adjusted incidence in African American men is about 30% higher than for Caucasian men. Lung cancer in African American women is at about the same rates as in Caucasian women. Figure 5.3 illustrates the American states with the highest and lowest cases of lung cancer, according to the American Lung Association. For example, Kentucky is the highest with 91.4 cases out of every 100,000 people, while Utah is the lowest with 26.3 cases per 100,000.

According to the World Cancer Research Fund, there were 2.1 million new cases of lung cancer throughout the world in 2018. Of these cases, about 1.8 million were fatal. Most people with lung cancer were older than age 60. On average, men were affected almost twice as often as women. Countries with the highest rates of lung cancer included the following: Hungary (56.7 cases out of every 100,000 people), Serbia (49.8 cases), the New Caledonia area of France (42.3), Greece (40.5), French Polynesia (39.8), Montenegro (39.7), Belgium (39.0), Guam (37.9),

Turkey (36.9), and Denmark (36.6) – see Figure 5.4). Because of these statistics, Caucasians are most often affected by lung cancer in countries outside of the United States.

Etiology and Risk Factors

Approximately 85% of cases of lung cancer are related to cigarette smoking. It should be understood that all types of tobacco products that are smoked increase the chance for developing lung cancer. The risks for lung cancer differ by age, the number of cigarettes smoked per day, and the number of years that smoking occurred. Risks are increased if a smoker or former smoker was also exposed to toxins. Risk factors include air pollution, exposure to second-hand smoke, marijuana smoking, and carcinogen exposure. Carcinogens related to lung cancer include asbestos, radiation, arsenic, radon, chromates, chloromethyl ethers, nickel, mustard gas, polycyclic aromatic hydrocarbons, coke-oven emissions, heating huts, and primitive methods of cooking. Lung cancer risks are also linked to electronic nicotine delivery systems, known as e-cigarettes, though this is believed to be to a

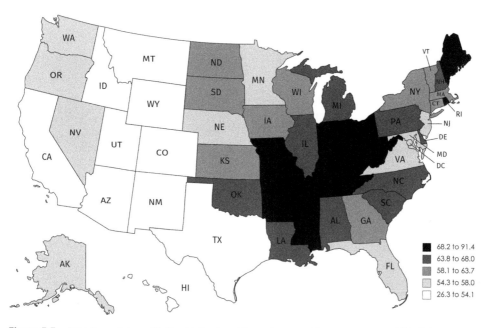

Figure 5.3 American states with the highest and lowest cases of lung cancer, per 100,000 people.

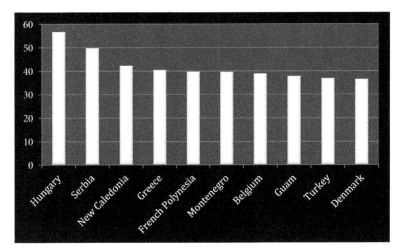

Figure 5.4 Countries with the highest rates of lung cancer, per 100,000 people.

much lesser degree than with cigarettes, cigars, or pipes.

Risks are reduced after a person quits smoking, but never achieves the risk level of people that have never smoked. Between 15% and 20% of people developing lung cancer have either never smoked or only smoked to a small degree. Exposure to radon within the home environment is still being debated as to the likeliness of developing lung cancer. Chronic inflammation also increases the risk of developing lung cancer, exemplified by conditions such as alpha-1 antitrypsin deficiency, chronic obstructive pulmonary disease (COPD), and pulmonary fibrosis. Lung scarring from tuberculosis or other lung diseases also increases the risks for lung cancer. Active smokers that take beta-carotene supplements have an increased risk as well.

Genetic factors are also causative. There is an effect called **field carcinogenesis**, in which the epithelial cells of the lungs require prolonged exposure to cancer-promoting agents, plus multiple genetic mutations to accumulate, prior to becoming cancerous. For some lung cancer patients, additional or secondary gene mutations, in genes that stimulate cell growth, result in abnormalities in growth factor receptor signaling. They inhibit apoptosis and can contribute to uncontrolled proliferation of cells that are abnormal. Examples of these genes that may become mutated include:

- *Kirsten rat sarcoma (K-ras)* and *myelocytomatosis (MYC)* – which stimulate cell growth
- *Epidermal growth factor receptor (EGFR)* and *human epidermal growth factor 2 (HER2)/neural (neu)* – which are involved in growth factor receptor signaling

Mutations that inhibit the tumor-suppressor genes *adenomatosis polyposis coli (APC)* and *tumor protein p53* can also cause cancer. Also, mutations may involve the *echinoderm microtubule associated protein-like-4 (EML-4)-anaplastic lymphoma kinase (ALK)* translocation, and mutations in *v-raf murine sarcoma viral oncogene homolog B (BRAF), phosphoinositide 3-kinase catalytic subunit alpha (PI3KCA),* and the *ROS-1 proto-oncogene – receptor tyrosine kinase.* Gene mutations such as these are called *oncogenic driver mutations,* which can cause or contribute to lung cancer in people that smoke. However, these mutations are very likely to be a lung cancer cause in people that have never smoked. According to the Lung Cancer Mutation Consortium, driver mutations are present in about 64% of lung cancers regardless of smoking history. Of these driver mutations, 25% are K-ras mutations, 17% are EGFR mutations, 8% are EML-4-ALK mutations, and 2% are BRAF mutations. Other mutations are being found, and clinical studies are ongoing about focusing on oncogenic driver mutations as a targeted-therapy treatment method.

Clinical Manifestations

Of all lung cancers, about 25% are asymptomatic, and are found incidentally during chest imaging for other reasons. When signs and symptoms develop, it may be from localized tumor progression, regional spreading, or distant metastasis. At any stage, **paraneoplastic syndrome** and constitutional manifestations may occur. The symptoms are not specific to the histological features, but some complications are more likely to occur with certain histologies. Complications of adenocarcinoma, squamous cell carcinoma, and large cell carcinoma include airway obstruction, hemoptysis, pleuritic involvement with pain, pneumonia, pleural effusion, shoulder or arm pain due to a **pancoast tumor**, superior vena cava (SVC) syndrome, hoarseness because of laryngeal nerve involvement, neurologic symptoms due to brain metastasis, jaundice due to liver metastasis, and pathologic fractures due to bone metastasis. Complications of small cell carcinoma include paraneoplastic syndromes and SVC syndrome.

Localized lung cancer may cause coughing, dyspnea because of airway obstruction, pneumonia or post-obstructive atelectasis, and parenchymal loss because of lymphangitic spread. Post-obstructive pneumonia may cause a fever. As many as 50% of patients have chest pain. Hemoptysis is not as common, with minimal loss of blood – except rarely, when the tumor invades a major artery. This causes massive hemorrhaging, and often death occurs from exsanguination or asphyxiation. While 20% of patients have hemoptysis at some point, only 10% have it as the initial symptom.

With regional spread of lung cancer, there may be pleuritic chest pain or dyspnea, caused by a pleural effusion. There can be hoarseness if the tumor encroaches the recurrent laryngeal nerve. Dyspnea and hypoxia can be caused by diaphragmatic paralysis because of the phrenic nerve being affected. Compression or invasion of the superior vena cava causes SVC syndrome, and sometimes, headache or head fullness, breathless when lying down, facial or arm swelling, **plethora**, and dilated veins of the face, neck, and upper trunk. Non-small cell lung cancer is also referred to as *pancoast tumor*, and *pancoast syndrome* occurs if this tumor or another apical tumor invades the brachial plexus, pleura, or ribs. This causes shoulder and upper arm pain and weakness, or ipsilateral hand atrophy. Pancoast syndrome can include Horner syndrome – anhidrosis, miosis, and ptosis. This occurs if the paravertebral sympathetic chain or the cervical stellate ganglion is involved. Tumor spread to the pericardium can be asymptomatic or result in cardiac tamponade or constrictive pericarditis. Rarely, dysphagia is caused by the tumor compressing the esophagus.

Metastasis of lung tumors causes different symptoms because of the metastatic site, as follows:

- Adrenal glands – adrenal insufficiency occurs in rare cases
- Bones – severe pain occurs, with pathologic fractures
- Brain – behavioral changes, aphasia, confusion, paralysis or paresis, seizures, nausea, vomiting, coma, and death
- Liver – nausea, pain, early satiety, and eventually, hepatic insufficiency

Paraneoplastic syndromes occur at sites that are far from a tumor or its metastases. With lung cancer, common paraneoplastic syndromes include the following:

- Cushing's syndrome
- Finger clubbing – with or without hypertrophic pulmonary osteoarthropathy
- Hypercalcemia – occurring when a squamous cell carcinoma produces parathyroid hormone-related protein, or if extensive bone metastases result in production of osteoclast-activating factors

- Hypercoagulability accompanied by migratory superficial thrombophlebitis – this is known as **Trousseau syndrome**
- Myasthenia-like symptoms – known as **Eaton–Lambert syndrome**
- Neurologic syndromes – such as encephalopathies, neuropathies, encephalitides, cerebellar disease, and myelopathies – neuromuscular syndromes develop because of tumor expression of autoantigens, plus production of autoantibodies – however, most other neurologic syndromes are of unknown cause
- Syndrome of inappropriate antidiuretic hormone (SIADH) secretion

Pathology

The two major pathological classifications of lung cancer are as follows:

Non-small cell lung cancer (NSCLC) and small cell lung cancer (SCLC). About 85% of cases are NSCLC and 15% of cases are SCLC. NSCLC has various amounts of aggressiveness, based on histology; approximately 40% of patients have metastasis outside of the chest upon diagnosis. SCLC is highly aggressive and nearly always occurs in people that smoke or have smoked; it grows quickly, with about 80% of patients already having metastatic disease at the time it is diagnosed.

The features of the various lung cancer subtypes can be broken down further. Adenocarcinomas make up 37.5% of lung cancers, followed by squamous cell carcinoma (27.5%), small cell carcinoma (14%), and large cell carcinoma (12.5%) (see Figure 5.5). Adenocarcinomas and large cell carcinomas are peripheral nodules or masses. Squamous cell carcinomas are centralized and endobronchial in location. Small cell carcinomas are perihilar masses in the submucosa of the airways.

Diagnosis

Initial diagnosis is often by chest X-ray, which can show clear abnormalities such as reticular shadows in the lungs (see Figure 5.6). These include one or multifocal masses, or a single pulmonary nodule. Other findings include an enlarged hilum, narrowing of the tracheobronchial areas, widening of the mediastinum, **atelectasis**, cavitary lesions, non-resolving parenchymal infiltrates, or pleural thickening or effusion that cannot be explained. These findings suggest lung cancer, but for confirmation, must be followed with CT or PET-CT scans as well as cytopathology. In a CT scan, an adenocarcinoma can present as solid lesions (see Figure 5.7). When a lesion is seen in a plain X-ray that is suggestive based on tobacco use, age, and symptoms, a PET-CT can assist with

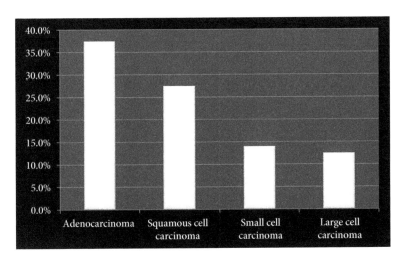

Figure 5.5 Percentages of occurrence of various lung cancer subtypes.

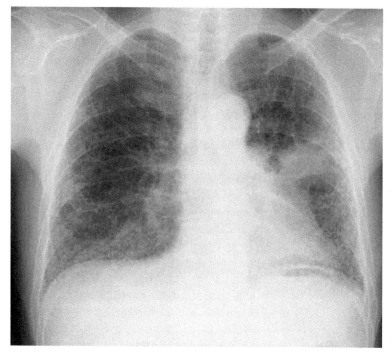

Figure 5.6 Chest X-ray showing reticular shadows in both lung fields and a mass lesion in the center of the left lung. *Source*: Shiratori et al. (2020).

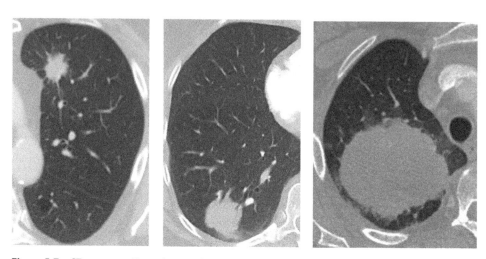

Figure 5.7 CT scan revealing adenocarcinoma presenting as solid lesions. (a) Solid peripheral nodule with lobulated margins; (b) peripheral spiculated nodule; (c) large solid mass. *Source*: Pascoe et al. (2018).

the diagnosis and tumor staging. The PET-CT combines anatomic CT images with functional PET images that help differentiate between inflammation and malignancy. CT as well as PET-CT aid in directing core needle biopsy of lesions that cannot be biopsied via the bronchoscopic technique. The PET images can also detect metastasis.

The location of the lesions and accessibility of tissues determines which cytological method can be used. The least invasive method is cytology of the sputum or pleural fluid. If the patient has a productive cough, a sputum specimen obtained upon awakening may contain large amounts of malignant cells. However, the yield from using this method is less than 50%. If the pleural fluid is used, a malignant effusion will indicate advanced stage disease and a poor outlook. Generally, false-negative cytology results can be reduced by obtaining as much sputum or pleural fluid as possible in the early morning. The sample must be sent to the laboratory immediately to reduce any processing delays, since they lead to cell breakdown. Molecular studies can be performed on tumor cell pellets embedded in paraffin, using pleural fluid that is spun down in a centrifuge, if the cell pellets are preserved quickly. The next least invasive method is percutaneous biopsy, which is more useful for metastatic sites than for lung lesions. These sites include the pleura, supraclavicular or other peripheral lymph nodes, adrenal glands, and liver. However, there is a 20–25% chance of pneumothorax, especially if the patient has severe emphysema, and risks for false-negative results.

For most cases of lung cancer, bronchoscopy is the diagnostic procedure done. This is often performed along with or in place of less invasive procedures because of its accuracy and the fact that it is required for staging. A tissue diagnosis is often achieved by combining brushings, washings, and biopsies of visible endobronchial lesions as well as hilar, mediastinal, paratracheal, and **subcarinal** lymph nodes. Bronchoscopy advances have improved diagnostic accuracy as well as the ability to sample more peripheral lesions. During bronchoscopy, endobronchial ultrasound-guided biopsy (EBUS) can be done, which is the preferred method for staging the mediastinum – except if the lymph nodes cannot be sampled because of anatomic factors.

For evaluating mediastinal lymph nodes, mediastinoscopy was the standard test, but is of high risk. It is usually done before more extensive thoracic surgeries, to confirm or exclude a tumor, if the patient has enlarged mediastinal lymph nodes unable to be sampled via EBUS. An open lung biopsy via open thoracotomy or with video assistance is indicated when the less

invasive methods are not diagnostic, and there are clinical or radiographic features indicating a high likelihood of resectability. A core biopsy is preferred over a fine-needle biopsy because it can retrieve enough tissue for an accurate genetic evaluation via genomic sequencing. The lung cancer can then be staged – see Figure 5.8.

There are two stages of SCLC: limited and extensive. Limited-stage disease is confined to one lung, along with the ipsilateral lymph nodes. It is encompassed in one tolerable radiation therapy port – except if there is pleural or pericardial effusion. Extensive-stage disease is outside of one lung, or is diagnosed if malignant cells are present in pleural or pericardial effusions. Less than 33% of patients have limited-stage disease, unfortunately, and the rest often have many distant metastases. There are four stages of NSCLC, I–IV, using the TNM staging system, based on tumor size and location, lymph node location, and any distant metastases. SCLC is sometimes called *oat cell cancer*. The

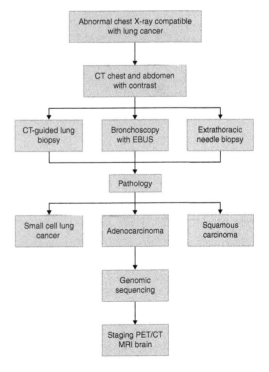

Figure 5.8 Diagnosis of lung cancer. *Source*: Oh and Chari [43].

International Staging System for Lung Cancer is summarized in Table 5.1.

The stage groupings used for lung cancer are as follows:

- Stage 0 – Tis, N0, M0
- Stage IA1 – T1mi to T1a, N0, M0
- Stage IA2 – T1b, N0, M0
- Stage IA3 – T1c, N0, M0
- Stage IB – T2a, N0, M0
- Stage IIA – T2a, N0, M0
- Stage IIB – T1a to T2b, N1, M0 or T3, N0, M0
- Stage IIIA – T1a to T2b, N2, M0 or T3, N1, N0 or T4, N0 to N1, M0
- Stage IIIB – T1a to T2b, N3, M0 or T3 to T4, N2, M0
- Stage IVA – any T, any N, M1a to M1b
- Stage IVB – any T, any N, M1c

Table 5.1 The International Staging System for Lung Cancer

Category	Description
Primary tumor (T)	
Tis	Carcinoma in situ
T1	Tumor 3 cm or less with no invasion more proximal than the lobar bronchus
T1mi	Minimally invasive adenocarcinoma
T1a	Tumor is 1 cm or less
T1b	Tumor is larger than 1 cm but not as large as 2 cm
T1c	Tumor is larger than 2 cm but not as large as 3 cm
T2	Tumor is larger than 3 cm but not as large as 5 cm, or involves the main bronchus 2 cm or larger distal to the carina, or invades the visceral pleura, or is associated with atelectasis or obstructive pneumonia extending to the hilar region, involving part or all of the lung
T2a	Tumor is larger than 3 cm but not as large as 4 cm
T2b	Tumor is larger than 4 cm but not as large as 5 cm
T3	Tumor is larger than 5 cm but not as large as 7 cm, or invades the chest wall (including superior sulcus tumors), phrenic nerve, or parietal pericardium; or there are separate tumor nodules in the same lobe
T4	Tumor is larger than 7 cm, or invades the diaphragm, mediastinum, heart, great vessels, trachea, recurrent laryngeal nerve, esophagus, vertebral body, or carina; or there are one or more satellite tumors in a different ipsilateral lobe
Regional lymph nodes (N)	
N0	No regional lymph node metastasis
N1	Metastasis to the ipsilateral peribronchial or ipsilateral hilar lymph node, or both, and to intrapulmonary nodes, including that by direct extension of the primary tumor
N2	Metastasis to the ipsilateral mediastinal or subcarinal lymph node, or both
N3	Metastasis to the contralateral mediastinal, contralateral hilar, ipsilateral or contralateral scalene, or supraclavicular lymph node, or a combination
Distant metastasis (M)	
M0	No distant metastasis
M1	Distant metastasis
M1a	Tumor with one or more tumor nodules in the contralateral lung, or with pleural or pericardial nodules, or with malignant pleural or pericardial effusion
M1b	One extrathoracic metastasis in one organ
M1c	Multiple extrathoracic metastases in one or more organs

Lymph node staging is further described as the following:

- Single station N1 (N1a)
- Multiple station N1 (N1b)
- Single station N2 without N1 (N2a1)
- Single station N2 with N1 (N2a2)
- Multiple station N2 (N2b)
- N3

A patient with metastatic disease is characterized by the number and location of metastasis into malignant pleural or pericardial effusion, a separate tumor nodule in a contralateral lobe (M1a), one extrathoracic metastasis in one organ (M1b), and more than one extrathoracic metastasis (M1c) – see Figure 5.9.

Endobronchial ultrasonography can sample enlarged lymph nodes while a lung lesion is biopsied. Some diagnostic tests are routine, while others are performed based on whether results would impact treatment. The PET scan is highly accurate and noninvasive, able to identify malignant mediastinal lymph nodes and other distant metastases as part of metabolic staging. With PET-CT, the scanners, giving even more accuracy for NSCLC, combine separate images.

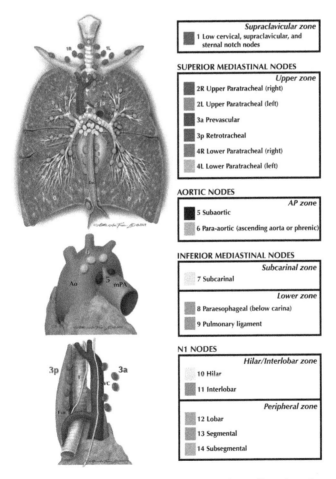

Figure 5.9 Lymph node map, including groupings of lymph node stations into zones for prognostic analysis (from the International Association for the Study of Lung Cancer, IASLC). *Source*: Rusch, V. W., Asamura, H., Watanabe, H., Giroux, D. J., Rami-Porta, R., & Goldstraw, P. (2009). The IASLC Lung Cancer Staging Project: A Proposal for a New International Lymph Node Map in the Forthcoming Seventh Edition of the TNM Classification for Lung Cancer. Journal of Thoracic Oncology, 4(5), 568–577. Reproduced with permission of Elsevier.

However, PET as well as PET-CT are of higher cost, less available, and vary in terms of specificity. The PET-CT is very sensitive, with an excellent negative predictive value, but with a lower positive predictive value. A replacement method is thin-section high-resolution CT (HRCT) from the neck to upper abdomen. This detects adrenal, cervical, hepatic, and supraclavicular metastases. It is one of the preliminary staging tests for SCLCs and NSCLCs. Often, CT is unable to identify post-inflammatory changes caused by malignant intrathoracic lymph node enlargement. Also, CT may not be able to identify benign lesions from malignant liver or adrenal gland lesions, which are distinctions needed for staging. If there are abnormalities in these areas, other tests are usually done. If a PET scan is not diagnostic, other options include the following:

- Bronchoscopy with endobronchial ultrasound
- Mediastinoscopy
- Video-assisted thoracoscopic surgery (VATS)

These are all able to biopsy mediastinal lymph nodes. However, without PET scanning, liver or adrenal gland lesions must be needle-biopsied. A chest MRI is a slightly more accurate method than upper chest HRCT to stage pancoast tumors and cancers near the diaphragm, such as mesothelioma. An MRI also provides a way to evaluate the vasculature around the tumors.

Blood tests are common. They include alkaline phosphatase and calcium levels. When high, this suggests bone metastases. While having no role in staging, CBC, AST, ALT, serum albumin, total bilirubin, creatinine, and electrolyte levels are important prognostically, concerning the patient's toleration of treatment. They may also reveal paraneoplastic syndromes. Once lung cancer is diagnosed, the patient must have brain imaging – usually MRI instead of CT – and this is highly necessary if the patient has a headache or any neurologic abnormalities. If there is bone pain or high serum calcium or alkaline phosphatase levels, a PET-CT or radionuclide bone scan should be performed.

Treatment

The treatment of lung cancer is based on the cell type and stage. Treatment choices are also influenced by poor cardiopulmonary reserve, frailty, poor physical performance status, undernutrition, and other coexisting conditions, and any psychiatric or cognitive illness. These factors can result in decisions on the type of treatment that will be best for the individual patient. With radiation therapy, there is a risk of radiation pneumonitis if large lung areas are exposed to high doses over time. Radiofrequency ablation involves the use of high frequency electrical current to treat small, early-stage tumors or small tumors recurring after chest radiation therapy. The ablation can preserve more lung function than with open surgery. Its less invasive nature may be excellent for patients who cannot receive open surgery. Immunotherapy is another option, for advanced stage IV NSCLC. Targeted-therapy drugs include the following, for specific subtypes of lung cancer:

- Adenocarcinoma with ALK mutation – alectinib, brigatinib, ceritinib, crizotinib
- Adenocarcinoma or squamous cell carcinoma with BRAF mutation – dabrafenib, trametinib
- Adenocarcinoma or squamous cell carcinoma with EGFR mutation – afatinib, erlotinib, gefitinib, necitumumab
- Adenocarcinoma with EGFR (T790M mutation) – osimertinib
- Adenocarcinoma with inhibited blood vessel growth – bevacizumab, ramucirumab
- Adenocarcinoma or squamous cell carcinoma with immune activation (checkpoint inhibitors) – atezolizumab, durvalumab, ipilumimab, nivolumab, pembrolizumab

For SCLC, there is usually an early response to treatment, but this does not continue. Based on stage, chemotherapy is given, with or without radiation therapy. Chemotherapy often prolongs survival and improves the patient's quality of life. Chemotherapies include etoposide with a platinum compound such as carboplatin or cisplatin. Other drugs include irinotecan, topotecan, vinblastine, vincristine, vinorelbine, cyclophosphamide, ifosfamide, doxorubicin, docetaxel, paclitaxel, and gemcitabine.

For NSCLC, treatment usually starts with evaluation of the patient for being able to have surgery of various types. Based on tumor type and stage, chemotherapy, radiation therapy, or combinations of these may be used. For stage I or II, surgical resection is usually via lobectomy or **pneumonectomy**, along with sampling of the mediastinal lymph nodes, or complete dissection of them. If the patient has poor pulmonary reserve, less intensive surgeries such as *segmentectomy* or wedge resection may be done. For stage I patients, surgery is curative 55–70% of the time. For stage II patients, it is curative 35–55% of the time. Results are usually better when a thoracic oncologic surgeon that has expertise in lung cancer performs surgery. If the patient has early-stage disease and high surgical risks, localized non-surgical treatment may be done, which includes conventional or stereotactic radiation therapy or radiofrequency ablation.

Adjuvant chemotherapy following surgery is regularly done for patients with stage II or stage III. It is also sometimes given to patients with stage IB disease and tumors larger than 4 cm. Via clinical trials, there has been increased five-year survival rates when adjuvant chemotherapy was used. Deciding on adjuvant chemotherapy for a patient is based on any assessed risks and other comorbid conditions. Cisplatin is often combined with docetaxel, paclitaxel, or vinorelbine.

Stage III NSCLC is treated with chemotherapy, radiation therapy, surgery, or combinations of these. Each patient's comorbidities and the area of the disease determine the order that the treatments are given. For unresectable stage IIIA disease, chemotherapy and radiation therapy are used concurrently, though survival will still only average 10–14 months. If a patient has stage IIIB disease, along with supraclavicular lymph node or contralateral mediastinal lymph node disease, radiation therapy and chemotherapy are used alone or together.

Stage IV NSCLC is treated with the goals of palliation and prolonged survival. Chemotherapy, radiation therapy, and targeted drugs are used.

Targeted therapy for NSCLC is also used. For adenocarcinomas, molecular analysis is performed to find certain mutations that can help guide therapy. This is a quickly advancing field of medicine, with new drugs being assessed. Immune oncology drugs such as atezolizumab, durvalumab, nivolumab, and pembrolizumab are used. Targeted-therapy drugs are used when a tumor progresses even with chemotherapy.

Prevention and Early Detection

There are no active methods of preventing lung cancer except for stopping smoking. If a home environment has radon, which is known to be causative of cancer, steps must be taken to eradicate the gas. However, reducing lung cancer incidence by removing radon from a home is of unknown effectiveness. Preventive measures also involve a good dietary intake of fruits and vegetables that are high in retinoids and beta-carotene. For smokers, vitamin supplementation with vitamin E is of unproven benefit, but beta carotene supplements must be avoided. Former smokers may or may not benefit from taking nonsteroidal anti-inflammatory drugs or vitamin E supplements. Chemopreventive interventions are only undertaken in clinical trials. Also under study are molecular methods that target cell signaling, cell cycle pathways, and tumor-associated antigens, which is known as *precision chemoprevention*.

For early detection, screening is important – especially for early NSCLC that can be surgically resected. Screening is recommended for people at high risk. Annual screening with low-dose helical CT (LDCT) has provided a 20% decrease in lung cancer deaths compared with only using chest X-rays. High-risk people are those generally between 55 and 74 years of age that were former smokers that quit in the last 15 years or still actively smoke, with at least 30 pack-years of smoking. The LDCT screening method has improved survival, based on nodule volume and volume-doubling time. Low-risk patients may not need this type of screening. The United States Preventive Services Task Force recommends that LDCT should be performed for asymptomatic smokers between ages 55 and 80 that have a 30 + pack-year history, whether they have quit in the last 15 years or continue to smoke. Physicians and patients should discuss options and utilize *shared decision-making*, with LDCT screening done at experienced facilities with good adherence regarding follow-up diagnosis and treatments. Future screening may combine molecular analysis for genetic markers with sputum cytometry, and exhaled breath detection of volatile organic compounds that are related to cancer. The genetic cancer markers include *EGFR*, *K-ras*, and *p53*. The volatile organic compounds include alkane and benzene. Trained dogs are now being used to discriminate lung cancer patients from those without cancer, using exhaled gas samples.

Prognosis

With treatment, the overall five-year survival for NSCLC is based on the type and the stage. For adenocarcinoma, squamous cell carcinoma, and large cell carcinoma, the five-year survival is as follows:

- Stage I – 60–70%
- Stage II – 39–55%
- Stage III – 5–25%, though stage IIIB disease has only a 5% prognosis
- Stage IV – less than 1%, and if a patient does not have a gene mutation that can be treated with a targeted drug, median survival is 9 months, with fewer than 25% of patients surviving for 12 months

Usually, an untreated patient with metastases will survive for just six months, and a treated patient with metastasis will survive for nine months. Early- and later-stage patients have survived longer because of newer treatment methods. For stage IB–IIIB patients, the use of platinum-based chemotherapies after surgical resection is improving survival. The overall five-year survival rate is 18%. Especially in later-stage

disease, targeted therapies and better sequential treatments are slightly prolonging survival times. For SCLC, if the disease is limited in its spread, the five-year survival with treatment is only 20%. If spread is extensive, the rate is less than 1% of patients. The median survival time for limited-stage small cell carcinoma is only 20 months.

Significant Point

Lung cancer causes more deaths per year than any other type of cancer, and more deaths than breast, prostate, and colon cancer combined. It kills nearly twice as many women as breast cancer, and more than three times as many men as prostate cancer. Less than one in seven lung cancer patients will be diagnosed in the earliest stage, when the disease is most able to be treated.

Clinical Case

1. Which type of tumors makes up the majority of lung cancers?
2. How significant is the link between cigarette smoking and lung cancer?
3. What are the complications of lung cancer?

A 68-year-old man was hospitalized because of SVC syndrome. During preliminary evaluation, suspicious tissue was found in his right lung. Histopathology revealed it to be a stage IV adenocarcinoma. There was no possibility for surgery. The patient was given a chemotherapy regimen of cisplatin with gemcitabine, which he tolerated fairly well. The disease progressed, and a second line of chemotherapy with docetaxel was administered. The disease still progressed. Even though no EGFR gene mutation was confirmed, the patient was given erlotinib. The disease began to stabilize, so the agent was continued. Palliative radiation was also done. The patient's overall condition improved. CT scans with contrast were done every three months, and the disease remained stable. There was no metastasis. Several years later, with the patient still taking erlotinib, his overall health remained good.

Answers:

1. **The majority of lung cancers are adenocarcinomas, which develop in the alveoli and other mucus-secreting glands. Adenocarcinomas make up 37.5% of lung cancers, followed by squamous cell carcinoma (27.5%), small cell carcinoma (14%), and large cell carcinoma (12.5%)**

2. **Approximately 85% of cases of lung cancer are related to cigarette smoking. All types of tobacco products that are smoked increase the chance of developing lung cancer. The risks differ by age, number of cigarettes smoked per day, and the number of years that smoking occurred. Risks are increased if a smoker or former smoker was also exposed to toxins.**

3. **Complications of lung cancer include airway obstruction, hemoptysis, pleuritic involvement with pain, pneumonia, pleural effusion, shoulder or arm pain due to a pancoast tumor, SVC syndrome, hoarseness because of laryngeal nerve involvement, neurologic symptoms due to brain metastasis, jaundice due to liver metastasis, pathologic fractures due to bone metastasis, and paraneoplastic syndromes.**

Clinical Case

1. How common is SCLC in comparison with NSCLC?

2. What are the differences between limited and extensive SCLCs?

3. What are the chemotherapies used for SCLC?

A 70-year-old woman who had smoked for 20 pack-years was diagnosed with small cell carcinoma of the lung. The disease was in a limited stage. She experienced a regular cough, slight chest pain, fatigue, and loss of appetite. The patient was treated for one month with carboplatin + etoposide, with no response. She was then treated with carboplatin + paclitaxel for four months. A parotid tumor was then discovered – a benign tumor, so radiation therapy was delayed for five months. The patient then underwent radiation therapy for about 70 days. The disease went into remission, and the patient's condition has overall improved.

Answers:

1. **SCLC is less common, making up approximately 15% of cases, with NSCLC making up 85%. SCLC is highly aggressive and nearly always occurs in people that smoke or have smoked; it grows quickly, with about 80% of patients already having metastatic disease at the time it is diagnosed.**

2. **Limited-stage SCLC is confined to one lung, along with the ipsilateral lymph nodes. Extensive-stage SCLC is outside one lung, or is diagnosed if malignant cells are present in pleural or pericardial effusions. Less than 33% of patients have limited-stage disease, unfortunately.**

3. **The chemotherapies used for SCLC include etoposide, carboplatin, cisplatin, irinotecan, topotecan, vinblastine, vincristine, vinorelbine, cyclophosphamide, ifosfamide, doxorubicin, docetaxel, paclitaxel, and gemcitabine.**

Bronchial Carcinoma

Bronchial carcinoma originates from the respiratory epithelium of the bronchi, bronchioles, and alveoli. This malignant tumor is related to the inhalation of tobacco smoke in the vast majority of cases. Though sometimes described as a form of lung carcinoma, this form is discussed separately because of where it originates. *Bronchioloalveolar carcinoma* makes up approximately 3% of pulmonary malignancies. It is believed to start in the **type II pneumocytes** of the alveoli, growing slowly along the alveolar and bronchial wall.

Epidemiology

The prevalence and incidence of bronchial carcinoma are not well documented, partly because this form of cancer is not always documented with the word *bronchial*, and is often simply diagnosed as lung cancer. Most people with bronchial cancer are over age 65, and men are diagnosed slightly more often than women. In 90% of men and 80% of women, bronchial carcinoma is directly linked to cigarette smoking. Like lung cancer, African American men are at highest risk for bronchial cancer. Global statistics are poor for bronchial carcinoma, but estimated to be similar to the statistics available from the United States.

Etiology and Risk Factors

Smoking tobacco products is the primary cause of bronchial carcinoma. About 95% of cases occur in smokers or former smokers. Mutations of DNA occur because of the inhalation of carcinogens such as benzopyrene and tar. There is a direct link between the number of cigarettes smoked and deaths from bronchial cancer. The term *pack-year* has been previously used in this chapter, and should be understood as a year in which an individual smoked at least one pack of cigarettes per day. Therefore, smoking one pack of cigarettes per day for 40 years = 40 pack-years of smoking. If two packs were smoked per day for a 40-year period, it would equal 80 pack-years of smoking. Once a person is at 40 pack-years,

the risk of death from bronchial carcinoma is 60–70 times higher than for a person who does not smoke. If a person stops smoking, the risk for bronchial carcinoma decreases continuously over time. Risks for bronchial carcinoma, aside from smoking, include asbestos, polycyclic hydrocarbons, radon, chromates, nickel, inorganic arsenic compounds, and lung scarring from silicosis or tuberculosis.

Clinical Manifestations

Bronchial carcinomas are often found incidentally during imaging studies for other conditions. Symptoms are usually not severe, but when they develop, the carcinoma has become advanced. Common symptoms include hemoptysis, persistent cough, chest pain, shortness of breath, decreased appetite, unexplained weight loss, chronic bronchitis, and wheezing. Once the carcinoma has spread, there may be bone pain, jaundice, blood stools, or constipation.

Hilar tumors have endobronchial growth, which may result in bronchial stenosis. Then, emphysema may develop. If there is complete closure atelectasis, the patient is likely to develop retention-pneumonia. Abscesses may then form, which antibiotics may not be able to treat. Peripheral nodules may disintegrate into tumor cavities, causing typical hemoptysis. If these caverns collapse, malignant effusion or empyema results. Pancoast syndrome is defined by tumors at the lung apex, growing into the brachial plexus and vessels. **Stokes-collar** is an outbreak of tumors into the upper mediastinum, with relocation of the SVC, and upper inflow congestion. Diffuse bronchial carcinomas arise in alveolar tumors that can resemble pneumonia. *Bronchioloalveolar carcinomas* cause diffusion disorder with hypoxia and restrictive ventilatory disorder. There may be large amounts of mucous sputum.

Pathology

Bronchial carcinomas are of monoclonal origin, meaning that just one cell mutates into a tumor cell, and then multiplies. Dominant oncogenes activate these mutations, while tumor-suppressor genes deactivate them. The dominant oncogenes require a mutation of just one allele. Point mutations of the *KRAS* gene or *myelocytomatosis (MYC) family oncogenes* are present in bronchial carcinomas. Both alleles must be inactivated at tumor-suppressor genes for the mutation to be effective. The most common mutations occur in the *p53* and *retinoblastoma (RB)* genes. There may be a familial disposition for bronchial carcinoma if a tumor-suppressor allele has already mutated in the germline. Bronchial carcinomas express nicotine receptors. If these bind onto a cancer cell, they inhibit apoptosis, enabling growth of the cell. Therefore, patients with bronchial carcinoma must not smoke at all. Regardless of this requirement, about half of all patients with bronchial carcinoma are documented as smoking to some degree. Squamous dysplasia at the bronchus may evolve into squamous cell carcinoma of the lungs. Metastasis of a bronchial carcinoma will be to the regional lymph nodes, liver, adrenal glands, bones, and brain.

Diagnosis

Bronchial carcinomas have either small cell or non-small cell features, based on their biological behavior. The distinction will influence treatment and prognosis. *Bronchioloalveolar carcinoma* may be considered a form of adenocarcinoma, diagnosed from a papillary structure and broncho-alveolar pattern, with differentiated cellular mucin and glandular cells. When poorly differentiated cells are present, they have a micropapillary pattern, and are more aggressive. Bronchioloalveolar carcinoma grows along the alveoli, with no invasion. When it appears as hazy infiltrates in X-rays, appearing like consolidation, the carcinoma is less aggressive. These tumors are diagnosed via bronchoscopy and cytological examination. Localization and spread of the various bronchial carcinomas help to determine treatments. On CT, bronchial carcinomas may have significant homogeneous contrast enhancement, and less often, calcification (see Figure 5.10).

The staging of bronchial carcinoma, like cancers beginning in the lung lobes, uses the TNM system. This is summarized as follows:

- T1 – the tumor is 3 cm or smaller in diameter, surrounded by lung or visceral pleura that is distal to the main bronchus
- T2 – the tumor is larger than 3 cm in diameter or there is involvement of the main bronchus of 2 cm or more, distal to the carina, or related to atelectasis of the hilus, but not of the whole lung
- T3 – there is tumor invasion of the chest wall, diaphragm, mediastinal pleura, or pericardium, or there is a tumor in the main bronchus of less than 2 cm, distal to the carina, or atelectasis of the entire lung
- T4 – there is tumor invasion into the mediastinum, heart, large blood vessels, esophagus, spine or carina, or the intralobular tumor nodules or malignant pleural effusion
- N0 – no regional lymph node metastasis
- N1 – ipsilateral peribronchial or hilar lymph node involvement
- N2 – ipsilateral mediastinal lymph node or subcarinal lymph node involvement
- N3 – contralateral mediastinal lymph node, scalenes lymph node, or supraclavicular lymph node involvement
- M0 – no distant metastases
- M1 – distant metastases

Treatment

Treatments for bronchial carcinomas are varied based on the subtype, staging, and metastasis. The most commonly used treatments include surgery, chemotherapy, and radiation therapy. Surgery is performed when there is only one tumor or when the cancer has not spread to the nearby lymph nodes or beyond. Surgery, when indicated, usually has a relatively high success rate. Unfortunately, bronchial cancer has often already metastasized by the time it is diagnosed. Chemotherapy for bronchial cancer is usually given intravenously, but sometimes is orally administered. Radiation therapy may be used before or after surgery, or along with chemotherapy. Radiation therapy is most often used if the cancer has spread into the lymph nodes or brain, but can be used prior to this occurring.

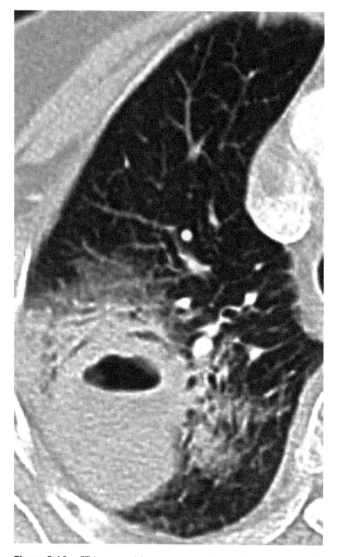

Figure 5.10 CT image, with contrast, of a bronchial carcinoma. *Source*: Pascoe et al. (2018).

Solitary bronchioloalveolar carcinomas can be surgically resected, but they are resistant to radiation therapy and chemotherapy.

Prevention and Early Detection

There is no known prevention for bronchial cancer, but stopping or avoiding smoking reduces the likelihood of its development. Other preventive measures include avoiding exposures to asbestos, arsenic-containing compounds, nickel dust, air pollution, radon, and some viruses. A diet rich in vitamins, such as from fruits and vegetables, is recommended. Preventing lung-scarring diseases such as tuberculosis is also helpful. Early detection of bronchial cancer is often not possible, and it is often found when a patient is being evaluated for COPD or chronic bronchitis. Screening may be performed for patients at high risk.

Prognosis

Overall, bronchial carcinoma has a poor prognosis and is often found after it is already extremely advanced, and no longer likely to be cured. Prognosis is improved for people who have never smoked, or for those who have quit. The five-year relative survival rate is only about 20.5% of patients. Unfortunately, only about 17% of patients are diagnosed when this cancer is localized. If still localized, the five-year relative survival rate is 59%. For regional disease, 31.7% will live for five years. For distant disease, only 5.8% will survive for five years.

Significant Point

Special types of bronchial carcinomas include bronchioloalveolar and semi-malignant tumors. Bronchioloalveolar carcinomas are also called bronchioalveolar carcinomas, and make up about 3% of all pulmonary malignancies. Bronchial adenomas are nearly always carcinoid tumors that progress from endocrine cells of the bronchial mucosa.

Clinical Case

1. What is death risk level in relation to bronchial carcinoma?
2. What are the common symptoms of bronchial carcinoma?
3. What is the prognosis for bronchial carcinoma?

A 72-year-old man with a 40 pack-year history of smoking went to his physician because of chronic bronchitis, which had not resolved over 2 months. He had begun coughing up a bloody sputum and was almost always short of breath. A chest X ray revealed a lesion on the right side of the carina. Bronchoscopy revealed a tumor that almost totally occluded the right mainstem bronchus, and a diagnosis of bronchial carcinoma was made. Specifically, the tumor was an adenocarcinoma. Surgery was decided against, and the patient was started on a chemotherapy regimen with adjuvant radiation therapy. He asked about enrolling in a clinical trial and was interested in trying experimental treatments, so he was put in touch with a clinical trial of nivolumab and ipilimumab for bronchial adenocarcinoma.

Answers:

1. **Once a person is at 40 pack-years of smoking, the risk of death from bronchial carcinoma is 60–70 times higher than for a person who does not smoke. If a person stops smoking, the risk for bronchial carcinoma decreases continuously over time.**
2. **The common symptoms of bronchial carcinoma include hemoptysis, persistent cough, chest pain, shortness of breath, decreased appetite, unexplained weight loss, chronic bronchitis, and wheezing.**
3. **Overall, bronchial carcinoma has a poor prognosis and is often found after it is already extremely advanced, and no longer likely to be cured. The five-year relative survival rate is only about 20.5% of patients.**

Carcinoid Tumors

Carcinoid tumors, also called **carcinoids** or *bronchial carcinoids*, develop from neuroendocrine cells in the pulmonary bronchi. However, carcinoids can also form in the gastrointestinal tract, pancreas, and genitourinary tract. Carcinoids are often benign or only locally invasive in these areas, but in the bronchus, they are often malignant. There may be endocrinological activity, based on their site of origin. This activity is less likely in tumors of the bronchi.

Epidemiology

Bronchial carcinoids make up only 1–2% of all lung cancers in adults. There are about 4,500 new diagnoses in the United States annually. Incidence is about 0.2 of every 100,000 people. These tumors affect patients most often between ages 40 and 70. For the typical bronchial carcinoids, average age at diagnosis is 45 years, but for the atypical subtype, it is 55 years. Women develop bronchial carcinoids just slightly more often than men. Caucasians develop them more than any other racial or ethnic group. The global prevalence of bronchial carcinoids is uncertain due to lack of documentation. Caucasians have more bronchial carcinoids globally, though individual statistics on a country-by-country basis are lacking.

Etiology and Risk Factors

The cause of bronchial carcinoids is not well understood. Some oncologists believe that these tumors may develop from small clusters of neuroendocrine cells and called *carcinoid tumorlets*. These tumorlets resemble carcinoid tumors but are much smaller – less than 5 cm across. They usually do not grow, but can evolve into carcinoid tumors. Risk factors for bronchial carcinoids include the female gender, Caucasian racial group, age over 40, multiple endocrine neoplasia type 1 (MEN1), and family history. Though typical bronchial carcinoids do not appear to be linked with smoking or exposure to chemicals, studies have found them to be more common in people that smoke.

Clinical Manifestations

About 50% of patients with bronchial carcinoids are asymptomatic. However, symptoms include dyspnea, wheezing, shortness of breath, and cough. Recurring chest pain – often when breathing deeply, hemoptysis, and pneumonia are often seen. Complications include paraneoplastic syndromes such as acromegaly due to ectopic growth hormone-releasing factor, Cushing's syndrome due to ectopic ACTH, and **Zollinger–Ellison syndrome** due to ectopic gastrin production. Less often, carcinoid syndrome develops, but only in less than 3% of cases of bronchial carcinoids. Symptoms of carcinoid syndrome include bronchospasm, diarrhea, wheezing, tachycardia, and flushing. Chronic sequelae include retroperitoneal fibrosis, right-sided valvular heart disease, and **telangiectasias**. In rare cases, a left-sided heart murmur develops because of serotonin-related valvular damage. The murmur may be described as mitral stenosis or regurgitation. There may be shortness of breath and weakness. If a large carcinoid causes partial or total blockage of an air passage, pneumonia can occur. The tumor may only be discovered after antibiotics are ineffective against the pneumonia, and additional evaluation is done. Bleeding from carcinoid tumors is rare but can be serious.

Pathology

Bronchial carcinoids grow slowly after arising from the bronchial mucosa. *Central carcinoids* form in the walls of the bronchi, and are the most common type. Nearly all central carcinoids are of the typical subtype. *Peripheral carcinoids* develop in the bronchioles, and are also usually of the typical subtype. The typical carcinoids grow slowly and rarely spread beyond the lungs. About 90% of all carcinoids are of the typical subtype. They do not appear to be pathologically influenced by smoking. Atypical carcinoids grow faster, and are more likely to spread to other organs. They have a large number of dividing cells and resemble other fast-growing tumors. Atypical carcinoids are more common in smokers than in non-smokers. When tumorlets are in the bronchi or bronchioles with an overgrowth of neuroendocrine cells, the condition is known as *diffuse idiopathic pulmonary neuroendocrine cell hyperplasia (DIPNECH)*. This can suggest that an actual bronchial carcinoid is likely to develop, though they can develop without DIPNECH.

Diagnosis

Diagnosis begins with medical history and physical examination. Because the symptoms of bronchial carcinoids mimic those of asthma, misdiagnoses often occur. Diagnosis is based on bronchoscopic biopsy, though an early chest CT can reveal tumor calcifications (see Figure 5.11). These calcifications are present in up to 33% of cases. However, bronchial brushing and washing techniques are not as helpful to diagnose carcinoids as they are for other types of lung cancer. Chest X-rays can be done, but small carcinoids do not always appear. If an imaging study reveals enlarged lymph nodes on either side of the trachea or in the carina,

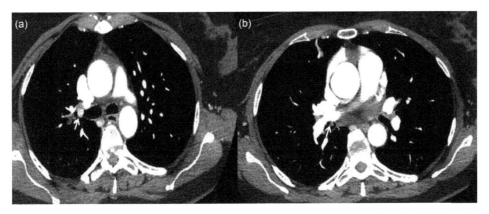

Figure 5.11 Contrast-enhanced CT showing (a) a vascularized round bronchial carcinoid with sub-occlusion of the upper right bronchus; (b) a triangular lesion on the intermedius bronchus. *Source*: Caterino et al.

endobronchial ultrasonography (EBUS) with biopsy can be performed to assess the nodes for cancer. A bronchoscope is fitted with an ultrasound transducer and passed through the trachea, using local anesthesia and light sedation. A hollow needle is passed through the bronchoscope to biopsy enlarged lymph nodes or abnormal tissues. Fine-needle aspiration or core biopsy methods are sometimes used. Passing the needle through the trachea or bronchi during bronchoscopy or EBUS does Transtracheal fine-needle aspiration or transbronchial fine-needle aspiration. Sometimes, a fine-needle aspiration biopsy is done during endoscopic esophageal ultrasound, with the scope passed down the esophagus instead of the trachea. The needle is then passed through the wall of the esophagus to biopsy the lymph nodes in the area. Diagnosis is supported by increased levels of urinary 5-hydroxyindoleacetic acid and serotonin, though in most cases these substances are not elevated. Blood tests can also reveal carcinoid-related features such as **chromogranin A**, cortisol, neuron-specific enolase, and substance P.

Treatment

Treatment for bronchial carcinoids is surgical resection, which may or may not be accompanied by adjuvant chemotherapy, radiation therapy, or both. For a bleeding tumor, such as after a biopsy is performed, drugs can be injected through a bronchoscope directly into the carcinoid to narrow its blood vessels or they can be sealed with a laser. Resectable carcinoids have not spread far beyond their site of origination, and can be completely removed. This is true for most stage I, II, and IIIA carcinoid tumors. Atypical carcinoids may require more extensive surgery than typical carcinoids, and nearby lymph nodes are also usually removed. If required, chemotherapy, radiation therapy, or both will be used as well.

However, some stage IIIA, and most stage IIIB and IV carcinoid tumors cannot be completely removed via surgery. Also, some people are simply not healthy enough to withstand surgery. For stage IIIA typical carcinoid tumors, radiation therapy is usually given, and radiation plus chemotherapy is given for atypical carcinoids. For stage IIIB and IV carcinoids, systemic treatments are often indicated, sometimes with radiation therapy. If a carcinoid tumor has spread to the liver and cannot be removed via standard surgery, a liver transplant is another option. If a liver metastasis is causing symptoms, ablation or hepatic artery embolization may be done, though these methods are unlikely to be curative. External radiation therapy also relieves bone pain. If the disease is more widespread, radioactive drugs may be successful.

Prevention and Early Detection

There is no known method of preventing bronchial carcinoids. Some studies have shown that atypical carcinoids are linked to smoking.

Therefore, quitting the habit or never starting it may reduce risks. There is no screening method for the early detection of bronchial carcinoids. However, people with MEN1 are at an increased risk, so physicians may recommend that these individuals have chest CT scans every 2–5 years. Since carcinoids usually grow and spread slowly, they are usually found at an early, localized stage, even if symptoms have persisted. Asymptomatic carcinoids are often found in an X-ray or CT scan done for another medical reason.

Prognosis

The prognosis of bronchial carcinoids depends on the actual type of tumor. For well-differentiated carcinoid tumors, the five-year survival rate is over 90%, but for poorly differentiated carcinoid tumors, it is only 50–70%. There is an overall five-year survival rate of 78–95%, and a 10-year survival rate of 77–90% for the typical carcinoid tumors. However, the overall five-year survival rate is 40–60% and the 10-year survival rate is 31–60% for the atypical carcinoid tumors.

Significant Point

Bronchial carcinoids are primary malignant neoplasms of the bronchi, bronchioles, and alveoli in the lungs. They arise from neuroectodermal cells, and are hormonally active. About 75% arise in the lobar bronchi, 15% in the periphery of the lung, and 10% in the mainstem bronchi. These tumors tend to spread locoregionally and should be resected by formal lobectomy if possible.

Clinical Case

1. What are the potential complications of bronchial carcinoid tumors?
2. What is the difference between central and peripheral bronchial carcinoid tumors?
3. What is the prognosis for the typical and atypical bronchial carcinoid tumors?

A 41-year-old woman was hospitalized because of recent history of persistent wheezing and coughing that were not related to any physical exertion. There had been a few episodes of hemoptysis. There was no significant family history. The patient had smoked for 10 pack-years but had quit at age 31, and consumed alcohol occasionally. Bronchoscopy revealed a tumor in the left main bronchus that completely occluded the lumen. A biopsy was performed, resulting in a diagnosis of a bronchial carcinoid tumor. Thoracic CT revealed the tumor to be about 22 mm in diameter, with very high enhancement after contrast medium was administered. Surgical resection of the tumor was performed, confirming the diagnosis. The patient was discharged within 10 days, and over several years of follow-up had no serious health problems or recurrence.

Answers:

1. **Complications of bronchial carcinoid tumors include paraneoplastic syndromes such as acromegaly due to ectopic growth hormone-releasing factor, Cushing's syndrome due to ectopic ACTH, and Zollinger–Ellison syndrome due to ectopic gastrin production. Less often, carcinoid syndrome develops, but only in less than 3% of cases of bronchial carcinoids.**
2. **Central carcinoid tumors originate in the walls of the bronchi, and are the most common type. Nearly all central carcinoids are of the typical subtype. Peripheral carcinoid tumors develop in the bronchioles, and are also usually of the typical subtype.**
3. **There is an overall five-year survival rate of 78–95%, and a 10-year survival rate of 77–90% for the typical bronchial carcinoid tumors. However, the overall 5-year survival rate is 40–60% and the 10-year survival rate is 31–60% for the atypical bronchial carcinoids.**

Mesothelioma

Mesothelioma is the only known cancer of the pleura. It is usually always caused by exposure to asbestos. The term *asbestos* actually refers to a group of natural silicates that are used in construction and many other industries because they resist heat and have strong structural properties. The three primary types of asbestos that are linked to mesothelioma include *amosite* (or *amphibole*, while has straight fibers), *chrysotile*, which has serpentine-like fibers, and *crocidolite*, which has very thin and sharp fibers. Use of asbestos is still not officially banned in the United States. However, the government has severely restricted its use since the 1970s. This means that incidence of mesothelioma likely has already peaked in the country. Today, most workers are exposed to asbestos when homes and buildings built before the 1980s are demolished or renovated. Occupations with high levels of asbestos exposure include mining, factory work, manufacturing or installing insulation, railroads, automotive manufacturing, shipbuilding, manufacturing of gas masks, plumbing, and construction.

Epidemiology

There are approximately 3,200 new cases of mesothelioma in the United States every year. Incidence rates were at their highest in the 1980s and 1990s, at 1.49 cases out of every 100,000 people. There is now about 1 new case per every 100,000 people. It is important to understand that people exposed to asbestos several decades before continued to develop the mesothelioma. Asbestos workers have as much as a 10% lifetime risk of developing mesothelioma. Most patients are diagnosed at age 65 or older, though people of ages 80–84 have the highest mesothelioma incidence (8.9 new cases per 100,000), followed by ages 85 and older (8.5 new cases per 100,000). Men are diagnosed in 75% of all cases. Women are, for some reason, nearly twice as likely to be diagnosed before age 65 as men. While African Americans have the same incidence rates as Caucasians before age 65, older African Americans have about half the incidence rate of Caucasians. There is another consideration – incidence by the *type* of mesothelioma, as follows:

- Pleural mesothelioma – 3.05 cases per 100,000
- Peritoneal mesothelioma – 0.21 cases per 100,000
- Pericardial mesothelioma – very rare
- Tunica vaginalis mesothelioma – very rare

The states with the highest mesothelioma incidence include: Alaska, New Jersey, Washington, Maine, West Virginia, Montana, California, Nevada, North Dakota, and Pennsylvania.

Globally, in many industrialized countries, workplace exposure to asbestos has already peaked, and is declining. Many countries banned mining, manufacturing, and use of asbestos-containing products. For example, all European Union countries have banned the importation, production, and use of asbestos or asbestos-containing products. Though *blue* and *brown* asbestos was banned in the United Kingdom in 1999, heavy use of brown asbestos is a factor in the highest rates of mesothelioma being seen in the United Kingdom and Australia. In 2017, there were 2,523 deaths from mesothelioma in the United Kingdom, and incidence rates nearly doubled between 1995 and 2017. In Australia in 2017, there were more than 700 new diagnoses of mesothelioma. Highest incidence rates were in Western Australia, with 4.9 cases per 100,000 people. Canada banned asbestos in 2018. Prior to that, incidence rates increased from 1.4 to 2.1 per 100,000 people. Developing countries that still use asbestos, and have increasing rates of exposure, include China, Kazakhstan, India, Russia, Mexico, Pakistan, Indonesia, and Thailand (see Figure 5.12). In many countries, accurate data on the use of asbestos and cases of mesothelioma are not available. Most affected people are over age 65, with men outnumbering women about 3:1. There is no specific racial or ethnic predilection.

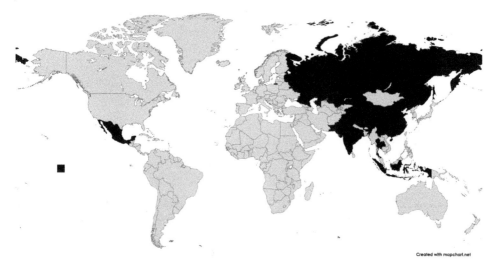

Figure 5.12 Countries with increasing rates of asbestos exposure.

Etiology and Risk Factors

The cause of mesothelioma is usually asbestos exposure, and this is independent of whether an individual smokes or not. Approximately 8 out of 10 people with mesothelioma have been exposed to asbestos. In some studies, radiation treatments for other types of cancer have been linked to mesothelioma. This is because radiation can also damage cellular DNA and result in unregulated cell growth. Risk factors for mesothelioma include asbestosis and lung cancers. Risks are related to the amount of asbestos exposure and the length of time exposed. There may be genetic factors related to mesothelioma. Other risk factors include exposure to minerals called **zeolites**, such as erionite, aging, male gender, and a rare mutation of the *ubiquitin carboxy-terminal hydrolase (BAP1)* gene.

Clinical Manifestations

Most patients with mesothelioma have dyspnea and non-pleuritic chest pain. When a patient presents for evaluation, constitutional symptoms are usually not seen. When there is invasion of other nearby structures, this may result in hoarseness, severe pain, dysphagia, brachial plexopathy, or Horner syndrome. Pleural mesothelioma may cause pleural effusion. Peritoneal mesothelioma may cause ascites. Pericardial mesothelioma may cause pericardial effusion. All of these conditions may be found during physical examination, or auscultation. Additional signs and symptoms of pleural mesothelioma include pain in the side of the chest or lower back, coughing, shortness of breath, and swelling of the face and arms. Peritoneal mesothelioma may cause abdominal pain, constipation, nausea, vomiting, and ascites. Pericardial mesothelioma may cause chest pain, heart murmur, irregular heart rhythm, and shortness of breath. The general symptoms of mesothelioma can also include excessive sweating, fever, fatigue, unintended weight loss, blood clots, and loss of appetite.

Pathology

In asbestos workers, mesothelioma usually takes 25–30 years to develop. Mesothelioma arises from the mesothelial surface of the pleural cavity. It can spread locally or metastasize to the hilar and mediastinal lymph nodes, diaphragm, pericardium, liver, peritoneum, adrenal glands, kidneys, and in rare cases, to the tunica vaginalis of the testis. The breathing in of asbestos fibers allows them to travel to the ends of small air passages, and reach the pleura, causing inflammation and scarring. This can result in damage to cellular DNA, and in changes that cause uncontrolled cell growth. When fibers are swallowed, they can reach the lining of the abdomen, and play a part in the development of peritoneal mesothelioma.

However, some people that are exposed to asbestos, even significantly, never develop mesothelioma. Over 50% of mesotheliomas have epithelioid cells, which offers a better prognosis than the other types. Approximately 10–20% of mesotheliomas have sarcomatoid cells, also described as *fibrous*. The remaining 20–30% of mesotheliomas are called mixed (biphasic), and have epithelioid and sarcomatoid areas.

Diagnosis

Diagnosis begins with medical history and physical examination, imaging, blood tests, and pleural biopsy or fluid cytology. The pleural form of mesothelioma is found in more than 90% of all cases. The disease appears in X-rays as diffuse unilateral or bilateral thickening of the pleura, with the lungs appearing to be encased. This usually causes the **costophrenic angles** to appear blunted. There may be calcium deposits on the pleura, fluid between the lungs and chest wall, or actual lung changes. In 95% of patients, there are pleural effusions that are usually hemorrhagic, large in size, and unilateral. Increased levels of **hyaluronidase** in the pleural fluid suggest mesothelioma but are not diagnostic. When diagnosis is not confirmed a biopsy by video-assisted thoracoscopic surgery (VATS) or thoracotomy is performed. Positive tumor markers include soluble mesothelin-related proteins that are released into the serum by mesothelial cells. However, these have a high false-positive rate. Based on the location of any present fluid, it is removed by either thoracentesis, paracentesis, or pericardiocentesis. If a needle biopsy is performed for mesothelioma, it is extremely important that a large enough sample is taken to make an accurate diagnosis, often with a more invasive biopsy method. Risks of needle biopsy include pneumothorax and a collapsed lung.

Endoscopic biopsies are commonly needed for diagnosing mesothelioma. In thoracoscopy, a thoracoscope can see inside the pleura and biopsy tissues. It is performed under general anesthesia and also allows the removal of lymph nodes and fluid. It can also be used as part of pleurodesis, to keep fluid from building up in the chest. In laparoscopy, a laparoscope is used to examine the abdomen and biopsy tumor tissues, also under general anesthesia. If imaging suggests that mesothelioma may have spread to the lymph nodes between the lungs, an endoscope is used to perform a mediastinoscopy under general anesthesia. This procedure also allows for biopsies. In endobronchial ultrasound needle biopsy, a bronchoscope with an ultrasound device in its tip is passed down into the trachea to assess nearby lymph nodes and take biopsy samples. This can be done under general anesthesia, or with local anesthesia and light sedation. When an endoscopic biopsy is insufficient for diagnosis, open surgical biopsy can be performed. Sometimes, removal of the entire tumor is indicated.

Staging is based on chest CT, mediastinoscopy, and MRI. CT imaging allows the fissures of the tumors to be visualized (see Figure 5.13). The CT

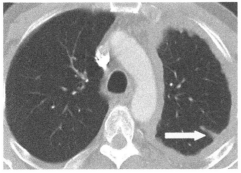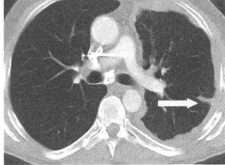

Figure 5.13 CT imaging of pleural mesothelioma involving both the mediastinal and parietal pleura. The arrows show fissural involvement of disease. *Source*: Courtesy: Norbet et al. (2015). Reproduced with permission from Elsevier.

and MRI techniques are almost equally sensitive and specific for mesothelioma. However, MRI helps to assess tumor extension into the chest wall, diaphragm, mediastinal structures, spinal cord, or spine. A PET scan may be preferred to visualize benign from malignant thickening of the pleura. This scan is also useful for assessing possible spread of the disease. A PET/CT scan allows comparison of areas of higher radioactivity with detailed CT images. Bronchoscopy can exclude concurrent endobronchial lung cancers. An echocardiogram may be performed if a pericardial effusion is suspected.

The stages of malignant pleural mesothelioma are listed as follows:

- *Stage IA* – T1, N0, M0 – mesothelioma in the pleura lining the chest wall on one side; may or may not affect the pleura lining the diaphragm, mediastinum, or pleura covering the lung; no spread to nearby lymph nodes or distant metastasis.
- *Stage IB* – T2, N0, M0 – mesothelioma in the pleura lining the chest wall on one side, and in the pleura coating the diaphragm, mediastinum, and lung; there is growth into the diaphragm or lung itself; no spread to nearby lymph nodes or distant metastasis, OR: mesothelioma has grown into nearby structures but still may be resectable; it is in the pleura lining the chest wall on one side, and in the pleura coating the lung, diaphragm, and mediastinum on the same side; it has grown into at least one of these: **endothoracic fascia**, fatty tissue in mediastinum, one place in deeper chest wall, or surface of the pericardium; no spread to nearby lymph nodes or distant metastasis.
- *Stage II* – T1 or T2, N1, M0 – mesothelioma is in the pleura lining the chest wall on one side; it may have grown into the diaphragm or lung itself; it has spread to nearby lymph nodes on the same side as the main tumor; no distant metastasis.
- *Stage IIIA* – T3, N1, M0 – mesothelioma has grown into nearby structures but may still be resectable; it is in the pleura lining the chest wall on onside side, and in the pleura coating

the lung, diaphragm, and mediastinum on the same side; it has also grown into at least one of these: endothoracic fascia, fatty tissue in mediastinum, one place in deeper chest wall, or surface of the pericardium; it has spread to nearby lymph nodes on the same side as the primary tumor; no distant metastasis.
- *Stage IIIB* – T1 to T3, N2, M0 – mesothelioma may or may not have grown into nearby structures, may still be resectable; has spread to nearby lymph nodes on opposite side, or to supraclavicular lymph nodes on either side; no distant metastasis, OR: mesothelioma can no longer be resected; it is in the pleura lining the chest wall on onside side, and in the pleura coating the lung, diaphragm, and mediastinum on the same side; it has also grown into at least one of these: more than one place in deeper chest wall including muscle or ribs, through diaphragm and into peritoneum, any organ in mediastinum, spine, across pleura to other side of chest, through pericardium or into the heart itself; it may or may not have spread to nearby lymph nodes; no distant metastasis.
- *Stage IV* – any T, any N, M1; mesothelioma may or may not have grown into nearby structures, may or may not have spread to nearby lymph nodes; it has spread to distant organs (bones, liver, opposite lung or pleura, peritoneum).

A simplified illustration of the staging of pleural mesothelioma is shown in Figure 5.14. Note that other abbreviations are also used, and include the following:

- TX = primary tumor cannot be evaluated because of insufficient information
- T0 = no evidence of a primary tumor
- NX = nearby lymph nodes cannot be evaluated because of insufficient information

Treatment

Surgical options include removal of the pleura, ipsilateral lung, hemidiaphragm, phrenic nerve, and pericardium. This may be combined with chemotherapy or radiation therapy, but survival

Stage Ia   Stage II

Stage III   Stage IV

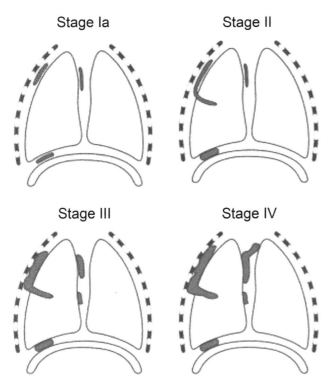

Figure 5.14 Simplified pictorial representation of pleural mesothelioma staging. *Source*: Oh and Chari [45]. Courtesy: https://www.mesothelioma.com/mesothelioma/stages).

time and prognosis are seldom improved. The primary focus of treatment is supportive care and relief of dyspnea and pain. Radiation therapy is usually not effective for local pain or needle-tract metastases because the disease is so diffuse. Radiation is also not usually used for treating nerve root pain. To reduce dyspnea from pleural effusions, pleurectomy or pleurodesis can be performed. Sufficient pain relief is difficult to achieve. In most cases, transdermal opioids and opioids via **indwelling epidural catheters** are required. Most stage I and II mesotheliomas, and some stage III mesotheliomas, may be resectable. Most physicians believe that only the epithelioid and mixed/ biphasic tumors can be resected. Unfortunately for many mesotheliomas, some cancer cells are left behind after surgery, and recurrence is common.

Suffering and deaths are more common with extrapleural pneumonectomy, but it may be able to remove all of the cancer from the patient. It is usually indicated for resectable epithelioid mesothelioma that has not spread to the lymph nodes. The lung on the side of the cancer is removed, along with the pleura lining the chest wall on that side, the diaphragm on that side. Approximately 33% of patients have major complications after surgery. These include bleeding, blood clots, changes in heart rhythm, wound infections, fluid build-up in the chest, pneumonia, and loss of lung function. The patient will have only limited activities after the surgery since the ribs often must be spread during the procedure.

Prevention and Early Detection
The only methods of prevention of mesothelioma are to use all protective equipment and safety procedures designed for working with asbestos. Air tests can be performed to assess levels of asbestos in a structure prior to any work

being done within it. There are experienced contractors available that can remove asbestos from buildings in a safe manner. There are no screening guidelines for mesothelioma in people that are exposed to asbestos. Serum biomarkers may have the ability to assist in diagnosis and monitoring, but are not yet proven. While early detection is difficult, for anyone known to have been exposed to asbestos, regular imaging tests, including chest X-rays or CT scans, may be performed to look for signs of mesothelioma or lung cancer. It is uncertain about how useful these methods are for finding mesothelioma early in its course of development. The disease is usually detected when a person goes to a physician because of chest pain or shortness of breath.

Prognosis

Since mesothelioma is incurable, long-term survival is rare. Most surgeries or other treatments do not greatly change prognosis or survival time. From the time of diagnosis, median survival time is 9–12 months, based on tumor location and cell type. Imaging and histopathologic staging provides the most accurate prognosis. The worst prognosis is for patients over age 75 with poor performance status, chest pain, lactate dehydrogenase levels over 500 units per liter, non-epithelial histology, and a platelet count over 400,000 per microliter. Additional factors linked to longer survival and a better prognosis include being female and of a younger age, being able to carry out normal tasks of daily living, and normal blood cells.

Significant Point

Mesothelioma is a rare and aggressive cancer caused mostly by asbestos exposure. The pleural and peritoneal subtypes are by far the most common. Life expectancy has increased due to more research, but most patients die within 18 months of diagnosis. Pleural mesothelioma causes symptoms that are similar to those of more common illnesses of the respiratory system, which may be mistaken for influenza or pneumonia.

Clinical Case

1. How common is mesothelioma in the United States today?
2. What are the clinical manifestations of pleural mesothelioma?
3. As in this case, how common is epithelioid mesothelioma?

A 66-year-old man who had worked in the construction industry, refurbishing old houses, went to the hospital because of chest and back discomfort. A chest X-ray, CT scan, and PET scan found right-sided pleural effusion with thickening of the pleura around the effusion. The diagnosis was of epithelioid mesothelioma of the right pleura. An extended pleurectomy was performed with adjuvant chemotherapy (pemetrexed + cisplatin), to improve the patient's survival time and quality of life. Additionally, IMRT was used over six weeks, because early clinical studies have indicated its ability to aid in treatment. After the radiation therapy, the patient complained of chest pain, shortness of breath, nausea, and lack of appetite. This eventually resolved. However, CT scans every 3 months, over 2.5 years, revealed that the disease was in remission, with no recurrence. This is remarkable considered that most cases of mesothelioma are fatal in much less time.

Answers:

1. **There are not about 3,200 new cases of mesothelioma in the United States every year. There is now about 1 new case per every 100,000 people.**
2. **Pleural mesothelioma causes pleural effusion, pain in the side of the chest or lower back, coughing, shortness of breath, dysphagia, hoarseness, and swelling of the face and arms.**
3. **Over 50% of mesotheliomas have epithelioid cells, which offers a better prognosis than the other types.**

Key Terms

Atelectasis	Oncolytic virotherapy
Carcinoids	Pancoast tumor
Carina	Paraneoplastic syndrome
Chromogranin A	Pericardiocentesis
Costophrenic angles	Plethora
Dyskeratosis congenita	Pleurodesis
Eaton–Lambert syndrome	Pneumonectomy
Endothoracic fascia	Stokes-collar
Field carcinogenesis	Subcarinal
Indwelling epidural catheters	Telangiectasias
Laryngeal cancer	Trousseau syndrome
Mesothelioma	Type II pneumocytes
Nasopharyngeal angiofibromas	Zeolites
Nasopharyngeal carcinoma	Zollinger–Ellison syndrome
Nasopharyngeal hemangiomas	

Bibliography

1 Agrawal, A. and Rangarajan, V. (2018). *PET/CT in Lung Cancer (Clinicians' Guides to Radionuclide Hybrid Imaging – PET/CT)*. New York: Springer.

2 American Cancer Society. (2018). *The American Cancer Society's Oncology in Practice – Clinical Management*. Hoboken: Wiley-Blackwell. Figure 1.2 from Page 8.

3 American Lung Association. (2020). *Lung Cancer Fact Sheet*. https://www.lung.org/lung-health-diseases/lung-disease-lookup/lung-cancer/resource-library/lung-cancer-fact-sheet Accessed 2021.

4 American Lung Association. (2020). *State of Lung Cancer 2020*. https://www.lung.org/research/state-of-lung-cancer Accessed 2021.

5 Anttila, S. and Boffetta, P. (2020). *Occupational Cancers*, 2nd Edition. New York: Springer.

6 Attanoos, R.L., Allen, T.C., Galateau-Salle, F., and Gibbs, A. (2013). *Advances in Surgical Pathology: Mesothelioma*. Philadelphia: Lippincott, Williams, & Wilkins.

7 Baldeyrou, P.P., Hanna, A., and Crutu, A. (2018). *Normal and Pathological Bronchial Semiology: A Visual Approach*. Cambridge: Academic Press.

8 Bates, M. and Sellors, T.H. (2013). *Bronchial Carcinoma: An Integrated Approach to Diagnosis and Management*. New York: Springer.

9 Busson, P. (2013). *Nasopharyngeal Carcinoma: Keys for Translational Medicine and Biology (Advances in Experimental Medicine and Biology, 778)*. New York: Springer.

10 Cagle, P.T., Allen, T.C., Beasley, M.B., Chirieac, L.R., Dacic, S., Borczuk, A.C., Kerr, K.M., Sholl, L.M., Portier, B., and Bernicker, E.H. (2017). *Precision Molecular Pathology of Lung Cancer (Molecular Pathology Library)*, 2nd Edition. New York: Springer.

11 Castelijns, J.A., Snow, G.B., and Valk, J. (2012). *MR Imaging of Laryngeal Cancer (Series in Radiology Book 2)*. New York: Springer.

12 Ceresoli, G.L., Bombardieri, E., and D'Incalci, M. (2019). *Mesothelioma: From Research to Clinical Practice*. New York: Springer.

13 Chahinian, A.P., Robinson, B.W.S., and Dunitz, M. (2007). *Mesothelioma*. London: Dunitz.

14 Dedivitis, R., Peretti, G., Hanna, E., and Cernea, C.R. (2019). *Laryngeal Cancer (Clinical Case-Based Approaches)*. Stuttgart: Thieme.

15 Downey, R. (2020). *Lung Cancer: Advances in Diagnosis and Treatment*. Forest Hills: Foster Academics.

16 Downey, R. (2020). *Lung Cancer: Clinical Progress*. New York: Hayle Medical.

17 Farver, C., Fraire, A.E., Cagle, P.T., and Tomashefski, J.F., Jr. (2008). *Dail and Hammar's Pulmonary Pathology Volume II: Neoplastic Lung Disease*, 3rd Edition. New York: Springer.

18 Farver, C., Ghosh, S., Gildea, T., and Sturgis, C.D. (2020). *Pulmonary Disease: Pathology, Radiology, Bronchoscopy*. New York: Springer.

19 Fossella, F.V., Putnam, Jr., J.B., Komaki, R., Cox, J.D., and Hong, W.K. (2003). *Lung Cancer (M.D. Anderson Cancer Care Series)*. New York: Springer.

20 Gerald, L.B. and Berry, C.E. (2016). *Health Disparities in Respiratory Medicine*. Totowa: Humana Press.

21 Giordano, A. and Franco, R. (2019). *Malignant Pleural Mesothelioma: A Guide for Clinicians*. Cambridge: Academic Press.

22 Harris, L. (2013). *Geriatric Chest Disease*. Oxford: Butterworth-Heinemann.

23 Hasse, J. and Telger, T.C. (2012). *Surgical Treatment of Bronchial Carcinoma: Screening Methods, Early and Late Results*. New York: Springer.

24 Hayat, M.A. (2008). *Methods of Cancer Diagnosis, Therapy and Prognosis: General Methods and Overviews, Lung Carcinoma and Prostate Carcinoma*. Vol. 2. New York: Springer.

25 Hesdorfffer, M. and Bates-Pappas, G.E. (2019). *Caring for Patients with Mesothelioma: Principles and Guidelines*. New York: Springer.

26 Huang, Y.C.T., Ghio, A.J., and Maier, L.A. (2012). *A Clinical Guide to Occupational and Environmental Lung Diseases (Respiratory Medicine Book 6)*. Totowa: Humana Press.

27 Jones, K.D. and Hornick, J.L. (2020). *Pulmonary Pathology, an Issue of Surgical Pathology Clinics (The Clinics: Surgery, Volume 13–1)*. Amsterdam: Elsevier.

28 Journal of Medical Imaging and Radiation Oncology. (2018). *CT scan revealing adenocarcinoma presenting as solid lesions, in 3 views*. https://onlinelibrary.wiley.com/doi/full/10.1111/1754-9485.12779. Figure 2. Accessed 2021.

29 Journal of Medical Imaging and Radiation Oncology. (2018). *CT image, with contrast, of a bronchial carcinoma*. https://onlinelibrary.wiley.com/doi/full/10.1111/1754-9485.12779. Figure 8. Accessed 2021.

30. Kalemkerian, G.P., Donington, J.S., Gore, E.M., and Ramalingam, S.S. (2016). *Handbook of Lung Cancer and Other Thoracic Malignancies*. New York: Demos Medical.

31 Kirchner, J. (2011). *Chest Radiology: A Resident's Manual*. Stuttgart: Thieme.

32 Kiselevskiy, M.V., Abdulaev, A.G., and Davydov, M.M. (2019). *Malignant Mesothelioma and Pseudomyxoma*. New York: Springer.

33 Kloecker, G., Fraig, M., Arnold, S.M., and Perez, C.A. (2020). *Lung Cancer: Standards of Care*. New York: McGraw-Hill Education/Medical.

34 Latif-Hamdan, A., Sataloff, R.T., and Hawkshaw, M.J. (2020). *Non-Laryngeal Cancer and Voice*. San Diego: Plural Publishing, Inc.

35 Lee, A.W.M., Lung, M.L., and Ng, W.T. (2019). *Nasopharyngeal Carcinoma: From Etiology to Clinical Practice*. Cambridge: Academic Press.

36 Marcu, L.G., Toma-Dasu, I., Dasu, A., and Mercke, C. (2018). *Radiotherapy and Clinical Radiobiology of Head and Neck Cancer (Series in Medical Physics and Biomedical Engineering)*. Boca Raton: CRC Press.

37 Martinet, Y., Hirsch, F.R., Mulshine, J., and Vignaud, J.M. (2012). *Clinical and Biological Basis of Lung Cancer Prevention (Respiratory Pharmacology and Pharmacotherapy)*. Basel: Birkhauser.

38 Mehta, A. and Jain, P. (2013). *Interventional Bronchoscopy: A Clinical Guide (Respiratory Medicine Book 10)*. Totowa: Humana Press.

39 Moreira, A.L. and Saqi, A. (2014). *Diagnosing Non-small Cell Carcinoma in Small Biopsy and Cytology*. New York: Springer.

40 MSD Manual – Professional Version. (2020). *Lung Carcinoma (Lung Cancer) – Genetic*

Factors. https://www.msdmanuals.com/professional/pulmonary-disorders/tumors-of-the-lungs/lung-carcinoma Accessed 2021.

41 Nakano, T. and Kijima, T. (2020). *Malignant Pleural Mesothelioma: Advances in Pathogenesis, Diagnosis, and Treatments (Respiratory Disease Series: Diagnostic Tools and Disease Managements.* New York: Springer.

42 National Library of Medicine, National Center for Biotechnology Information. (2020). *Updates on larynx cancer epidemiology (Chin J Cancer Research).* 32(1): 18–25. https://pubmed.ncbi.nlm.nih.gov/32194301

43 Oh, W. and Chari, A. (2019). *Mount Sinai Expert Guides – Oncology – Potential Pitfalls/common Mistakes, Clinical Pearls, Management Algorithms, Evidence-based Guidelines.* New York: Icahn School of Medicine at Mount Sinai/Wiley Blackwell. Figure (Algorithm) 6.1 from Page 69.

44 Oh, W. and Chari, A. (2019). *Mount Sinai Expert Guides – Oncology – Potential Pitfalls/common Mistakes, Clinical Pearls, Management Algorithms, Evidence-based Guidelines.* New York: Icahn School of Medicine at Mount Sinai/Wiley Blackwell. Figure 7.2 from Page 87.

45 Oh, W. and Chari, A. (2019). *Mount Sinai Expert Guides – Oncology – Potential Pitfalls/common Mistakes, Clinical Pearls, Management Algorithms, Evidence-based Guidelines.* New York: Icahn School of Medicine at Mount Sinai/Wiley Blackwell. Figure 7.1 from Page 87.

46 Oury, T.D., Sporn, T.A., and Roggli, V.L. (2014). *Pathology of Asbestos-Associated Diseases,* 3rd Edition. New York: Springer.

47 Pass, H.I., Vogelzang, N., and Carbone, M. (2005). *Malignant Mesothelioma: Pathogenesis, Diagnosis, and Translational Therapies.* New York: Springer.

48 Popper, H., Murer, B., and Moinfar, F. (2020). *Pulmonary Pathology: A Practical Guide (Essentials of Diagnostic Pathology).* New York: Springer.

49 Respirology Case Reports. (2020). *Contrast-enhanced CT showing a bronchial carcinoid and a triangular lesion on the intermedius bronchus.* https://onlinelibrary.wiley.com/doi/full/10.1002/rcr2.585. Figure 1. Accessed 2021.

50 Scarantino, C.W., Choplin, R.H., Faulkner II, C.S., Kovacs, C.J., Mann, S.G., O'Connor, T., and Richards II, F. (2012). *Diagnostic Procedures and Therapeutic Management with Special Reference to Radiotherapy (Medical Radiology).* New York: Springer.

51 Scott, W.J. (2018). *Lung Cancer: From Diagnosis to Treatment,* 3rd Edition. Omaha: Addicus Books.

52 Stockley, R. (2012). *Molecular Biology of the Lung: Volume II: Asthma and Cancer (Respiratory Pharmacology and Pharmacotherapy).* Basel: Birkhauser.

53 Testa, J.R. (2017). *Asbestos and Mesothelioma (Current Cancer Research).* New York: Springer.

54 Verna, O. and Sharma, A. (2019). *Essentials of Lung Cancer: With Orthodox and Alternative Treatments.* Lucknow (India): Verna.

55 Warner, C. (2020). *Lung Cancer: Evaluation and Management.* New York: Hayle Medical.

56 Wiley Online Library – Thoracic Cancer. (2020). *Effect of nintedanib on non-small cell lung cancer in a patient with idiopathic pulmonary fibrosis: A case report and literature review.*11 (6): 1720–1723. https://onlinelibrary.wiley.com/doi/full/10.1111/1759-7714.13437

57 World Cancer Research Fund, American Institute for Cancer Research. (2018). *Lung cancer statistics – Lung cancer is the most common cancer worldwide.* https://www.wcrf.org/dietandcancer/cancer-trends/lung-cancer-statistics Accessed 2021.

58 Zhang, C. and Myers, J.L. (2018). *Atlas of Lung Pathology (Atlas of Anatomic Pathology).* New York: Springer.

6

Digestive Tumors

OUTLINE

Oral and Oropharyngeal Cancer

Oral cancer occurs between the **vermilion border** of the lips, the point at which the hard and soft palates meet, or the posterior 1/3 of the tongue. Most cases of *oral squamous cell carcinoma* are related to use of alcohol, tobacco, or both. Early in the disease course, the lesions are asymptomatic and curable, so the prevention of deaths from oral cancer can be achieved by early screening. *Oropharyngeal squamous cell carcinoma* affects the tonsil, base of the tongue, posterior 1/3 of the tongue, soft palate, and the posterior and lateral walls of the pharynx. The major risk factors are again alcohol and tobacco use, though the human papillomavirus (HPV) is now recognized as the cause of most of these tumors.

Epidemiology

In the United States, oral squamous cell carcinoma is diagnosed in about 34,000 people annually. About 10.5 adults per 100,000 develop oral cancer during their lifetimes. Most cases occur in people who are age 50 or older. There is a slight male prevalence, with this oral cancer being present in 3% of male cancer patients, and in 2% of female cancer patients, out of cancers of all types. Squamous cell carcinoma is the most common type of oral cancer. There appears to be no racial or ethnic predilection for oral cancer. The global prevalence of oral cancers was over 750,000 new cases in 2018. Incidence was the highest in the country of Papua New Guinea with 20.4 cases out of every 100,000 population – this figure along with those of other countries is shown in Figure 6.1.

Global Epidemiology of Cancer: Diagnosis and Treatment, First Edition. Jahangir Moini,
Nicholas G. Avgeropoulos, and Craig Badolato.
© 2022 John Wiley & Sons Ltd. Published 2022 by John Wiley & Sons Ltd.

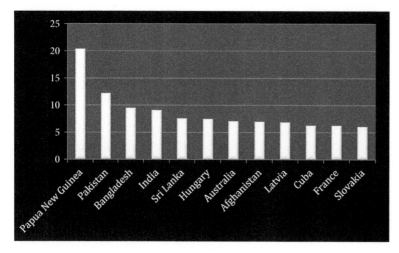

Figure 6.1 Countries with the highest rates of oral cancer, in cases out of every 100,000 people.

Globally, the peak ages of patients with oral cancer are between 60 and 70 years. As in the United States, the prevalence of oral cancer is slightly higher in men in comparison with women. There is no specific racial or ethnic predilection.

As of 2018 in the United States, there were more than 17,500 new cases of oropharyngeal cancer. However, estimates by the American Cancer Society are that over 53,300 people will develop either oropharyngeal or oral cancers annually. This is about 14.1 of every 100,000 people. Though incidence rates are increasing, rates of curative treatments are also higher than ever before. The median age of diagnosis is 57 years, though there are peaks at age 30 and age 55. The male-to-female ratio of oropharyngeal cancer is 3:1. However, oropharyngeal cancer that is not related to the human papillomavirus is more common in older men, with a median age of 61. The global prevalence of oropharyngeal cancers is estimated at over 500,000 cases annually, with over 290,000 deaths. Global incidence of oropharyngeal cancer was the highest in Cuba, with 9 cases out of every 100,000 people. The majority of affected individuals are over age 43, with men predominating. People from countries with a predominant Caucasian population have the highest rates of oropharyngeal cancers, most of which were associated with HPV, of 9.4 men per 100,000 and 1.8 women per 100,000. The lowest rates were found in people from Pacific Island nations.

Etiology and Risk Factors

The causes of oral cancer include smoking or chewing tobacco, drinking alcohol, chronic mouth irritation such as dental caries, using mouthwash excessively, or chewing **betel quid**, which is most common outside of the United States in southern Asia. Having oral–genital contact, which may spread the oral human papillomavirus (HPV) may be causative for some oral cancers, but HPV is not linked with oral cancer as much as it is with oropharyngeal cancer. Sun exposure can also develop cancer on the external surfaces of the lips. The chief risk factors for oral squamous cell carcinoma are drinking alcohol, and smoking – in most cases, more than two packs of cigarettes per day. For alcohol use, the risks are much higher if a person drinks more than 36 ounces of beer, more than 15 ounces of wine, or more than 6 ounces of distilled liquor per day. When alcohol is combined with smoking, the risks for oral cancer are 100 times higher in women and 38 times high in men.

Oropharyngeal cancer is mostly caused (60%) by HPV type 16. Numbers of sexual partners and participation in oral–genital sex are both implicated. If a patient has HPV, the risk for oropharyngeal cancer is about 16 times higher. Overall, the various types of HPV cause 70–80% of oropharyngeal cancers in many countries. Patients that drink 4 or more alcoholic beverages per day have a 7-times higher risk for this cancer, and patients that smoke 1.5 packs of cigarettes or more per day have a 3-times higher risk. If they drink alcohol and smoke heavily, there may be a 30-times higher risk.

Clinical Manifestations

At first, oral lesions are asymptomatic, and good oral screening can often detect them early. Dental professionals routinely examine the mouth and oropharynx as part of regular care. If there is an abnormal area or areas, a brush biopsy may be performed. The lesions may be areas of **leukoplakia** or **erythroplakia**. They may be ulcerated or **exophytic**. If oral cancer is present, it often is **indurated**, firm, and has a border described as having a "rolled" appearance. When the lesions grow, manifestations may include **dysarthria, dysphagia**, and pain. Lesions that appear on the middle tongue and buccal or gingival surfaces are often from tobacco and similar products contacting the mucosa for long periods of time. Anterior tongue cancers are usually due to smoking. Manifestations of oral cancer include: a painful mass or ulcer, a painless lump, or mucosal thickening. Small lesions on the lateral tongue may cause pain that is referred to the gums, mandible, and ear due to the sharing of sensory nerves. If the speech becomes affected, it may be from a tumor restricting motion of the tongue or cranial nerve XII dysfunction. If a tumor is in the gingiva, it can loosen teeth and invade the mandible near the tooth sockets. Tumors of the tonsil or base of the tongue may cause localized pain and referred ear pain. They are often asymptomatic, however, and can become very large before causing speech changes, **globus, trismus**, or restricted tongue movements. These

tumors may occur as solid or cystic neck masses. Oral cavity tumors spread to the submandibular and **submental** lymph nodes, usually in an orderly fashion, and to the midcervical nodes.

Oropharyngeal cancer symptoms can be varied, but usually, they include dysphagia, sore throat, dysarthria, **odynophagia**, and **otalgia**. The patient may develop extreme fatigue, loss of appetite and nausea, reduced taste sensations, **xerostomia**, weight loss, and flu-like symptoms. Often, there is a neck mass that in many patients is cystic. Unfortunately, since symptoms are similar to those of upper respiratory infections, diagnosis may be delayed by many months.

Pathology

Approximately 40% of intraoral squamous cell carcinomas start to form on the mouth floor, or on the tongue's lateral or ventral surfaces. About 38% of oral squamous cell carcinomas develop on the lower lip, and are usually related to sun exposure on the external lip surfaces. These cancers develop because of unregulated proliferation of mucous basal cells. One precursor cell is transformed into a clone that consists of many daughter cells with an accumulation of oncogenes. The pathology of oropharyngeal cancer involves three processes. First, the cancer invades the surrounding normal tissues. Then, it invades the lymphatic system, traveling through the lymph vessels to reach other body sites. Finally, it invades the veins and capillaries, traveling through the blood to other sites. At stage 0 (carcinoma in situ), abnormal cells are within the lining of the oropharynx. At stage 1, cancer has formed but not spread. At stage 2, the cancer has enlarged but still not spread. By stage 3, the cancer may or may not have spread to one adjacent lymph node. By stage 4, it has spread to one or more of many tissues near the oropharynx as well as one or more nearby lymph nodes. After this point, the pathological processes have become severe.

Diagnosis

Suspicious areas of the oral cavity must be biopsied. Brush biopsy or incisional biopsy is done based on the surgical preference. For all patients with oral cancer, direct laryngoscopy and esophagoscopy are performed so that a concurrent secondary primary cancer can be excluded from the diagnosis. Common procedures also include head and neck computed tomography (CT) scans and chest X-rays. Today, positron emission tomography with CT scan (PET/CT) is becoming more common for better evaluation of oral cancers. An MRI scan is useful for tumors of the base of the tongue and parapharyngeal spaces.

Oropharyngeal cancer patients first should have a direct laryngoscopy and biopsy to evaluate a primary lesion and search for secondary lesions. If carcinoma is confirmed, a CT scan with contrast is performed on the neck, and usually, a PET is done of the neck and chest. Diagnosis of HPV is via HPV DNA positivity in a polymerase chain reaction test. Another method is via immunohistochemical staining for the p16 protein, which is present in most HPV-positive cancers, and in some HPV-negative cancers.

Treatment

For the majority of oral cancers, surgery is the first treatment that is performed. If the disease is more advanced or its features are of high risk, radiation or chemoradiation will be added. If the risk of lymph node disease is greater than 15–20%, selective neck dissection will be performed. Usually, these dissections are done for any lesion that has more than 3.5 mm depth of invasion (DOI). Postoperative abnormalities of the mouth are reduced by routine surgical reconstruction, ranging from localized tissue flaps to free transfers of tissue. If the resections are extreme, therapy may be needed to achieve normal speech and swallowing. Radiation therapy is used alternatively. While chemotherapy is not regularly done as primary therapy, it is usually an adjuvant therapy, with radiation, for patients that have advanced lymph node disease. For squamous cell carcinoma of the lip, surgical excision is performed, with reconstruction, so that postoperative function is maximized. If large regions of the lip show premalignant changes, surgical shaving can be successful, or laser can remove all affected mucosa. Another option is **Mohs surgery**, in which thin skin layers that contain cancer are progressively removed and examined under a microscope. When only cancer-free tissue remains, the surgery is considered complete. After any type of surgery, the patient must apply adequate sunscreen whenever going outside.

Oropharyngeal cancer is often treated with surgery. For tumors of the tonsil and base of the tongue, **transoral laser microsurgery** (TLM) is being used via an endoscopic procedure. **Transoral robotic surgery** (TORS) is very popular for many lesions, and involves a surgical robot with a variety of adaptable "arms" that are controlled by a surgeon at a computerized console. Used along with an endoscopic camera, the arms are inserted through the patient's mouth while it is held open with a retractor. The TORS procedure allows for good visualization and causes fewer postsurgical problems. If it is used for more advanced tumors, postoperative radiation or chemoradiation is commonly administered. Radiation therapy or chemoradiation may be primary or postoperative treatment options. *Intensity-modulated radiation therapy* is a good way to spare surrounding tissue and reduce any long-term adverse effects. After treatment, if there is cervical lymph node metastasis, post-treatment neck dissection is an option.

Prevention and Early Detection

The prevention of oral cancer is based on avoiding the risk factors and increasing any possible protective cancers. This means quitting smoking or chewing tobacco, limiting alcohol intake, avoiding betel quid or **gutka** chewing, losing weight to prevent being overweight or obese, receiving the HPV vaccination, and getting regular exercise. For early detection, screening for oral cancer must include a thorough history and physical examination, with visual inspection and palpation of the head, neck, oral, and pharyngeal regions. Mouth mirrors are essential. Forceful protraction of the tongue with gauze helps completely visualize the tongue and its base. Any present risk factors are documented. There is a review of histories of head and neck radiotherapy, family history of head and neck cancer, and any personal cancer history. Any patient with symptoms lasting longer than 2–4 weeks must be referred promptly to a specialist. Diagnostic imaging of the oral cavity aids in early detection. Fine-needle aspiration is another useful tool.

Oropharyngeal cancer can be prevented by stopping smoking or chewing tobacco products, limiting alcohol intake, and avoiding the HPV infection. Early detection of precancerous changes in the oropharynx caused by HPV may help prevent the progression to cancer. Dental check-ups should be performed every 6–12 months, during which the oropharynx as well as the mouth can be examined for any abnormalities. Precancerous cells may appear as white, red, or a combination.

Prognosis

If there is carcinoma of the tongue that is localized, without lymph node involvement, the five-year survival percentage is above 75%. If there is localized carcinoma of the mouth floor, the five-year survival percentage is at 75%. With lymph node metastasis, the survival rate is about 37.5% over five years. The metastases reach the regional lymph nodes at first, and after that, the lungs. For lesions of the lower lip, the five-year survival is at 90%, with metastases being rare. However, carcinoma of the upper lip is usually more aggressive, with metastases.

For oropharyngeal cancer, the overall five-year survival rate is approximately 60%, though the cause of the disease affects prognosis. Patients with HPV have a three-year survival of nearly 90%, and a five-year survival of more than 75%. Patients without HPV have a five-year survival of less than 50%. The reasons that oropharyngeal cancers caused by HPV have a better survival rate is related to better tumor biology and the fact that patients are usually younger and healthier.

Significant Point

Cancer of the oral cavity is the 11th most common malignancy in the world. Though there has been a slight decrease, the incidence of cancers of the tongue is increasing. Most oropharyngeal cancers are associated with the human papillomavirus, and the excessive use of alcohol and tobacco products. The only known methods of prevention are to get the HPV vaccination, avoid potentially dangerous oral–genital sex and multiple partners, stopping smoking or chewing tobacco, and limiting alcohol intake.

Clinical Case

1. What are the epidemiological statistics concerning oral cancer?
2. What are the clinical manifestations of oral cancer?
3. What are the most common forms of treatment for oral cancer?

A 58-year-old man went to his dentist for a routine check-up. An ulcer was present on the right side of his tongue, which he stated had been there for about five months, and never healed. The patient also complained about pain and difficulty to swallow. He denied any use of alcohol or tobacco products. The ulcer was 1 cm in diameter, indurated, and firm. The man was referred to an oral surgeon. It was diagnosed as a squamous cell carcinoma, a malignancy of epithelial origin. The lesion was surgically removed and this was followed by radiation therapy. After treatment, the patient went for check-ups every other month during the first year, and then once every three months during the second year. He remained cancer-free and was scheduled for once yearly check-ups after that.

Answers:

1. The most common form of oral cancer is squamous cell carcinoma, which is diagnosed in about 34,000 people annually in the United States. About 10.5 adults per 100,000 develop oral cancer during their lifetimes, usually when they are age 50 or older. The global prevalence of oral cancers was over 750,000 new cases in 2018. Incidence was the highest in the country of Papua New Guinea with 20.4 cases out of every 100,000 population. However, globally, the peak ages of patients with oral cancer are between 60 and 70 years.

2. At first, oral lesions are asymptomatic. The lesions may be areas of leukoplakia or erythroplakia, and may be ulcerated or exophytic. If oral cancer is present, it often is indurated, firm, and has a border described as having a "rolled" appearance. When the lesions grow, manifestations may include dysarthria, dysphagia, and pain.

3. For the majority of oral cancers, surgery is the first treatment that is performed. If the disease is more advanced or its features are of high risk, radiation or chemoradiation will be added. If the risk of lymph node disease is greater than 15–20%, selective neck dissection will be performed.

Clinical Case

1. What is the prevalence and incidence of oropharyngeal cancer?
2. What is oropharyngeal cancer mostly caused by?
3. How does oral screening relate to oropharyngeal cancer?

A 59-year-old man had been diagnosed with left tonsillar squamous cell carcinoma, within his oropharynx. A CT scan of his chest and radiographs of his thoracic spine revealed no metastasis. The patient had quit smoking earlier in the year, after 35 years of one pack per day. He also admitted to drinking up to six alcoholic beverages per day for many years. He recently reduced his alcohol intake to three alcoholic beverages 3–4 days per week. The patient had not regularly had any dental treatment, was missing several teeth, and had periodontitis of his gums. This meant that he had to have all needed dental work completed before any surgery, radiation, or chemotherapy could be initiated. A modified radical neck dissection was then performed. The tumor was of 1.7 cm in diameter, with a depth of 6 mm. There was metastasis to three lymph nodes. The tumor was diagnosed as stage IV squamous cell carcinoma. Chemotherapy with radiation therapy was given. The patient developed extreme fatigue, loss of appetite and nausea, reduced taste sensations, xerostomia, weight loss, and flu-like symptoms. He also had difficulty swallowing. Over time, the symptoms began to resolve.

Answers:

1. As of 2018 in the United States, there were more than 17,500 new cases of oropharyngeal cancer. Though incidence rates are increasing, rates of curative treatments are also higher than ever before. Global prevalence is over 500,000 cases annually, with incidence being the highest in the country of Cuba.

2. Oropharyngeal cancer is mostly caused (60%) of HPV type 16. Numbers of sexual partners and participation in oral–genital sex are both implicated. If the patient has HPV, the risk for oropharyngeal cancer is about 16 times higher. Overall, the various types of HPV cause 70–80% of oropharyngeal cancers in many countries.

3. Good oral screening can often detect asymptomatic lesions early. Dental professionals routinely examine the mouth and oropharynx as part of regular care.

Esophageal Cancer

There are two primary forms of esophageal cancer, which include *squamous cell carcinoma* and *adenocarcinoma*. Approximately half of all esophageal cancers are squamous cell carcinomas, which usually occur in the middle and lower two-thirds of the esophagus. The remaining 50% are adenocarcinomas. Esophageal cancer begins at the inside lining of the esophagus and spreads outward.

Epidemiology

The prevalence of esophageal cancer in the United States is about 17,300 cases per year, with nearly 16,000 fatalities. The incidence of adenocarcinoma of the esophagus is increasing. Most people with esophageal cancer are of age 65 years or older upon diagnosis. Squamous cell carcinoma of the esophagus is 2–3 times more common in men than in women. For some reason, it is 4–5 times more common in African Americans than in Caucasians. There are 15 cases out of every 100,000 African American men, while there are only 3 cases out of every 100,000 Caucasian men. Adenocarcinoma of the esophagus occurs in 50% of all esophageal carcinomas in Caucasians, being four times more common in this racial group compared with African Americans.

Squamous cell carcinoma of the esophagus is more common in areas of Asia and South Africa, with rates as high as 100 cases per 100,000 people. There are also more cases in Iran, India, and in some Mediterranean countries. According to data from the Cancer Incidence in Five Continents study, an estimated 398,000 squamous cell carcinomas and 52,000 adenocarcinomas of the esophagus occur annually throughout the world. This translates to 5.2 esophageal squamous cell carcinomas per 100,000 people, and 0.7 esophageal adenocarcinomas per 100,000 people. As in the United States, most people with esophageal cancer are aged 65 or older. Men have esophageal squamous cell carcinomas at 2.7 times the rate seen in women, and for esophageal adenocarcinoma, the rate is 4.4 times the rate in women. Most esophageal squamous cell carcinomas occur in Southeastern and Central Asia, making up 79% of total global cases. However, most cases of esophageal adenocarcinomas occur in Northern and Western Europe, North America, and the Oceanic countries, collectively making up 46% of total global cases (see Figure 6.2).

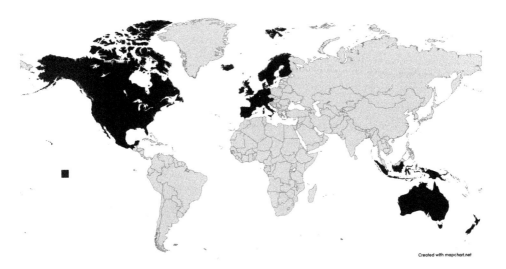

Figure 6.2 Countries with the highest rates of esophageal cancer.

Etiology and Risk Factors

The exact cause of esophageal cancer is unknown. It occurs when esophageal cells experience DNA mutations, and then begin to grow and divide without control, eventually forming a tumor in the esophagus. Cancers that are most likely to metastasize to the esophagus include melanoma and breast cancer, followed by head and neck cancers, and cancers of the bones, lungs, stomach, liver, kidneys, prostate gland, and testes.

The primary risk factors for esophageal cancer include excessive alcohol use and the use of any type of tobacco products, especially if an individual smokes more than 25 cigarettes per day, which causes the relative risk to be 6 times higher. Cigarette smokers that also drink beer or whiskey have a 10–25 times higher risk of developing esophageal squamous cell carcinoma. Additional risk factors include **achalasia**, HPV infection, ingestion of **lye**, esophageal webs caused by **Plummer–Vinson syndrome**, irradiation of the esophagus, and sclerotherapy. A genetic cause has not been proven. However, about half of all patients with **tylosis**, an autosomal dominant disorder, develop esophageal cancer by the age of 45 years. By age 55, about 95% of these individuals develop it.

Clinical Manifestations

In the early stages, esophageal cancer is usually asymptomatic. Dysphagia usually develops once the esophageal lumen constricts to less than about 14 mm. There is difficulty swallowing solid food, followed by semisolid food, and finally, liquid foods along with saliva. This suggests a growing malignancy. If chest pain is present, it usually radiates to the back. Weight loss occurs even if the patient still has a good appetite. Hoarseness and vocal cord paralysis may occur because of the compression of recurrent laryngeal nerve. If nerve compression is present, there may be hiccups, diaphragm paralysis, or spinal pain.

Pulmonary metastasis or malignant pleural effusions can cause dyspnea. When there is an intraluminal tumor, it may cause hematemesis, odynophagia, vomiting, iron deficiency anemia, melena, aspiration, and coughing. Additional manifestations include bone pain, malignant ascites, and superior vena cava syndrome. There is usually metastasis to the lungs and liver, and less often, to the bones, brain, heart, adrenal glands, kidneys, and peritoneum.

Pathology

Primary esophageal cancers begin in the mucosa or submucosa. Most esophageal adenocarcinomas arise in **Barrett esophagus**, because of chronic gastroesophageal reflux disease (GERD) and reflux esophagitis. A metaplastic, columnar and glandular mucosa has brush border and goblet cells, resembling the mucosa of the intestines. This replaces normal stratified squamous epithelia of the distal esophagus, as acute esophagitis is healing, but stomach acid is continually present. Esophageal adenocarcinoma is related to obesity, which causes a 16-times higher risk, likely because obesity can cause reflux. Primary esophageal cancers most commonly metastasize to the lymph nodes, lungs, liver, bones, adrenal glands, and brain. Less common esophageal malignancies include spindle cell carcinoma, pseudosarcoma, verrucous carcinoma, adenosquamous carcinoma, mucoepidermoid carcinoma, cylindroma, choriocarcinoma, primary oat cell carcinoma, carcinoid tumor, primarily malignant melanoma, and sarcoma. About 3% of esophageal cancers are metastatic. Tumors from other sites usually seed the loose connective tissue stroma that surrounds the esophagus.

Diagnosis

Diagnosis begins with physical examination to evaluate changes in skin, nails, and hair as results of malnutrition. Weight loss may cause generalized cachexia and wasting of muscles. Lymphadenopathy may be present in the supraclavicular and anterior cervical regions. If esophageal cancer is suspected, an endoscopy should be performed, with cytology and biopsy. This procedure is needed for tissue diagnosis, even though a barium X-ray can show obstructive lesions. If esophageal cancer is identified, a

CT scan of the chest and abdomen is performed to determine tumor spread. If metastasis is negative, an endoscopic ultrasound is done. This determines tumor depth in the esophageal wall, as well as regional lymph node involvement. Fine-needle aspiration is then used to analyze the cells. If there is bone pain, a bone scan may be needed. For some patients, PET is also performed. If there has been metastasis to the liver, hepatomegaly and complications of liver disease may be present. Also, basic blood tests include complete blood count, electrolytes, and liver function tests. Because of upper GI bleeding, there may be progressive iron deficiency anemia. Metabolic alkalosis may cause vomiting and hypernatremia, because of dehydration. Hepatocellular and cholestatic liver enzyme abnormalities are suggestive of liver metastasis. A summary of staging for esophageal cancer is as follows:

- Stage 0 – Tis (carcinoma in situ); no regional lymph node metastasis and no distant metastasis
- Stage I – T1 (lamina propria or submucosa affected); no regional lymph node or distant metastases
- Stage II – T2 (muscularis propria affected) or T3 (adventitia affected); no regional lymph node or distant metastases
- Stage III – T3 or T4 (adjacent structures affected), regional lymph node metastasis is present, but no distant metastasis
- Stage IV – any level of maximum tumor penetration, any level of regional lymph node metastasis, along with the presence of distant metastasis

Treatment

Treatments are determined by staging, tumor size, and location, and the patient's choices, since many do not want to undergo aggressive therapies. Surgical resection is usually successful for patients with stage 0, I, or IIa disease. Preoperative chemotherapy and radiation also improve outcomes. However, patients with stages IIb and III disease have poor results with only surgery. Therefore, preoperative radiation and chemotherapy can reduce tumor volume before surgery. If the patient cannot or does not want to have surgery, radiation with chemotherapy may be beneficial. However, radiation or chemotherapy alone is usually not beneficial. If the patient has stage IV disease, palliative care is required, and surgery should not be done.

After treatment, the patient is screened for recurrence. This is done via endoscopy and CT of the neck, chest, and abdomen every six months, over a three-year period, and then once per year after that. If Barrett esophagus is present, the patient receives aggressive long-term treatment for GERD and endoscopic monitoring for any malignant transformations. This occurs every 3 months, 6 months, or up to every 12 months based on metaplasia of the disease. Surgery may involve a variety of options, as follows:

- *Endoscopic mucosal resection or endoscopic submucosal dissection* – for early, superficial non-invasive cancers, if endoscopic ultrasound has confirmed the lesion to be superficial
- *En bloc resection* – for most patients, this is performed to achieve a cure; the entire tumor is removed along with the proximal and distal margins of normal tissues, all lymph nodes that might be malignant, and part of the proximal stomach that contains the distal draining lymphatics; gastric pull-up is required with esophagogastric anastomosis, and interposition of the small intestine or colon. **Pyloroplasty** ensures normal gastric drainage, since esophagectomy usually causes bilateral **vagotomy**. However, en bloc resection may not be suitable for patients over 75 years of age, especially if they have an ejection fraction of less than 40%, or forced expiratory volume in 1 s (FEV1) of less than 1.5 l per minute. Operative mortality is about 5% of patients.

Preoperative chemotherapy with radiation may improve survival following surgical resection of a thoracic esophageal cancer. Sometimes, chemotherapy is used on its own after surgery.

However, surgical complications include anastomotic leaking, fistulas, strictures, bilious gastroesophageal reflux, and **dumping syndrome**. The burning due to bile reflux may be worse than the original dysphagia. This may require a Roux-en-Y jejunostomy to divert the bile. Because an interposed segment of the small intestine or colon within the chest has a small blood supply, there can be resulting gangrene, ischemia, or torsion.

External beam radiation therapy is usually combined with chemotherapy if the patient is unlikely to be cured by surgery, even if the cancer is advanced. However, radiation is contraindicated with tracheoesophageal fistula since the fistula will be enlarged by shrinkage of the tumor. Also, if the patient has tumor encased blood vessels, tumor shrinkage can cause massive hemorrhaging. Early in the course of radiation therapy, edema can make dysphagia, esophageal obstruction, and odynophagia worse. This may require placement of a stent, pre-radiation dilation, or both. A temporary percutaneous gastrostomy feeding tube is sometimes required. Additional adverse effects of radiation include nausea, vomiting, anorexia, esophagitis, fatigue, and mucus production by the esophagus that becomes excessive, stricture, xerostomia, pericarditis, pneumonitis, myelitis, and myocarditis.

Chemotherapy on its own is not a good treatment for esophageal cancer. Tumor response rates are defined as a 50% or greater reduction in all measurable areas. These rates range from 10–40%, but usually, responses are not complete and are only temporary. The tumor may slightly shrink, but not as much as desired. Usually, cisplatin with 5-fluorouracil combination is used. Other effective drugs include doxorubicin, mitomycin, bleomycin, vindesine, and methotrexate.

Palliative care focuses on reducing esophageal obstruction to allow sufficient oral intake of foods and liquids. The obstruction may cause the patient to salivate and experience recurring aspiration. The methods used to relieve obstruction include manual dilation, stents inserted via the mouth, laser photocoagulation, radiation, and **photodynamic therapy**. Sometimes, there is a need for cervical esophagostomy with feeding jejunostomy. Using an endoscopic laser to burn a channel through the tumor, once or several times as needed may relieve dysphagia. In photodynamic therapy, porfimer sodium is injected, which is a derivative of hematoporphyrin. The tissues take up this substance, which functions as a photosensitizer. When a laser beam is directed on the tumor, it activates the porfimer sodium, releasing cytotoxic oxygen, destroying tumor cells. The patient must avoid sun exposure for 6 weeks, because the skin will also be sensitized to light.

For supportive care, enteral nutrition improves the results of all types of treatment. If there is an obstruction, an endoscopically or surgically placed feeding tube allows for a more distal feeding route. End-of-life care should focus on controlling pain, inability to swallow secretions, and any other present symptoms. The patient may eventually require large doses of opioids. Therefore, before these final stages, the patient should be advised to make end-of-life care decisions, recording them in an **advance directive**.

Prevention and Early Detection

Possible methods of preventing esophageal cancer include avoiding risk factors and increasing protective factors. Smoking and excessive alcohol use should be stopped, and nonsteroidal antiinflammatory drugs (NSAIDs) have protective effects. Gastric reflux should be treated to avoid development of adenocarcinoma. Another preventive measure is radiofrequency ablation of the esophagus. Unfortunately, there are no screening tests for early detection of esophageal cancer.

Prognosis

The prognosis of esophageal cancer is based on staging, but is usually poor since many patients present with advanced disease. The five-year prognosis is usually less than 5% survival. However, if the cancer is only within the mucosa, there is an approximate 80% survival rate. If there is submucosal involvement, survival is less than 50% survival. The rate is 20% if there is extension to the muscularis propria, 7% with extension to nearby structures, and less than 3% with distant metastases.

Significant Point

While relatively rare, esophageal cancer is the seventh leading cause of cancer death in men, globally. It is challenging to treat, especially if it has become advanced. Unfortunately, symptoms often do not appear until this has occurred, so the average five-year survival rate is only 19% of patient. In the United States, most esophageal cancer is linked to obesity.

Clinical Case

1. What are the differences in epidemiology for esophageal squamous cell carcinoma and esophageal adenocarcinoma?
2. To which other locations do primary esophageal cancers commonly metastasize?
3. What are the preventive methods for esophageal cancer?

A 65-year-old man visited his physician because of progressive dysphagia, accompanied by dyspnea and coughing. The man has a history of chewing tobacco of over 40 years. Imaging studies reveal a tapering of the esophageal lumen and significant narrowing of the middle portion of the esophagus, with slight mucosal abnormalities. There is abnormal heterogeneously enhancing thickening of the lower thoracic esophagus. A lymph node lesion has encroached the left main bronchus, and there is thrombosis of the left pulmonary artery. The diagnosis is of esophageal cancer, specifically squamous cell carcinoma. The patient is scheduled for surgery, and consideration is given to the use of chemotherapy and radiation therapy.

Answers:

1. **Squamous cell carcinoma of the esophagus is 2–3 times more common in men than in women. For some reason, it is 4–5 times more common in African Americans than in Caucasians. Adenocarcinoma of the esophagus occurs in 50% of all esophageal carcinomas in Caucasians, being four times more common in this racial group compared with African Americans. Globally, squamous cell carcinomas of the esophagus are more than five times common than adenocarcinomas of the esophagus. Men have esophageal squamous cell carcinomas at 2.7 times the rate seen in women, and for esophageal adenocarcinoma, the rate is 4.4 times the rate in women. Most esophageal squamous cell carcinomas occur in Southeastern and Central Asia, while most esophageal adenocarcinomas occur in Europe, North America, and the Oceanic countries.**
2. **Primary esophageal cancers most commonly metastasize to the lymph nodes, lungs, liver, bones, adrenal glands, and brain.**
3. **Possible methods of preventing esophageal cancer include avoiding the risk factors and increasing protective factors. Smoking and excessive alcohol use should be stopped, and nonsteroidal anti-inflammatory drugs have protective effects. Gastric reflux should be treated to avoid the development of adenocarcinoma. Another preventive measure is radiofrequency ablation of the esophagus.**

Stomach Cancer

Stomach cancer is also referred to as *gastric cancer*. Beginning in the stomach itself, it is a type of cancer that usually develops slowly, over years. Before actual cancer, precancerous changes often happen in the mucosa of the stomach. They are usually asymptomatic and undetected. The primary types of stomach cancers include adenocarcinomas, lymphomas, gastrointestinal stromal tumors, and carcinoid tumors. Rarely, stomach cancers may be squamous cell carcinomas, small cell carcinomas, or leiomyosarcomas.

Epidemiology

Stomach cancer prevalence in the United States is over 26,240 cases annually, with about 10,800 being fatal. Gastric adenocarcinoma is by far the most common type, making up 95% of malignant stomach tumors. Incidence has declined during recent decades, and stomach cancer is now the seventh most common cause of cancer death in the United States. Over 75% of patients are 50 years of age or older. Men are two times as likely to develop stomach cancer as women. It is most common in African Americans, Hispanics, and American Indians.

There are over 1 million new global cases of stomach cancer every year, and an estimated 783,000 deaths. Cases are increasing every year, and the burden of stomach cancer remains very high in many countries. Incidence ranges between 5 and 11 cases per 100,000 person/years, with a median of 8 cases per 100,000 person/years. Globally, the average age of diagnosis is 68 years, and about 60% of people diagnosed are older than 64 years. According to the World Cancer Research Fund, stomach cancer is the fourth most commonly occurring cancer in men and the seventh most commonly occurring cancer in men, though statistics are widely varying between different countries. Men develop stomach cancer two times more often than women. The countries with the most cases of stomach cancer included South Korea (39.6 per 100,000 people), Mongolia (33.1), Japan (27.5), China (20.7), Bhutan (19.4), Kyrgyzstan (18.6), Chile (17.8), Belarus (16.5), Peru (16.1), and Vietnam (15.9) – see Figure 6.3. Therefore, there is a distinct predilection for Asian ethnicities. For example, just in South Korea, about 41.8 people of every 100,000 will develop stomach cancer during their lifetimes. In all Asian countries, cases of stomach cancer are expected to continually increase, though deaths are now decreasing due to earlier detection and treatment.

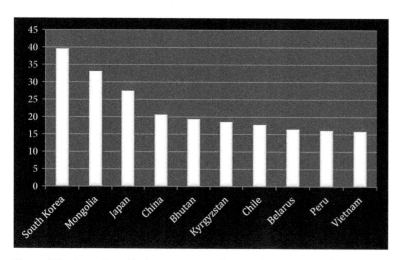

Figure 6.3 Countries with the most cases of stomach cancer, per 100,000 people.

Etiology and Risk Factors

While the actual cause of stomach cancer is uncertain, there are many different risk factors. These include *Helicobacter pylori* infection, autoimmune atrophic gastritis, gastric polyps, smoking, genetic factors, and excessive consumption of processed meat. Inflammatory polyps can develop from excessive use of NSAIDs. Also, proton pump inhibitors may cause **fundic foveolar polyps**. The most likely type of polyps to develop into stomach cancer is the *adenomatous polyps* – especially if there are more than one present. If one of these polyps is larger than 2 cm in diameter, or has a villous histology, cancer is especially likely. Since malignant transformation is undetectable via inspection, any polyps discovered during endoscopy should be removed. Additional risk factors for adenocarcinoma of the stomach include *N-nitroso compounds*, formed in the stomach by **nitrosation** of ingested nitrates, commonly found in the diet. Atrophic gastritis, pernicious anemia, *N-methyl-N'-nitro-N-nitrosoguanidine*, and achlorhydria are also implicated.

Clinical Manifestations

The symptoms of stomach cancer are at first nonspecific. Dyspepsia often is present, which mimics peptic ulcer. Often, the symptoms are dismissed, or the patient is treated to reduce stomach acid. With disease progression, early satiety may occur if the tumor obstructs the pylorus, or if the stomach has become **nondistensible**, due to linitis plastica. If a tumor in the cardia obstructs the esophageal outlet, this may cause dysphagia. A common manifestation is loss of weight or strength, usually due to dietary restriction. Though melena or serious hematemesis is uncommon, occult blood loss may cause secondary anemia. Sometimes, initial symptoms are due to metastasis, and include ascites, bone fractures, and jaundice. There may be stools that are heme-positive or unremarkable physical signs. Later in the course of stomach cancer, abnormalities include hepatomegaly, an epigastric mass, abnormalities of the left axillary, left supraclavicular, or umbilical lymph nodes, and ovarian or rectal masses. Also, there can be lesions of the central nervous, pulmonary, or skeletal systems.

Pathology

Adenocarcinomas of the stomach are classified by gross appearance, which may be described by the following terms:

- *Penetrating* – the tumor is ulcerated
- *Protruding* – the tumor is fungating or polypoid, and becomes symptomatic earlier, giving a better prognosis than the superficial spreading tumors
- *Linitis plastica* – the tumor has infiltrated the stomach wall, with a related fibrous reaction, causing rigidity of the stomach that is described as a "leather bottle"
- *Superficial spreading* – the tumor has spread along the mucosa or superficially infiltrated the stomach wall

There are also *intestinal* and *diffuse* classifications of stomach adenocarcinomas. The intestinal type is usually within the distal stomach, has ulcerations, often follows premalignant lesions, and is becoming less common in the United States. The diffuse type is characterized by thickening of the stomach – mostly in the cardia – often affecting younger patients, and may exist as *linitis plastica*. Genetic factors linked to the pathology of these tumors include: type A blood, having a first-degree relative with the disease, mutations of the *E-cadherin* or *alpha-catenin* genes, **Lynch syndrome**, and familial adenomatous polyposis. Loss of heterozygosity of the *adenomatous polyposis coli* gene is also implicated. The *p53* gene is also mutated in both stomach cancer and in precancerous lesions. For sporadic stomach carcinoma, microsatellite DNA changes or unstable dinucleotide repeats are common.

Diagnosis

Physical examination may reveal an epigastric mass, if the later stages of cancer development have occurred. If there has been metastasis to the liver, there may be hepatomegaly, jaundice, and ascites. Splenomegaly may be present, due to portal or splenic vein invasion and thrombosis. If stomach cancer is suspected, an endoscopy with multiple biopsies and brush cytology should be performed. Upper endoscopy with biopsy and cytologic examination is 95–99%

accurate for all stomach cancers. Sometimes, a biopsy of only the mucosa does not find tumor tissue located in the submucosa. Endoscopy is needed even if lesions are shown in X-rays such as double-contrast barium studies. Differential diagnoses include peptic ulcer and related complications. If stomach cancer is identified, there must be a CT scan of the chest and abdomen to determine how much tumor spread has occurred. If there is no metastasis, endoscopic ultrasonography can determine tumor depth and any regional lymph node abnormalities. This affects treatment and prognosis.

Blood tests include CBC, electrolytes, and liver function tests. These assess anemia, general health, hydration, and possible metastasis to the liver. Fecal occult blood tests may be positive. *Krukenberg's tumor* describes metastasis to the ovaries. Paraneoplastic syndromes may have previously or concurrently existed, such as **Trousseau syndrome, acanthosis nigricans**, and neuromyopathy affecting the sensory or motor pathways. There may be abnormal serology of carcinoembryonic antigen (CEA) and iron deficiency anemia, microangiopathic hemolytic anemia, and hypoalbuminemia.

Treatment

For stomach cancer, a cure can be achieved by surgical resection of most or all of the stomach via *total gastrectomy*, as well as nearby lymph nodes. This is usually successful when the disease is only within the stomach, or sometimes when it has reached the regional lymph nodes – however, this is in less than half of all patients. A total gastrectomy, with Roux-en-Y reconstruction to restore GI tract continuity is shown in Figure 6.4. This procedure allows for biliary and pancreatic drainage from the duodenum. The proximal jejunal "Y" limb is anastomosed to the distal jejunal "Roux" limb, approximately 40–60 cm from the esophagojejunal anastomosis, to avoid bile reflux. For tumors of the distal stomach, a distal subtotal gastrectomy is preferred. If the tumor can be resected, adjuvant chemotherapy or combined chemotherapy and radiation therapy may be helpful after surgery. If locally advanced regional disease is resected, the median survival is 10 months, in comparison with 3–4 months without any resection.

For metastasis or significant lymph node involvement, palliative treatments are usually given. It should be noted that actual tumor spread is often

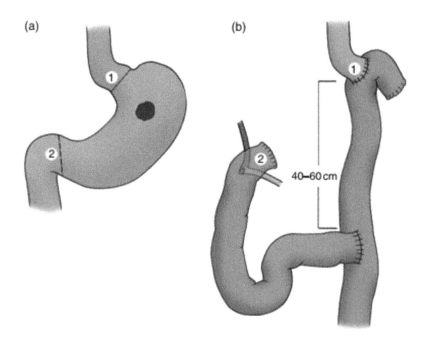

Figure 6.4 Total gastrectomy, with reconstructive Roux-en-Y procedure. *Source:* American Cancer Society [6].

not seen until curative surgery is performed. For palliative surgery, a **gastroenterostomy** is usually done, bypassing a pyloric obstruction. However, this is reserved only for cases in which quality of life will improve. If surgery is not indicated, combination chemotherapies may result in a temporary improvement yet do not greatly affect five-year survival. Chemotherapies include doxorubicin, 5-luorouracil, cisplatin, mitomycin, and leucovorin. Targeted therapies have become more common recently, trastuzumab along with chemotherapies for advanced disease are used. Immunotherapy may be used for patients that have programmed cell death ligand 1 (PD-L1)-positive stomach cancer that is advanced or metastatic. The agent used for this is called pembrolizumab. Radiation therapy on its own is of little benefit.

Prevention and Early Detection

According to the American Cancer Society, there is no proven way to prevent stomach cancer. However, risks can be lowered by regular physical activity to maintain a normal body weight, a diet high in fresh fruits and vegetables, and avoiding or limiting alcohol consumption. Other methods of possible prevention include avoiding tobacco products, treating *Helicobacter pylori* infections, using aspirin or other NSAIDs, and genetic testing for *hereditary diffuse gastric cancer syndrome*. Early detection of stomach cancer may be done for high-risk patients, such as in Japan, though in the United States, since the disease is much less common, routine screening is not performed. Screening is done for people with stomach cancer risk factors however, and includes medical history, physical examination, upper endoscopy, endoscopic ultrasound, biopsy, imaging, upper GI series, CT scans, MRI scans, PET scans, chest X-rays, laparoscopy, and a variety of blood tests.

Prognosis

The prognosis of stomach cancer is based on staging. However, the prognosis is poor, with less than 5–15% survival over five years. When a tumor is only within the mucosa or submucosa,

five-year survival is up to 80% of patients. If the local lymph nodes are involved, survival is 30%. Once the disease has become more widely spread, the patient usually does not survive 12 months. The best prognosis is for gastric lymphomas such as mucosa-associated lymphoid tissue (MALT) lymphoma or non-Hodgkin's lymphomas that affect the stomach.

Significant Point

In the more advanced stages of stomach cancer, the patient may experience some or all of the following: nausea, vomiting, blood in the stool or vomit, heartburn, loss of appetite, unexplained weight loss, pain in the abdomen close to the belly button, and feeling full after eating only a small amount of food.

Clinical Case

1. What is the most common type of stomach cancer?
2. What are the five general types of stomach adenocarcinomas?
3. Which methods may be helpful in preventing stomach cancer?

A 60-year-old Asian-American man went to his physician because of stomach pains. He also complained of having lost weight over the past 6 months even though he had made no changes in diet or exercise. Physical examination revealed a firm mass in the stomach area. Gastroscopy revealed a 5 cm malignant stomach tumor in the lower portions of the organ. Also, *Helicobacter pylori* infection was present. When questioned, the patient admitted to eating a large amount of processed meat every week. He had also recently quit smoking, a habit that he had continued for over 25 years, and took over-the-counter antacids because of chronic acid reflux. The patient was sent for chest X-rays and a PET-CT scan, which fortunately revealed that the cancer had not spread outside the stomach. The cancer was surgically resected, and chemotherapy and radiation therapy were used as adjuvant therapies, and the patient survived.

Answers:

1. **Gastric adenocarcinoma is by far the most common type, making up 95% of malignant stomach cancers.**
2. **Adenocarcinomas of the stomach are classified by their gross appearance, which may be described as penetrating (ulcerated), protruding (fungating or polypoid), linitis plastica (causing stomach rigidity), superficial spreading (along the mucosa, or with infiltration of the stomach wall), and miscellaneous (having characteristics of two or more of the other types).**
3. **Though there is no proven way to prevent stomach cancer, risks can be lowered by regular physical activity to maintain a normal body weight, a diet high in fresh fruits and vegetables, avoiding or limiting alcohol consumption, avoiding tobacco products, treating *Helicobacter pylori* infections, using aspiring of other NSAIDs, and genetic testing for hereditary diffuse gastric cancer syndrome.**

Small-Bowel Tumors

There are a variety of small-bowel tumors, also known as *small-intestine tumors*, which include benign and malignant forms. Benign tumors include leiomyomas, lipomas, fibromas, and neurofibromas. Polyps of the small bowel are less common than in the colon. Common manifestations include abdominal distention, bleeding, pain, and diarrhea. If an obstruction forms, vomiting usually occurs. Malignant tumors include primary malignant lymphoma, carcinoid tumors, Kaposi sarcoma, and adenocarcinoma. However, only about 1–2% of primary gastrointestinal tumors originate within the small intestine, and more often metastasize there from other GI sites.

Epidemiology

Small-bowel tumors make up 1–5% of all GI tumors. Small-bowel cancer is diagnosed in nearly 11,110 people annually in the United States, with nearly 1,700 of these being fatal. This means that small-bowel tumors make up 0.6% of all new cancer cases, and 0.3% of all cancer deaths. The rate of new cases of small-bowel cancer is 2.4 per 100,000 people annually. The death rate is 0.4 per 100,000 people annually. About 0.3% of men and women are diagnosed with small-bowel cancer at some point in their lives. As of 2017, there were about 70,229 people living with small-bowel cancer in the United States. The average age at diagnosis is about 67 years. Small-bowel tumors occur slightly more frequently in African Americans than in other racial or ethnic groups. Studies on the global prevalence and incidence of small-bowel tumors are lacking, but statistics are likely to be close to those of the United States. The most common ages for small-bowel tumors to develop, globally, are in the sixth and seventh decades of life. The male-to-female ratio is equal.

Etiology and Risk Factors

Most small-bowel cancers are of unknown cause, but they usually begin when healthy cells experience DNA mutations. The risk factors for small-bowel cancers include inherited gene mutations as part of Lynch syndrome, familial adenomatous polyposis, and **Peutz–Jeghers syndrome**. There is a link between small-bowel cancers and celiac disease, Crohn's disease, and inflammatory bowel disease. An increased risk also comes from a weakened immune system, such as in people with HIV/AIDS or those taking anti-rejection medications after organ transplantation.

Clinical Manifestations

Less than 33% of small-bowel carcinoid tumors cause bleeding, **carcinoid syndrome**, obstruction, and pain. Adenocarcinomas often cause abdominal pain and distention, nausea, vomiting, and unexplained weight loss. While usually asymptomatic, Kaposi sarcoma may cause bleeding, diarrhea, intussusception, and protein-losing enteropathy. General signs and symptoms of small-bowel cancer include occult blood, dark or black stools, a lump in the abdomen, abdominal pain or cramps, unexplained weight loss, and severe nausea or vomiting.

Pathology

Small-bowel lymphomas can cause chronic celiac disease that is often untreated. Primary malignant lymphoma in the ileum may cause rigidity of a long portion of this area. However, these lymphomas make up only 8% of all small-bowel neoplasms, usually forming in the ileum. Nearly all of these are non-Hodgkin's lymphomas. Carcinoid tumors are most common in the ileum as well as the appendix, and larger lesions may become malignant. In half of all cases, there are multiple tumors. For tumors larger than 2 cm in diameter, by the time of surgery about 80% have already metastasized to the liver. Small-bowel carcinoids make up 44% of all malignancies in this area. Kaposi sarcoma occurs aggressively when there are GI tract involvement in 40–60% of cases, most commonly in AIDS patients, transplant recipients, and African Americans. Lesions are most common in the small bowel, stomach, and distal colon. Adenocarcinoma of the small bowel usually forms in the duodenum or proximal jejunum, with few symptoms. It makes up 40% of all malignant small-bowel tumors, forming in the duodenum mostly (65% of all adenocarcinomas in the small bowel). If the patient has Crohn disease of the small bowel, the tumors are usually distal, and within loops of bowel that are bypassed or inflamed. Malignant connective tissue tumors make up 10–17% of all small-bowel neoplasms that mostly form in the duodenum.

Diagnosis

Diagnosis begins with medical history and physical examination, to search for abdominal swelling or sounds that may indicate a blockage of the bowel. Imaging tests include upper GI series with barium, lower GI series with barium enema, CT scan, MRI, and endoscopy. **Enteroclysis**, which may or may not be *CT enteroclysis*, is overall the most common diagnostic method for multiple small-bowel lesions. To visualize and biopsy tumors, *push endoscopy*, using an **enteroscope**, may be done. Small-bowel lesions – primarily sites of bleeding – can also be identified via *video capsule endoscopy*. This involves a capsule that is swallowed by the patient, which transmits two images every second to an external recorder. Blood tests including CBC and blood chemistry are helpful.

Treatment

The treatment of carcinoid tumors of the small bowel is surgical resection, as for many other small-bowel tumors, but this sometimes requires multiple operations. Alternatives to resection include *electrocautery, laser phototherapy*, and *thermal obliteration*. Treatment of Kaposi sarcoma of the small bowel is based on cell types, location, and the number of lesions that exist. Resectable cancers are surgically removed, along with some healthy surrounding tissues. If the cancer is in the duodenum, a pancreaticoduodenectomy (**Whipple procedure**) is usually done (see Figure 6.5). If the tumor is in another part of the small bowel, a segmental resection is more common. If the cancer is near the end of the small bowel, part of the colon also may need to be removed. Adjuvant chemotherapy or radiation therapy may be recommended if the cancer has grown through the bowel wall or spread to nearby lymph nodes. It is unknown if adjuvant therapies actually extend survival times.

For unresectable cancers, a large part of the tumor may still be resected, or it may be bypassed. This is palliative treatment, but can prevent abdominal pain, nausea, and vomiting.

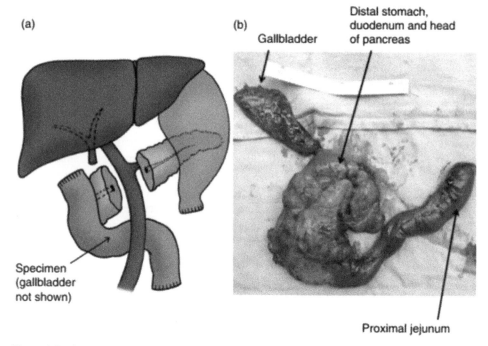

Figure 6.5 Organs removed in a Whipple procedure, with (a) depiction of the technique, and (b) the resected organs. *Source*: American Cancer Society [7].

Chemotherapy is usually part of this treatment, and may be given directly into the abdominal space after surgery, which is called *intraperitoneal chemotherapy*. Radiation therapy is used to treat cancer that has spread – primarily to the brain or bones. Also, immunotherapy is an option, to boost the body's immune response. *Checkpoint inhibitors* such as pembrolizumab may be helpful if the patient has changes such as mismatch repair gene mutations or microsatellite instability.

Prevention and Early Detection

There is no known way to prevent the majority of small-bowel adenocarcinomas. However, quitting smoking, limiting alcohol intake, and limiting dietary red meats may be helpful in preventing these cancers. Surgery can have some preventive value for those with familial adenomatous polyposis or duodenal polyps. No effective screening tests have been found for small-bowel cancers. For people at high risk, regular tests may be performed to detect the cancer early – especially in the duodenum. Tests include upper endoscopy, CT scans, and endoscopic ultrasound.

Prognosis

According to the National Cancer Institute, the five-year relative survival of small-bowel cancer is about 68.3% of patients. About 32% of patients are diagnosed at the localized stage, 35% at the regional stage, and 27% at the distant stage.

Significant Point

Overall, tumors of the small bowel are rare. Usually, they grow unnoticed for long periods of time. Most of them are found while the bowel is being examined for other reasons. Small-bowel adenocarcinoma is the most common *cancerous* form, and begins in the bowel lining, within the glandular cells. Tumors may cause intestinal blockage.

Clinical Case

1. What is the incidence of small-bowel tumors?
2. Where is the most common location of the adenocarcinoma in the small bowel?
3. What is the overall prognosis for small-bowel tumors?

A 57-year-old man was taken to the emergency department because of abdominal pain and distention, unexplained weight loss, and nausea and vomiting. He had begun to develop these symptoms two months earlier. There was no history of any abdominal problems in the patient's family. No signs of peritonitis were present. A CT scan revealed an obstructive area in the terminal ileum without significant distension. An exploratory laparotomy was performed with terminal ileum-right colectomy, with ileotransverse anastomosis because the lesion was stenotic. The diagnosis was of a stage III adenocarcinoma. The patient was referred to an oncology facility to begin follow-up chemotherapy. He survived without recurrence.

Answers:

1. **Small-bowel tumors make up 1–5% of all GI tumors. Small-bowel cancer is diagnosed in nearly 11,110 people annually in the United States, with nearly 1,700 of these being fatal. Small-bowel tumors make up 0.6% of all new cancer cases, and 0.3% of all cancer deaths. The rate of new cases is 2.4 per 100,000 people annually. About 0.3% of men and women are diagnosed with small-bowel cancer at some point in their lives.**
2. **Adenocarcinomas of the small bowel usually form in the duodenum or proximal jejunum, not in the ileum.**
3. **The 5-year relative survival rate of small-bowel cancer is about 68.3% of patients.**

Familial Adenomatous Polyposis

Familial adenomatous polyposis is a hereditary disorder. It involves the development of many polyps in the colon, and often become carcinoma by the age of 40 years. Though patients are usually asymptomatic, the stool may be heme-positive. The disease is classified as an *autosomal dominant* condition.

Epidemiology

Familial adenomatous polyposis occurs in 1 of every 8,000 to 14,000 people. By the age of 15 years, about half of all cases already have polyps. By age 35, nearly 95% of people have polyps. The disease makes up 0.5% of all cases of colorectal cancer. The cancer develops before age 40 in almost all patients who have the genetic predisposition but do not receive treatments. It affects males and females equally. There appears to be no specific racial or ethnic predilection. Global prevalence of familial adenomatous polyposis is similar to that of the United States, making up about 0.5% of all cases of colorectal cancer. Though it has been seen in teenagers, it is mostly a disease of younger adults, with males and females affected equally. No specific races or ethnicities appear to be affected in higher numbers.

Etiology and Risk Factors

Familial adenomatous polyposis is caused by a gene mutation of *adenomatous polyposis coli (APC)*, usually inherited from a parent, though some people develop the abnormal gene on their own. About 66% of cases are inherited, and if a parent has it, the children have a 50% of developing the disease. Nearly everyone with the gene mutation that causes the classic form of the disease will develop colorectal polyps by age 50 unless preventive measures are taken. Risk factors are increased if there is a first-degree relative with the condition.

Clinical Manifestations

Along with polyps, patients with familial adenomatous polyposis can also develop a variety of benign and malignant manifestations outside of the colon. These manifestations are collectively known as **Gardner syndrome** outside of the colon, include adenomas in other areas of the GI tract, desmoid tumors, osteomas of the mandible of skull, and sebaceous cysts. There is an increased risk of developing duodenal cancer, pancreatic cancer, thyroid cancer, and brain cancer. Many patients with familial adenomatous polyposis are asymptomatic, though rectal bleeding may occur, and is usually occult.

Pathology

In familial adenomatous polyposis, 100 or more polyps form in the colon and rectum. The APC gene is a tumor suppressor gene involved in control of the cell cycle. The APC protein usually is involved in apoptosis of epithelial cells in the colon. The APC gene mutation may cause an expansion of the crypt base cell counts, including **crypt stem cells**. Mutant crypt stem cells can expand clonally, forming adenomas and carcinomas. When beta-catenin is no longer downregulated, it can stimulate cell growth. Adenomatous polyps form when there is inactivation of the remaining normal APC allele. Colorectal adenocarcinomas form in similar ways to the sporadic-type colorectal adenocarcinomas, such as by *Kirsten rat sarcoma (KRAS)* or TP53 mutations. The more that there are adenomatous polyps, the higher the chance for developing colorectal adenocarcinoma.

Diagnosis

The diagnosis of familial adenomatous polyposis is based on the presence of more than 100 polyps, found during colonoscopy. They can also be recognized during sigmoidoscopy, but colonoscopy is able to find more proximal polyps. This is assessed for any metastasis prior to treatments. Genetic testing can reveal specific mutations and should be evaluated in first-degree relatives. If such testing cannot be performed, relatives must be screened via yearly sigmoidoscopy starting at the age of 12 years, and then less often as each decade passes. If there are no polyps by the age of 50, the screening frequency becomes the same as for people who are of average risk. When a parent has familial adenomatous polyposis, the children must be screened for hepatoblastoma from birth to the age of five years, utilizing yearly serum **alpha-fetoprotein** levels. Sometimes, liver ultrasound is also performed.

Treatment

Soon after diagnosis, a colectomy should be performed. Performing total proctocolectomy eliminates the risk of colorectal cancer. This utilizes **ileostomy** or mucosal proctectomy with ileoanal pouch. A *subtotal colectomy* is the removal of the majority of the colon, but leaves the rectum intact. If this procedure is done along with ileorectal anastomosis, the remaining rectum must be monitored regularly for any changes. Any new polyps must be resected or **fulgurated**. New polyp formation can be inhibited by the use of NSAIDs. If new polyps form too quickly or in large numbers, the rectum must be excised, with permanent ileostomy. Following colectomy, the patient must have upper endoscopy periodically. This includes duodenoscopy, beginning at 25–30 years of age, with repeated surveillance every 6 months to 4 years – depending upon staging of duodenal polyposis. Also, the thyroid gland should be screened with ultrasonography every year.

Prevention and Early Detection

There is no known way to prevent familial adenomatous polyposis. However, an individual with the condition can prevent cancer from developing via surgical removal of the large intestine. Genetic testing and counseling can help to raise awareness of the condition being present before choosing to have children. Surveillance guidelines have been proposed to help in the earliest possible detection of familial adenomatous polyposis and related hereditary polyposis syndromes.

Prognosis

The overall prognosis for familial adenomatous polyposis is fair to good. When the disease is found before it has become cancerous or when cancerous polyps are confined to the intestinal tract, surgical resection has a high success rate of preventing or removing the cancer, without recurrence. This is because the areas from which the cancer forms are completely removed. After surgery, if a partial colectomy has been done, regular monitoring can help find any new polyps, which is the best way to achieve a good prognosis and outlook.

Significant Point

Familial adenomatous polyposis is an inherited cancer syndrome. It predisposes patients to early-onset colorectal cancers. It is a dominant genetic disease, meaning that only one copy of the mutated APC gene is required for a person to have the syndrome. Most people with this gene mutation will eventually develop colorectal cancer.

Clinical Case

1. How common is familial adenomatous polyposis?
2. Which manifestations can occur outside of the colon?
3. What should be done when specific gene mutations are found?

A 32-year-old man visited his physician, complaining of changes in his bowel habits, intermittent rectal bleeding, and decreased appetite. None of his family has ever complained of the same symptoms. Physical examination found a polypoidal mass, and proctoscopy revealed many small polyps surrounding a larger polyp. A contrast-enhanced CT scan of the patient's abdomen showed the polyps to be located within the distal transverse colon. Colonoscopy revealed polyps of larger than 1 cm in size, throughout the rectum, and continuing up to the anal canal. Biopsies were taken of many different areas of the colon, and several showed significant signs of pre-malignancy. A permanent ileostomy was chosen to be the best surgical method, and the patient recovered well from the surgery. Screening was soon done for the patient's children, both of which were found to have multiple polyps as well. The children were followed up annually with sigmoidoscopy but, to date, have not needed surgery.

Answers:

1. **Familial adenomatous polyposis occurs in 1 of every 8,000 to 14,000 people. It makes up 0.5% of all cases of colorectal cancer, and develops before age 40 in almost all patients who have the genetic predisposition but do not receive treatments, affecting males and females equally.**
2. **The manifestations of Gardner syndrome, outside of the colon, include adenomas in other areas of the GI tract, desmoid tumors, osteomas of the mandible of skull, and sebaceous cysts. There is an increased risk of developing duodenal cancer, pancreatic cancer, thyroid cancer, and brain cancer.**
3. **Genetic testing can reveal specific gene mutations. If found, these must be evaluated in first-degree relatives, such as the children. When testing cannot be performed, relatives must be screened via yearly sigmoidoscopy, starting at the age of 12 years, and then less often as each decade passes.**

Colorectal Tumors

Colorectal tumors may begin as non-malignant polyps on the lining of the sigmoid colon or rectum. Untreated, polyps may become cancer. Polyps are classified by behavior and cause, and can be benign, premalignant, or malignant.

Colorectal cancer (CRC) is very common, ranking as the third most diagnosed type of cancer out of all types in the United States and most other countries.

Epidemiology

Colorectal cancer results in more than 140,000 cases and over 50,000 deaths annually in the United States, making it the third most common type of cancer, but the second most common cause of cancer-related deaths. About 5% of men and women will be diagnosed during their lifetimes. Lifetime risks average about 1 in every 18–20 people. The disease peaks significantly near the ages of 40 and 50 years, though the median age is 69 years, and is slightly more common in men compared with women. About 54 men of every 100,000 are diagnosed, and also about 40 women of every 100,000. Colorectal cancer disproportionately affects African Americans about 20% more than other racial or ethnic groups, and they are also about 40% more likely to die from the disease.

Globally, over 1 million people are diagnosed with colorectal cancer every year, and over 715,000 die. It makes up 9.2% of cancer diagnoses in women, and 10% in men. Global incidence varies, with the highest rates in Australia, New Zealand, Europe, and the United States (see Figure 6.6). In the United Kingdom, colorectal cancer is the fourth most common type of cancer. The lowest rates are in Africa and South-Central Asia. For unknown reasons, the disease is more common in Caucasians globally than in other races.

Etiology and Risk Factors

The exact cause of colorectal cancer is unknown. Approximately 80% cases are sporadic, with the remaining 20% being inherited. It may be predisposed by chronic ulcerative colitis and Crohn colitis. The longer these conditions last, the higher the risks of CRC. Adenocarcinoma of the colon is 10–20 times more common if the patient previously had ulcerative colitis. Incidence is 60% higher in those with inflammatory bowel disease. Other factors include advanced age, family history, and inherited syndromes. If there is a first-degree relative with CRC, the risk for malignancy is increased to two or three times,

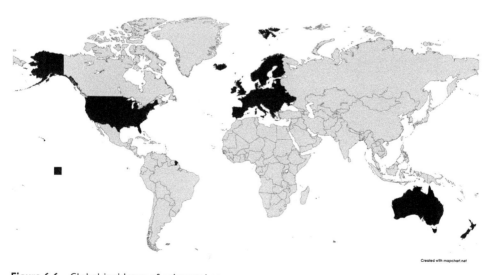

Figure 6.6 Global incidence of colorectal cancer.

and if there is more than one affected first-degree relative, it is increased to five or six times. Populations that have a higher incidence of CRC consume diets that are low in fiber but high in red meat, refined carbohydrates, and fat. Though carcinogens may exist in foods, bacterial effects upon substances in the diet more often produce them.

Clinical Manifestations

Because of the slow growth pattern, colorectal adenocarcinomas take a long time to cause symptoms, which are based on the tumor's site, subtype, size, and complications. Obstruction occurs late if the tumor is within the right colon because of its largeness, thin wall, and liquid contents. Bleeding usually occurs on an occult basis, and constipation as well as distention are common. Severe anemia may cause fatigue and weakness. Tumors may become so large that they can be felt through the abdominal wall prior to other symptoms starting. In the left colon however, the lumen is not as large, and the feces are semisolid. Therefore, obstruction by a tumor usually happens earlier. The first sign may be colicky abdominal pain with partial obstruction, or complete obstruction may be the first sign. There may be blood mixed or streaked through the stool. For some patients, there are signs that a perforation has occurred, which is usually focal pain and tenderness. Less often, there is diffuse peritonitis.

For rectal cancer, the most common symptom initially is bleeding during defecation. It is important for everyone to be aware that whenever there is rectal bleeding – even when hemorrhoids are known to exist or diverticular disease has been diagnosed – cancer must be ruled out since it can coexist. There may be a feeling of incomplete evacuation of the bowel, or tenesmus. If the perirectal area is affected, pain often occurs. For some patients, the first manifestations may indicate metastasis – such as ascites, hepatomegaly, or supraclavicular lymph node enlargement.

Pathology

Approximately, over 96% of colorectal cancers are adenocarcinomas. They develop from columnar glandular epithelium in the mucosa. In about 5% of patients, there may be several lesions, which are described as **synchronous cancer**. In most cases, the pathology of CRC begins as changes in adenomatous polyps. Colorectal cancer spreads via direct extension through the colon wall, metastasis through the blood, perineural spreading, and regional lymph node metastasis. There is slow growth of colorectal adenocarcinomas. Most adenocarcinomas are non-mucinous, yet the mucinous phenotype makes up 20% of all colorectal cancers. Epidermoid carcinomas make up to 25% of all colorectal cancers, mostly located in the rectum. Primary colorectal lymphomas make up only 10–20% of all GI lymphomas, yet lower than 1% of CRCs.

Diagnosis

For patients of average risk, colorectal cancer screening should start at age 50 and continue until age 75. However, the American Cancer Society recommends that adults who are of average risk should start being screened at age 45. This is because of increasing rates of CRC in people under age 50. The decision to be screened between ages 76 and 85 is based on each patient's health status and previous screening history. Screening options include a colonoscopy once every 10 years, a CT colonography every 5 years, an annual fecal occult blood test (with fecal immunochemical test [FIT] being preferred), flexible sigmoidoscopy every 5 years (or every 10 years if done with FIT), and fecal DNA testing with FIT every 3 years.

According to the *American Journal of Gastroenterology*, colonoscopy should be done every 10 years, or a yearly FIT should be done. However, if a patient has a family history, with a first-degree relative having had CRC before the age of 60 years, a colonoscopy should be done every 5 years starting at age 40 – or 10 years prior to the age that the relative was diagnosed – whichever is earlier.

Fecal immunochemical tests to find blood in the stool are better than the older guaiac-based tests since many different substances in the diet affected those. Even so, a positive test for blood in the stool can occur because of non-malignancies such as diverticulosis and ulcers. Also, negative test results do not mean that cancer is not present, since continuous bleeding does not occur. Fecal DNA testing finds methylation markers and DNA mutations that come from tumors in the colon. This type of testing is usually combined with FIT, which is approved for average-risk patients. Almost 10% of patients that have a positive fecal DNA-FIT test result have a colonoscopy that has normal results.

Virtual colonoscopy uses CT to generate 2D and 3D images of the colon. **Multidetector row CT** is used, combined with an orally administered contrast agent, and gas that distends the colon. The high-resolution 3D images can slightly simulate the views seen in an optical endoscopy. This test may be good for people who cannot tolerate or are unwilling to have an endoscopic colonoscopy. However, it is not as sensitive and requires a skilled person to interpret the results. The patient does not need to be sedated, but the bowel preparation procedures still must occur. Also, gas distension is uncomfortable for some patients. Lesions, however, can obviously not be biopsied during the procedure. **Video capsule endoscopy** is not currently an acceptable screening test due to technical problems. Blood-based tests such as the **Septin 9 assay** is used for patients of average risk, but lack sensitivity.

When a fecal occult blood test is positive, a colonoscopy is required. A colonoscopy is also required after a lesion is seen in an imaging study or during sigmoidoscopy. All lesions are completely removed and examined. When a lesion is **sessile** or cannot be removed during colonoscopy for some reason, surgical excision may be required. Less accurate than colonoscopy is barium enema X-ray.

If colorectal cancer is diagnosed, the patient must have routine laboratory tests, an abdominal CT scan, and chest X-rays to determine whether there is metastasis. In 70% of patients with CRC, elevated serum CEA levels exist. However, the CEA test is not sensitive or specific, so it is not a recommended screening method. When the CEA level is high before an operation and low after a colon tumor is removed, it should be monitored so that any recurrence can be found sooner rather than later. Other tumor markers that are used include *carbohydrate antigens 19-9* and *125*. Today, surgically resected colon tumors are tested for gene mutations that cause Lynch syndrome. Anyone with relatives that had colon, endometrial, or ovarian cancer at a young age, or with multiple relatives with these cancers must be tested for Lynch syndrome.

The staging for colorectal cancer uses the tumor (T) maximum penetration, regional lymph node (N) metastasis, and distant metastasis (M) classification. This TNM classification is broken down as follows:

- Stage 0 – Tis (carcinoma in situ), N0 = no regional lymph node metastasis, and M0 = no distant metastasis
- Stage I – T1 (submucosa) or T2 (muscularis propria), N0, and M0
- Stage II – T3 (penetrates all layers; for rectal cancer, this includes the perirectal tissue), N0, and M0
- Stage III – any T or T4 (adjacent organs or peritoneum), N0, and M0
- Stage IV – any T, any N, and M1 (distant metastasis is present)

It should be noted that "any N" describes N1 (one to three regional nodes), N2 (four or more regional nodes), and N3 (apical or vascular trunk nodes)

Treatment

For 70% of patients without metastatic disease, surgery can be curative. There is wide tumor resection, regional lymphatic drainage, and reanastomosis of colon segments. When there is 5 cm or less of normal colon tissue between the lesion and the **anal verge**, an abdominoperineal resection is usually performed, with a permanent colostomy. For some patients that are not debilitated, subsequent resection of 1–3 liver metastases is recommended. After primary tumor resection, criteria for this include those with liver metastases in one hepatic lobe, without any extrahepatic metastases. A small number of patients with liver metastases qualify, but five-year survival after surgery is 25%. Surgical procedures may involve laparotomy with hemicolectomy, lymph node dissection, and for some patients, appendectomy.

For rectal cancer with 1–4 positive lymph nodes, combined radiation and chemotherapy are used. When there are more than four positive lymph nodes, this combination is not as effective. Pre-surgical radiation therapy and chemotherapy improve resectability rates of rectal cancer, or can decrease incidence of lymph node metastasis.

Following curative surgery for colorectal cancer, a surveillance colonoscopy one year later is essential. This can also be done one year after the preoperative colonoscopy. Another surveillance colonoscopy is done three years after the one-year surveillance colonoscopy when no tumors or polyps are found. After that, surveillance colonoscopy is done every five years. When a pre-surgical colonoscopy was not complete due to an obstructing cancer, a "completion colonoscopy" is done 3–6 months after surgery, to find synchronous cancers, and to find and remove any precancerous polyps. Further screening for recurrence must include patient history, physical examination, and measurement of CEA levels every three months, for three years. After that, it is done every six months, for two years. A CT or MRI is recommended once per year, though these are of unproven benefit for regular follow-up when there are no abnormalities during examinations or blood tests.

When surgery will not be curative or there are extreme surgical risks, limited palliative surgery may be performed, such as to resect an area of perforation or relieve an obstruction. The median survival time is only seven months, however. **Electrocoagulation** can debulk some obstructive tumors, or the colon can be held open by stents. Chemotherapy has the ability to reduce tumor size and extend life for several months. Newer medications can be used alone or combined with others, and include capecitabine, irinotecan, and oxaliplatin. The monoclonal antibodies are sometimes effective, and include bevacizumab, cetuximab, and panitumumab. There is no "best" regimen for metastatic colorectal cancer, though some chemotherapy can delay progression. If colon cancer is advanced, a highly experienced person manages the chemotherapy, with access to drugs that are under investigation.

Prevention and Early Detection

There is no proven method of preventing colorectal cancer. However, some of the risk factors can be controlled by regular colorectal cancer screening, maintaining a normal body weight via physical activity and a good diet, limiting red and processed meats, and increasing intake of fruits, vegetables, and whole grains. Avoiding or limiting alcohol intake is also suggested, and smoking should be avoided. Some studies indicate that daily multi-vitamins that contain folic acid, plus calcium and magnesium supplements, may be helpful. Studies have also shown that people who regularly take aspirin and other nonsteroidal anti-inflammatory drugs (NSAIDs) have lower risks of colorectal polyps and cancer. Estrogen and progesterone replacement therapy after menopause may be helpful for women in reducing risks for colorectal cancer. Early detection of colorectal polyps or cancer can occur via regular screening methods. If found earlier, this can improve treatment and prognosis, and regular screening may even prevent the disease, since a polyp may take 10–15 years to become cancerous.

Prognosis

The prognosis for colorectal cancer is greatly dependent upon the staging. If the cancer is limited only to the mucosa, the 10-year survival rate is close to 90%. If there is extension through the colon wall, this rate is 70–80%. However, if there are positive lymph nodes, the rate is 30–50%, and for metastasis, the rate is less than 20% for 10-year survival.

Significant Point

Colorectal cancer is the third most commonly diagnosed cancer in men and women in the United States. The general population has a lifetime risk of about 5%. Colorectal cancer affects about 4.5% of men and about 4.2% of women. However, anyone with a family history of colorectal cancer has a 10–15% chance of developing the disease.

Clinical Case

1. How common is colorectal cancer in relation to other types of cancer?
2. Do symptoms of colorectal adenocarcinomas occur quickly or slowly?
3. When should screening for colorectal cancer begin?

A 63-year-old man went to his physician complaining of left-sided abdominal pain, distention, and constipation. An endoscopic examination revealed an ulcerated tumor of the descending colon. Liver function tests were normal. An abdominal X-ray revealed findings consistent with bowel obstruction. A CT scan revealed thickening of the descending colon wall, indicating advanced descending colon cancer. During colonoscopy, a biopsy revealed the tumor to be adenocarcinoma. A laparotomy procedure was performed, with left hemicolectomy, lymph node dissection, and appendectomy completed. There were no metastatic regional lymph nodes, but there were some carcinoma cells found in the lymphatic vessels and veins.

Answers:

1. **Colorectal cancer results in more than 140,000 cases and over 50,000 deaths annually in the United States, making the third most common type of cancer, and the second highest cause of cancer death. About 5% of men and women will be diagnosed during their lifetimes. Globally, over 1 million people are diagnosed with colorectal cancer every year, and over 715,000 die. It makes up 9.2% of cancer diagnoses in woman, and 10% in men.**

2. **Because of the slow growth pattern, colorectal adenocarcinomas take a long time to cause symptoms, which are based on the tumor's site, subtype, size, and complications. As in this case study, if the tumor is in the left colon, with the lumen not being as large and the feces being semisolid, obstruction by a tumor usually happens earlier.**

3. **For patients of average risk, colorectal cancer screening should start at age 50 and continue until age 75. However, the American Cancer Society recommends that adults who are of average risk should start being screened at age 45. This is because of increasing rates of CRC in people under age 50. The decision to be screened between ages 76 and 85 is based on each patient's health status and previous screening history. However, if a patient has a family history, with a first-degree relative having had CRC before age 60, a colonoscopy should be done every 5 years starting at age 40 – or 10 years prior to the age that the relative was diagnosed – whichever is earlier.**

Anorectal Cancer

Anorectal cancer, also referred to simply as *anal cancer*, is much less common than colorectal cancer. Squamous cell carcinoma of the anorectum makes up 3–5% of distal cancers of the large intestine. Subtypes of squamous cell carcinoma include basaloid carcinoma or nonkeratinizing squamous cell carcinoma. Less common forms of anorectal cancer include basal cell carcinoma, Bowen disease (also called intraepidermal squamous cell carcinoma), **cloacogenic carcinoma**, and malignant melanoma.

Epidemiology

In 2020, there were about 8,590 cases of anorectal cancer in the United States, with about 1,350 deaths. The disease has been increasing in occurrence for many years. The incidence of anorectal cancer is about 1 in 500 people, though the risk is higher in those who have risk factors for the disease. It is rare in people under age 35, and is primarily a disease of older adults, with the mean age being in the early 60s. Anorectal cancer is more common in women (5,900 cases) than in men (2,690 cases). It is also more fatal in women (810 deaths) than in men (540 deaths). For some reason, anorectal cancer is most common in Caucasian women and in African American men.

There are about 48,500 cases of anorectal cancer annually diagnosed throughout the world, making the disease just 0.3% of all diagnosed cancers. Again, women are more frequently diagnosed, with over 28,300 cases per year, with men having just over 20,100 cases per year. Aside from the United States, incidence of anorectal cancer is the highest in Canada, Denmark, Sweden, England, Scotland, and Australia (see Figure 6.7). The incidence rates, combined, result in about 5 cases per 100,000 people, globally. About 90% of patients with anorectal cancer are older than 40 years of age. The racial or ethnic statistics are not as clear as in the United States, but generally appear to be similar.

Etiology and Risk Factors

The exact cause of anorectal cancer is not known. Risk factors for anorectal cancer include chronic fistulas, HPV infection, leukoplakia, anal warts, *Condyloma acuminatum* infection, **Lymphogranuloma venereum** infection, and smoking. There is an increased risk for anorectal cancer in people who receive anal intercourse. Having multiple sex partners also increases risks because this is associated with higher risks for HIV and HPV. Also, women who previously had cancer of the cervix, vagina, or vulva have an increased risk for anorectal cancer. Anyone with reduced immunity,

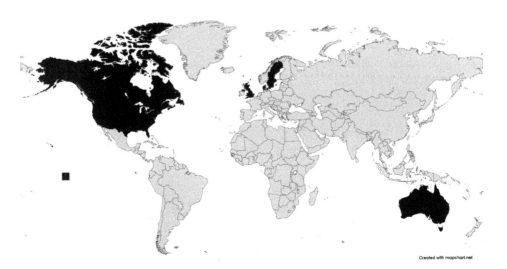

Figure 6.7 Countries with the highest incidence of anorectal cancer.

including patients recovering from organ transplantation, have a higher risk for developing anorectal cancer.

Clinical Manifestations

The most common initial manifestation of anorectal cancer is bleeding during defecation. There may also be pain in the area of the anus, a sensation of incomplete evacuation, or tenesmus. In some cases, there is a palpable mass present, found during digital rectal examination. Some patients also complain of persisting anal itching.

Pathology

When an individual has HPV infection, he or she may have dysplasia in normal-appearing or slightly abnormal-appearing anal epithelium. This is referred to as *anal intraepithelial neoplasia*, graded as I, II, or III disease. These changes occur more often in people with HIV. The higher grades of the disease can become invasive carcinoma. According to the American Cancer Society, the following are the stages of anorectal cancer:

- Stage 0 – pre-cancer cells are only within the mucosa and have not reached deeper layers, nearby lymph nodes, or distant sites
- Stage I – the cancer is approximately 2 cm or less in size and has not spread to nearby lymph nodes or distant sites
- Stage IIA – the cancer is 2–5 cm across, but has not spread to nearby lymph nodes or distant sites
- Stage IIB – the cancer is larger than 5 cm across, but has not spread to nearby lymph nodes or distant sites
- Stage IIIA – the cancer is 2 cm across or smaller, and *has* spread to nearby lymph nodes, but has not spread to distant sites
- Stage IIIB – the cancer is of any size and is growing into nearby organs, including the vagina, urethra, prostate gland, or bladder; it has not spread to nearby lymph nodes or distant sites
- Stage IIIC – the cancer is larger than 5 cm across, and *has* spread to lymph nodes close to the rectum, but not to distant sites
- Stage IV – the cancer is of any size, and *has* spread to distant organs –such as the lungs or liver

Diagnosis

Diagnosis of anorectal cancer is via use of a flexible sigmoidoscopy, or a rigid anoscopy or sigmoidoscopy. For lesions close to the **squamocolumnar junction** (Z line), skin biopsy by a surgeon or dermatologist may be required. Coexisting cancer must be ruled out if there is rectal bleeding, even if the patient has visible hemorrhoids or is known to have diverticular disease. Using CT, MRI, or PET may assist staging. Screening tests include the digital rectal examination and the *anal Pap test*. Additional methods used for diagnosis include endoscopy, blood tests, ultrasound, and chest X-rays to assess metastasis.

Treatment

For most patients, combination chemotherapy and radiation therapy is done first. There is a high cure rate when the cancer involves anal squamous or cloacogenic tumors. If chemotherapy and radiation do not result in total tumor regression, or the disease recurs, abdominoperineal resection must be performed. Stage 0 tumors can often be totally removed via local resection, along with a margin of healthy tissue surrounding them. Radiation or chemotherapy is rarely needed. For stage I or II tumors, local resection may remove smaller tumors that do not involve the sphincter muscle, and may be followed with chemotherapy or radiation. The standard treatment for anal cancers that cannot be removed without harming the anal sphincter is *external beam radiation therapy (EBRT)* combined with chemotherapy. This *chemoradiation* method involves two treatments, usually of 5-fluorouracil with mitomycin. The EBRT is given daily, Monday through Friday, for 5–7 weeks. It can take months for the full effects of chemoradiation to appear. At six months, more treatment is often needed if the cancer is still present. At this point, abdominoperineal resection is often recommended.

For stage III disease, chemoradiation usually occurs first. If some cancer remains, it is monitored closely for up to six months. Abdominoperineal resection then may or may not be done. If cancer has reached the lymph nodes, they may be surgically resected or treated with radiation therapy. For stage IV disease, treatment is palliative – usually with chemotherapy, with or without radiation. Immunotherapy is another option. There are also clinical trials of newer treatments that can be tried. In the case of anorectal malignant melanoma, which does not respond well to chemotherapy or radiation, surgery is indicated. If it has spread to other organs, immunotherapy or targeted therapy drugs are used.

Prevention and Early Detection

There is no known method to prevent anorectal cancer. However, methods that can reduce the risks for the disease include the HPV vaccine, avoiding or quitting smoking, treating HIV, and in some studies, using condoms during all forms of intercourse. Regarding early detection, it is uncertain if early detection and treatment can improve the long-term outcome of anorectal cancer. Therefore, there are no clear recommendations for screening.

Prognosis

The majority of cases of anorectal cases are cured by chemoradiation. Follow-up visits usually occur every 3–6 months, for 2 years after chemoradiation is completed. According to the Surveillance, Epidemiology, and End Results Program, the five-year relative survival rates for anorectal cancer are as follows:

- Localized – 82% survival over five years
- Regional – 65%
- Distant – 32%

Clinical Case

1. What is the incidence of anorectal cancer?
2. What is the description of stage IIIb anorectal cancer, including malignant melanoma?

3. How does the treatment of anorectal squamous cell carcinoma differ from that of anorectal malignant melanoma?

A 72-year-old man went to his physician complaining of an anal region mass. He was then referred to the local hospital because a malignant melanoma was suspected. Examination revealed a 25-mm-black type 1 tumor that was 33% the size of the anal canal circumference, and located externally to it. A transanal resection was performed, and the diagnosis was confirmed. Multiple macular black lesions were observed, from the tumor to the pectinate line. A biopsy also confirmed malignant melanoma, so an abdominoperineal resection was performed. The patient was diagnosed with stage IIIb malignant melanoma and followed on an outpatient basis, with no recurrence over three months.

Answers:

1. **Anorectal cancer is much less common than colorectal cancer. In 2020, there were about 8,590 cases in the United States, with about 1,350 deaths. The disease has been increasing in occurrence for many years, with incidence about 1 in 500 people, though the risk is higher in those who have risk factors for the disease. It is primarily a disease of older adults. There are about 48,500 cases of anorectal cancer annually diagnosed throughout the world, making the disease just 0.3% of all diagnosed cancers. Malignant melanoma is one of the less common forms of anorectal cancer.**
2. **In stage IIIb cancer, it is of any size and is growing into nearby organs, which may include the vagina, urethra, prostate gland, or bladder, but has not spread to nearby lymph nodes or distant sites.**
3. **For squamous cell carcinoma of the anorectal region, combination**

chemotherapy and radiation therapy is done first. In the case of anorectal malignant melanoma, which does not respond well to chemotherapy or radiation, surgery is indicated. If it has spread to other organs, immuno-therapy or targeted therapy drugs are used.

Pancreatic Cancer

Pancreatic cancer is an extremely invasive malignant tumor of the digestive system. The most common form of pancreatic cancer is *ductal adenocarcinoma*. The majority of pancreatic cancers are exocrine tumors, forming from the ductal and acinar cells. Pancreatic endocrine tumors originate from the islet and gastrin-producing cells, and often secrete several hormones. This type of tumor can also appear in the duodenum, jejunum, and lungs. They are generally either functioning or nonfunctioning.

Epidemiology

Pancreatic cancer affects about 55,500 people annually in the United States, and is unfortunately fatal in over 43,300 of these. It accounts for 3% of all cancers in the United States, and about 7% of all cancer deaths. Incidence is about 13.2 per 100,000 people, with 11 of these cases being fatal. Pancreatic cancer is the 9th most common cancer in men, and the 10th most common cancer in women. About 93% of pancreatic cancers are exocrine adenocarcinomas, which occur at a mean age of 55 years, and are 2 times more common in men than in women. Pancreatic cancer incidence and mortality is the highest in African Americans, compared with all other racial or ethnic groups.

Globally, pancreatic cancer is the 12th most common cancer in men and the 11th most common cancer in women. There are more than 460,000 new cases throughout the world every year. The incidence of pancreatic cancer comprises 2.5% of all types of cancer, worldwide. On average, about 47% of new cases of pancreatic cancers occur in people aged 75 and older. Age-specific incidence rates increase sharply at age 50–54. Throughout the world, men develop pancreatic cancer slightly more than women (1.1–2 times higher). The countries with the highest rates of pancreatic cancer include Hungary (10.8 cases out of every 100,000 people), Uruguay (10.7 cases), Moldova (10.5), Latvia (10.3), Japan (9.7), Slovakia (9.6), Estonia (9.2), Czech Republic (9.0), Armenia (8.9), the metropolitan areas of France (8.9), Serbia (8.8), and Austria (8.7) – see Figure 6.8.

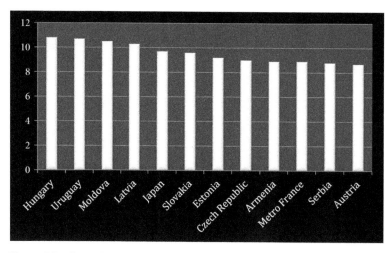

Figure 6.8 Countries with the highest rates of pancreatic cancer, per 100,000 people.

Etiology and Risk Factors

The exact cause of pancreatic cancer is not known. The most common risk factors for pancreatic cancer include smoking, chronic pancreatitis, the male gender, obesity, and the African American ethnicity. Heredity is also slightly implicated. Alcohol and caffeine use do not appear to be risk factors, though some studies have revealed that heavy alcohol use can lead to chronic pancreatitis, which can influence the development of pancreatic cancer.

Clinical Manifestations

In most cases, pancreatic cancer's initial symptoms, including pain and weight loss, are not specific, meaning that a diagnosis is usually achieved late in the disease course. Upon diagnosis, about 90% of patients have locally advanced tumors that have affected the retroperitoneal structures, regional lymph nodes, or even the lungs or liver. Severe upper abdominal pain is common, usually radiating to the back. An adenocarcinoma of the head of the pancreas causes obstructive jaundice and itching in 80–90% of patients. If the cancer is located in the pancreatic body or tail, there may be obstruction of the splenic vein that causes splenomegaly, esophageal and gastric varices, and GI hemorrhage. In 25–50% of patients, pancreatic cancer causes diabetes and glucose intolerance, resulting in polydipsia and polyuria. The cancer can alter production of digestive enzymes, known as *pancreatic exocrine insufficiency*, resulting in malabsorption of food and nutrients. This causes bloating, gas, and a foul-smelling diarrhea that may also be watery or greasy. Weight loss continues, and vitamin deficiencies occur.

Pathology

Adenocarcinomas of the exocrine pancreas usually originate from duct cells – in fact, nine times more often than those forming from the acinar cells. About 80% of these adenocarcinomas develop in the head of the pancreas. Over 90% of pancreatic tumors have a ductal origin. The pathological subtypes, each with different morphologies, may have the same molecular background as the classical form, while others have a distinct molecular pathogenesis. In general, ductal adenocarcinomas are firm and poorly defined. They can range from poor- to well-differentiated, having glandular structures within desmoplastic stroma. This stroma, plus varying amounts of mucin are thought to contribute to the common hypodense appearance during CT scans. The tumors do not stain with endocrine markers. Serum levels of pancreatic enzymes are usually not elevated.

Microscopically, diagnosis is confirmed by visualizing a stained, thin tissue section via bright-field microscopy. There is progressive accumulation of somatic mutations in epithelial cells. There is disorganization of the extracellular matrix, and its cells, using hematoxylin and eosin or other dyes, show strong multi-photo excitation fluorescence and third harmonic generation (THG) signals. Quantification of nuclei shape and size can be performed using THG microscopy. Similar conditions that can develop into pancreatic ductal adenocarcinoma include *intraductal papillary mucinous neoplasia* and *mucinous cystic neoplasia*.

Diagnosis

Magnetic resonance cholangiopancreatography, endoscopic ultrasonography, and abdominal CT with contrast enhancement are indicated to diagnose pancreatic cancer (see Figure 6.9). If a patient with obstructive jaundice, *endoscopic retrograde cholangiopancreatography* may be the initial procedure performed for diagnosis. For all patients, routine laboratory tests are performed. If there is elevated alkaline phosphatase and bilirubin, this can indicate liver metastasis or bile duct obstruction. If pancreatic carcinoma is diagnosed, *pancreas-associated antigen, carbohydrate antigen (CA) 19-9* may be part of monitoring the patient. It is also used to screen high-risk patients, such as those with hereditary pancreatitis, *breast cancer 2 (BRCA2)* or *hereditary nonpolyposis colorectal cancer (HNPCC)* gene mutations, two or more

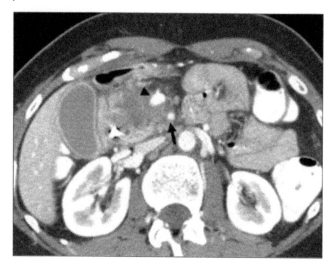

Figure 6.9 Contrast-enhanced CT showing an advanced pancreatic adenocarcinoma, which has encased the superior mesenteric artery (arrow and arrowhead). *Source*: From Dr. Matthew et al. (2008).

first-degree family members with pancreatic cancer, or Peutz–Jeghers syndrome. The levels of amylase and lipase are normal in most patients.

Treatment

Unfortunately, 80–90% of pancreatic cancers are considered to be unresectable when they are diagnosed, due to metastases or major blood vessel invasion. Based on tumor location, a Whipple procedure is usually performed. Adjuvant therapy is often given with gemcitabine-based combinations. EBRT is usually used. The chemotherapy and radiation combinations are also used for localized yet unresectable tumors, resulting in median survival of about 12 months. There is no drug, either used alone or in combination, that provides superior results, but gemcitabine and others may be more effective than chemotherapies based on 5-fluorouracil. If the patient has liver or distant metastases, chemotherapy may be done on an investigational basis, but this does not improve prognosis.

If during surgery an unresectable tumor is found, and GI or bile duct obstruction is present or may soon develop, a double gastric/biliary bypass operation can relieve the obstruction. If there is an inoperable lesion and the patient has jaundice, a bile duct stent or biliary drain may be placed in an endoscopic procedure. Duodenal stenting is also common. Surgical bypass is considered in patients with unresectable lesions if the life expectancy is more than 6–7 months, due to the complications of using stents.

For moderate to severe pain, oral opioids are given in sufficient dosages. Pain control is more important than any concern about addiction. Long-acting preparations are good for chronic pain, and include transdermal fentanyl, oxycodone, or oxymorphone. If pain is intolerable, opioids may be given by subcutaneous, intravenous, or epidural.

Exocrine pancreatic insufficiency is treated with oral pancrelipase, which contains pancreatic enzymes derived from pigs. There are many varieties of this available. Dosage is based on symptoms, amount of steatorrhea, and dietary fat content. Usually, patients must take between 5,000 and 40,000 IU of these products between snacks or meals. Proton pump inhibitors or H2-blockers may also be needed. If diabetes mellitus is present, it must be monitored and controlled with care.

Prevention and Early Detection

There is no known method of preventing pancreatic cancer. However, steps that can be taken to reduce risks of its development include avoiding or quitting smoking, eating a healthy diet, maintaining a normal body weight, getting regular physical activity, avoiding heavy use of alcohol, and avoiding exposure to chemicals in the workplace. Pancreatic cancer is difficult to detect early. Tumors in the organ cannot be seen or felt during routine physical examinations. No screening test has been proven to lower the risk of dying from pancreatic cancer. However, for people with family history, genetic testing may be able to find gene changes that increase the risks of contracting the disease. For those at high risk, endoscopic ultrasound or MRI may help to detect early pancreatic cancer.

Prognosis

The prognosis for pancreatic cancer is usually poor, but can be varied. For most patients, the five-year survival rate is less than two years, since so many have advanced disease by the time it is diagnosed. The survival rates for various stages of pancreatic cancer are as follows:

- Localized – 39.4% survival over 5 years
- Regional – 13.3%
- Distant – 2.9%

Significant Point

Pancreatic cancer is increasing in prevalence and incidence, and is hard to diagnose when it is early in its development. This is also when the disease is more treatable. The disease is often ignored early because its symptoms are so vague and nonspecific. About 93% of pancreatic tumors are exocrine tumors, and the most common type of pancreatic cancer is adenocarcinoma.

Clinical Case

1. How common is pancreatic cancer in men compared with women?
2. Upon diagnosis, what have pancreatic tumors usually done in regard to their growth and development?
3. What steps can be taken to reduce risks of developing pancreatic cancer?

A 68-year-old man was diagnosed with pancreatic cancer – specifically, ductal adenocarcinoma, and treatment options were discussed. He had lost about 15 pounds over a few months. Upon examination, the patient had abdominal pain and jaundice. Imaging revealed a mass within the head of the pancreas. It was biopsied and identified as a low-grade pancreatic adenocarcinoma. A biliary drain was placed, and the patient was discharged. One week later, a Whipple procedure was performed. The tumor was moderately differentiated, with negative margins, and 16 nearby lymph nodes were negative. Within 8 days, the biliary drain was removed, and the patient was discharged to a skilled nursing facility. Though at high risk for recurrence, the low grade of the tumor was likely to respond well to adjuvant chemotherapy (gemcitabine or 5-fluorouracil). He was started on gemcitabine, which he tolerated well, and has been followed for 6 months without recurrence.

Answers:

1. **In the United States, pancreatic cancer is the 9th most common in men and the 10th most common cancer in women. For some reason, the global statistics are different. It is the 11th most common cancer in women and the 12th most common cancer in men.**
2. **Upon diagnosis, about 90% of patients have locally advanced tumors that**

have affected the retroperitoneal structures, regional lymph nodes, or even the lungs or liver. An adenocarcinoma of the head of the pancreas causes obstructive jaundice and itching in 80–90% of patients.

3. Steps that can be taken to reduce risks of developing pancreatic cancer include avoiding or quitting smoking, eating a healthy diet, maintaining a normal body weight, getting regular physical activity, avoiding heavy use of alcohol, and avoiding exposure to chemicals in the workplace.

Liver and Biliary Tract Cancers

Liver and biliary tract cancers include hepatocellular carcinoma, liver metastases, and gallbladder cancer. Most malignant tumors that arise from the liver parenchyma and ductal epithelium of the biliary tract have a poor prognosis. Collectively, these cancers constitute the third leading cause of global cancer deaths. They are increasing in incidence.

Hepatocellular Carcinoma

Hepatocellular carcinoma is also referred to as *hepatoma*. It is most common in patients who have cirrhosis of the liver, and in areas of the world where hepatitis B and C viruses occur most often. Hepatocellular carcinoma is the most common form of primary liver cancer.

Epidemiology

There are over 42,000 cases of primary liver cancer annually in the United States, and nearly 32,000 are fatal. About 75% of cases are hepatocellular carcinoma. The incidence of hepatocellular carcinoma has more than tripled in the United States since 1980. It is the most rapidly increasing cancer in both men and women – primarily due to the rise in cases of hepatitis C virus

(HCV)-induced cirrhosis. Most people that are diagnosed with hepatocellular carcinoma are over 50 years of age. Liver cancers are about 3 times more common in men compared with women. The disease disproportionately affects people of lower socioeconomic status. Death rates are higher in these people due to the disease not being discovered as early in its course as in people of higher socioeconomic status, since they generally can afford better health care. On a racial or ethnic basis, people with higher rates of cirrhosis and hepatitis generally have higher rates of hepatocellular carcinoma. African American men are the group with the highest mortality rates from hepatocellular carcinoma.

However, liver cancers are more common outside the United States – especially in East Asia and sub-Saharan Africa. There are more than one million people diagnosed with hepatocellular carcinoma every year throughout the world. Hepatocellular carcinoma is the sixth most common cancer worldwide, and the fourth major cause of cancer-related death. The incidence of liver cancers is similar to the incidence of chronic hepatitis B virus (HBV) infection in East Asia and sub-Saharan Africa. However, there is an overall average of about 9 cases per 100,000 men throughout the world, which is about 4 times higher than it was 20 years previously. Also, there are about 2.2 cases per 100,000 women throughout the world – also 4 times higher than 20 years previously. As in the United States, most diagnoses occur after age 50, and about 3 times more men than women are diagnosed. The countries with the highest rates of hepatocellular carcinoma include: Mongolia (93.7 cases per 100,000), Egypt (32.2 per 100,000), Gambia (23.9), Vietnam (23.2), Laos (22.4), Cambodia (21.8), Guinea (21.8), Thailand (21.0), China (18.3), South Korea (17.3), North Korea (16.5), and Ghana (15.4) – see Figure 6.10.

Therefore, the global cases definitely favor people from Asian or African racial backgrounds.

Etiology and Risk Factors

The cause of hepatocellular carcinoma is primarily cirrhosis. However, the presence of the

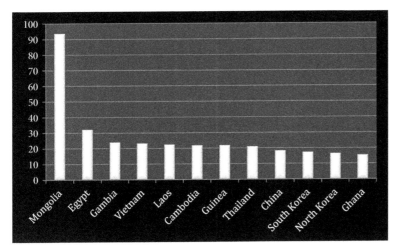

Figure 6.10   Countries with the highest rates of hepatocellular carcinoma, out of every 100,000 people.

hepatitis B virus increases risks by 100 times in people who carry HBV. If HBV-DNA is incorporated into the genome, this may trigger malignant transformation, even if there is no cirrhosis or chronic hepatitis. Other risk factors include alcoholic cirrhosis, hemochromatosis, and chronic HCV infection. Like HBV infection, hepatocellular carcinoma can form in patients that have non-cirrhotic non-alcoholic steatohepatitis. Increased risks are present if cirrhosis is caused by any other conditions. In subtropical areas of the world, the high incidence of hepatocellular carcinoma is believed to occur from ingesting food that has been contaminated with fungal **aflatoxins**.

Clinical Manifestations

Usually, a patient with cirrhosis that was previously stable will develop abdominal pain, a right upper quadrant mass, weight loss, and deterioration of health that cannot otherwise be explained. Fever is sometimes present. For a small number of patients, the initial signs and symptoms of hepatocellular carcinoma include bloody ascites, peritonitis, or shock – caused by tumor hemorrhage. There can also be **bruit** or a hepatic friction rub. Clinical complications may include systemic metabolic abnormalities, such as erythrocytosis, hypoglycemia, hypercalcemia, and hyperlipidemia. Other potential outcomes

include portal hypertension, encephalopathy, GI bleeding, jaundice, cachexia, fatigue, caput medusae, splenomegaly, and **asterixis**.

Pathology

Hepatocellular carcinoma is a heterogeneous tumor. The pathology of this cancer comprises multiple nodules, often with irregular borders or satellite nodules. Larger tumors have macroscopic venous invasion, with or without a fibrous capsule. Smaller tumors usually lack venous invasion, necrosis, or hemorrhage. The origin of this cancer is related to recurring cycles of necrosis and regeneration. The HBV and HCV genomes have genetic material that can predispose cells to accumulate mutations, or to experience disrupted growth. The gross pathology is of a pale mass in the liver that can be unifocal, multifocal, or diffusely infiltrative. The growth subtypes are nodular, massive, and infiltrative. The microscopic appearance ranges from well-differentiated to undifferentiated.

Diagnosis

Diagnosis of hepatocellular carcinoma can occur prior to symptoms developing, by palpating the area of the liver, if an imaging test detects an upper right quadrant mass and the patient has cirrhosis, or if there is unexplainable decompensation attributable to chronic liver disease. Along with imaging, AFP test is performed, which can reveal dedifferentiation of hepatocytes – a strong indicator of hepatocellular carcinoma. Lower AFP values are not as specific, and may occur along with hepatocellular regeneration, such as in hepatitis.

The initial imaging test may be contrast-enhanced CT, MRI, or ultrasound. Contrast imaging is ordered as a *triple-phase protocol* since the delayed-contrast (third) phase is required for a radiographic diagnosis. Hepatic arteriography may be helpful for some cases, to outline vascular anatomy if surgery or ablation is being considered. Diagnosis is clear when the AFP is elevated and there are characteristic features. Screening patients with cirrhosis is a good method, but is somewhat under debate and does not reduce the number of deaths. Ultrasound may be performed every 6–12 months. In obese people, ultrasound is not as sensitive, and should be alternated with CT or MRI. Screening is often advised for patients with chronic hepatitis B, even without cirrhosis.

Treatment

Staging of the disease influences treatment choices, as does the level of liver disease. If the patient has just one tumor of less than 5 cm in size, or up to 3 tumors that are all 3 cm in size or less, confined to the liver without microvascular invasion, and the AFP is less than 500 mcg/L, liver transplantation provides just as good a prognosis as when the procedure is done for non-cancerous disorders. It has been curative for many patients. These criteria are referred to as the "Milan criteria," to determine hepatocellular carcinoma patients that will be good candidates for liver transplantation. If the patient has one tumor of less than 5 cm in size and no portal hypertension, surgical resection can be curative. The 5-year survival rates are between 60% and 80%.

Ablative treatments include hepatic arterial chemoembolization, selective internal radiation therapy, and radiofrequency ablation. All of these provide for palliation and cause tumor growth to become slower. They are done for patients awaiting a new liver. The radiofrequency ablation technique can be curative for tumors smaller than 2 cm. For tumors larger than 5 cm that are multifocal, have invaded the portal vein, or are metastatic, radiation therapy is usually ineffective, with a 5-year survival rate of 5% or less. Sorafenib may slightly improve the outlook, extending survival by about three months. Newer agents can prolong survival for a longer time and/or cause fewer side effects. They include lenvatinib, regorafenib, and the immunotherapy agent called nivolumab. Levatinib is an alternative first-line therapy, providing progression-free survival that is better than with sorafenib.

Prevention and Early Detection

The HBV vaccine is preventive in that it decreases incidence of hepatocellular carcinoma – primarily in endemic areas of the world. Preventing cirrhosis from any cause is important, and can be achieved by methods such as treating alcoholism, detecting hemochromatosis early, or treating chronic hepatitis C. Hepatocellular carcinoma is usually not detected early in its development. By the time a tumor can be felt, it is often quite large. At this time, there are no widely recommended screening tests for people at average risk. For a person with long-term cirrhosis, physicians may test for liver cancer if there is a sudden worsening of health condition for no obvious reason. Some experts recommend screening with AFP blood tests and ultrasonography every six months for high-risk patients.

Prognosis

Overall prognosis for hepatocellular carcinoma is poor, with a 5-year relative survival rate of 18%. For localized disease, this rate is 33%; for regional disease it is 11%, and for distant disease, it is only 2.4%. Survival time is based on the amount of cirrhosis that is present. A shorter survival time is predicted if there is also portal vein occlusion – a common occurrence. About the same number of patients die of liver failure as do from tumor progression. Patients with diabetes, poor glycemic control, or obesity have a poorer prognosis than those without.

Significant Point

Hepatocellular carcinoma is the most common type of liver cancer. For some reason, it affects men three times more often than women. More than 80% of patients have pre-existing cirrhosis of the liver. Untreated, life expectancy with hepatocellular carcinoma is under 4 months, and with treatment, only about 50% of patients will survive for 2 years.

Clinical Case

1. Has the incidence of hepatocellular carcinoma changed over time?
2. How influential is cirrhosis upon development of hepatocellular carcinoma?
3. Which pathological factors are related to hepatocellular carcinoma?

A 65-year-old African American man was referred by his physician to a hepatology clinic because the patient had positive hepatitis C antibody test, cirrhosis of the liver, and a possible liver tumor. The patient reported right upper quadrant abdominal pain. A CT scan was performed, which revealed a liver lesion that was large and solid, located in the right lobe, and measuring 8 cm in diameter. A follow-up CT scan of the chest, abdomen, and pelvis showed the presence of multifocal hepatocellular carcinoma. The tumor had seeded into the right hepatic vein, inferior vena cava, and right atrium. The disease was staged as "advanced." The patient was started on the chemotherapy agent called sorafenib, along with radiation therapy. Follow-up CT showed good improvement of the tumor with the right atrium, but otherwise the liver

tumor was unchanged. Radioembolization was then performed to the right hepatic artery, with did not succeed in stopping disease progression. Transarterial chemoembolization was performed to the other locations, again without success. Additional radiation therapy was performed, but the patient died within one year.

Answers:

1. **The incidence of hepatocellular carcinoma has more than tripled in the United States since 1980. It is the most rapidly increasing cancer in both men and women – primarily due to the rise in cases of HCV-induced cirrhosis. Globally, the incidence of liver cancers is similar to the incidence of chronic HBV in East Asia and sub-Saharan Africa.**
2. **The cause of hepatocellular carcinoma is primarily cirrhosis. Increased risks are present if cirrhosis is caused by any other conditions.**
3. **Hepatocellular carcinoma is a heterogeneous tumor. Factors related to its development include chronic infections with hepatitis B or C, cirrhosis, metabolic syndrome, and alcohol consumption.**

Liver Metastases

Common cancers that metastasize to the liver include those of the gastrointestinal tract, breasts, colon, lungs, and pancreas. Metastatic liver cancer is more common than primary liver cancer. It is also called *secondary liver cancer.* Advanced leukemia and other blood disorders often affect the liver.

Epidemiology

According to the journal called *Cancer Epidemiology*, about 5.14% of all cancer patients present with concurrent liver metastases.

Metastatic tumors in the liver are 20 times more common than primary liver tumors. Incidence of liver metastases is less than 5 cases per 100,000 for patients under age 40, but over 100 per 100,000 for patients aged 70 or older. Incidence increases with age, and is based on the incidence of the primary type of cancer. For men, the most common primary site was the colon, and for women, it was the breasts. Though actual racial or ethnic statistics are more in relation to the type of primary cancer, it has been documented that African Americans with cancer are 14% more likely to have metastatic disease upon presentation. This is likely due to poorer access to early health care.

The global statistics about prevalence and incidence of metastatic liver cancer are not readily available for most countries. However, some countries have published data. For example, similar to the United States, metastatic liver cancer is 20 times more common in Australia than primary liver cancer, and this situation is believed to be very similar around the world. The vast majority of cases occur in people that are 70 years of age or older, with a nearly equal predilection between men and women. There is no distinct global difference regarding racial or ethnic groups, since this type of cancer spreads because of many other cancers.

Etiology and Risk Factors

The causes of metastatic liver cancer are obvious – other cancers from different body areas. Risk factors for metastatic liver cancer include the male gender, obesity, anaplastic steroid use, diabetes mellitus, inherited metabolic diseases, alpha-1-antitrypsin deficiency, **tyrosinemia**, and **Wilson's disease**.

Clinical Manifestations

In early stages, liver metastases are often asymptomatic. The nonspecific symptoms of cancer often appear initially. These include anorexia, fever, and weight loss. The liver can increase in size and become hard or tender. Signs and symptoms can include abdominal pain or pain near the right shoulder, nausea, abdominal bloating or swelling, and continuing fatigue or weakness. Advanced disease is signified by extreme hepatomegaly and palpable nodules. Uncommon but definitive signs are liver bruits and pain that mimics pleuritis, with a friction rub. If a tumor has obstructed the biliary duct, jaundice can develop. Otherwise, jaundice is initially absent or only slight. Once the patient reaches the terminal stages, progressive jaundice and hepatic encephalopathy signify that death is imminent.

Pathology

When another cancer has spread to the liver, it is usually already in stage IV. There is often macroscopically visible peritoneal dissemination. In some patients, there can be multiple necrotic lesions that may be hemorrhagic. Liver metastases from colorectal cells macroscopically have characteristic structures that resemble villi. Microscopically, there may be antibodies against microtubulin-associated protein 2 (MAP2) in the cytoplasm and cell processes. Poorly differentiated carcinoma may diffusely infiltrate hepatic sinusoids. The microenvironment of stroma surrounding the tumor cells is made up of a three-dimensional extracellular matrix, along with stromal cells such as fibroblasts and inflammatory cells.

Diagnosis

Blood chemistry tests may reveal an increase in alkaline phosphatase, gamma-glutamyl transpeptidase, and lactate dehydrogenase. Levels of aspartate aminotransferase can be varied. Serum calcium, CEA and CA 15-3 tumor markers is often increased. Imaging tests are usually assistive, with contrast CT or contrast MRI being more accurate than ultrasound. Image-guided liver biopsy confirms diagnosis. It is performed when other tests are not diagnostic or when histologic information could help in the treatment decision.

Treatment

Treatment is based on the amount of metastasis. Surgical resection can lengthen survival if there is only one or just a few metastases related to colorectal cancer. Surgical options include minimally invasive and laparoscopic techniques. Systemic chemotherapy can sometimes shrink tumors and prolong life, but not achieve a cure. Agents include 5-fluorouracil, cyclophosphamide, interferon-alpha, and epirubicin. Hepatic intra-arterial chemotherapy is also good, and offers less systemic adverse effects, as well as milder effects. Severe pain from advanced metastases can be sometimes helped by radiation therapy, though this will not extend life. Once the disease is extensive, palliative care is indicated, along with support for the patient's family. For patients with a hematologic cancer that has metastasized to the liver, the treatment is focused on the initial cancer. Even when a primary cancer has been removed, liver metastasis can occur, even years later. Radiofrequency ablation is also commonly used to treat liver tumors. *Radioembolization* is used for tumors that cannot be surgically removed, in which tiny radioactive beads are delivered directly into the tumor.

Prevention and Early Detection

There is no method of preventing metastatic liver cancer, except for preventive efforts to stop the primary form of cancer that initiates its development. Liver metastases that are larger than 1–2 cm in size can be detected by high level CT and MRI techniques. Microscopic metastases are not often detected via anatomic imaging, and are only rarely discovered during surgery or biopsy. Radionuclide or Doppler perfusion techniques may be able to detect alterations in perfusion that are caused by angiogenesis in microscopic lesions. Fortunately, recent developments in CT and MRI are improving methods of early detection.

Prognosis

In nearly all cases, when a primary cancer has metastasized to the liver, there is no possible cure. Current treatments focus on relieving symptoms and improve the patient's life expectancy. Unfortunately, life expectancy and prognosis are usually poor. Overall five-year survival rates are based upon the primary type of cancer, age, gender, and overall health. For example, the 5-year survival rates for patients with liver metastases originating in the colon are less than 8 months without treatment, and only an 11% chance of survival with treatment.

Significant Point

End-stage liver metastasis can be signified by serious problems, including persistent vomiting, blood in the vomit, recent and unexplained weight loss, black bowel movements, difficulty swallowing, new swelling in the legs or abdomen, and jaundice.

Clinical Case

1. Are metastatic liver tumors common in younger patients?
2. What are the treatment options for liver metastases?
3. What is the overall prognoses for liver metastases?

A 39-year-old Asian-American woman had been diagnosed with a primary breast tumor. She underwent a radical left mastectomy, with diagnosis suggesting a papillotubular carcinoma. There was vascular and lymphatic invasion, and estrogen and progesterone receptors in the primary tumor were positive. The patient underwent radiotherapy and received medroxyprogesterone acetate, but developed fatigue and skin eruptions. Physical examination then revealed liver dysfunction, and a CT revealed liver metastasis from the breast cancer. The patient had palpable lymph node swelling. There were multiple diffuse foci throughout the liver. There were increased levels of aspartate aminotransferase, alkaline phosphatase, lactate dehydrogenase, gamma-glutamyl transpeptidase, serum calcium, and the CA 15-3 and CEA tumor markers. Large lesions were present at the hepatic portal, with the tumor making up 50% or more of the liver volume. The patient received intra-arterial infusion of 5-fluorouracil followed by continuous IV infusion of cyclophosphamide, tumor necrosis factor, and interferon-alpha. The patient slowly improved over time. She was transferred to a local clinic, undergoing arterial injections of epirubicin and IV injection of cyclophosphamide. She has survived for seven years without recurrence.

Answers:

1. **Metastatic tumors in the liver occur in less than 5 cases per 100,000 for patients under age 40, but over 100 per 100,000 for patients at age 70 or older. Metastatic breast cancer is the most common primary tumor in women with liver metastases.**
2. **Treatment options include surgical resection that may be minimally invasive or laparoscopic, systemic chemotherapy, hepatic intra-arterial chemotherapy, radiation therapy, biological response modifiers, tumor necrosis factor, targeted therapies, hormonal therapies, radiofrequency ablation, and radioembolization.**
3. **In nearly all cases, when a primary cancer has metastasized to the liver, there is no possible cure. Unfortunately, life expectancy and prognosis are usually poor. Overall five-year survival rates are based upon the primary type of cancer, age, gender, and overall health. For example, the 5-year survival rates for patients with liver metastases**

originating in the colon are less than 8 months without treatment, and only an 11% chance of survival with treatment.

Gallbladder Cancer

Gallbladder cancer is an uncommon form of cancer that, along with bile duct tumors, may cause extrahepatic biliary obstruction. *Gallbladder carcinoma* and *gallbladder polyps* both occur, with polyps being much more common. Even though gallbladder carcinoma is overall rare, it is still the most common type of cancer of the biliary system. It is also the fifth most common type of gastrointestinal cancer. Gallbladder carcinoma can only be cured if it is found before it spreads.

Epidemiology

Gallbladder carcinoma occurs in 2.5 of every 100,000 people. According to the American Cancer Society, there were about 11,980 new cases diagnosed in 2020, with 4,090 deaths. The median age for gallbladder cancer to develop is 67 years. Gallbladder cancer is more common in women than in men, with 6,380 of the 2020 cases in the United States being women and 5,600 being men. Also, there were 2,390 female deaths from the disease and 1,700 male deaths. The racial or ethnic group most commonly affected is American Indians.

Globally, gallbladder cancer is the 17th most common cancer in men and the 18th most common cancer in women, with almost 220,000 new cases reported in 2018. Incidence affects about 11% of the world population, with cases ranging between 12.3 and 27.3 out of every 100,000 people. Older adults are most likely to develop gallbladder cancer, with those in their late 60s most affected. The countries with the most cases of gallbladder cancer are as follows: Bolivia (14.0 cases out of every 100,000 people), Chile (9.3 cases), Thailand (7.4), South Korea (6.8), Nepal (6.7), Bangladesh (5.1), Peru (4.8), Japan (4.5),

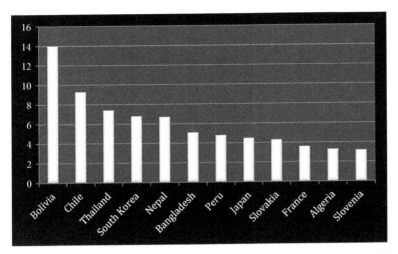

Figure 6.11   Countries with the highest rates of gallbladder cancer, per 100,000 people.

Slovakia (4.3), France (3.6), Algeria (3.3), and Slovenia (3.2) – see Figure 6.11. The wide range of people affected includes all racial and ethnic groups, with no specific prevalence.

Etiology and Risk Factors

Though the actual cause is not fully understood, gallbladder carcinoma is related to the presence of gallstones larger than 3 cm in size, and to extensive gallbladder calcification because of *chronic cholecystitis*, which is also known as *porcelain gallbladder*. Between 70% and 90% of cases of gallbladder carcinoma also involve gallstones. Genes that may be implicated in the development of this cancer include the *KRAS*, and *homolog B v-raf murine sarcoma (BRAF)*. Risk factors include chronic gallbladder inflammation, such as from gallstones, along with ductal defects that cause pancreatic juices to reflux into the gallbladder and bile ducts.

Clinical Manifestations

Gallbladder carcinoma may cause biliary pain (in 80% patients upon presentation), cholelithiasis, or advance to cause constant pain, weight loss (40% of patients), an abdominal mass, or obstructive jaundice (30%). Additional signs and symptoms may include nausea and vomiting (50% of patients), loss of appetite, fever, itchy skin, dark urine, and stools that are light in color or greasy. Gallbladder polyps are usually asymptomatic, benign projections of the mucosa within the lumen of the gallbladder.

Pathology

Gallbladder carcinoma begins in the mucosal layer of the organ, and moves outward. More than 90% of cases are adenocarcinomas, with most related to chronic inflammatory **metaplasia** and dysplasia. Of the adenocarcinomas, the subtypes include scirrhous (90%), papillary (5%), and colloid (5%). Squamous cell carcinoma makes up only 3% of all primary gallbladder malignancies. The majority of gallbladder polyps are less than 10 mm in diameter. They are made up of cholesterol ester and triglycerides, and when present, the condition is called **cholesterolosis**. The primary types of polypoid growths in the gallbladder also include *cholesterosis with fibrous dysplasia*, adenomyomatosis, *hyperplastic cholecystosis*, and adenocarcinoma. Most polyps that are less than 1 cm in size are not cancerous and may not change for years. However, polyps that occur along with primary sclerosing cholangitis are more likely to be malignant, and larger polyps more often develop into adenocarcinomas.

Diagnosis

Gallbladder carcinoma is often found incidentally during a cholecystectomy. It is suspected when there is unexplained extrahepatic biliary obstruction. The amount of cholestasis present is reflected in laboratory tests. If there is *primary sclerosing cholangitis*, there should be periodic measurement of serum CEA and CA levels 19-9. Diagnosis is based on ultrasound, and magnetic resonance cholangiopancreatography (MRCP). A CT scan is sometimes performed since it may provide better information than ultrasound. If still inconclusive, an endoscopic retrograde cholangiopancreatography is required to detect the tumor. Also, a diagnosis can be obtained via the tissue brushings that are performed, which sometimes means that ultrasound-guided or CT-guided needle biopsies are unneeded. Other options for diagnosis include blood chemistry tests, liver function tests, chest X-rays, and percutaneous transhepatic cholangiography (PTC). The stages of gallbladder carcinoma are as follows:

- Stage 0 – carcinoma in situ – the cancer is only within the mucosal layer
- Stage I – the cancer has spread to the muscularis layer
- Stage II – the cancer has spread beyond the visceral peritoneum to the liver, stomach, small intestine, pancreas, bile ducts, muscles, connective tissues, or lymph nodes
- Stage III – the cancer has moved to the liver or organs near it, and sometimes, to the lymph nodes
- Stage IV – the cancer has moved to nearby lymph nodes and/or the organs located far from the gallbladder

Treatment

The primary treatments for gallbladder carcinoma include surgery, radiation therapy, chemotherapy, targeted therapies, and immunotherapy. If the carcinoma is completely resectable, this may be curative. Only a small number are resectable when they are detected, however. The surgery is usually done at a major cancer center due to its complexity. If the tumor is not fully resectable, palliative surgery is done to treat or prevent complications such as bile duct blockage. It can reduce symptoms and prolong life somewhat. Often, a laparoscopy is first performed to assess the potential for resection.

Radiation may be used as an adjuvant treatment after surgery, but also as part of main therapy for certain advanced cancer, or as palliative therapy. The types of radiation used include EBRT, three-dimensional conformal radiation therapy (3D-CRT), intensity-modulated radiation therapy (IMFT), and chemoradiation. While chemotherapy can help some patients, it is not clear as to how effective it is against gallbladder cancer. Chemotherapy may be used after surgery, as part of primary treatment.

Prevention and Early Detection

There is no known method of prevention for gallbladder cancer, but reducing risk factors may be preventive. Maintaining a healthy weight, staying physically active, eating a healthy diet, and reducing or avoiding alcoholic beverages are suggested. Since gallstones are a major risk factor, surgery to remove the gallbladder from any person with gallstones may prevent cancer from developing. However, most physicians do not recommend this surgery unless the gallstones are causing serious problems. For porcelain gallbladder, the organ should be removed. Gallbladder cancer is not easy to detect early in its development. There are no reliable testing methods to screen for this cancer. The disease is often discovered when the gallbladder is removed because of gallstones.

Prognosis

The median survival with gallbladder carcinoma is only three months, though this is for distant metastasis of the disease. Only 2% of people with distant metastases will survive for five years. For localized cancer, the five-year survival rate is 62% and for regional cancer, it is 27%.

Significant Point

Gallbladder cancer is rare, and is difficult to detect or diagnose since there are often no noticeable signs during the early stages. An important factor in treating gallbladder cancer is that the organ is hidden behind the liver, making surgery more complicated.

Clinical Case

1. What is the incidence rate of gallbladder cancer?
2. How common are gallstones along with gallbladder cancer?
3. When gallstones are present, can surgery actually prevent gallbladder cancer?

A 79-year-old woman was hospitalized because of right upper quadrant abdominal pain and suspected acute cholecystitis. She had been being treated for hypertension, diabetes mellitus, and dyslipidemia, but did not drink alcohol or smoke. She had undergone a right mastectomy 25 years previously for breast cancer. Her levels of white blood cells, bilirubin, aspartate aminotransferase, alanine aminotransferase, and C-reactive protein were abnormal. Ultrasound revealed small gallstones and CT revealed the gallbladder to have thickened walls. Multiple nodular lesions were seen in the areas of the pancreas, suggestive of metastatic lymph nodes. Endoscopic ultrasound-guided fine-needle aspiration resulted in a diagnosis of small cell carcinoma or adenocarcinoma, but the primary lesion could not be identified. A radical cholecystectomy with partial liver resection was performed, along with lymph node dissection. Pathology revealed the entire gallbladder to contain tumors, which also invaded the liver. Histopathology revealed them to be small cell neuroendocrine carcinomas, and the patient was staged at IV. After surgery, the patient developed progressive jaundice that could not be relieved by biliary stenting. She died 3 months after surgery.

Answers:

1. **Gallbladder cancer is more common in women than in men, with 6,380 of the cases in 2020, in the United States, being women, and 5,600 being men. There were 2,390 female deaths from the disease and 1,700 male deaths. The disease also affects more women globally than men.**
2. **Gallbladder carcinoma is related to the presence of gallstones larger than 3 cm in size. Between 70% and 90% of cases of gallbladder carcinoma also involve gallstones. Risk factors include chronic gallbladder inflammation, such as from gallstones, along with ductal defects that cause pancreatic juices to reflux into the gallbladder and bile ducts.**
3. **Since gallstones are a major risk factor, surgery to remove the gallbladder from any person with gallstones may prevent cancer from developing. However, most physicians do not recommend this surgery unless the gallstones are causing serious problems.**

Key Terms

Acanthosis nigricans
Achalasia
Advance directive
Aflatoxins
Alpha-fetoprotein
Anal verge
Anorectal cancer
Asterixis
Barrett esophagus
Betel quid
Bruit
Carcinoid syndrome
Cholesterolosis
Cloacogenic carcinoma
Crypt stem cells
Dumping syndrome
Dysarthria
Dysphagia
Electrocoagulation
Enteroclysis
Enteroscope
Erythroplakia
Exophytic
Fulgurated
Fundic foveolar polyps
Gardner syndrome
Gastroenterostomy
Globus
Gutka
Hepatocellular carcinoma
Ileostomy
Indurated
Leukoplakia

Lymphogranuloma venereum
Lynch syndrome
Metaplasia
Mohs surgery
Multidetector row CT
Nitrosation
Nondistensible
Odynophagia
Otalgia
Pancreatic cancer
Peutz–Jeghers syndrome
Photodynamic therapy
Plummer–Vinson syndrome
Pyloroplasty
Septin 9 assay
Sessile
Squamocolumnar junction
Submental
Synchronous cancer
Tenesmus
Transoral laser microsurgery
Transoral robotic surgery
Trismus
Trousseau syndrome
Tylosis
Tyrosinemia
Whipple procedure
Wilson's disease
Vagotomy
Vermilion border
Video capsule endoscopy
Xerostomia

Bibliography

1 Agbanashi, L. (2020). *Liver Cancer: A Comprehensive and Perfect Guide on Liver Cancer*. New York: Agbanashi.

2 Ahuja, N. and Coleman, J. (2011). *Johns Hopkins Patients' Guide to Pancreatic Cancer*. Burlington: Jones & Bartlett Learning.

3 American Cancer Society. (2021). *Can Stomach Cancer Be Prevented?* https://www.cancer.org/cancer/stomach-cancer/causes-risks-prevention/prevention.html Accessed 2021.

4 American Cancer Society. (2021). *Treatment of Anal Cancer, by Stage*. https://www.cancer.org/

cancer/anal-cancer/treating/by-stage.html Accessed 2021.

5 American Cancer Society. (2021). *Key Statistics for Gallbladder Cancer*. https://www.cancer.org/cancer/gallbladder-cancer/about/key-statistics.html Accessed 2021.

6 American Cancer Society, The. (2018). *The American Cancer Society's Oncology in Practice – Clinical Management*. Hoboken: Wiley-Blackwell. Figure 4.1 from Page 57.

7 American Cancer Society, The. (2018). *The American Cancer Society's Oncology in Practice – Clinical Management*. Hoboken: Wiley-Blackwell. Figure 6.6 from Page 91.

8 American Cancer Society. (2008). *A Cancer Journal for Clinicians- Tumor-Node-Metastasis Staging of Pancreatic Adenocarcinoma*. 58 (2): 111–125. https://acsjournals.onlinelibrary.wiley.com/doi/10.3322/ca.2007.0012 http://CAonline.AmCancerSoc.org. Figure 3. Accessed 2021.

9 American Journal of Gastroenterology. (2021). *ACG Clinical Guidelines: Colorectal Cancer Screening 2021*. Wolters Kluwer Health, Inc. https://journals.lww.com/ajg/Fulltext/2021/03000/ACG_Clinical_Guidelines__Colorectal_Cancer.14.aspx

10 Arias, I.M., Alter, H.J., Boyer, J.L., Cohen, D.E., Shafritz, D.A., Thorgersson, S.S., and Wolkoff, A.W. (2020). *The Liver: Biology and Pathobiology*. 6th Edition. Hoboken: Wiley-Blackwell.

11 Beger, H.G., Warshaw, A.L., Hruban, R.H., Buchler, M.W., Lerch, M.M., Neoptolemos, J., Shimosegawa, T., and Whitcomb, D. (2018). *The Pancreas – An Integrated Textbook of Basic Science, Medicine, and Surgery*, 3rd Edition. Hoboken: Wiley-Blackwell.

12 Benjamin, L. (2020). *Stomach Cancer: The Complete Cure Guide on Everything You Need to Know about Stomach Cancer*. New York: Benjamin.

13 Bishop Pitman, M. and Layfield, L.J. (2015). *The Papanicolaou Society of Cytopathology System for Reporting Pancreaticobiliary Cytology – Definitions, Criteria and Explanatory Notes*. New York: Springer.

14 Boardman, L.A. (2016). *Intestinal Polyposis Syndromes: Diagnosis and Management*. New York: Springer.

15 Cancer Epidemiology. (2020). *Epidemiology of liver metastases*. ResearchGate GmbH. https://www.researchgate.net/publication/342257824_Epidemiology_of_liver_metastases Accessed 2021.

16 Clavien, P.A., Sarr, M.G., Fong, Y., and Miyazaki, M. (2015). *Atlas of Upper Gastrointestinal and Hepato-Pancreato-Biliary Surgery*, 2nd Edition. New York: Springer.

17 Delaini, G.G. and Goldberg, S.M. (2006). *Inflammatory Bowel Disease and Familial Adenomatous Polyposis: Clinical Management and Patients' Quality of Life*. New York: Springer.

18 Del Chiaro, M., Haas, S.L., and Schulick, R.D. (2016). *Cystic Tumors of the Pancreas: Diagnosis and Treatment*. New York: Springer.

19 Duncan, M.D., Shockney, L.D., and Shapiro, G.R. (2010). *Patients' Guide to Cancer of the Stomach and Esophagus (Johns Hopkins Medicine)*. Burlington: Jones & Bartlett Learning.

20 Engin, O. (2020). *Colon Polyps and Colorectal Cancer*, 2nd Edition. New York: Springer.

21 Esophageal Cancer Education Foundation. (2019). *Esophagectomy Post-Surgical Guide: Questions and Answers*, 2nd Edition. Bloomington: AuthorHouse.

22 Guillem, J.G. and Friedman, G. (2020). *Management of Hereditary Colorectal Cancer: A Multidisciplinary Approach*. New York: Springer.

23 Herman, J.M., Pawlik, T.M., and Thomas, Jr., C.R.. (2014). *Biliary Tract and Gallbladder Cancer: A Multidisciplinary Approach*, 2nd Edition. New York: Springer.

24 Hohenberger, W. and Parker, M. (2017). *Lower Gastrointestinal Tract Surgery: Volume 2, Open Procedures (Surgery Atlas Series)*. New York: Springer.

25 International Association of Cancer Registries, International Agency for Research on Cancer, World Health Organization. (2015). *Cancer Incidence in Five Continents Volume XI*.

https://www.iarc.who.int/wp-content/
uploads/2018/07/CI5-XI-Call_For_Data-1.pdf
Accessed 2021.

26 Jarnagin, W.R. (2012). *Blumgart's Surgery of
the Liver, Biliary Tract and Pancreas: Expert
Consult*, 5th Edition. Philadelphia: Saunders.

27 Lepori, L.R. (2011). *Oncology: Tumors of the
Digestive System – Miniatlas*. London: Letbar
Associates S.A.

28 Monteiro Correia, M., Choti, M.A., Rocha,
F.G., and Wakabayashi, G. (2020). *Colorectal
Cancer Liver Metastases: A Comprehensive
Guide to Management*. New York: Springer.

29 Myers, J.N. and Sturgis, E.M. (2013). *Oral
Cavity and Oropharyngeal Cancer, an Issue of
Otolaryngologic Clinics of North America (The
Clinics: Internal Medicine)*. Amsterdam:
Elsevier.

30 National Cancer Institute, Cancer.net. (2021).
Small Bowel Cancer: Statistics. https://www.
cancer.net/cancer-types/small-bowel-cancer/
statistics Accessed 2021.

31 National Cancer Institute – Surveillance,
Epidemiology, and End Results Program.
(2020). *Cancer Stat Facts: Anal Cancer – 5-Year
Relative Survival*. U.S. Department of Health
and Human Services/National Institutes of
Health/National Cancer Institute/USA.gov.
https://seer.cancer.gov/statfacts/html/anus.
html Accessed 2021.

32 Posner, M.C., Vokes, E.E., and Weichselbaum,
R.R. (2002). *Cancer of the Upper
Gastrointestinal Tract (American Cancer
Society Atlas of Clinical Oncology)*. Atlanta:
American Cancer Society.

33 Raymond, E., Faivre, S., and Ruszniewski, P.
(2014). *Management of Neuroendocrine
Tumors of the Pancreas and Digestive Tract
– From Surgery to Targeted Therapies: A
Multidisciplinary Approach*. New York:
Springer.

34 Roberts, L.R., Yang, J.D., and Venkatesh, S.K.
(2020). *Evaluation and Management of Liver
Masses*. New York: Springer.

35 Russo, P., Ruchelli, E.D., and Piccoli, D.A.
(2014). *Pathology of Pediatric Gastrointestinal
and Liver Disease*, 2nd Edition. New York:
Springer.

36 Saba, N.F. and El-Rayes, B.F. (2019).
*Esophageal Cancer: Prevention, Diagnosis
and Therapy*, 2nd Edition. New York:
Springer.

37 Santoro, G.A., Di Falco, G., and Cola, B.
(2012). *Atlas of Endoanal and Endorectal
Ultrasonography: Staging and Treatment
Options for Anorectal Cancer*. New York:
Springer.

38 Scholefield, J.H. and Eng, C. (2014). *Colorectal
Cancer: Diagnosis and Clinical Management*.
Hoboken: Wiley-Blackwell.

39 Shah, J.P. and Johnson, N.W. (2018). *Oral and
Oropharyngeal Cancer*, 2nd Edition. Boca
Raton: CRC Press.

40 Shami, V.M. and Kahaleh, M. (2010).
*Endoscopic Ultrasound (Clinical
Gastroenterology)*. Totowa: Humana Press.

41 Sharma, P., Sampliner, R., and Ilson, D. (2015).
Esophageal Cancer and Barrett's Esophagus,
3rd Edition. Hoboken: Wiley-Blackwell.

42 Tewari, M. (2018). *Surgery for Pancreatic and
Periampullary Cancer: Principles and Practice*.
New York: Springer.

43 Thomas, C.R. and Fuller, C.D. (2008). *Biliary
Tract and Gallbladder Cancer: Diagnosis &
Therapy*. New York: Demos Medical.

44 Tsai, S., Ritch, P.S., Erickson, B.A., and Evans,
D.B. (2019). *Management of Localized
Pancreatic Cancer: Current Treatment and
Challenges*. New York: Springer.

45 WHO Classification of Tumours Editorial
Board. (2019). *Digestive System Tumors: WHO
Classification of Tumors*, 5th Edition. Geneva:
World Health Organization.

46 World Cancer Research Fund, American
Institute for Cancer Research. (2018). *Stomach
cancer statistics*. https://www.wcrf.org/
dietandcancer/cancer-trends/stomach-cancer-
statistics Accessed 2021.

47 Zimmermann, A. (2017). *Tumors and
Tumor-Like Lesions of the Hepatobiliary Tract:
General and Surgical Pathology*. New York:
Springer.

7

Lymphatic and Blood Cancer

Lymphomas

Lymphomas are heterogeneous tumors that form in the lymphatic and **reticuloendothelial** systems. The primary forms are NHL and Hodgkin's lymphoma. The differences between these two forms include their lymph node involvement, how they spread, their effect upon the **Waldeyer ring** and the mesenteric lymph nodes, extranodal involvement, the stage at diagnosis, and in children, their histologic classification. These qualities are discussed in the separate pathology sections below. Lymphomas were previously believed to be completely different from leukemias, but we now know that distinctions between the two diseases are not always clear. This is based on advanced knowledge of cell markers and how they can be evaluated. Lymphomas are not always contained entirely within the lymphatic system, and leukemias in their early stages are not always confined to the bone marrow. Malignant lymphoma cells can be found in the bone marrow and blood, along with the lymph nodes. This feature is most common in low-grade or indolent NHLs, including *chronic lymphocytic leukemia/small lymphocytic lymphoma (CLL/SLL)*, *marginal zone lymphoma*, and *mantle cell lymphoma*, which is a more aggressive form.

Non-Hodgkin's Lymphoma

Non-Hodgkin's lymphoma (NHL) is actually a heterogeneous group of disorders. All NHLs develop from malignant lymphocytes, and there are more than 70 subtypes, with unique biological and clinical features. More than 89% of NHLs are derived from B-cells, with the rest coming from T-cells and natural killer (NK) cells. Classifications of NHL derived from B-cells or T-cells are based on clinical, genetic, immunophenotypic, and genetic features. Other

Global Epidemiology of Cancer: Diagnosis and Treatment, First Edition. Jahangir Moini, Nicholas G. Avgeropoulos, and Craig Badolato.
© 2022 John Wiley & Sons Ltd. Published 2022 by John Wiley & Sons Ltd.

methods of classification include resemblances to normal B-cells and T-cells, and the stage of differentiation.

Epidemiology

NHLs are the most common hematologic malignancy in the United States. There are about 72,000 cases diagnosed every year, and 20,000 of these are fatal. NHL accounts for about 4% of new cancers in the United States. They result in 3% of cancer deaths. Overall, NHL is the seventh most common cancer in the United States. Incidence increases with every decade of life between ages 20 and 80, and the median age is 66 years. The disease is slightly more common in men (1 of every 42) than women (1 of every 54). *Hepatosplenic T-cell lymphoma* is seen in younger men that have had solid-organ transplants or other conditions that cause immune deficiency. Caucasians have the highest rates of NHL compared with African Americans, Latino Americans, and Asian Americans. The lowest rates are in Native Americans and Alaska natives.

Globally, there are over 510,000 new annual cases of NHL. Rates are the highest in Israel, with 17.6 of every 100,000 people affected, and followed by the United States, Canada, Portugal, Lebanon, Greece, and Montenegro (see Figure 7.1). Incidence appears to be slowly increasing worldwide, but statistics from many countries are either not available or out of date. As in the United States, the median age is 66 years. The disease is also slightly more common in males throughout the world. As in the United States, Caucasian people from various countries are most affected.

Etiology and Risk Factors

The exact cause of NHLs is not fully understood. Genetics and environmental exposures may be implicated because studies have shown a slightly increased risk of developing NHL between first-degree relatives. Also, a patient's level of immunity is involved if there is exposure to organic solvents. Congenital and acquired immunodeficiencies are also related to a higher risk for NHLs of the B-cell type. The T-cell type is related to ataxia–telangiectasia. Post-transplant lymphoproliferative disorders are related to both the T-cell and NK-cell types. Loss of cellular immunity or impaired cellular immunity – especially of the T-cell type – results in unregulated proliferation of B-cells in lymphoid tissues. Extranodal T-cell lymphomas are rare, and linked to defects in immunity. Risk factors for NHLs include age

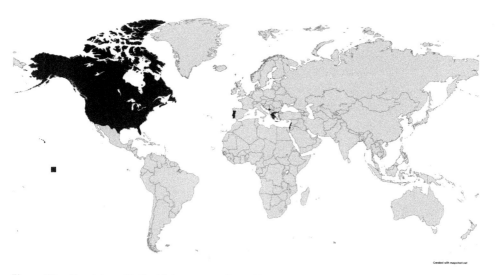

Figure 7.1 Countries with the highest rates of non-Hodgkin's lymphoma.

over 60 years, gender, Caucasian race, infections, benzene exposure, herbicide exposure, insecticide exposure, chemotherapies for other cancers, radiation exposure, weakened immunity, autoimmune diseases, and obesity. Table 7.1 summarizes factors that are related to the development of NHL.

Clinical Manifestations

The most common presentation of NHL is lymphadenopathy. Patients notice cervical, axillary, or inguinal adenopathy. The lymph nodes are firm and painless. Lymphadenopathy may occur in the mediastinum or retroperitoneum, causing chest pain, cough, superior vena cava syndrome,

Table 7.1 Factors related to the development of non-Hodgkin's lymphoma.

Factors	Examples
Inherited immune disorders	Ataxia–telangiectasia
	Autoimmune lymphoproliferative syndrome
	Common variable immunodeficiency disease
	Severe combined immunodeficiency disease
	Wiskott–Aldrich syndrome
	X-linked lymphoproliferative disorder
Acquired immune disorders	Acquired immunodeficiency syndrome (AIDS)
	Hashimoto thyroiditis
	Methotrexate therapy for autoimmune disorders
	Rheumatoid arthritis
	Sjögren syndrome
	Solid-organ transplantation
	Systemic lupus erythematosus
Infectious agents	*Borrelia burgdorferi*
	Campylobacter jejuni
	Chlamydia psittaci
	Epstein–Barr virus
	Helicobacter pylori
	Hepatitis C virus
	Human herpesvirus type 8
	Human T-lymphotropic virus type 1
Occupational and environmental exposures	Diet
	Drugs
	Hair dyes
	Herbicides
	Organic solvents
	Smoking
	Ultraviolet light

abdominal pain, back pain, and spinal cord compression. Systemic symptoms include fever, night sweats, unintended weight loss, or symptoms of localized compression that cause pain.

Pathology

The pathology of NHL is very different from Hodgkin's lymphoma. With NHL, there is usually dissemination to lymph nodes, and it spreads in an interrupted pattern. The two most common growth patterns are follicular, which is also called *nodular*, and diffuse. In follicular growth, the lymphoma mimics the follicular center structures. In diffuse growth, the lymphoid cells proliferate in a rather unorganized fashion. Sometimes, the lymph is distributed within lymph node sinuses. Knowledge of specific molecular markers is useful for understanding the pathogenesis of these lymphomas.

Diagnosis

The diagnosis of NHLs is based on enough tissue via core needle biopsy that can be evaluated. An excisional lymph node biopsy is usually done, though multiple core needle biopsies may be performed. Only rarely is fine-needle aspiration sufficient for an initial diagnosis, due to the fact that it is not informative about the structure of the lymph nodes, and provides insufficient material for complete immunohistochemical or molecular study. Sometimes, an initial biopsy is ambiguous or non-diagnostic. It is important that biopsies be confirmative, because inflammatory or infectious diseases can mimic lymphomas in radiographic imaging and in behavior. Follicular or marginal zone lymphomas are able to transform into more aggressive disease as they progress. The staging of NHLs is as follows:

- Stage I – the lymphoma is only in one lymph node area or a lymphoid organ such as the tonsils; or the lymphoma is only in one area of a single organ outside of the lymphatic system
- Stage II – the lymphoma is in two or more groups of lymph nodes on the same side

(above or below) of the diaphragm, such as the nodes of the armpit and neck, but not in a combination of the armpit and groin; or the lymphoma is in a group of lymph nodes and in one area of a nearby organ, and may also affect other groups of lymph nodes on the same side of the diaphragm
- Stage III – the lymphoma is in lymph node areas on both sides of the diaphragm; or the lymphoma is in lymph nodes above the diaphragm, as well as in the spleen
- Stage IV – the lymphoma has spread into at least one organ outside the lymphatic system, such as the bone marrow, liver, or lungs

"Bulky disease" is a term often used to describe large tumors in the chest. This is very important for stage II lymphomas, since more intensive treatment may be required.

Diagnosis focuses on careful history and physical examination, laboratory tests include CBC with differential, serum chemistry for lactate dehydrogenase levels, routine electrolyte assessment – including calcium, and both kidney and liver function. Imaging studies include computed tomography (CT) scan of chest, abdomen, and pelvis (see Figure 7.2). Positron emission tomography is also useful.

Treatment

Treatment of the various subtypes of NHLs can be quite varied. For indolent B-cell lymphomas, which are basically considered to be incurable, adequate treatment is intermittent, over the course of the patient's life. It is often able to control the clinical manifestations of the disease and usually provides a long lifespan. Treatments that are extremely effective include the alkylating agents, anthracyclines, anti-CD20 monoclonal antibodies, purine analogs, immunomodulators, and tyrosine kinase inhibitors. These drug classes include cyclophosphamide/hydroxydaunorubicin/oncovin/prednisone (CHOP therapy), rituximab, obinutuzumab, ibritumomab tiuxetan, lenalidomide, ibrutinib, idelalisib, and ifosfamide–carboplatin–etoposide (ICE chemotherapy). Antibiotic therapy is helpful for

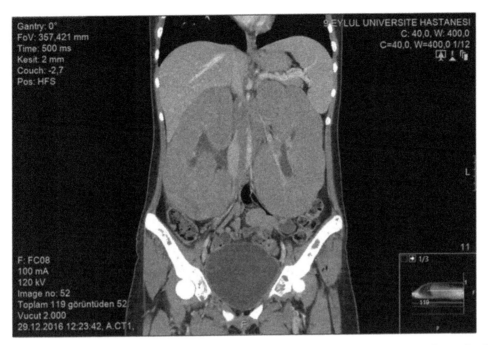

Figure 7.2 CT scan of chest, abdomen, and pelvis showing non-Hodgkin's lymphomas. *Source*: Deniz Kizmazoglu et al. (2018).

extranodal marginal zone lymphoma of the stomach, which is related to *Helicobacter pylori*.

Prevention and Early Detection

There is no known way to prevent NHL. However, certain risk factors can be avoided, which can lower the risk of developing the disease. The human immunodeficiency virus (HIV) is known to increase the risk of developing NHL, so intravenous drug use and unprotected sex with multiple partners must be avoided. The same is true for the human T-cell lymphotropic virus (HTLV-1). Preventing *Helicobacter pylori* infection with antibiotics and antacids may also lower the risks of developing NHL. Since some studies have indicated that being overweight or obese can increase risks for the disease, maintaining a healthy weight with regular physical activity, and eating a healthy diet may lower risks for NHL.

There are no widely recommended screening tests available. The best way to detect the disease early is to be aware of possible signs and symptoms: enlargement of one or more lymph nodes on the side of the neck, in the armpit, or in the groin. Additional symptoms include chills, fever, night sweats, weight loss, tiredness, and abdominal swelling. Regular medical check-ups are important for individuals with known risk factors, which include HIV infection, autoimmune diseases, organ transplants, or prior cancer treatments.

Prognosis

Prognosis depends on the subtype of the disease, staging, age, and overall health. For all subtypes, the five-year survival is 71%, in a range of 81% (for stage I disease) to 61% (for stage IV disease). For follicular lymphoma, the five-year survival rates are 96% (localized), 89% (regional), and 85% (distant). For diffuse large B-cell lymphoma, the five-year survival rates are 73% (localized), 72% (regional), and 55% (distant). This means that the follicular subtype has an overall five-year survival of 88%, and the diffuse subtype has an overall five-year survival of 63%.

Significant Point

There are actually more than 60 types of NHL, which are determined by the type of lymphocyte involved, the microscopic appearance, and the speed of growth. Non-Hodgkin's lymphomas are the most common type of white blood cell cancer. Fortunately, ongoing research is studying new vaccinations as future treatment options, to trigger the immune response.

Clinical Case

1. From which cells do most cases of NHLs develop?
2. How common are NHLs?
3. What is the primary difference between non-Hodgkin's and Hodgkin's lymphomas?

A 75-year-old man was diagnosed with stage I NHL, after discovering a lump in his right groin. The full diagnosis was of an aggressive diffuse B-cell lymphoma. The patient received cyclophosphamide, hydroxydaunorubicin, oncovin, and prednisone – collectively known as "CHOP chemotherapy." He was also given immunotherapy with monoclonal antibodies, and remained cancer-free for 15 years. Unfortunately, the lymphoma eventually recurred, and the patient was treated with rituximab as immunotherapy and ifosfamide–carboplatin–etoposide (ICE) chemotherapy every 14 days, in 3 cycles, and the patient was cured.

Answers:

1. **More than 89% of NHLs are derived from B-cells, with the rest coming from T-cells and NK cells.**
2. **Non-Hodgkin's lymphomas are the most common hematologic malignancy in the United States. There are** about 72,000 cases diagnosed every year and 20,000 of these are fatal. NHL accounts for about 4% of new cancers in the United States. Overall, NHL is the seventh most common cancer in the United States. Globally, the prevalence of NHL is over 510,000 new cases annually. Incidence rates are the highest in Israel, followed by the United States, Canada, and Portugal. Incidence appears to be slowly increasing worldwide.
3. **These two types of lymphomas are very different. With NHL, there is usually dissemination to lymph nodes, and it spreads in an interrupted pattern. The two most common growth patterns are follicular (nodular) and diffuse. Hodgkin's lymphoma is usually localized to a specific group of lymph nodes.**

Hodgkin's Lymphoma

Hodgkin's lymphoma is also known as *Hodgkin's disease.* It is a localized or disseminated proliferation of malignant B lymphocytes from the lymphoreticular system. It mostly affects the lymph nodes, bone marrow, liver, and spleen. There is an excellent response to treatment, with the majority of patients being cured.

Epidemiology

In the United States, approximately 8,500 new cases of Hodgkin's lymphoma are diagnosed every year. Of these cases, about 970 fatalities occur. The relative 5-year survival rate is 87.4% of patients. There are 2.6 new cases per 100,000 people, and the death rate is 0.3 per 100,000. Hodgkin's lymphoma is most common in early adulthood, in people who are in their 20s. Risks increase again after age 55. Overall, the average age at diagnosis is 39. It is also commonly diagnosed in teenagers from 15 to 19. The disease is slightly more common in males than females, and is most common in non-Hispanic Caucasians, followed by Hispanic Caucasians.

Hodgkin's lymphoma is least common in Asian Americans and Pacific Islanders.

According to the International Agency for Research on Cancer, there are about 83,000 global cases of Hodgkin's lymphoma per year, with over 23,000 deaths (see Figure 7.3). The disease is rare before the age of 10 years, and most common between 20 and 40, with another peak in occurrence in adults over 60. Males are affected more than females, in a 1.4:1 ratio. Hodgkin's lymphoma occurs more often in countries with a high socio-demographic index, for unknown reasons. Regions of the world with the most cases include the United States, Canada, Switzerland, Denmark, Finland, Iceland, Norway, and Sweden. Intermediate rates are occurring in eastern and southern Europe. The lowest rates are seen in eastern Asia (see Figure 7.4). These statistics mean that Hodgkin's lymphoma is most common in Caucasian people in comparison with any other racial groups throughout the world, and least common in Asians throughout the world.

Etiology and Risk Factors

The cause of Hodgkin's lymphoma is unknown. Family history, occupations such as woodworking, use of phenytoin, radiation therapy, chemotherapy, the Epstein–Barr virus, herpesvirus type 6, the HIV, and *Mycobacterium* tuberculosis – these are all implicated. Risk factors include certain immunosuppressants, such as used after organ transplantation. Other risk factors include congenital immunodeficiency disorders, which include ataxia–telangiectasia, **Chédiak–Higashi syndrome, Klinefelter syndrome**, and **Wiskott–Aldrich syndrome**. Also, autoimmune disorders and their treatments may be risk factors, including celiac disease, rheumatoid arthritis, **Sjögren syndrome**, and systemic lupus erythematosus.

Clinical Manifestations

The signs and symptoms of Hodgkin's lymphoma most often include lymphadenopathy. Painless cervical or axillary adenopathy or mediastinal areas are present in most patients. In rare cases, pain occurs in areas of the body where the disease has manifested, immediately after consuming alcoholic beverages. This can be an early indication of the diagnosis. Sometimes, there is **Pel–Ebstein fever**, night sweats, intense and unrelieved pruritus due to a rash, and unintentional weight loss due to loss of appetite, splenomegaly, and more rarely, hepatomegaly. These manifestations develop as the disease spreads through the reticuloendothelial system, usually to sites that are continuous. Some patients lose more than 10% of their body weight over six months, which can signify that the mediastinal or retroperitoneal lymph nodes have become affected, along with the liver or bone marrow. As the disease advances, cachexia is common as well as bacterial infections, fungal, protozoal, and viral infections.

Bone marrow involvement often proceeds without symptoms. However, there can be vertebral osteoblastic lesions known as **ivory vertebrae**. In rare cases, there is pain, with osteolytic lesions and compression fractures. Other rare features include cutaneous, gastric, and intracranial lesions. If they are present, they indicated uncontrolled disease that is related to HIV. Death can occur because of progressive disease or an infection. Local compression of tissues by tumor masses may cause jaundice, lymphedema in the legs, and severe dyspnea and wheezing. If epidural invasion compresses the spinal cord, it may cause paraplegia. When enlarged lymph nodes compress the recurrent laryngeal or cervical sympathetic nerves may cause paralysis of the larynx.

Pathology

Hodgkin's lymphoma is usually localized to a specific group of lymph nodes. There is usually no effect upon the Waldeyer ring or mesenteric lymph nodes. Hodgkin's lymphoma develops from clonal transformation of cells that originated as B-cells, forming **pathognomic** cells of which each contains two nuclei, known as **Reed–Sternberg cells** (see

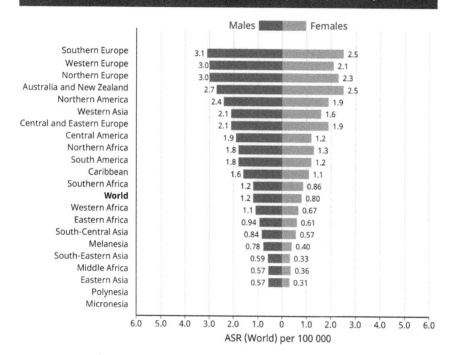

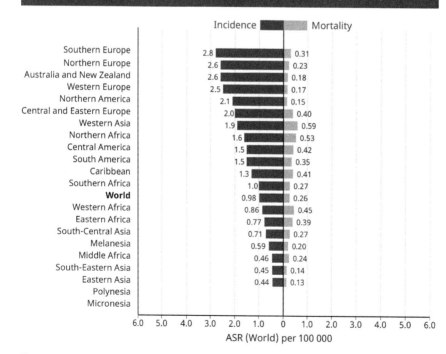

Figure 7.3 Age-standardized (world) incidence rates of Hodgkin's lymphoma by gender, and its incidence and mortality rates. *Source*: The Global Cancer Observatory (part of International Agency for Research on Cancer 2020 and World Health Organization) [17].

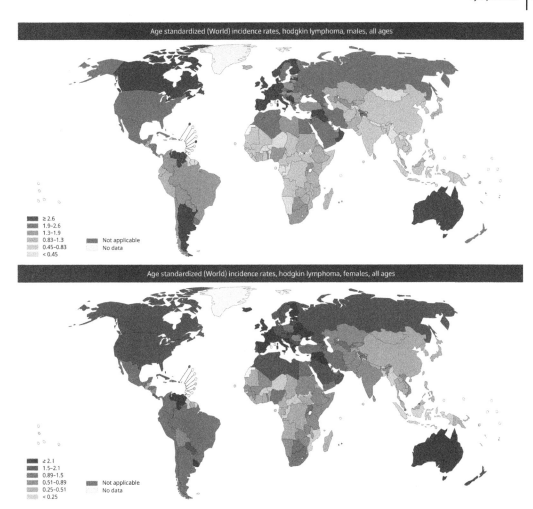

Figure 7.4 Age-standardized (world) incidence rates of Hodgkin's lymphoma for males and females. *Source*: The Global Cancer Observatory (part of International Agency for Research on Cancer 2020 and World Health Organization) [17].

Figure 7.5). Extranodal involvement is infrequent. Hodgkin's lymphoma is usually early in its development when it is diagnosed, and in children, the histologic classification mostly carries a favorable diagnosis. Most patients develop a slowly progressing defect in their cell-mediated immunity, which involves T-cell function.

Diagnosis

The diagnosis of classic Hodgkin's lymphoma is based on lymph node biopsy and painless lymphadenopathy. A similar type of lymphadenopathy can be related to viral infections, including cytomegalovirus infection or infectious mononucleosis. It can also be caused by leukemia, NHL, or toxoplasmosis. Chest X-rays may appear similar to those seen with lung cancer, sarcoidosis, or tuberculosis. Abnormalities are confirmed by chest X-rays, CT scans, or positron emission tomography (PET) scans. When the mediastinal nodes are the only ones enlarged, the following may be done: **mediastinoscopy**, a **Chamberlain procedure**, or **video-assisted thoroscopy**.

The biopsy will reveal the characteristic Reed–Sternberg cells in a heterogeneous cellular infiltrate. This is made up of eosinophils, histiocytes, lymphocytes, monocytes, and plasma cells.

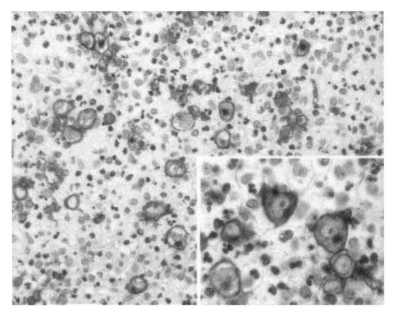

Figure 7.5 Cluster of Reed–Sternberg cells and variants. Original magnification 400×, with inset showing 600× magnification. *Source*: Portlock et al. (2004).

Antigens on the Reed–Sternberg cells help to differentiate Hodgkin's lymphoma from NHL. The antigens also help to differentiate classic Hodgkin's lymphoma from the nodular lympho-cyte-predominant form. The disease greatly increases the amounts of neutrophils and plate-lets, while lowering the lymphocytes and hemo-globin. The staging of Hodgkin's lymphoma is as follows:

- Stage I – the lymphoma is only in one lymph node area or a lymphoid organ such as the thymus; or the lymphoma is only in one part of one organ outside the lymphatic system
- Stage II – the lymphoma is in two or more lymph node areas on the same side (above or below) of the diaphragm; or the lymphoma extends locally from one lymph node area into a nearby organ
- Stage III – the lymphoma is in lymph node areas on both sides of the diaphragm; or the lymphoma is in lymph nodes above the dia-phragm, and in the spleen
- Stage IV – the lymphoma has spread to at least one organ outside of the lymphatic system, such as the liver, bone marrow, or lungs

Like NHLs, there is also a "bulky disease" description of Hodgkin's lymphomas. This means there are chest tumors at least one-third as wide as the entire chest, or tumors in other areas that are at least 10 cm across. Bulky dis-ease is usually labeled by adding the letter "X" to the stage. This is very important for stage II lym-phomas, because bulky disease may mean that more intensive treatment is needed. Every stage of Hodgkin's disease may have a letter "B" added if any of the following symptoms are present:

- Loss of 10% of body weight or more over the past six months without dieting
- An unexplained fever of 100.4°F (38°C) or more
- Drenching night sweats

The above symptoms usually mean that the lymphoma is more advanced. Treatment will often have to be more intensive. When none of the above symptoms is present, the stage will have a letter "A" added.

Treatment

Fortunately, the available treatments for Hodgkin's lymphoma are usually curative. They consist of chemotherapy, immunotherapy, and radiation therapy. Treatment choices are complicated, based on the precise disease stage. The initial treatment of limited-stage disease involves abbreviated chemotherapy known as ABVD: Adriamycin (doxorubicin), bleomycin, vinblastine, and dacarbazine. This is given with or without radiation therapy. If the patient has bulky mediastinal disease, the chemotherapy may need to be different or longer in duration, and radiation therapy is often used.

However, there are complications of Hodgkin's lymphoma treatments. Within 3–10 years, chemotherapies may increase the risk of developing leukemia. The drugs most implicated include the alkylating agents such as cyclophosphamide, mechlorethamine, and procarbazine; and other drugs such as doxorubicin and etoposide. Doxorubicin and mediastinal radiation increase risks for valvular heart disease, cardiomyopathy, and coronary atherosclerosis. Bleomycin can cause lung damage that may be severe and, in rare cases, fatal.

Prevention and Early Detection

Since few of the known risk factors for Hodgkin's lymphoma can be changed, it is not possible to prevent most cases of the disease at this time. There is no widely recommended screening test for Hodgkin's lymphoma, but some cases are still detected early in the disease course. The best way to find it early is to watch for possible symptoms – usually enlargement or swelling of one or more lymph nodes. These are most often on the side of the neck, in the armpit, or in the groin. It is important to have any lymph node changes evaluated by a physician. Careful and regular medical check-ups may be useful for people with known risk factors for the disease, such as a family history.

Prognosis

For limited-stage classic Hodgkin's lymphoma, 85–90% of patients are cured. With advanced-stage disease, 75–80% are cured. The limited-stage disease is often divided into *favorable* and *unfavorable* prognoses. Unfavorable disease is based on the risk factors, which include the presence of bulky disease, age over 50 years, four or more nodal sites involved, and an ESR of more than 50 mm/h. For advanced-stage Hodgkin's lymphoma, prognosis is worsened if the patient is male, over 45 years of age, and has signs of inflammation such as anemia, leukocytosis, low albumin, and lymphopenia. There is some disagreement as to which of these is most prognostic. There is a poor prognosis for patients that do not receive remission after treatment, or that relapse within 12 months.

Significant Point

Hodgkin's lymphoma was first described in 1666, but was later named by a physician named Thomas Hodgkin. The largest group of patients (31.4%) are diagnosed between the ages of 20 and 34, yet the most deaths (22.3%) occur in the 75–84 age group. Though treatments can last for six months or more, the disease is highly curable.

Clinical Case

1. How do you describe the epidemiology of Hodgkin's lymphoma?
2. From which cells does Hodgkin's lymphoma develop?
3. How successful are the treatments for Hodgkin's lymphoma?

A 25-year-old woman was hospitalized because of experiencing night sweats, fever, an itchy rash, and 15% weight loss over three months. Imaging studies revealed a large soft tissue mass in the patient's neck, and biopsy established a diagnosis of Hodgkin's lymphoma. Her white blood cell count was extremely high, with twice the number of neutrophils, very low lymphocytes, low hemoglobin, and excessively large amounts of platelets. The patient was given six cycles of Adriamycin (doxorubicin), bleomycin, vinblastine, and dacarbazine (collectively known as ABVD chemotherapy). At three years of follow-up, the patient has no signs of recurrence or metastasis.

Answers:

1. In the United States, about 8,500 new cases of Hodgkin's lymphoma are diagnosed every year, with about 970 fatalities. The prevalence rate of new cases is 2.6 per 100,000 people, and the death rate is 0.3 per 100,000. It is the most commonly diagnosed type of cancer in teenagers from 15 to 19. It is most common in non-Hispanic Caucasians. Globally, there are about 83,000 cases per year, with over 23,000 fatalities. For unknown reasons, the disease occurs more often in countries with a high socio-demographic index. It is most common in the United States, Canada, Switzerland, Denmark, Finland, Iceland, Norway, and Sweden.

2. Hodgkin's lymphoma develops from clonal transformation of cells that originated as B-cells, forming pathognomic cells, of which each contains two nuclei, known as Reed–Sternberg cells.

3. Fortunately, the available treatments for Hodgkin's lymphoma are usually curative. They consist of chemotherapy, immunotherapy, and radiation therapy.

Multiple Myeloma

Multiple myeloma is a malignancy of the plasma cells, with infiltration of the bone marrow and widespread skeletal breakdown. It causes anemia, bone pain, and fractures. The disease is often also referred to simply as *myeloma*. There must be 10% or more clonal plasma cells in the bone marrow, or a plasmacytoma found during biopsy.

Epidemiology

Multiple myeloma makes up over 10% of all hematologic malignancies and about 1% of all types of malignancies. In the United States, there are about 4.3 cases per 100,000 people. More than 30,000 new cases occur annually, and more than 11,000 are fatal. In the United States, the lifetime incidence of multiple myeloma is 1 in every 132 people, or 0.76% of the population. Median age is 66 years, and just 2% of cases occur in people younger than 40 years of age. It affects males slightly more often than females. The disease is twice as common in African Americans compared with Caucasians. It has been seen in families, affecting two or more first-degree relatives as well as identical twins.

Globally, there are more than 160,000 new cases of multiple myeloma per year, with over 106,000 cases being fatal. Incidence is increasing, and from 1990 to 2016, cases of multiple myeloma increased by 126% throughout the world, and deaths increased by 94%. The age-standardized incidence ratio is 1.5 per 100,000 people. Multiple myeloma mostly affects older adults, often around the age of 60 years, with another peak in occurrence between the ages of 85 and 89. As in the United States, the disease affects males slightly more than females. The highest rates of multiple myeloma outside of the United States occur in New Zealand, Australia, Iceland, the United Kingdom, Israel, and Norway (see Figure 7.6). The disease is least common in Egypt, the Philippines, and Thailand.

Etiology and Risk Factors

The cause of multiple myeloma is not clear. Risk factors include radiation exposure, as well as exposure to benzene, other organic solvents, insecticides, and herbicides. Nearly every case follows a pre-malignant phase that utilizes a random "two-hit" genetic process of malignant transformation.

Clinical Manifestations

Multiple myeloma is most often manifested with bone pain, fatigue, and pallor. Osteolytic

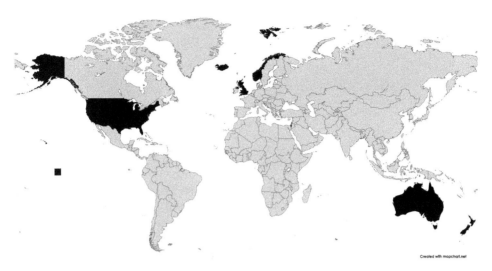

Figure 7.6 Countries with the highest rates of multiple myeloma.

bone lesions, compression fractures, or both are common. They can be seen in standard X-rays, CT scans, MRI, or FDG-PET scans. Bone pain may occur in a persistent or "migratory" manner – usually in the pelvis and lower back. The pain can occur suddenly if it is related to a fracture, and often follows movement. If there is extramedullary expansion of bone lesions, there can be nerve root or spinal cord compression. Anemia is present in 70% of cases, and the main cause of fatigue. Hypercalcemia is present in 25% of cases, and nearly half of all cases involve elevated serum creatinine. In about 5% of patients, the liver is palpable, and the spleen may be palpable in about 1%.

Pathology

In nearly 100% of cases, multiple myeloma likely evolves from an asymptomatic stage that is premalignant. It occurs in more than 3% of people who are 50 years or older, progressing to multiple myeloma or a related malignancy at 1% per year. There is genomic instability found in molecular genetic testing. This may be triggered by antigenic stimulation. Myeloma cell lines as well as primary myeloma cells have many different toll-like receptors (TLRs), which come from B lymphocytes, and are needed for the cells to be recognized by infectious agents and pathogen-associated molecular patterns. This initiates the host–defense response. Abnormal expression of TLRs by the plasma cells may allow them to respond to ligands that are specific for TLRs. There is then an abnormal and sometimes sustained infection response. These ligands cause increased myeloma cell proliferation and survival, along with resistance to apoptosis caused by dexamethasone. Autocrine interleukin (IL)-6 production somewhat mediates these effects. Interleukin-6 is a major plasma cell growth factor. Therefore, abnormal TLR expression, overexpression, or both of IL-6 receptors in plasma cells may cause early initiation of events leading to abnormal infection response. Plasma cells are believed to acquire a cytogenetic abnormality that causes limited clonal plasma cell proliferative processes.

Diagnosis

Diagnosis of multiple myeloma is based on the presence of 10% or more clonal plasma cells in the bone marrow, a plasmacytoma found on biopsy, or both. Additionally, according to the International Myeloma Working Group, there must be one or more of the following:

- Evidence of end-organ damage – anemia, bone lesions, hypercalcemia, or renal insufficiency;

this is attributed to the underlying plasma cell abnormalities

- 60% or more clonal plasma cells in the bone marrow
- More than one focal lesion of 5 mm or greater in size seen in MRI

New criteria allow for CT and PET-CT to be used to diagnose myeloma bone disease, and allow for early diagnosis plus treatments that can prevent end-organ damage in extremely high-risk patients. Radiologic imaging reveals punched-out lytic lesions, osteoporosis, or fractures in most patients.

Additional diagnostic methods include CBC, serum creatinine, calcium, albumin, C-reactive protein, lactate dehydrogenase levels, and urinalysis. Blood tests will reveal low hemoglobin, low neutrophils, and high platelet levels. Peripheral blood flow cytometry should be performed if it is available, to assess circulating plasma cells. Other tests include identification and counting of monoclonal proteins, tests for bone disease, and tests for bone marrow abnormalities. The bone marrow can also be assessed for disease risks. Multiple myeloma is signified by the presence of monoclonal immunoglobulins in the serum, urine, or both. These are usually referred to as **monoclonal proteins**. The staging for multiple myeloma is as follows:

- Stage I – serum beta-2 microglobulin is less than 3.5 mg / L, albumin is 3.5 g /dL or more, cytogenetics are considered "standard risk," and LDH levels are normal; note that "high-risk" cytogenetics include loss of a piece of chromosome 17, a translocation of material between chromosomes 4 and 14, and a translocation of material between chromosomes 14 and 16
- Stage II – only diagnosed when the patient's condition does not meet the criteria for Stage I or Stage III
- Stage III – serum beta-2 microglobulin is 5.5 mg / L or more, cytogenetics are considered "high risk," and/or LDL levels are high

Treatment

In about half of newly diagnosed patients under age 65, autologous peripheral blood stem-cell transplantation (ASCT) with high doses of chemotherapy will improve survival, compared with traditional chemotherapy treatments. The drugs used for treatment include lenalidomide, dexamethasone, bortezomib, thalidomide, and cyclophosphamide. The ASCT technique is performed with melphalan, used as a conditioning regimen. Sometimes, ASCT is repeated if needed. Stem cells can be cryopreserved for future use. The reasons that ASCT may not be possible include patient age, lack of a matched sibling donor, or insufficient cardiac, pulmonary, or renal function. Treatment-related deaths occur in 20% of cases. If a patient is ineligible for ASCT, treatments combine melphalan, prednisone, and the addition of thalidomide or bortezomib. Patients are assessed on an individual basis regarding the choice of drug regimens.

Palliative radiation is only used if the patient has disabling pain and an obvious focal process that has not responded to chemotherapy, and for those with spinal cord compression because of a plasmacytoma. Management of complications such as hypercalcemia, renal insufficiency, infection, skeletal lesions, hyperviscosity, and anemia may be required.

Prevention and Early Detection

There is no known way to prevent multiple myeloma. However, research is underway about treating *high-risk smoldering multiple myeloma* to keep it from becoming active multiple myeloma. It is unfortunately difficult to diagnose multiple myeloma early. It often causes no symptoms until it has become advanced, or causes vague symptoms that mimic those of other diseases. It can be found early if a routine blood test shows a very low amount of albumin. After a diagnosis of a solitary plasmacytoma, the patient has regular bloodwork done to monitor for the development of multiple myeloma, so the disease can be diagnosed sooner in these patients, compared with those that did not have the predisposing factors.

Prognosis

Because of new therapies, prognosis for multiple myeloma has greatly improved over the past decade. Survival rates are varied based on several factors: overall health, ability to tolerate treatment, staging, aggressiveness of the disease, and how susceptible the myeloma cells are to the drugs used. Patients younger than 65 years of age may have ASCT, improving prognosis. Patients with multiple myeloma considered to be of "standard risk" have an overall survival of 7–10 years, and often longer. Those with a high-risk form have a median overall survival of less than three years. However, some high-risk patients have increased survival if treated with bortezomib in combination with other medications, as well as with ASCT. For those with a "late-stage" diagnosis, less than 50% survive for five years.

Significant Point

The reason that myeloma is referred to as "multiple myeloma" is that most patients have tumors in several areas of their bodies. When the disease becomes active, known as "symptomatic myeloma," such as hypercalcemia, kidney problems, anemia, and/or bone damage. Staging is based on the amount of myeloma cells, and the amount of damage they have caused.

Clinical Case

1. How do you describe the epidemiology of multiple myeloma?
2. What is the characteristic of bone pain in multiple myeloma?
3. How can multiple myeloma be diagnosed early?

A 67-year-old man complained to his physician of extreme fatigue whenever he tried to exercise or do yard work. Blood tests revealed low hemoglobin, low neutrophil levels, and high platelet levels. Skeletal imaging revealed occult lytic skull lesions and also lesions in both of his humerus bones. Bone marrow biopsy revealed 65% involvement by abnormal plasma cells, which was confirmed by immunohistochemical staining. The diagnosis was of symptomatic multiple myeloma. Because of the spread of the cancer to the patient's skull and arm bones, he was unfortunately given a late-stage diagnosis. Treatments began with chemotherapy and corticosteroids, and immunomodulators were considered for the future. However, less than half of patients with late-stage multiple myeloma will survive for five years.

Answers:

1. **In the United States, there are about 4.3 cases of multiple myeloma per 100,000 people. More than 30,000 new cases occur annually, and more than 11,000 are fatal. Globally, there are over 160,000 new cases per year, and more than 106,000 fatalities.**
2. **With multiple myeloma, bone pain may occur in a persistent or "migratory" manner – usually in the pelvis and lower back. The pain can occur suddenly if it is related to a fracture, and often follows movement.**
3. **It is unfortunately difficult to diagnose multiple myeloma early. It often causes no symptoms until it has become advanced, or causes vague symptoms that mimic those of other diseases. It can be found early if a routine blood test shows a very low amount of albumin.**

Leukemias

Leukemia is a malignant condition, in which there is excessive production of immature or abnormal white blood cells (leukocytes). This eventually will suppress production of normal blood cells and cause symptoms that are related to various types of cytopenia. At the **pluripotent stem-cell** level, malignant transformation is most common. Sometimes, committed stem cells that are not highly self-renewing are involved. Normal blood elements are replaced with malignant cells because of processes that include abnormal proliferation, aberrant differentiation, clonal expansion, and reduced **apoptosis**. According to the World Health Organization, leukemias are classified based on clinical, genetic, immunophenotypic, and morphologic factors. Another method is the French–American–British (FAB) system, which mostly focuses on the morphology of abnormal leukocytes. Leukemias may be acute or chronic, and myeloid or lymphoid. Acute or chronic leukemias are determined by the percentage of blasts or leukemia cells in the blood or bone marrow. Myeloid or lymphoid classifications are based on the primary lineage of malignant cells. The leukemias discussed below collectively make up 98% of all leukemias. Figure 7.7 illustrates the percentages of occurrence of the various types of leukemias.

Acute Lymphoblastic Leukemia

Acute lymphoblastic leukemia (ALL) affects adults of all ages, yet is the most common childhood cancer. It is also called *acute lymphocytic leukemia*. There is uncontrolled proliferation and malignant transformation of abnormally differentiated hematopoietic progenitor cells. They have long life spans and their presence results in a significant number of circulating blasts. Malignant cells replace the normal bone marrow, and there is potential for infiltration of the central nervous system, and in males, the testes.

Epidemiology

ALL makes up 10% of all new cases of leukemia, according to the National Cancer Institute. In the United States, there are about 6,150 new cases per year, with about 1,520 being fatal. Lifetime incidence is approximately 1 of every 1,000 people. Approximately 60% of cases occur in children, peaking between two and five years of age. There is a second peak after age 50. In children under age 15, ALL makes up 75% of leukemias and is the second most common cause of death. It makes up about 20% of adult acute leukemias. Males are slightly more affected than females, and also have a slightly higher mortality rate. For some reason, Hispanic populations within the United States have a higher incidence, partly because of polymorphisms of the *ARID5B* gene.

The global incidence of ALL is increasing, with prevalence ranging from 0.37 to 1.6 per 100,000, and lifetime incidence ranging from 0.4 to 2 of every 100,000 people. There are a total of over 56,000 cases, worldwide every year. The global statistics about the age of people affected

Figure 7.7 Percentages of occurrence of the various types of leukemias.

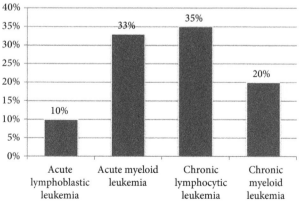

by ALL are the same as in the United States, and males are also slightly more affected than females, with a 1.4:1 ratio. The countries with the highest rates of ALL include Honduras, Mexico, and Dominica, while those with the lowest rates included Namibia, South Africa, and Botswana. Again, this indicates that ALL is most likely to affect people with Hispanic ethnicity.

Etiology and Risk Factors

ALL is caused by a group of acquired genetic changes. Mutations in various genes can be found in ALL cells, though larger changes in several chromosomes are also common. Translocations are the most common chromosomal changes that may be causative. The most common translocation in adults is the **Philadelphia chromosome** (Ph chromosome), a swap of DNA between chromosomes 9 and 22. Risk factors for ALL include exposure to radiation or benzene, the human T-cell lymphoma/ leukemia virus-1 (HTLV-1), the Epstein–Barr virus, Down syndrome, Klinefelter syndrome, **Fanconi anemia, Bloom syndrome**, ataxia-telangiectasia, neurofibromatosis, Li–Fraumeni syndrome, age, Caucasian race, male gender, and having an identical twin with ALL. Unproven risk factors include exposure to electromagnetic fields, smoking, exposure to hair dyes, and workplace exposures to diesel fuel, gasoline, and pesticides.

Clinical Manifestations

The signs and symptoms of ALL may be present for days to weeks prior to diagnosis, and the patient usually presents with anemia, granulocytopenia, and thrombocytopenia. Symptoms of anemia include fatigue and lethargy, pallor, weakness, dyspnea upon exertion, malaise, exertional chest pain, abdominal or chest pain found during examination, and tachycardia. Granulocytopenia as well as neutropenia can result in a high risk of a variety of bacterial, fungal, or viral infections that cause a fever. The infections can be severe, and commonly recur. Thrombocytopenia may cause easy bruising, mucosal bleeding, epistaxis,

petechiae or purpura, bleeding gums, and heavy menstrual bleeding. Rarely, there is G.I. bleeding and hematuria. Spontaneous hemorrhages can occur, which include intra-abdominal or intracranial hematomas. If leukemic cells are infiltrative, there can be enlargement of the lymph nodes, liver, and spleen. In children with ALL, there is often bone and joint pain caused by bone marrow and periosteal infiltration. This can also occur in adults. Meningeal infiltration and CNS penetration are common, which may cause auditory symptoms, cranial nerve palsies, headache, visual symptoms, mental changes, and stroke or transient ischemic attack.

Pathology

Malignant transformation usually occurs at the pluripotent stem-cell level. Precursor lymphoid neoplasms are widely categorized, based on lineage. The categories are: B-lymphoblastic leukemia/lymphoma or T-lymphoblastic leukemia/lymphoma. The B-lymphoblastic leukemia/ lymphoma tumors are derived from pre-germinal center naïve B-cells with unmutated *variable-heavy (VH)* region genes. There are many immunophenotyping abnormalities relative to normal B-cell precursors known as **hematogones**. When relapse occurs, 73% of cases show a loss of one or more abnormality, and 60% have new abnormalities. The T-lymphoblastic leukemia/ lymphoma tumors develop from T-lineage lymphoblasts into lymphomatous masses that involve the blood and bone marrow. It may be derived from a T-cell progenitor of the bone marrow. The T-lymphoblastic leukemia/lymphoma makes up 85–95% of cases that usually develop as a mediastinal mass with no or minimal bone marrow involvement.

Diagnosis

ALL is sometimes diagnosed after some type of infection persists chronically, and the patient is lethargic. When bone marrow cells are unavailable or insufficient, using a peripheral blood sample and the same criteria can help make a diagnosis. A complete blood count and peripheral smear are done first. Leukemia is suggested by the presence of **pancytopenia** and peripheral blasts. The blast cells in the peripheral smear may be close to 90% of the WBC count. The differential diagnosis of severe pancytopenia should consider aplastic anemia, folate deficiency, infectious mononucleosis and other viral infections, and vitamin B12 deficiency. High blast counts are not seen with leukemoid reactions to infectious disease. Leukemoid reactions are signified by extreme granulocytic leukocytosis, such as white blood cells being more than 50,000 per microliter (over 50×10^9 per liter). **Auer rods** are not present in ALL like they are in acute myeloid leukemia (AML). These rods are linear **azurophilic** inclusions in blast cell cytoplasm (see Figure 7.8).

Bone marrow aspiration and needle biopsy is regularly performed for ALL diagnosis. The blast cells are usually found to be between 25% and 95% in the bone marrow. The blasts of ALL can be distinguished via cytogenetics, histochemical studies, and immunophenotyping. Other diagnostic

findings include hyperphosphatemia, hyperkalemia, hyperuricemia, hypocalcemia, and elevated lactate dehydrogenase. These findings likely mean that a **tumor lysis syndrome** is present. There can also be elevated serum hepatic transaminases or creatinine, and hypoglycemia. Hyperleukocytosis is often seen in patients with Philadelphia chromosome positive ALL. If there are CNS symptoms, a CT of the head is performed. A spinal tap may reveal that the CSF contains many lymphoblasts. CT of the chest and abdomen may detect mediastinal masses, lymphadenopathy, and hepatosplenomegaly. Baseline cardiac function is usually assessed via echocardiography or multi-gated acquisition scans.

Treatment

Treatments for ALL usually start with 3–4 cycles of non-cross-resistant chemotherapies for 9–12 months. This is followed by 2.5–3 years of maintenance chemotherapies. The four general phases include: remission

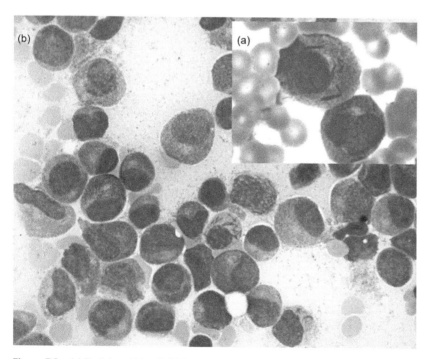

Figure 7.8 (a) Peripheral blood; (b) bone marrow in a patient with acute myeloid leukemia, showing cells that contain multiple splinters known as Auer rods. *Source*: Merino et al. (2018).

induction, post-remission consolidation, interim maintenance with intensification, and maintenance. Goals of induction treatment focus on complete remission. With complete remission, the most important factor for prognosis is a low measurable residual disease. Induction therapy is based on high-dose corticosteroids, anthracyclines, and vincristine. Corticosteroids can reduce disease before intensive induction begins. For younger adults, asparaginase with or without cyclophosphamide is used for induction, which is similar to how children are treated. Sometimes, a second induction course is needed to get the patient to complete remission prior to consolidation. Chemotherapeutic drugs with different dosing and schedules are given, which are less intensive than during induction or consolidation. The majority of chemotherapeutic regimens include maintenance therapy, using vincristine once per month, methotrexate once per week, mercaptopurine once per day, and corticosteroids for five days per month. Maintenance therapy usually lasts for 2.5–3 years.

If the patient has a matched brother or sister who can donate, stem-cell transplantation after re-induction chemotherapy or immunotherapy has the highest chance of a cure or long-term remission. Transplantation is mostly used for people under age 65 due to the chance of success and the adverse effects. If there is a CNS relapse, intrathecal methotrexate, with or without corticosteroids or cytarabine, may be used. If a male experiences a testicular relapse, biopsy is required, and radiation therapy or systemic re-induction therapy may be needed.

For supportive care, transfusions of red blood cells or platelets may be needed. Antimicrobials may be needed because of immunosuppression. General prophylaxis is provided for all patients by *acyclovir* or *valacyclovir*. It is also important that the patient remains hydrated.

Prevention and Early Detection

There is no known method of prevention for ALL. However, avoiding proven cancer-causing chemicals such as benzene could lower the risk of developing ALL. Unfortunately, there are no special tests recommended for the early detection of ALL.

Prognosis

The prognosis for ALL is varied by many factors. A good prognosis is given for patients between three and nine years of age. No matter what the prognosis is, initial remission occurs in more than 95% of childhood cases, and 70–90% of adult cases. More than 80% of affected children have disease-free survival for five years, and appear cured. Patients with poorer prognoses often receive more intense therapy, since increased risks and possible toxicities of treatment are still preferred to using less intense treatments, due to the likelihood of death.

Significant Point

ALL quickly worsens without treatment, so it is very important to begin treatment soon after it is diagnosed. The subtypes are determined by the cells they develop from, cell maturity, and if there are cellular chromosomal abnormalities. Most people have the B-cell subtype.

Clinical Case

1. How common is ALL in children?
2. How do most patients with ALL present to a physician?
3. As part of diagnosis, what do bone marrow aspiration and needle biopsy usually reveal?

A 6-year-old boy was brought back to see his pediatrician after having a streptococcal throat infection because he continued to have a sore throat and was lethargic. The boy's skin was pale, and when the pediatrician examined him and pressed upon his sternum, it caused significant pain. Further examination revealed an enlarged spleen and lymph nodes. The boy's mother told the pediatrician that the boy had been also having nosebleeds. A throat culture and CBC were performed. There was no sign of any streptococcal bacteria. The CBC revealed pancytopenia, with low RBCs, low hemoglobin, low hematocrit, and low platelets. A diagnosis of leukemia was made, along with anemia and thrombocytopenia. The boy was hospitalized, and a bone marrow aspiration was performed. The final diagnosis was of ALL. A spinal tap revealed many lymphoblasts in the CSF. Chemotherapy was started, along with several blood transfusions. Three weeks later, the boy developed a fever, accompanied by abnormal breath sounds, so chest X-rays were ordered. There was a right upper lob infiltrate. Further tests revealed that he had gram-negative pneumonia, which was successfully treated with antibiotics. Six more weeks of chemotherapy were successful in curing the leukemia, though the boy's anemia and thrombocytopenia only improved slightly.

Answers:

1. **Approximately 60% of cases of ALL occur in children, peaking between two and five years of age. In children under age 15, ALL makes up 75% of leukemias and is the second most common cause of death.**
2. **Patients with ALL usually present with anemia, granulocytopenia, and thrombocytopenia. Symptoms of anemia include fatigue and lethargy, pallor, weakness, dyspnea upon exertion, malaise, exertional chest pain, abdominal or chest pain found during examination, and tachycardia. Granulocytopenia or neutropenia can cause many different infections, and a fever. Thrombocytopenia may cause easy bruising, mucosal bleeding, epistaxis, petechiae or purpura, bleeding gums, and heavy menstrual bleeding.**

3. **Bone marrow aspiration and needle biopsy, as part of diagnosis for ALL, usually reveal blast cells that are between 25% and 95% in the bone marrow.**

Acute Myeloid Leukemia

Acute myeloid leukemia (AML) is also known as *acute myelogenous leukemia* and *acute myelocytic leukemia*. Malignant transformation and uncontrolled proliferation of abnormally differentiated myeloid progenitor cells occurs. They have a long life span, and cause high circulating amounts of immature blood cells, with malignant cells replacing normal bone marrow.

Epidemiology

AML makes up 33% of all new cases of leukemia. There are about 20,000 new cases of AML in the United States every year, and nearly 11,200 deaths – mostly in adults. Average lifetime risk for both sexes is approximately 1 of every 200 Americans. This disease makes up 25% of all childhood leukemias, and often develops during infancy. Incidence increases with age, and AML is the most common adult acute leukemia. The median age of onset is 68 years. AML is slightly more common in males than in females, with a 1.3:1 ratio. It may develop secondarily after chemotherapy or radiation therapy for another cancer. AML mostly affects non-Hispanic Caucasians, non-Hispanic African Americans, and Hispanic Americans.

Globally, the prevalence of AML ranges between 0.6 and 11.0 per 100,000 people. The median age of patients, as in the United States, is 68 years. The global lifetime incidence of AML is approximately 0.53% of men and 0.5% of women, while the highest rates of AML occur in North America, followed by India and China (see Figure 7.9). The total number of cases of AML, has the potential to increase by 31% between 2017 and 2027. Differences in the rates of AML between continents may be based on environmental factors, population genetics, or both.

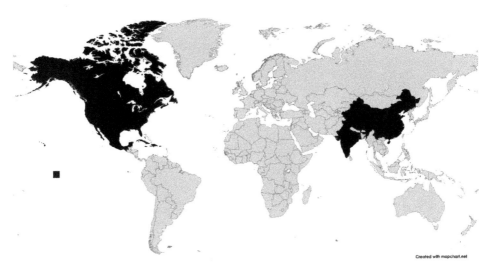

Figure 7.9 Countries with the highest rates of acute myeloid leukemia (AML).

Overall, AML is common in darker-skinned people from different countries, likely due to more cytogenetic abnormalities. Developed countries have an overall higher age-standardized rate of AML. Countries with the lowest number of cases include Malawi, Cote D'Ivoire, and Gambia.

Etiology and Risk Factors

AML is also caused by specific genetic abnormalities involving the pluripotent stem cells or committed stem cells. Patients with chromosomal abnormalities including trisomy 21 (Down syndrome), Klinefelter's syndrome, Fanconi anemia, Bloom syndrome, and ataxia–telangiectasia have a higher risk of developing AML. Risk factors may include exposure to smoking, hair dyes, diesel fuel, gasoline, and pesticides. However, the roles of these risk factors are not clear.

Clinical Manifestations

Like ALL, the signs and symptoms of AML may be seen only days to weeks prior to diagnosis, and usually include anemia, thrombocytopenia, and granulocytopenia. Anemia causes fatigue, pallor, weakness, and dyspnea on exertion, malaise, exertional chest pain, and tachycardia. Thrombocytopenia may cause easy bruising, mucosal bleeding, epistaxis, petechiae or purpura, bleeding gums, oral ulcers, and heavy menstrual bleeding. Gastrointestinal bleeding and hematuria are sometimes seen. The patient may have spontaneous hemorrhages that include intra-abdominal or intracranial hematomas. Granulocytopenia leads to high risk of bacterial, fungal, and viral infections. There may be a fever that is often of unknown cause, and the infections can be severe, recurrent, or both. Bacterial infections can rapidly progress to become life-threatening. **Leukemia cutis** may appear as nodules, papules, or plaques. It can be brown, erythematous, hemorrhagic, or a **violaceous** and grayish-blue appearance (see Figure 7.10). In AML, the leukemic cell infiltration of other organs is less common or severe than with ALL. When infiltration does occur, the liver, lymph nodes, and spleen may become enlarged. Bone and joint pain may be caused by bone marrow and periosteal infiltration. Meningeal infiltration can cause cranial nerve palsies, headache, altered mental status, transient ischemic attack or stroke, and auditory or visual abnormalities.

Pathology

AML develops from mutations of a gene located on chromosome 13. These mutations occur in all types of AML. It is the most frequent molecular

Figure 7.10 Leukemia cutis on the trunk, of the hemorrhagic subtype. *Source*: Wagner et al. (2011).

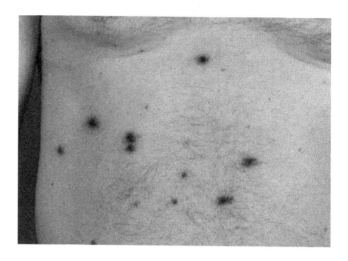

abnormality, occurring in 20–40% of all cases. There is usually peripheral leukocytosis and normal cytogenetics.

Diagnosis

The diagnosis of AML is based on the peripheral blood tests. Complete blood count and peripheral smear are the first tests. AML is suggested by pancytopenia and peripheral blasts. Blast cells in the peripheral smear may be close to 90% of the leukocyte count. The differential diagnosis of severe pancytopenia should consider aplastic anemia, folate deficiency, infectious mononucleosis, and vitamin B12 deficiency. Leukemoid reactions to infections do not manifest with high blast counts. These reactions are exemplified by significant granulocytic leukocytosis, such as a WBC count of more than 50,000 per microliter. Bone marrow examination via aspiration and needle biopsy is commonly performed. The blast cells in the bone marrow are usually between 25% and 95%.

Treatment

The treatment of AML is based on the patient's overall health status. The continually improving treatment of AML is best performed at specialized facilities, especially in the remission induction phase. Initial treatment is induction chemotherapy to induce complete remission. Consolidation therapy then occurs, which may

include allogeneic hematopoietic stem-cell transplantation. Complete remission means that there are less than 5% blast cells in the bone marrow.

Basic induction is continuous IV infusion of cytarabine for seven days, with daunorubicin or idarubicin given IV for three days. Significant myelosuppression usually occurs, along with bleeding or infections. There is a long latency before recovery of the bone marrow, so close preventive and supportive care is essential. Allogeneic stem-cell transplantation during the first complete remission generally improves results if the patient has intermediate or adverse-risk cytogenetics. About 6–12 weeks are needed to prepare for a stem-cell transplant. Standard high-dose cytarabine consolidation chemotherapy usually continues during this period. A patient may be ineligible for the stem-cell transplantation however, due to poor overall performance, and because of moderate to severe cardiac, kidney, liver, or pulmonary impairment.

Prevention and Early Detection

There is no known method of preventing AML. However, the most significant controllable risk factor may be smoking, so quitting this habit offers the greatest chance to reduce the possible development of AML. There are no screening tests that have been proven to be helpful in finding AML early. The best way to detect this disease is to report any possible symptoms to a physician as soon as they occur.

Prognosis

The remission induction rate is between 50% and 85%. Overall, long-term disease-free survival is 20–40%. In younger patients receiving intensive chemotherapy or stem-cell transplantation, the long-term disease-free survival is 40–50%. Patients with extremely negative prognostic features usually receive intense therapies that are followed by allogeneic stem-cell transplantation. The potential benefits are believed to outweigh the increased treatment toxicities. The strongest predictor of results is the leukemia cell karyotype. The normal karyotype provides an intermediate prognosis. A poorer prognosis is also given if there is a previous myelodysplastic phase, a high WBC count, and therapy-related AML. Adverse factors include a patient age of 65 years or older, comorbidities, and poor performance status. If the patient is older, high-risk cytogenetic abnormalities are more likely.

Significant Point

The symptoms of AML can be slight, and are often unnoticed or thought of as being caused by lack of sleep or influenza. Any person experiencing fatigue, weight loss, and fever should see their physician to avoid disease progression. The disease was first documented in the 1890s, yet still is of uncertain cause.

Clinical Case

1. How common is AML in adults?
2. How do you differentiate leukemic cell infiltration of other organs between AML and ALL?
3. What is the initial treatment for AML?

A 54-year-old man went to his physician after 2 weeks of a low fever and malaise. A blood test revealed that his WBC count was elevated and contained 80% blast cells. Acute myeloid leukemia was diagnosed. Chemotherapy with cytarabine and idarubicin was started, and the patient's temperature returned to normal. However, 3 days later, the fever returned and reached 103 degrees Fahrenheit. Ulcers developed in his mouth, which tested negative for cytomegalovirus and herpes simplex virus. It was determined that he had a neutropenic fever, which was treated with cefepime, but this only reduced his temperature slightly. In two days, the patient developed diarrhea, caused by *Enterococcus faecium*, so the cefepime was replaced with imipenem/vancomycin. The temperature increased again and the diarrhea worsened, so fluconazole was added. It was discovered that the patient also had a yeast infection in his blood, so the fluconazole was replaced with anidulafungin. A CT scan revealed diffuse thickening of the patient's small intestine and ascending colon walls. By the 17th day of treatment, the patient became hypotensive, and it was discovered that a gram-negative bacteria (*Acinetobacter baumanii*) was also present, which was treated. By the 22nd day, the fever, diarrhea, and leukemia had resolved, and the patient was discharged.

Answers:

1. **Mostly in adults, there are about 20,000 new cases of AML in the United States every year, and nearly 11,200 deaths. Incidence increases with age, and AML is the most common adult leukemia. The median age of onset is 68 years. In adults, the disease occurs most often in North America, Europe, and the Oceanic countries.**
2. **In AML, the leukemic cell infiltration of other organs is less common or severe than with ALL. When infiltration does occur, the liver, lymph nodes,**

and spleen may become enlarged. Bone and joint pain may be caused by bone marrow and periosteal infiltration.

3. The initial treatment for AML is chemotherapy to induce complete remission. Consolidation therapy then occurs, which may include allogeneic hematopoietic stem-cell transplantation. The treatment of AML must be performed at specialized facilities, especially in the remission induction phase.

Chronic Lymphocytic Leukemia

Chronic lymphocytic leukemia (CLL) involves progressive accumulation of malignant B lymphocytes that are phenotypically mature. The main sites of CLL include the bone marrow, peripheral blood, lymph nodes, and spleen. This disease usually progresses more slowly than other types of leukemia.

Epidemiology

CLL makes up 37% of all new cases of leukemia, according to Cancer.net. It is the most common type of leukemia in the western parts of the world and is twice as common as chronic myeloid leukemia (CML). There are more than 21,000 new cases annually, and nearly 4,100 deaths. The incidence rate is 20 cases per 100,000 persons each year. This is much lower than the prevalence because of earlier diagnosis and better treatments, which have prolonged survival. Average lifetime risk is about 0.57% of the American population. The majority of cases and nearly all of the deaths occur in adults. This disease occurs rarely in those younger than 30 years. A peak age group is in individuals between 30 and 39 years. However, the average patient age at diagnosis is 70 years. The male to female ratio is about 2:1. Incidence does not appear to be higher in Japanese people who have moved to the United States, which suggests that genetic components are present. Intermediate incidence rates are shown in persons of Hispanic origin. CLL is more common in Jewish people who come from Eastern European lineages. The disease is much more common in non-Hispanic Caucasians than any other group, followed by Hispanic Americans and non-Hispanic African Americans.

Globally, the prevalence is quite varied – for example, in the United Kingdom, CLL is the most common form of leukemia, making up 38% of all leukemia cases. It is also common in most of Europe and in Australia. The incidence of CLL among Asians in China, Japan, and Korea is only 10%. It is also of low incidence in African countries. Also similarly, about twice as many as men throughout the world develop CLL compared with women. The disease mostly affects non-Hispanic Caucasians from various countries, and is seen in lower amounts in Hispanics and Africans.

Etiology and Risk Factors

The exact cause of CLL is unknown. However, it has been linked to genetics. In most cases of CLL, a change can be found in at least one chromosome, with deletions being the most common type of change. The loss of a part of chromosome 13 is the most common deletion. There can also be an extra chromosome 12. Risk factors for CLL include age over 50 years, exposure to herbicides, pesticides, or the gas called *radon*; history of CLL in a parent, brother, sister, or children; male gender (in which CLL is just slightly more common); and a family background originating in North America or Europe. Farmers have a higher incidence of CLL than do those in other population, which is raising the possibility of an etiologic role for herbicides or pesticides.

Clinical Manifestations

Most patients with CLL are often asymptomatic initially. There is an insidious onset of symptoms that are nonspecific. These include fatigue, lethargy, anorexia, weight loss, weakness, fever, and night sweats. Over half of all cases have enlarged lymph nodes. This may be localized or generalized. If localized, the cervical and supraclavicular nodes are the most involved.

Leukemia cutis is rare. Abnormal hematopoiesis causes anemia, neutropenia, decreased immunoglobulin production, and thrombocytopenia. In as many as 66% of patients, hypogammaglobulinemia develops, which increases the risk of infections. There is more susceptibility to autoimmune hemolytic anemia and autoimmune thrombocytopenia. Splenomegaly or hepatomegaly may also be present.

Pathology

CLL develops as CD5 + B-cells experience malignant transformation. They are continuously activated by acquired gene mutations, resulting in monoclonal B-cell lymphocytosis (MBL). As genetic abnormalities and oncogenic changes of the monoclonal B-cells occur, CLL manifests. Lymphocytes accumulate first in the bone marrow, spreading to the lymphoid tissues, which include the lymph nodes. The disease can evolve into B-cell prolymphocytic leukemia and a high-grade NHL. Approximately 2–10% of cases develop into diffuse large B-cell lymphoma, which is known as **Richter's transformation**.

Diagnosis

Diagnosis of CLL is based on an absolute lymphocytosis count that typically ranges from 5,000 to 600,000 cells per microliter in the peripheral blood. Clonality in the circulating B-cells can be confirmed by using peripheral blood flow cytometry. Diagnosis of CLL does not require bone marrow aspiration and biopsy. If these are performed, however, more than 30% of the bone marrow will be lymphocytes. Other diagnostic findings include elevated LDH, hypogammaglobulinemia in fewer than 15% of cases, elevated hepatic enzymes, and elevated uric acid. In rare cases, hypercalcemia is present. The anemia is usually normochromic and normocytic, and reticulocyte count is normal unless the patient has autoimmune hemolytic anemia, which usually results from the development of a warm-reacting IgG antibody. Scintigraphy may be performed to assess persistent symptoms, and can reveal inflammatory osteometabolic reactions in the bones. Total body CT scans can reveal calcifications, lymph node enlargement, and prostate changes.

Treatment

CLL is currently incurable, and treatments focus on reducing symptoms. Treatment begins when the patient has one of the following manifestations: symptoms related to the disease, a lymphocyte doubling time of less than six months, or progressive lymphocytosis, with an increase of 50% or more in two months. Other symptoms that require treatment include: extreme fatigue, fever, night sweats, weight loss, recurrent infections; extreme hepatomegaly, lymphadenopathy, or splenomegaly; and symptomatic anemia, thrombocytopenia, or both. Based on the extent of the disease, treatment options include chemoimmunotherapy, radiation therapy, and targeted therapy. Supportive care includes antimicrobials for infections, platelet transfusions for thrombocytopenia-related bleeding, and transfusion of packed red blood cells to treat anemia. Antibiotic therapy should be bactericidal since hypogammaglobulinemia and neutropenia reduce bacterial death. For patients with hypogammaglobulinemia and refractory infections, or as prophylaxis when two or more severe infections occur in six months, gammaglobulin infusions may be used.

Chemotherapy regimens are wide ranging. As initial therapy, they include the purine analogs and alkylating agents, used in combination with rituximab. Combinations of fludarabine, cyclophosphamide, and rituximab are also used. Older patients may have better toleration of medications such as bendamustine and rituximab. If the patient has a 17p deletion, ibrutinib is the most successful drug. For older patients with comorbidities, obinutuzumab is used with chlorambucil. For relapsed or refractory CLL, which must be histologically confirmed, drugs include ibrutinib, idelalisib, venetoclax, rituximab, obinutuzumab, and ofatumumab. Some patients may benefit from allogeneic stem-cell transplantation. Radiation therapy is used palliatively for lymphadenopathy, and for liver or spleen involvement that does not respond well to chemotherapy. It is also used if chemotherapy causes chronic thrombocytopenia. Temporary symptoms relief may be achieved by small doses of total body irradiation.

Prevention and Early Detection

There is no known way to prevent CLL. There are no screening tests routinely recommended for this disease. Often, it is discovered when routine blood tests are performed for other reasons. Any symptoms that could be caused by CLL should be reported to a physician immediately.

Prognosis

The prognosis of CLL may be determined via cytogenetic and molecular studies of the peripheral blood. Survival ranges from approximately 2 to 20 years, but can be longer. The median survival time is about 10 years. *Lymphocyte doubling time* is used to determine prognosis, and is the number of months required for the absolute lymphocyte count to double. In an untreated patient with a lymphocyte doubling time of less than 12 months, the disease is more aggressive.

Significant Point

Most cases of CLL begin in the B lymphocytes. It is the most common form of leukemia in adults. Known risk factors include exposure to herbicides and pesticides, or having an immediate family member with the disease, or with any type of lymphoma.

Clinical Case

1. What are the statistics on fatalities caused by CLL?
2. What are the global variances in the commonality of CLL?
3. What do treatments for CLL focus upon?

A 66-year-old man went for a regular check-up and was found to have lymphocytosis via a CBC. A flow cytometry test revealed that the patient had CLL. Since the patient was asymptomatic, he was merely observed for a few months. However, once he developed acute anemia, he was hospitalized. A bone marrow biopsy confirmed the diagnosis of CLL, and there was 90% infiltration of the marrow. The patient also had slight splenomegaly. Within one month, persistent symptoms resulted in a scintigraphy procedure being performed. It revealed an extreme inflammatory osteometabolic reaction of the right tibia, fibula, and ankle. The next month, a total body CT scan revealed two nodular calcifications of the right lung lobe, aortopulmonary and axillary lymph node enlargement, and increased prostate size. Two cycles of chemotherapy were performed, but the patient developed chronic thrombocytopenia, so radiation therapy replaced the chemotherapy. The patient's condition improved, and he continues to be closely monitored as additional radiation procedures occur.

Answers:

1. **In the United States, nearly 4,100 deaths occur annually from CLL, out of more than 21,000 new cases. Earlier diagnosis and better treatment methods have prolonged survival. The majority of cases and nearly all of the deaths occur in adults.**
2. **Globally, the prevalence is quite varied. In the United Kingdom and Western parts, it is the most common form of leukemia, and is also common in most of Europe and in Australia. Yet, the incidence of CLL among Asians in China, Japan, and Korea is only 10%. It is also of low incidence in African countries.**
3. **CLL is currently incurable, and treatments focus on reducing symptoms. Treatment begins when the patient**

has one of the following manifestations: symptoms related to the disease, a lymphocyte doubling time of less than six months, or progressive lymphocytosis, with an increase of 50% or more in two months.

Chronic Myeloid Leukemia

Chronic myeloid leukemia (CML) is also called *chronic myelogenous leukemia*, and begins in pluripotent stem cells of the bone marrow, eventually invading the blood. There is a large overproduction of cells of the myeloid series, resulting in marked leukocytosis and splenomegaly. Basophilia and thrombocytosis are common.

Epidemiology

CML makes up 20% of all cases of leukemia, which causes nearly 8,500 new cases every year in the United States, and over 1,100 of these are fatal. The incidence of CML increases with age. Average lifetime risk is about 0.19% of the American population. The median age at diagnosis is 50–55 years. The disease is slightly more common in men than in women. It is also most common in Caucasians compared with any other racial or ethnic group.

Globally, there are more than 34,200 cases of CML every year, with over 24,000 fatalities. Global incidence is between 0.7 and 1.0 cases out of every 100,000 people. The median age at diagnosis is 57–60 years, and for some reason, unlike in the United States, there is a female prevalence of 1.7 compared with a male prevalence of 1.2. While the disease is most common in North America, it is also relatively common in Europe and the Asian Pacific countries. Therefore, statistics reveal that Caucasians are most affected. Though Asians are less affected, when they do develop CML, it is usually in somewhat younger people.

Etiology and Risk Factors

Usually, no etiologic agent is known in CML. Exposure to ionizing radiation in survivors of the atomic bomb explosions in Japan in 1945 increased the risk for CML. The peak incidence occurs 5–12 years after exposure and is dose related. Radiologists working without adequate protection before 1940 were more likely to develop myeloid leukemia. No increase in the risk for CML has been shown among people working in the nuclear facility. The incidence of CML increases with age.

Clinical Manifestations

Approximately 40–50% of patients have no symptoms at the diagnosis. The disease is found on routine physical examination or blood tests. Most patients, about 85%, first present with signs and symptoms with CML when they are in the chronic phase. The symptoms of CML include fatigue, anorexia, weight loss, weakness, night sweats, gouty arthritis, and abdominal fullness or pain, usually in the left upper quadrant. At first, bleeding, pallor, easy bruising, and lymphadenopathy are uncommon. However, moderate to extreme splenomegaly occurs in 60–70% of cases. As the disease progresses, splenomegaly may worsen, and bleeding and pallor are common. Symptoms such as fever, significant lymphadenopathy, and maculopapular skin lesions are signs of severe disease.

Pathology

The Philadelphia chromosome is present in 90–95% of patients with CML. This chromosome develops a balanced translocation of genetic material between the long arms of chromosomes 9 and 22. Part of chromosome 9 results in translocation of the cellular oncogene ABL1 to a region on chromosome 22 coding for the major breakpoint cluster region. It fuses to the BCR gene. The BCR-ABL gene is a chimeric fusion gene, causing the production of oncoproteins known as *bcr-abl tyrosine kinase*, which has uncontrolled activity. It causes deregulation of cellular proliferation, less adherence of leukemia cells to bone marrow stroma, and also protect leukemic cells from apoptosis. CML develops as abnormal pluripotent hematopoietic progenitor cells produce all cells of the myeloid lineage – mostly in the bone marrow, but also in the spleen and liver. Aside from granulocytes, neoplastic clones include megakaryocytes, monocytes, red blood cells, and even B-cells and T-cells. Normal stem cells remain and are able to emerge if drugs suppress the CML clones.

Diagnosis

CML is usually suspected because of an abnormal complete blood count performed for another reason, or as part of the evaluation of splenomegaly. The granulocyte count is high, usually less than 50,000 per microliter when the patient is asymptomatic, but between 200,000 and 1,000,000 per microliter in symptomatic patients. Common manifestations include basophilia, eosinophilia, and neutrophilia. The platelet count is normal or slightly increased. Thrombocytosis may be a presenting sign. Hemoglobin levels are usually more than 10 grams per deciliter. A peripheral smear may differentiate CML from other diseases. They usually show immature granulocytes, plus absolute basophilia and eosinophilia. If the white blood cell count is 50,000 per microliter or less, or occasionally in patients with higher WBC counts, immature granulocytes may not appear. Bone marrow examination is required to evaluate cellularity, myelofibrosis, and the karyotype.

Diagnosis of CML is confirmed by the presence of the Ph chromosome, though about 5% of patients do not have the classic Ph chromosome cytogenetic abnormality. Diagnosis can be confirmed via fluorescence in situ hybridization (FISH) or reverse transcription polymerase chain reaction (RT-PCR). When the patient is in the accelerated phase, anemia and thrombocytopenia are common. There may be defective maturation of granulocytes, and increased basophils. Immature cells may increase in number. Myelofibrosis may develop in the bone marrow, and sideroblasts may be found.

Treatment

Treatment of CML is based on disease stage. The tyrosine kinase inhibitors are very effective in the chronic phase and are the first treatment of choice if the patient is in this phase and has no symptoms. They include bosutinib, dasatinib, imatinib, nilotinib, and ponatinib. These drugs are sometimes used during the accelerated or blast phase.

Allogeneic hematopoietic stem-cell transplantation is only done in patients with accelerated or blast-phase CML, or if the disease does not respond to the tyrosine kinase inhibitors (TKIs). Treatment is curative only when stem-cell transplantation is successful. Some patients eventually can discontinue TKIs and remain in remission. Drugs used for palliation include busulfan, hydroxyurea, and pegylated or recombinant interferon. Hydroxyurea reduces severe splenomegaly and adenopathy, and also gout and tumor lysis syndrome. Interferon produces remission in 19% of patients.

Prevention and Early Detection

There is no known way to prevent most cases of CML. The only possibly avoidable risk factor is exposure to high doses of radiation, which affects very few people. No screening tests are commonly recommended to detect CML early.

Prognosis

Before the use of TKIs, 5–10% of patients with CML died within two years after diagnosis – regardless of the treatments used. Another 10–15% of patients died each year after that, and median survival was 4–7 years. About 90% of deaths occurred after the blast phase or accelerated phase. The median survival after a blast crisis was usually 3–6 months, but sometimes longer if remission occurred. Today, because of the TKIs, survival is more than 90% of patients within five years following diagnosis of the chronic phase of the disease. The response to TKI therapy is the main prognostic factor.

Significant Point

CML in the early phase is usually asymptomatic or only slightly symptomatic until the WBC count becomes very high. Accelerated-phase CML is symptomatic and requires targeted therapy, chemotherapy, and bone marrow transplantation. Blast-phase CML acts aggressively, but is rare. It most often occurs after targeted therapy for chronic-phase CML, and bone marrow transplantation is often done.

Clinical Case

1. What is the prevalence and incidence of CML, in the United States, and globally?
2. When do symptoms of CML usually appear?
3. How commonly is the Philadelphia chromosome implicated in CML?

A 58-year-old woman had been diagnosed with CML, positive for the Philadelphia chromosome. A peripheral blood smear showed increased amounts of neutrophils and their precursors, basophilia, occasional blasts, and inconspicuous nucleoli. The RBCs had slight anisocytosis and poikilocytosis. A bone marrow aspirate and biopsy was performed, revealing excessive amounts of blasts and basophils, and a high myeloid-to-erythroid precursor ratio. There was marked cellularity of nearly 100%. Flow cytometry showed cells of a B-cell lineage that made up 19% of the total cells. The CML was in an accelerated phase. The patient was started on chemotherapy with hydroxyurea, which helped to resolve the leukemia for a while, but then the disease worsened, and the patient died seven months later.

Answers:

1. **CML makes up 20% of all cases of leukemia, which causes nearly 8,500 new cases every year in the United States, and over 1,100 of these are fatal. The incidence of CML increases with age. The average lifetime risk is about 0.19% of the American population. Globally, there are more than 34,200 cases of CML every year, with over 24,000 fatalities. Global incidence is between 0.7 and 1.0 cases out of every 100,000 people.**
2. **About 85% of patients first present with signs and symptoms of CML when they are in the chronic phase. The symptoms include fatigue, anorexia, weight loss, weakness, night sweats, gouty arthritis, and abdominal fullness or pain, usually in the left upper quadrant.**
3. **The Philadelphia chromosome is present in 90–95% of patients with CML. This chromosome develops a balanced translocation of genetic material between the long arms of chromosomes 9 and 22. The Philadelphia chromosome is also implicated in ALL.**

Key Terms

Acute lymphoblastic leukemia
Acute myeloid leukemia
Apoptosis
Ataxia–telangiectasia
Auer rods
Azurophilic
Bloom syndrome
Chamberlain procedure
Chédiak–Higashi syndrome
Chronic lymphocytic leukemia
Chronic myeloid leukemia
Fanconi anemia
Hematogones
Hodgkin's lymphoma
Ivory vertebrae
Klinefelter syndrome

Leukemia
Leukemia cutis
Lymphomas
Mediastinoscopy
Monoclonal proteins
Multiple myeloma
Non-Hodgkin's lymphoma
Pancytopenia
Pathognomic
Pel–Ebstein fever
Philadelphia chromosome
Plasma cells
Pluripotent stem cell
Reed–Sternberg cells
Reticuloendothelial
Richter's transformation

Sjögren syndrome
Tumor lysis syndrome
Video-assisted thoroscopy

Violaceous
Waldeyer ring
Wiskott–Aldrich syndrome

Bibliography

1 Batchelor, T. and DeAngelis, L.M. (2012). *Lymphoma and Leukemia of the Nervous System*, 2nd Edition. New York: Springer.

2 Bhushan, B. (2020). *CLL (Chronic Lymphocytic Leukemia): A Survival Guide for Patients*. Jaipur: Bhushan.

3 Blanchett, O. (2012). *Coping with Lymphoma: Symptoms, Diagnosis and Treatment of Lymphatic Cancer*. New York: Blanchett.

4 British Journal of Haematology. (2018). *Bilateral renomegaly: Diagnosed as Non-Hodgkin lymphoma*. https://onlinelibrary.wiley.com/doi/full/10.1111/bjh.15536. Figure 1. Accessed 2021.

5 British Journal of Haematology. (2004). *Cluster of Reed-Sternberg cells and variants*. https://onlinelibrary.wiley.com/doi/full/10.1111/j.1365-2141.2004.04964.x. Figure 1. Accessed 2021.

6 Cancer.net. (2020) *Leukemia – Chronic Lymphocytic – CLL: Statistics*. American Society of Clinical Oncology (ASCO) / Conquer Cancer – The ASCO Foundation. https://www.cancer.net/cancer-types/leukemia-chronic-lymphocytic-cll/statistics Accessed 2021.

7 DeVita, V.T., Jr., Lawrence, T.S., and Rosenberg, S.A. (2015). *Lymphomas and Leukemias: Cancer – Principles & Practice of Oncology*, 10th Edition. Philadelphia: Lippincott, Williams, and Wilkins.

8 Drexler, H.G. (2000). *The Leukemia-Lymphoma Cell Line Factsbook*. Cambridge: Academic Press.

9 Duffield, A.S., Song, J.Y., and Venkataraman, G. (2020). *Atlas of Lymph Node Pathology: A Pattern Based Approach*. Philadelphia: Lippincott Williams, and Wilkins.

10 Engert, A. and Younes, A. (2020). *Hodgkin Lymphoma: A Comprehensive Overview (Hematologic Malignancies)*, 3rd Edition. New York: Springer.

11 Faderl, S.H., Kantarjian, H.M., and Estey, E. (2021). *Acute Leukemias (Hematologic Malignancies)*, 2nd Edition. New York: Springer.

12 Ferry, J.A. (2011). *Extranodal Lymphomas: Expert Consult*. Philadelphia: Saunders.

13 Gasparetto, C. and Sivaraj, D. (2017). *Understanding Multiple Myeloma*. Burlington: Jones & Bartlett Learning.

14 Global Cancer Observatory, The (part of the International Agency for Research on Cancer and World Health Organization). (2020). *Age-standardized (world) incidence rates of Hodgkin's lymphoma by gender, and its incidence and mortality rates*. https://gco.iarc.fr/today/data/factsheets/cancers/33-hodgkin-lymphoma-fact-sheet.pdf (bottom two graphs on Page 2). Accessed 2021.

15 Global Cancer Observatory, The (part of the International Agency for Research on Cancer and World Health Organization). (2020). *Age-standardized (world) incidence rates of Hodgkin's lymphoma for males and females*. https://gco.iarc.fr/today/data/factsheets/cancers/33-hodgkin-lymphoma-fact-sheet.pdf (top two maps on Page 2). Accessed 2021.

16 Gorczyca, W. (2017). *Flow Cytometry in Neoplastic Hematology: Morphologic-Immunophenotypic Correlation*, 3rd Edition. Boca Raton: CRC Press.

17 International Agency for Research on Cancer, World Health Organization. (2020). *Hodgkin lymphoma – Number of ne cases in 2020, both sexes, all ages*. The Global Cancer Observatory. https://gco.iarc.fr/today/data/factsheets/cancers/33-Hodgkin-lymphoma-fact-sheet.pdf Accessed 2021.

18 International Journal of Laboratory Hematology. (2018). *Peripheral blood and bone marrow in a patient with acute myeloid leukemia, showing cells that contain multiple splinters known as Auer rods.* https://onlinelibrary.wiley.com/doi/full/10.1111/ijlh.12831. Figure 2. Accessed 2021.

19 International Myeloma Working Group (IMWG). (2020). *Criteria for the Diagnosis of Multiple Myeloma.* International Myeloma Foundation. https://www.myeloma.org/international-myeloma-working-group-imwg-criteria-diagnosis-multiple-myeloma Accessed 2021.

20 Journal of the German Society of Dermatology. (2011). *Leukemia cutis on the trunk, of the hemorrhagic subtype.* https://onlinelibrary.wiley.com/doi/full/10.1111/j.1610-0387.2011.07842.x. Figure 6. Accessed 2021.

21 Kaspers, G.J.L., Coiffier, B., Heinrich, M.C., and Estey, E.H. (2008). *Innovative Leukemia and Lymphoma Therapy.* Boca Raton: CRC Press.

22 Kaushansky, K., Lichtman, M., Prchal, J., Levi, M., Burns, L., and Linch, D.C. (2021). *Williams Hematology,* 10th Edition. New York: McGraw-Hill Education/Medical.

23 Leukemia and Lymphoma Society, The. (2019). *Non-Hodgkin Lymphoma.* Rye Brook: The Leukemia and Lymphoma Society.

24 Maziarz, R.T. and Schubach Slater, S. (2021). *Blood and Marrow Transplant Handbook: Comprehensive Guide for Patient Care,* 3rd Edition. New York: Springer.

25 Medeiros, L.J. and Miranda, R.N. (2017). *Diagnostic Pathology: Lymph Nodes and Extranodal Lymphomas,* 2nd Edition. Amsterdam: Elsevier.

26 Medifocus. (2018). *Guidebook on Chronic Lymphocytic Leukemia: A Comprehensive Guide to Symptoms, Treatment, Research, and Support.* Scotts Valley: CreateSpace Independent Publishing Platform.

27 Mughal, T., Goldman, J., and Mughal, S. (2009). *Understanding Leukemias, Lymphomas, and Myelomas,* 2nd Edition. Boca Raton: CRC Press.

28 National Cancer Institute – Surveillance, Epidemiology, and End Results Program. (2020). *Cancer Stat Facts: Leukemia – Acute Lymphocytic Leukemia (ALL) – How Common Is This Cancer?* U.S. Department of Health and Human Services, National Institutes of Health, National Cancer Institute, USA.gov. https://seer.cancer.gov/statfacts/html/alyl.html Accessed 2021.

29 National Comprehensive Cancer Network (NCCN). (2020). *Guidelines for Patients – Chronic Myeloid Leukemia.* Plymouth Meeting: National Comprehensive Cancer Network (NCCN).

30 NetCE. Alexander, L. (2018). *Childhood Leukemias and Lymphomas.* Sacramento: NetCE.

31 Palsson, B.O. and Masters, J. (2002). *Cancer Cell Lines: Part 3: Leukemias and Lymphomas, Volume III.* New York: Springer.

32 Pezzella, F., Tavassoli, M., and Kerr, D. (2019). *Oxford Textbook of Cancer Biology (Oncology).* Oxford: Oxford University Press.

33 Reaman, G.H. and Smith, F.O. (2010). *Childhood Leukemia: A Practical Handbook (Pediatric Oncology).* New York: Springer.

34 Sekeres, M.A. (2020). *When Blood Breaks Down: Life Lessons from Leukemia.* Cambridge: The MIT Press.

35 Smith, G.H. and Smith, F.O. (2010). *Childhood Leukemia: A Practical Handbook (Pediatric Oncology).* New York: Springer.

36 Tamkin, J. and Visel, D. (2017). *The Myeloma Survival Guide: Essential Advice for Patients and Their Loved Ones,* 2nd Edition. New York: Demos Health.

37 Tariman, J.D. and Faiman, B. (2015). *Multiple Myeloma (A Textbook for Nurses),* 2nd Edition. Pittsburgh: Oncology Nursing Society.

38 Ultmann, J.E., Griem, M.L., Kirsten, W.H., and Wissler, R.W. (2012). *Current Concepts in the Management of Lymphoma and Leukemia (Recent Results in Cancer Research 36).* New York: Springer.

39 Verma, O. and Sharma, A. (2019). *Multiple Myeloma New Horizon: With Orthodox and Alternative Treatments.* Kota (India): Verma-Sharma.

40 Wapner, J. (2014). *The Philadelphia Chromosome (A Genetic Mystery, a Lethal Cancer, and the Improbable Invention of a Livesaving Treatment)*. New York: The Experiment.

41 Wiernik, P.H., Dutcher, J.P., and Gertz, M.A. (2018). *Neoplastic Diseases of the Blood*, 6th Edition. New York: Springer.

42 Williams, J.R. (2019). *The Immunotherapy Revolution: The Best New Hope for Saving Cancer Patients' Lives*. Atlanta: Williams.

43 Woelfel, R. (2017). *Leukemia: From Diagnosis to Winning the Battle – Perspective – Family – Bliss*. Plano: Kouba Graphics Inc.

44 World Health Organization, National Library of Medicine, and National Center for Biotechnology Information. (Originally 2010). *Classification of tumors of the hematopoietic and lymphoid tissues: An overview with emphasis on the myeloid neoplasms (revised 2017 by WHO)*. National Library of Medicine. https://pubmed.ncbi.nlm.nih.gov/32719169. https://pubmed.ncbi.nlm.nih.gov/19857474 Accessed 2021.

45 Zavaleta, B.A. (2019). *Braving Chemo: What to Expect, How to Prepare and How to Get through It*. Brownsville: Sugar Plum Press, LLC.

46 Zhang, L., Shao, H., and Alkan, S. (2020). *Diagnostic Pathology of Hematopoietic Disorders of Spleen and Liver*. New York: Springer.

8

Male Reproductive Tumors

OUTLINE

Benign Prostatic Hyperplasia
Prostate Cancer
Testicular Cancer
Penile Cancer
Key Terms
Bibliography

Benign Prostatic Hyperplasia

Benign prostatic hyperplasia (BPH) occurs in the periurethral portion of the prostate gland, and is a nonmalignant adenomatous overgrowth of tissue. It is also referred to as *benign prostatic hypertrophy*. The condition results in symptoms that constitute bladder outlet obstruction, which along with digital rectal examination, prompt the diagnosis. It is often first noticed because of changes in urination. The condition is treated with a variety of medications as well as surgery. The average weight of the prostate gland is 25–30 g between ages 40 and 49 and 40 g between ages 50 and 59, as well as 45 g after age 60. If the gland becomes heavier than these weights during their specific age ranges, BPH may be developing.

Epidemiology

The prevalence of BPH in men between 40 and 74 years of age is 19% of the American male population. The incidence of BPH increases greatly with age, and every year, there are more than 27 million men over age 50, affected. For unknown reasons, African American men have the highest number of cases of BPH, followed by Caucasians and Hispanic Americans. Asian American men have the lowest rates. Globally, BPH affects over 6% of the male population. Prevalence is 2.7% of men aged 45–49, but 24% by the age of 80. Incidence rates are 3 out of every 1,000 men aged 45–49, and 38 cases per 1,000 men aged 75–79 year. Though studies have been limited, countries with the highest rates of BPH have included the Czech Republic, Romania, former Yugoslavia, Hungary, Cuba, Mexico, and Uruguay.

Etiology and Risk Factors

The cause of BPH is unknown, but likely involves age-related hormonal changes. Men produce less testosterone in proportion to their small amounts of naturally produced estrogen. It may be that the estrogen triggers further growth of the prostate gland. Also, when testosterone levels fall, another male hormone called *dihydrotestosterone* (DHT) may still remain high. Not all men produce DHT, and those that

Global Epidemiology of Cancer: Diagnosis and Treatment, First Edition. Jahangir Moini, Nicholas G. Avgeropoulos, and Craig Badolato.
© 2022 John Wiley & Sons Ltd. Published 2022 by John Wiley & Sons Ltd.

do not produce it do not develop BPH, suggesting a link between high DHT levels and BPH. Risk factors for BPH include older age, family history of a close relative with BPH, obesity, cardiovascular problems, type 2 diabetes, erectile dysfunction, and a lack of exercise.

Clinical Manifestations

The symptoms of BPH are often progressive, and patients complain hesitancy, intermittency, nocturia, urgency, and urinary frequency. Incomplete emptying and fast refilling of the bladder cause frequency, nocturia, and urgency. There is usually no pain or dysuria. Some patients have sensations of incomplete emptying; overflow incontinence, terminal dribbling, or complete urinary retention. If the patient strains to urinate, this can result in congestion of the superficial veins of the prostatic urethra and trigone, which can rupture, resulting in hematuria. Straining may cause acute **vasovagal syncope**. Over time, straining may cause hemorrhoidal vein dilation or inguinal hernia dilation.

Sometimes, there is sudden and complete urinary retention, with extreme abdominal discomfort and distention of the bladder. Prior to urinary retention, there may have been continued attempts to postpone urination, immobilization, exposure to cold temperatures, or the use of anesthetics, anticholinergics, opioids, alcohol, or sympathomimetics. The symptoms are assessed by using the American Urological Association Symptom Score, allowing for monitoring of the progression of the symptoms.

According to the American Urological Association, BPH is evaluated by symptoms that occur over the past 30 days before the questions are answered by each patient. The questionnaire that is used asks the following questions, and if they have never occurred, happened in ranges between less than 20% and over 50% of the time, or if they almost always occurred:

- How often have you had a sensation of not emptying your bladder completely after you finish urinating?
- How often have you had to urinate again less than two hours after you finished urinating?
- How often have you stopped and started again several times when urinating?
- How often have you found it difficult to postpone urination?
- How often has your urinary stream been weak?
- How often have you had to push or strain to begin urination?
- How many times did you most typically get up to urinate between going to bed at night and waking in the morning?

The score is then added up to make the evaluation. The patient has severe symptoms of BPH if the total score is 20–35 points; moderate symptoms if the score is 8–19 points; and minimal symptoms if the score is 0–7 points. Lower urinary tract symptoms may also be related to infections, overactive bladder, and prostate cancer. In some patients, BPH and prostate cancer coexist.

Pathology

In the periurethral region of the prostate gland, multiple fibroadenomatous nodules form. They likely originate in the periurethral glands, instead of the actual fibromuscular prostate, known as the *surgical capsule*, which is peripherally displaced as the nodules increase in size. With the lumen of the prostatic urethra becoming thinner and longer, there is progressive urine outflow obstruction. With increased pressure in relation to urination and bladder distention, there may be a progression to hypertrophy of the bladder detrusor muscles, formulation of **cellules**, trabeculation, and diverticula. If there is incomplete bladder emptying, stasis develops, predisposing the patient to the formation of calculi and also infections. Incomplete or complete urinary tract obstruction, over time, causes hydronephrosis and reduced kidney function.

Diagnosis

Upon digital rectal examination (DRE) for suspected BPH, the prostate is usually enlarged, but not tender. The consistency feels "rubbery," ad often, the **median furrow** cannot be palpated. The size of the prostate gland during DRE is not completely an accurate consideration, since even a small prostate is able to cause obstruction. The urinary bladder may also be palpable or **percussible** during abdominal examination if it is distended. Hard or firm areas in the prostate gland may indicate prostate cancer. Though palpable tenderness of the prostate is suggestive of an infection, there is often an overlap between the DRE results between BPH and prostate cancer. While cancer may cause a very hard, nodular, and irregularly enlarged prostate, a majority of patients with BPH or prostate cancer (or both at the same time), have only an enlarged prostate that "feels" as if it is benign. Therefore, testing is required if there are palpable abnormalities or symptoms.

Urinalysis and urine culture is usually performed, and serum prostate-specific antigen (PSA) levels are measured. If there are moderate or severe obstructive symptoms, **uroflowmetry** is performed to test urine volume and flow rate, and bladder ultrasound is used to measure post-void residual volume. Obstruction is indicated if the flow rate is less than 15 mL per second, and retention is suggested if the post-void residual volume is higher than 100 mL. Interpretation of PSA levels can be difficult. In 30–50% of BPH patients, the PSA levels are moderately elevated. This is based on the size of the prostate and the level of obstruction. The PSA is elevated in 25–92% of patients with prostate cancer, based on the volume of the tumor. In patients without prostate cancer, the serum PSA levels, if over 1.5 ng/mL (or 1.5 mcg/L) usually reveal a prostate volume of 30 mL or more. When the PSA level is above 4 ng/mL (4 mcg/L), there must be a discussion on having other tests or a biopsy. For a man under age 50 that has a high risk of prostate cancer, a lower threshold may be used, which is a PSA of higher than 2.5 ng/mL (2.5 mcg/L). There may be other needed measurements, including the rate of PSA increase, and the free-to-bound PSA ratio.

If prostate cancer is suspected, a transrectal biopsy is often done with ultrasound guidance.

Transrectal ultrasound accurately measures prostate volume. Further testing is decided upon clinically. Unless the patient has had a urinary tract infection with obstructive symptoms or fever that were prolonged and severe, CT or intravenous urography (IVU) is rarely needed. Upper urinary tract abnormalities often develop because of bladder outlet obstruction. These include upward displacement of the terminal parts of the ureters (known as *fish hooking*), dilation of the ureters, and hydronephrosis. If there is pain or elevated serum creatinine, ultrasound may be ordered since it avoids radiation and exposure to IV contrast agents.

Men with suspicious PSA levels may undergo *multiparametric MRI* since it is more sensitive, but less specific, than transrectal biopsy. Biopsies should be restricted to areas discovered during multiparametric MRI, reducing the extent of these procedures as well as diagnosis of prostate cancers that are clinically insignificant. Restricting these biopsies also offers the possibility of increasing diagnosis of prostate cancers that are clinically significant. To decide which type of surgery will be best, and to rule out obstructive strictures, cystoscopy may be preferred.

Treatment

The treatment of BPH includes many different medications; avoiding anticholinergics, opioids, and sympathomimetics; and surgery. For extreme urinary retention, immediate decompression is needed. A standard urinary catheter is passed if possible – if not, a catheter with a **coudé tip** may be successful. If this also is not possible, there may be a requirement for flexible cystoscopy, or the insertion of **filiforms** and **followers**, which progressively open the urinary passageway, performed by a urologist. If transurethral approaches will not work, suprapubic percutaneous decompression of the bladder is performed.

All anticholinergics, opioids, and sympathomimetics (even those present in OTC medications) must be stopped. Infections must be treated with antibiotics. For men with mild to moderate obstructions, alpha-adrenergic blockers may decrease urination problems. These include doxazosin, terazosin, alfuzosin, and tamsulosin. Prostate size may reduce with 5 alpha-reductase inhibitors such as dutasteride or finasteride. These decrease urination problems over months – primarily for patients with prostate glands that are 30 mL or larger. Both classes of drugs, when combined, usually give better results than when either is used alone. If the patient also has concurrent erectile dysfunction, tadalafil may help relieve both conditions when it is taken daily. Many OTC complementary and alternative agents such as *saw palmetto*, are being promoted for successful treatment of BPH, but have not been proven to be any better than a placebo.

When medications fail, or the patient develops recurrent UTIs, urinary calculi, severe bladder dysfunction, or upper urinary tract dilation, surgery is indicated. Transurethral resection of the prostate (TURP) is preferred. For most patients, continence and erectile function are preserved. However, 5–10% of patients experience retrograde ejaculation. Incidence of erectile dysfunction following TURP is in 1–35% of patients. Incidence of incontinence is 1–3%. Use of a **bipolar resectoscope**, which includes the use of saline irrigation, has improved the safety of performing TURP, since it avoids hemolysis and hyponatremia. Approximately 10% of TURP patients require a repeat of the procedure within 10 years due to continued prostate growth. Alternatives to TURP include various laser ablation techniques. Prostates over 75 g usually require open surgery, using a retropubic or suprapubic approach. However, newer techniques such as **holmium laser enucleation of the prostate** (HoLEP) can be performed transurethrally (see Figure 8.1). All of these surgeries require post-operative catheter drainage over 1–7 days.

Alternative treatments include **electrovaporization**, microwave thermotherapy, laser therapies, high-intensity focused ultrasonography, radiofrequency vaporization, transurethral needle ablation, pressurized heated water injection therapy, steam injection therapy, urethral life, and intraurethral stents. Determination of which technique to use is not firmly established. However, since microwave thermotherapy and radiofrequency procedures can be done in a physician's office without general or regional anesthesia, they are becoming more popular. Their ability to change the natural course of BPH over time is still being studied.

Prevention and Early Detection

There is no actual prevention for BPH. The gland will continue to grow in some men. For early detection, men should monitor for changes in urination that include dribbling, difficult beginning urination, excessive urination, waking up several times per night to urinate, a weak urine stream, or urination that stops and starts. Immediate medical attention must be sought if a man cannot urinate at all, feels extreme pain or discomfort in the lower abdomen, finds blood in the urine, repeatedly needs to urinate immediately, experiences pain while urinating, or if fever or chills develop in relation to any of these other factors.

Prognosis

The prognosis for BPH is generally excellent. Treatment is not even always needed, but can help control symptoms and prevent complications. As long as instructions of the physician are followed, BPH is usually managed quite well and does not seriously compromise activities of daily living.

Significant Point

In younger men, the prostate gland is about the size of the walnut, but it increases in size with aging. Enlargement of the gland squeezes the urethra, making it more difficult to urinate. BPH is common after age 50, though treatment is often not required. When symptoms become significant or cause infections, treatments include medications and various types of surgery.

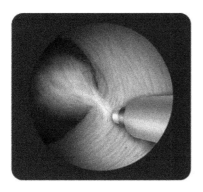

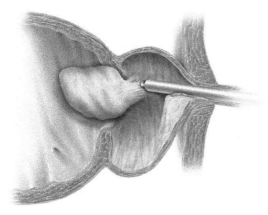

Figure 8.1 Holmium laser enucleation of the prostate (HoLEP) showing (a) the laser close to the prostate; (b) a lateral view. *Source*: Peter Gilling et al. (2007) / with permission of John Wiley & Sons, Inc.

Clinical Case

1. How does the prostate gland change in weight with aging?
2. What is the prevalence and incidence of benign BPH in the United States and globally?
3. As performed in this clinical case, what is TURP and why is it used?

A 75-year-old man sees his physician because of the need to urinate almost every hour due to a feeling of incomplete bladder emptying. He also sometimes has to strain to urinate. A DRE is performed, and the patient's prostate gland is smooth, non-tender, and does not have any nodules. The PSA is normal and there are no indications of prostate cancer.

After completing a questionnaire about his symptoms, the patient is diagnosed with BPH. Urinalysis reveals no evidence of infection or hematuria. The patient's post-void residual urine is low. The drug terazosin is prescribed, to relax the prostatic smooth muscle and allow for opening of the prostatic urethra. There is a gradual improvement in the patient's condition. A urologist determines that a TURP would be effective in relieving the prostatic obstruction. The surgery is performed with no difficulties, and the patient's condition improves dramatically.

Answers:

1. **The average weight of the prostate gland is 25–30 g between ages 40 and**

49, and 40 g between ages 50 and 49, as well as 45 g after age 60. If the gland becomes heavier than these weights during their specific age ranges, BPH may be developing.

2. **The prevalence of BPH in men between 40 and 74 years is 19% of the American male population. The incidence of BPH increases greatly with age, and every year, there are more than 27 million men over age 50, affected. Globally, prevalence is 2.7% of men aged 45–49, but 24% by age 80. Incidence rates are 3 out of every 1,000 men aged 45–49, and 38 cases per 1,000 men aged 75–79 years.**

3. **Transurethral resection of the prostate is the preferred surgery for relieving prostatic obstruction. For most patients, continence and erectile function are preserved. About 10% of TURP patients require a repeat of the procedure within 10 years due to continued prostate growth.**

Prostate Cancer

Adenocarcinoma of the prostate is the most common type of prostate cancer in men in the United States. The disease is the second leading cause of cancer death, after lung cancer. Ninety-five percent of prostate cancers are adenocarcinomas, and the remaining types are transitional cell carcinoma, squamous cell carcinoma, sarcoma, and ductal carcinoma.

Epidemiology

Over 240,000 men are diagnosed with prostate cancer every year in the United States. There is a 1-in-7-lifetime risk of developing it, and a 1-in-38 risk of dying from the disease. Obviously, most men with prostate cancer do not die from the disease. According to the American Cancer Society, the estimated incidence of new cases of prostate cancer in 2021 is 248,530, with an estimated 34,130 deaths. The average age at diagnosis is 66. African American men have the most cases of prostate cancer, as well as higher rates of death from the disease.

Globally, there were 1,414,259 new cases of prostate cancer in 2020, with 375,304 deaths from the disease. This means that prostate cancer made up 7.3% of all cases of cancer, and the deaths from prostate cancer made up 3.8% of all cancer deaths. The highest number of cases occurred in Northern America, Western and Northern Europe, and the Caribbean. The lowest rates were found in South-Central Asia, Northern Africa, and Southeastern and Eastern Asia. However, the highest number of deaths occurred in Barbados, Trinidad and Tobago, Cuba, South Africa, Lithuania, Estonia, and Latvia. The lowest death rates occurred in Thailand and Turkmenistan. Figure 8.2 illustrates areas of the world with the highest rates of prostate cancer.

Etiology and Risk Factors

The exact cause of prostate cancer is unknown, but it is believed to be hormone-related. Inherited gene changes may implicate in about 10% of cases. The mutated genes that have been linked to hereditary prostate cancer. Risk factors for prostate cancer combine the patient's age, family history, race, and factors such as diet and smoking. Family history of prostate cancer increases the risks, which almost doubles when a man has any affected family member, and almost triples if a brother has prostate cancer. While smoking plays a role in prostate cancer, it is not as significant as in lung cancer. There is a link between smoking at the time of diagnosis and poorer outcomes, including death. Smoking is also related to more aggressive prostate cancers, plus a higher risk of recurrence. Another risk factor is age, over 50 years.

Clinical Manifestations

Prostate cancer is usually of slow progression, and does not often cause symptoms until it has

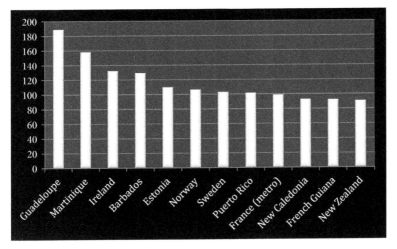

Figure 8.2 Areas of the world with the highest rates of prostate cancer (number of cases per 100,000 population).

become advanced. Hematuria, hesitancy, straining, weak or intermittent urine stream, a feeling of incomplete emptying, and terminal dribbling may occur. Other manifestation includes anorexia, weight loss, bone pain, or neurologic deficits from spinal compression (with metastasis). Prostate cancer commonly metastasizes to the bones – usually the pelvis, ribs, and vertebral bodies, causing bone pain, pathologic fractures, or spinal cord compression (see Figure 8.3).

Pathology

Under the microscope, prostate cancer is evaluated and graded by using the *Gleason score*, a number that indicates the aggressiveness of the disease. This is based on the structural pattern of the cancer cells in the biopsied tissues. Today, the *Gleason scoring system* has been somewhat modified, using five grades. It assigns the cellular patterns a grade of one through five, with five being the highest risk. However, due to the newness of this grading system change, sometimes the classic Gleason scoring is also reported, in which two different malignant patterns are given a score, and then the scores are added together, with 10 being the highest score possible. For example, a patient could have a classic Gleason score of 4 + 3 = 7, as well as a new

Gleason score of "Grade 2." A higher Gleason grade plus increased PSA levels and a more advanced stage of the tumor are linked to higher numbers of prostate cancer deaths. The pathological grading is broken down further as follows:

- High risk – PSA higher than 20 ng/mL, or a Gleason score of 8–10, or clinical stage of T2c
- Intermediate risk – PSA between 10 and 20 ng/mL, or a Gleason score of 7, or clinical stage T2b without qualifying for "high risk"
- Low risk – PSA less than 10 ng/mL, and a Gleason score of 6 or less, and clinical stage T1c or T2a

---

Significant Point

To better understand the new scoring system for prostate cancer, which has been adopted by the World Health Organization, the new "grade groups" are compared here with the traditional Gleason scores: Grade group 1 = Gleason 3 + 3; Grade group 2 = Gleason 3 + 4; Grade group 3 = Gleason 4 + 3; Grade group 4 = Gleason 8; and Grade group 5 = Gleason 9 and 10.

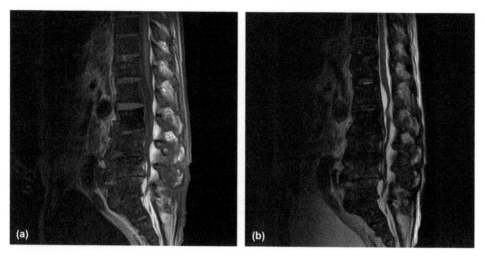

Figure 8.3 (a) Contrast-enhanced MRI; (b) MRI without contrast, showing multiple low-intensity spinal metastases from prostate cancer. *Source*: Figure 02 from Ogushi et al. (2018).

Diagnosis

Prostate cancer may be asymptomatic at the time of diagnosis. The early detection include DRE and the PSA test. Age, race, and family history need to be considered when interpreting PSA results. However, new diagnostic methods include the **Prostate Health Index** and the *4Kscore* (both blood tests), as well as the *PCA3*, a urine test. According to the American Urological Association, screening for PSA is not recommended in men under age 40, and routine screening for those 40–45 at average risk is also not recommended. For men 55–69, deciding to have PSA screening is based on benefits versus risks of screening and treatment. Shared decision-making between the patient and physician is recommended, based on the values and preferences of the patient. A routine screening interval of two years or more may be preferred over annual screening. This two-year screening offers most of the benefits and reduces false positive and overdiagnosis of the disease. Routine PSA screening is not recommended for any man over 70, or for anyone with a life expectancy of less than 10–15 years.

A prostate biopsy is usually recommended based on higher patient risk factors, the DRE, and the PSA results. The procedure is performed with ultrasound guidance, and often, local anesthesia and antibiotics. Patients usually need to stop taking any anticoagulants before the biopsy. The patient lies on his side as a urologist passes the ultrasound probe into the rectum and injects lidocaine into the nerves around the prostate gland. A hollow core needle is directed into the prostate to acquire about 12 biopsy cores – 6 from each side of the gland – in the peripheral zone, which is the most likely area for cancer to develop. The entire procedure takes only about 10 minutes, and the patient is able to drive himself to and from the urology office. Sometimes, there is minor bleeding from the rectum or blood in the urine, which resolves soon. A pathologist then analyzes the biopsied cores. The patient is instructed to report any fever or signs of infection after the biopsy.

The 12-core biopsy method can miss clinically significant prostate cancer in 20–30% of cases. A re-biopsy is sometimes ordered, with sampling of other areas of the prostate gland. The use of MRI can be used to identify suspicious areas, guiding the re-biopsy. When prostate cancer is diagnosed, other imaging test may be ordered by the urologist to ensure that the cancer has not spread outward to other body structures. These options are summarized in Table 8.1.

Table 8.1 Imaging options to assess spread of prostate cancer.

Imaging	
Bone scan	Performed if the PSA is higher than 20, clinical stage is T3 or T4, Gleason score is 8 or higher, serum alkaline phosphatase is elevated, or new bone pain suggests metastatic disease
Pelvic CT or MRI	Searches for cancer extension in the form of enlarged lymph nodes or other organ spread, which is less common than prostate cancer spreading to the bones; MRI is becoming very accurate for diagnosis and better tumor staging

The "TNM" system is used to stage prostate cancers. This is further summarized as follows:

- T1a – prostate cancer is found incidentally during *TURP*; it is present in no more than 5% of the tissues
- T1b – prostate cancer is found during TURP and present in more than 5% of the tissues
- T1c – prostate cancer is found by needle biopsy performed because of increased PSA
- T2a – prostate cancer is palpable on DRE in half or less of the left or right side of the gland
- T2b – prostate cancer on DRE is more than half of the left or right side of the gland
- T2c – prostate cancer on DRE is found in both sides of the gland
- T3a – prostate cancer extends outside of the gland but not to the seminal vesicles
- T3b – prostate cancer has spread to the seminal vesicles
- T4 – prostate cancer has grown into tissues next to the gland, besides the seminal vesicles, including the urethral sphincter, rectum, bladder, and/or wall of the pelvis
- N0 – no positive regional lymph nodes
- N1 – metastasis in regional lymph nodes
- M0 – no distant metastasis
- M1a – metastasis to non-regional lymph nodes
- M1b – metastasis to bones
- M1c – metastasis to other sites, with or without the bones being affected

Treatment

When prostate cancer is contained within the capsule of the gland, treatment options include **active surveillance**, surgery to remove the entire prostate gland and its capsule, radiation therapy, cryotherapy, and hormonal therapy. Active surveillance is used more often when the patient is of low risk, and allows for other interventions if the tumor progresses. Urologists prefer it when the patient's "low risk" consists of the following:

- PSA 10 ng/mL or lower
- Gleason score of 6 or less
- Clinical stage of T2a or lower
- Less than three positive biopsy cores
- Less than 50% cancer in each biopsy core

The *Prostate Cancer Intervention versus Observation Trial* (PIVOT) revealed that for men with low to intermediate risks, there were no differences in death rates from prostate cancer compared with death from any cause within 12 years of active surveillance. In active surveillance, the patient undergoes serial DRE, serum PSA tests, and consideration of repeat MRI-guided prostate biopsies every one to three years. When surgery is indicated, known as *radical prostatectomy*, the entire prostate gland and seminal vesicles are removed, often with removal of the local pelvic lymph nodes. In the open retropubic radical prostatectomy, an incision is made below the navel. After the prostate gland is resected, the neck of the bladder is reconnected to the urethra. The patient usually remains in the hospital for two to four days. A **Foley catheter** is left to drain the bladder for 1–2 weeks so that the new connection between bladder and urethra can heal.

Today, at least in the United States, over 80% of radical prostatectomies are performed laparoscopically, using **robotic surgery** techniques (see Figure 8.4). The patient's abdomen is filled with carbon dioxide gas. Robotic arms, instruments, and a camera are passed through five small incisions surrounded by a **port cannula**. Robotic-assisted surgery has resulted in shorter hospitalizations, by one to two days, and less overall blood loss during surgery. The catheter is still required as the patient heals. However, robotic surgery has not shown any improved cancer recurrence rates or mortality rates. Complications after traditional or robotic surgery include the need for blood transfusions, pain, infection, and blood clot formation in the legs, but these are standard complications of many other types of surgery. Some men experience prostate cancer surgery specific complications, which include erectile dysfunction and urinary incontinence (which is usually stress-induced, related to coughing, physical exertion, or sneezing). The incontinence is usually worse soon after surgery when the catheter is removed, but improves over six months to one year. If the incontinence persists beyond this, an artificial urinary sphincter can be put in place. For erectile dysfunction, the patient's age, pre-surgical erection function, and surrounding nerve damage must be assessed before any treatments can occur.

External beam radiation therapy (EBRT) can be delivered to the prostate and pelvis instead of surgery, and is used for low-risk patients, or along with hormone therapy androgen deprivation therapy (ADT), if the patient is of intermediate or high risk. When CT is used for guidance, the radiation can be precisely

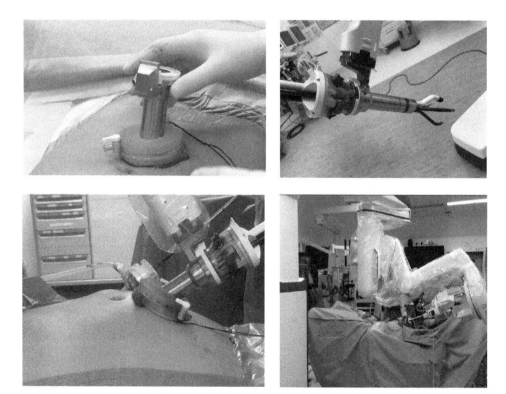

Figure 8.4 Robotic laparoscopic radical prostatectomy procedure. (a) Port cannula covering incisions; (b) the robotic arms, instruments, and camera; (c) placement of the robotic components through the port cannula; (d) the position of the patient during the robotic surgery. *Source*: Figure 02 from Ng et al. (2019).

directed toward the prostate gland. The standard of care is now **Conformal Radiation Therapy**, in which the radiation beam assumes the shape of the gland. This reduces the dose of radiation that is delivered to other nearby organs, resulting in fewer complications. In most cases, up to 50 separate daily doses of radiation are performed, 5 days per week. **Gamma radiation** is usually used, though other options include proton or neutron beam radiation, but they are more expensive and not proven to be significantly better. Adverse effects and complications of radiation therapy include erection abnormalities, urinary frequency, urgency, and burning upon urination. However, for high-risk patients, better outcomes occur when ADT is added, from 6 to 24 months, based on the actual level of risk. **Brachytherapy** delivers radiation via small radioactive seeds inserted directly into the prostate gland with ultrasound guidance. It can be a monotherapy if the patient is of low or intermediate risk, or can be combined with external beam radiation for higher-risk patients. Brachytherapy is usually done as an outpatient procedure. If the patient previously had a TURP procedure for benign prostate enlargement, he usually will not be given brachytherapy due to increased rates of urinary complications. If brachytherapy is performed, urinary frequency and burning upon urination are common, but resolve eventually. Sometimes, the patient requires a catheter being left in place for a while to urinate. Erectile dysfunction is less common with brachytherapy.

When the patient is of low or intermediate risk, but is a poor candidate for surgery or radiation, cryotherapy may be performed. Probes are placed in the prostate gland, with ultrasound guidance. Argon gas is pumped into the probes and the nearby tissue temperature lowers to about −40°C. A ball of ice is therefore created, and cell death begins immediately, continuing over time. A catheter is placed through the urethra to the bladder, which allows for warming, preventing urethral damage. The freezing procedure is repeated again, maximizing cancer cell destruction. If urethral damage occurs even with the warming catheter, this may cause urinary retention, incontinence, pain, and the formation of fistulas – abnormal connections between the urethra and rectum. However, fistulas develop in less than 1% of cases. Most men do report some degree of erectile dysfunction after cryotherapy. If the prostate is large, the patient is not a good candidate for cryotherapy because it will be difficult to achieve uniform freezing of all prostate tissue. Cryotherapy is usually performed on an outpatient basis. Most patients must have a Foley catheter in place for one week after the procedure. If a patient has a life expectancy of less than 10 years, watchful waiting is preferred unless there is symptomatic disease progression.

Prevention and Early Detection

Regarding the prevention of prostate cancer, a 1993 trial began to test the drug called *finasteride*, since this 5-alpha-reductase inhibitor stops the enzyme that converts testosterone into the highly potent *dihydrotestosterone*. Finasteride has long been used to treat BPH since it causes the gland to reduce in size. Since prostate cancer is influenced by testosterone, it was believed that finasteride could stop the disease from developing. The trial lasted for 10 years. Finasteride was shown to reduce the overall relative risk of "low-risk" prostate cancer cases by 25%. This proved that there may be higher-risk cases as well, and the Food and Drug Administration (FDA) refused to approve finasteride as prevention against prostate cancer. A different trial studied a similar drug, *dutasteride*, and the results were similar. Additional preventive trials for vitamin E and selenium also failed, and vitamin E was actually found to increase risks for prostate cancer.

The early detection of prostate cancer requires a DRE and a PSA test. PSA is a serine protease enzyme. It causes the seminal fluid to be liquefied upon ejaculation, which aids in sperm motility, and is secreted by the prostate and found in semen as well as blood. In the 1980s, PSA was first measured quantitatively in the blood, as a tumor marker for prostate cancer. Since then, along with a DRE, it has become the screening test of choice. There is still controversy, however. The United States Preventive Services Task Force argued that a large number of men with asymptomatic prostate cancer found during PSA screening would never develop symptoms. This means they would then have to undergo additional testing and treatment that was unneeded. However, most urologists feel that PSA is useful for detecting prostate cancer in its earliest stages, and the screening has resulted in fewer deaths from the disease. Also, if the PSA changes quickly in velocity over time, this can indicate a more aggressive cancer. The density of the PSA compares it with the volume of the prostate measured at the time of biopsy. DRE is very important since most cancers develop in the peripheral zone – the outside edge of the gland. The physician's gloved and lubricated finger can feel this zone to detect nodular cancer, even if the PSA proves not to be elevated.

Prostate cancer does recur, with high-risk patients most likely to experience this. Higher rates of recurrence are seen when there are positive margins and positive lymph nodes after surgery, if the patient continues to smoke, or if he is obese. After a radical prostatectomy, if the tumor extended beyond the surgical margins or outside the gland, the PSA may never become undetectable, or can increase after surgery. Therefore, the patient may need to be considered for further EBRT. If the PSA was never undetectable, the therapy is called *adjuvant radiation*. If the PSA became undetectable but then increased, the therapy is called **salvage radiation**. If a patient previously had radiation therapy without surgical removal of the gland, the PSA may never become undetectable. Usually, if the PSA increases by 2 ng/mL or more above the lowest recorded level, the patient may be considered for a salvage radical prostatectomy, or salvage cryotherapy. These are technically difficult procedures, linked to higher rates of complications.

If prostate cancer is locally advanced, extending outside the capsule, radical prostatectomy is probably not a good choice. Radiation therapy is likely to be the chosen procedure. When combined with ADT, it can be curative, or at least is able to control cancer progression. For metastatic prostate cancer, ADT is the primary treatment, destroying cancer deposits by removing the effects of testosterone. This usually causes no adverse effects, but bone pain, anemia, kidney obstruction, and fatigue may occur. Stopping testosterone production by the testes can be done via their surgical removal, or by injecting the drugs called *leuprolide, triptorelin,* or *goserelin*. These drugs work by causing the body to make more androgens – known as *testosterone flair*. After the first injection, an oral medication is given that blocks the testosterone receptors, and the flair cannot affect the cancer. The most common oral medication used is *bicalutamide*. Within 1 month, serum testosterone levels are usually less than 50 ng / dL – considered "castration level." If the cancer cells respond to the ADT, tumor burden shrinks, symptoms improve, and the PSA is lowered. While ADT is usually not used as monotherapy for localized disease, it can be used along with radiotherapy, and less often, surgery for more advanced local disease. It is the first-line treatment for metastatic prostate cancer.

Significant adverse effects are related to ADT that intensify the longer that treatment occurs. There may be **gynecomastia**, testicular atrophy, loss of skeletal muscle mass, and weight gain. Most patients develop fatigue, hot flashes, erectile dysfunction, and loss of libido. Over longer periods of time, there may be weakening of the bones, osteoporosis, and cardiac abnormalities. Though ADT controls many cases of advanced and metastatic prostate cancer, the cancer cells can still grow and divide again. This is known as *castration-resistant prostate cancer*. Newer treatment options are then attempted. These include oral medications such as abiraterone and enzalutamide. Immune system therapies to eradicate tumor cells are available. For example, sipuleucel-T is a therapy that uses the patient's own immune cells, which are withdrawn, combined with a medication that stimulates immune action, and then reinjected. External radiation can be directed specifically at metastatic bone lesions to relieve some symptoms. Also, radium 223 can be injected, which targets prostate cancers in bones.

Prognosis

Most cases of localized or regional prostate cancer carry a very good prognosis. For older men, life expectancy may not be very different from age-matched men that do not have prostate cancer – based on age and other concurrent diseases. Long-term localized control, or even a cure, is often possible. The potential for a cure is based on the tumor's grade and stage, even when it is clinically localized. However, without early treatment, high-grade and poorly differentiated tumors have a poor prognosis. Conventional therapies are often not effective against ductal transitional carcinoma, squamous cell carcinoma, or undifferentiated prostate cancer. If the cancer has metastasized, there is no cure. Though some patients live for a long time with prostate cancer, the median life expectancy with metastatic disease is only 1–3 years.

Significant Point

According to the Centers for Disease Control and Prevention (CDC), prostate cancer is one of the types of cancer that is most likely to metastasize to the bones. This occurs in over 60% of patients with advanced prostate cancer. From one 2017 study, it was found that 35% of these patients have a 1-year survival rate, 12% have a 3-year survival rate, and only 6% have a 5-year survival rate.

Clinical Case

1. What are the lifetime risks of developing prostate cancer?
2. To which areas of the body does prostate cancer most often metastasize?
3. What are the factors of the pathological grading for high-risk, intermediate-risk, and low-risk prostate cancers?

A 57-year-old African American man was referred to a urologist because of increased PSA. His family history was positive for breast cancer, in his mother and one sister. One of his brothers had pancreatic cancer. The patient's DRE was normal, but an MRI of the prostate revealed that the gland was slightly enlarged, with a lesion in the left peripheral zone. It was scored as grade 5, and there were questionable invasions into the left seminal vesicle. A transrectal ultrasound fusion biopsy was performed, showing 4 positive cores out of 12. They were all Gleason Group 3. A whole-body one scan plus CT of the chest, abdomen, and pelvic region were all negative for metastatic disease. Considered treatments included external beam radiation with hormone therapy, external beam radiation plus brachytherapy with hormone therapy, and radical prostatectomy. Since the patient was otherwise healthy, it was decided that external beam radiation plus hormone therapy would be the initial treatment.

Answers:

1. **There is a 1-in-7 lifetime risk of developing prostate cancer, and a 1-in-38 risk of dying from the disease.**
2. **Prostate cancer commonly metastasizes to the bones – usually the pelvis, ribs, and vertebral bodies, causing bone pain, pathologic fractures, or spinal cord compression.**
3. **High-risk prostate cancer: PSA higher than 20 nanograms per mL, or a**

Gleason score of 8 to 10, or clinical stage of T2c. Intermediate-risk: PSA between 10 and 20 ng/mL, or a Gleason score of 7, or clinical stage T2b without qualifying for "high risk." Low risk: PSA less than 10 ng/mL, and a Gleason score of 6 or less, and clinical stage T1c or T2a.

Testicular Cancer

Testicular cancer is the most common in men between 15 and 35 years of age. They are divided into nonseminomas and seminomas. Nonseminomas are usually more aggressive than seminomas. Seminomas make up 40–45% of all germ cell tumors. Nonseminomas can be differentiated from seminomas in that they contain undifferentiated embryonic stem cells. The subcategories of nonseminomas include: embryonal carcinomas, yolk sac carcinomas, and choriocarcinomas. *Embryonal carcinomas* usually occur in 20–30-year-old men, and make up 87% of nonseminomas. *Yolk sac carcinomas* are most common in infants and children below three years of age, in which there is a very good prognosis; however, yolk sac carcinomas in adults can be life-threatening. *Choriocarcinomas* are extremely rare tumors that are highly aggressive; they make up less than 1% of all testicular tumors; choriocarcinomas do not cause testicular enlargement, but can be palpated as nodules; the two cell types found in choriocarcinomas include *cytotrophoblasts* and *syncytiotrophoblasts*.

Epidemiology

Testicular seminomas account for 1–3% of all male malignancies in Western populations, and are the most common non- hematologic malignancy in males between 15 and 35 years of age. Incidence of seminomas is increasing in the United States, as well as throughout the world.

Seminomas are the most common type of germ cell tumors in men between ages 40 and 50. All types of germ cell tumors are very rare after the age of 50. Seminomas occur 6–10 times more often in Caucasians than in any other racial group, across men of all ages. For unknown reasons, seminomas occur mostly in people of a high socioeconomic status.

Though statistics throughout the world are difficult to ascertain, annual incidence of testicular seminomas is 1 of every 62,000 men, accounting for 40% of testicular cancer cases. Several European countries have the highest number of cases of testicular cancer. These countries include Denmark, Norway, Germany, Switzerland, and the Czech Republic. It is also more common in Australia. Incidence is increasing mostly in younger men. As in the United States, Caucasian men are most often affected, and the incidence is rising.

Nonseminomas are the most prevalent testicular malignancy, accounting for about 60% of all cases. These tumors are most common in younger men – those between 15 and 35 years of age, though there is a peak in incidence in the late teens to 20s. Nonseminomas, like seminomas, are most common in Caucasians than in any other racial group, doubling in incidence over the past 40 years. The annual increase in cases, within the Caucasian group, is 3–6%. According to a 2017 study, Hispanic American men are showing increases in recent years, and are estimated to surpass Caucasian men in incidence by 2026.

Etiology and Risk Factors

The cause of testicular cancer is unknown, but believed to be from an embryonic germ cell that leads to testicular intraepithelial neoplasia. The most firmly established risk factor for a seminoma is *cryptorchidism*. Personal history of testicular cancer, positive family history for testicular cancer, testicular dysgenesis, Klinefelter syndrome, HIV infections, and belonging to the Caucasian race are other risk factors.

Clinical Manifestations

A painless mass is the most common presenting sign, and tumors are slightly more common in the right testicle. Less often, the patient develops gynecomastia because of hormones from the tumor. Based on metastases, different symptoms may be present. A chronic hydrocele may be discovered, causing the testicle to feel "heavy."

Pathology

Testicular seminomas arise from germ cell neoplasia in situ (GCNIS) cells that are believed to form from delayed maturation of primordial germ cells or gonocytes, with **polyploidization**. This results in transformed germ cells. This continues after puberty to develop into seminomas. Most likely, GCNIS cells evolve into intratubular seminomas and then invasive seminomas. The tumors are well-demarcated, homogeneous, and solid cream or gray in color. There is surface nodularity and lobulation. Multiple nodules may be present. Necrosis or hemorrhage is usually only minimal. With regression, only a scar may be seen. The tumors are usually confined to the testis, in 90% of cases.

Nonseminomas are pathologically divided into the previously discussed subtypes. They tend to be more heterogeneous than seminomas and often have cystic areas or calcifications. Nonseminomas often invade the tunica, but may be quite varied in their actual appearance. They may be variegated due to a mixture of different components. Embryonal carcinomas have solid cellular sheets, tubular papillary architecture, primitive cells with indistinct borders, and significant nuclear atypia. Choriocarcinomas may have areas of hemorrhage and necrosis, plus a plexiform admixture of syncytiotrophoblasts, cytotrophoblasts, and intermediate trophoblasts. Yolk sac carcinomas may be focally cystic, with mucinous cut surfaces. They may have varied histologic patterns, with a microcystic/reticular pattern being most common. The stroma is myxoid, with Schiller–Duval bodies, and both extracellular and intracellular hyaline globules. All nonseminomas develop when a GCNIS or a seminoma cell becomes reprogrammed. Testicular cancer metastasizes beyond the retroperitoneal lymph nodes, and reaches the liver, lungs, bones, and brain.

Diagnosis

Diagnosis of a seminoma is usually confirmed by ultrasound. Measurement of tumor markers such as alpha-fetoprotein (AFP), **beta human chorionic gonadotropin** (ß-hCG), and lactate dehydrogenase (LDH) are useful when the tumor is very small. Classical seminomas do not secrete AFP. Men with raised levels of AFP are diagnosed with a nonseminoma. Following radical orchiectomy, staging is assigned by histopathological characteristics of the tumor. Nonseminomas must be excluded for an accurate diagnosis.

The diagnosis of nonseminomas is highly related to their secretion of tumor markers, since 85% secrete at least one tumor marker. Since seminomas and the choriocarcinoma subtype of nonseminomas do not secrete AFP, its presence helps to narrow down the diagnosis of a nonseminoma to embryonal carcinoma, yolk sac carcinoma, or a benign teratoma. Diagnosis of testicular choriocarcinomas is aided by finding a heterogeneous appearance, cystic components, and calcifications during imaging studies.

Treatment

The initial treatment is orchiectomy. For the radical orchiectomy surgery, the testicle and spermatic cord are removed through an inguinal incision, soon after the mass is confirmed. The procedure is curative for many patients. The procedure is usually done in an outpatient setting. A scrotal incision is not used because it can affect predictable lymphatic spread of testicular tumors. The inguinal incision allows the entire spermatic cord to also be removed with the testicle

(Figure 8.5). About 85% of seminomas managed by active surveillance after orchiectomy will not relapse. If relapse occurs, most happen in the first year. Increased risk of relapse is with tumors larger than 4 cm or with **rete testis** invasion. Relapse occurs 97% of the time in the high iliac or retroperitoneal lymph nodes. Metastasis is rare, but can reach the lungs, liver, bones, and central nervous system. Seminomas, unlike nonseminomas, are very sensitive to radiation. Therefore, external beam radiotherapy (EBRT) is very successful for treatment of testicular cancer. Adverse effects of EBRT include fatigue, bone marrow suppression, and nausea. There can be long-term toxicities, including bowel inflammation, infertility, and secondary malignancies. In young patients with a longer life expectancy, EBRT greatly increases risks for other cancers, as well as heart disease, later in life.

Stage I seminomas can be treated with single-agent carboplatin, in one or two cycles. Higher stages require bleomycin plus etoposide and cisplatin in three or four cycles based on risk classification. For patients with reduced lung capacity, emphysema, or for heavy smokers, ifosfamide is used instead of bleomycin – primarily when there is already lung damage. Long-term adverse effects of chemotherapy include interstitial pneumonitis, pulmonary fibrosis, atherosclerosis, bone marrow suppression, infertility, heart disease, and secondary cancers.

Cisplatin-based chemotherapy has greatly improved prognosis for testicular cancers. Because of it, increased use of active surveillance has proven to be effective since relapses are usually effectively cured with the chemotherapy. For clinical stage I tumors, chemotherapy reduces relapses to less than 5% of cases. For stage II diseases, chemotherapy can treat retroperitoneal lymph nodes successfully. Chemotherapy is also standard for patients with extensive lymph node involvement or stage III diseases.

Prevention and Early Detection

There are no proven methods of preventing testicular cancer. However, there are generalized things that can be done to improve overall

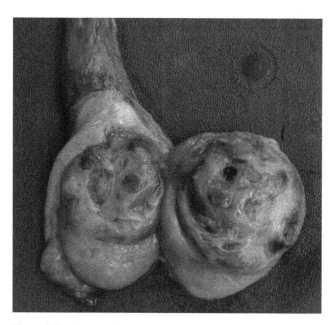

Figure 8.5 A resected testicle that has been cut partially through (bivalved), showing a mixed nonseminoma replacing most of the testicular parenchyma. *Source*: Stein and Luebbers [48]. with permission of John Wiley & Sons.

health and strengthen the immune system. These include: reducing exposure to chemical toxins, eating a cancer-fighting diet, engaging in regular exercise, reducing stress, detoxifying and protecting the liver, and taking nutritional supplements that include turmeric, **boswellia**, and medicinal mushrooms. Early detection of testicular cancer is extremely important in better treatment outcomes. Any signs of swelling, lumps, pain, or pressure should be described to a physician for evaluation. There are no known methods of preventing for testicular tumors. Regular monthly self-examination at age 15 may assist early diagnosis of a mass in the testis. Earlier detection may help improve outlook.

Prognosis

Prognosis has improved greatly over the past decades because of much-improved treatment options. Most patients with testicular cancer are cured. The five-year survival rate is more than 95% for seminomas localized to the testis. Relapse rates at five years are based on risk factors such as invasion of the rete testis, and a tumor size larger than 4 cm. However, the relapse rate is only 12% in patients without risk factors. The prognosis of nonseminomas is varied, based on the biological behavior of the individual tumor subtype. Tumor markers are highly important in assessing outlook. If tumor markers are low, there is a non-mediastinal location of the primary tumor, and there are no non-pulmonary metastases, prognosis is good after orchiectomy and chemotherapy. If the tumor markers are in the intermediate range, there is a non-mediastinal location of the primary tumor, and there are no non-pulmonary metastases, prognosis is intermediate after chemotherapy, and sometimes after adjuvant surgery. However, when tumor markers are high, the primary tumor is within the mediastinum, and there are non-pulmonary metastases present, the prognosis is poor. Aggressive chemotherapy is usually the only treatment method that may improve this prognosis.

Clinical Case

1. What are the basic differences between testicular seminomas and nonseminomas?
2. What are the signs and symptoms of testicular cancer?
3. What usually confirms diagnosis of testicular seminomas?

A 56-year-old man presented with right testicular pain and swelling. Physical examination revealed an enlarged and rigid right testicle that was tender when palpated. Ultrasound revealed a hypoechoic heterogeneous well-circumscribed lesion, with nodularity and vascularity. A CT scan of the chest, abdomen, and pelvis revealed multiple enlarged retroperitoneal, para-aortic, and aortocaval lymphadenopathies. Tumor marker testing revealed slightly elevated ß-hCG and significantly increased LDH. A right radical inguinal orchiectomy was performed. Diagnosis was of a classic seminoma, stage pT2, with lymphovascular invasion and negative spermatic cord margins. The staging was IIB, and the patient was started on cytotoxic chemotherapy, with one cycle of bleomycin – etoposide – cisplatin, followed by three cycles of etoposide – cisplatin, since the patient experienced pulmonary toxicity from the bleomycin. The patient was at risk for pulmonary complications because he was still smoking cigarettes. The patient responded well, and there were significant shrinkages of the lymph nodes. Over two years of follow-up, there has been no recurrence.

Answers:

1. **Testicular seminomas are usually less aggressive than nonseminomas. Seminomas make up 40% of all cases. Nonseminomas can be differentiated from seminomas in that they contain undifferentiated embryonic stem cells.**

2. **A painless mass is the most common presenting sign, and tumors are slightly more common in the right testicle. Less often, the patient develops gynecomastia because of hormones from the tumor. Based on metastases, different symptoms may be present. A chronic hydrocele may be discovered, causing the testicle to feel "heavy."**

3. **Diagnosis of a seminoma is usually confirmed by ultrasound. Measurement of tumor markers such as AFP, beta human chorionic gonadotropin (ß-hCG), and lactate dehydrogenase (LDH) are useful when the tumor is very small.**

Significant Point

Stage I nonseminomas are limited to the testis and are curable in over 95% of cases. For adults with this form of testicular cancer, surgical orchiectomy and retroperitoneal lymph node dissection are considered to be the standard treatments. Nearly all patients that relapse after orchiectomy can be cured with combination chemotherapy, so retroperitoneal lymph node dissection is sometimes not needed.

Clinical Case

1. How is a testicular nonseminoma different from a seminoma, on a cellular basis?
2. How prevalent are nonseminomas among various testicular malignancies?
3. What is the prognosis for testicular nonseminomas?

A 46-year-old hypertensive man discovered a mass in his left testicle, and after examination by his physician, was sent to a urologist for further evaluation. The urologist ordered an ultrasound, but the patient became very anxious and had no interaction for four months. He noticed his vision was becoming much worse very quickly, and an ophthalmologist assessed his condition, finding retinal hemorrhages and a blood pressure of 220/110 mm Hg. The patient was hospitalized. He had anemia, hypercalcemia, and acute renal failure. The left testicular mass had enlarged further. Several CT scans showed the mass to be about 15 cm in diameter, and there was a retroperitoneal mass obstructing the left kidney, causing hydronephrosis. Additionally, there was a large, calcified pelvic mass. A chest CT showed mediastinal adenopathy and a right upper lung lobe nodule. The hydronephrosis was treated successfully. Tumor markers revealed increased levels of LDH, AFP, and ß-hCG. The retroperitoneal mass was found to be a malignant seminoma. There was no metastasis of the seminoma. Further testing confirmed the testicular mass to be a nonseminoma, of intermediate risk. Cisplatin-based chemotherapy was initiated, with etoposide and cisplatin. Significant hydration was used to offset any nephrotoxicity from the cisplatin. Over time, the treatments were successful, and the patient was released, followed-up for one year with no recurrence.

Answers:

1. **Nonseminomas can be differentiated from seminomas in that they contain undifferentiated embryonic stem cells. Subcategories of nonseminomas include: embryonal carcinomas, yolk sac carcinomas, and choriocarcinomas.**

2. **Nonseminomas are the most prevalent testicular malignancy, accounting for about 60% of all cases.**

3. **The prognosis of nonseminomas is varied, based on the biological behavior of the individual tumor subtype. Tumor markers are highly important in assessing outlook. If they are low, there is a non-mediastinal location of the primary tumor, and there are no non-pulmonary metastases, prognosis is good after orchiectomy and chemotherapy. As in this case, however, if intermediate, with a non-mediastinal location of the primary tumor, and no non-pulmonary metastases, prognosis is likewise intermediate after chemotherapy, and sometimes after adjuvant surgery.**

Penile Cancer

Penile cancer is a rare malignancy of the penis genesrally occurring in uncircumcised men and associated with genital herpesvirus infection and poor hygiene. There are several types, which include *basal cell carcinoma, melanoma, sarcoma*, and *adenocarcinoma*. Basal cell carcinoma of the penis accounts for less than 0.03% of all basal cell carcinomas, with less than 25 cases ever reported, worldwide. An even smaller number of penile cancers are melanomas. There have been only 11 cases ever reported of sarcoma of the connective tissues and smooth muscles of the penis.

Epidemiology

Carcinoma of the penis is very rare in the United States. It makes up less than 1% of all cancers in men. Rates of penile cancer are much less in men that are circumcised, since there is a better ability to maintain genital hygiene. Only about 1 in 100,000 American men are affected. There are about 1,600 cases and 350 deaths annually. About 80% of cases are diagnosed in men over age 55 and about 66% are diagnosed in those over age 65. Men circumcised at birth have less than 50% the chance of developing carcinoma of the penis compared with uncircumcised men. There is no racial or ethnic preference.

Globally, it is also rare, accounting for 0.2% of all cancers and 0.1% of cancer deaths in men. However, in Africa and South America, penile cancer accounts for as much as 10% of all cancers. Incidence is generally the same throughout the world, with no geographical preferences, though carcinoma of the penis is slightly more common in parts of Asia, Africa, and South America.

Etiology and Risk Factors

Carcinoma of the penis is potentially caused by sexually transmitted infections with the human papillomavirus (HPV), chronic inflammation due to tropical or desert climates, and psoriasis that is treated with *psoralen* plus ultraviolet light. Penile cancer is more common in men that have phimosis or AIDS.

Poor immunity, HPV infection, and high-risk sexual practices are implicated, with older men most often affected. Other factors in the development of squamous cell carcinoma of the penis include organ transplantation, HIV/AIDS infection, immunosuppressant drugs, smoking tobacco products, and chronic ulcerative **lichen planus**.

Clinical Manifestations

The development of carcinoma of the penis includes precancerous signs such as leukoplakia. Genital warts from HPV may be implicated in the precancerous lesions. There may be reddened and inflamed areas of Paget's disease, and soft, red, ulcerative masses of **erythroplasia of Queyrat**. Concurrent, invasive penile carcinoma may accompany leukoplakia or erythroplasia of Queyrat. These lesions usually involve the glans. There can also be large, scaly, and invasive growths of **Buschke–Lowenstein tumor**; red and encrusted plaques of **Bowen's disease**, and in situ carcinoma – usually of the penile shaft. Late signs of penile cancer include pain and bleeding (see Figure 8.6). Also, metastatic solid tumors can spread to the penis from the bladder, kidneys, prostate, or rectum.

Pathology

About 95% of cases are *squamous cell carcinoma*. It affects the skin or mucosal membranes, and when it spreads, the inguinal lymph nodes are usually affected. Once carcinoma of the penis has become locally invasive, there is a significant change of it spreading to local lymph nodes, and then metastasizing. Before the disease develops, there are signs of premalignant cancer or epidermal cancer in situ.

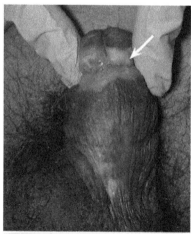

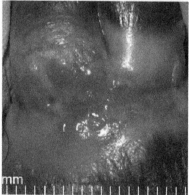

Figure 8.6 Penile squamous cell carcinoma in late stages. *Source*: Kravvas et al. (2017). With permission of John Wiley & Sons, Inc.

Diagnosis

After examination, biopsy documents the locations, sizes, and fixations of the lesions are required. Ultrasound, CT, or MRI assesses the extent of cancer spread. A fine-needle aspiration of lymphatic tissue confirms any regional adenopathy. Before diagnosis, about 30% of penile cancers have already reached the lymph nodes. Though distant metastasis occurs in less than 10% of patients, it can reach the lungs, liver, bones, or brain. Staging of carcinoma of the penis is as follows:

- Stage 0 – carcinoma in situ; the cancer is only in the top layer of the skin, has not spread to nearby lymph nodes; and has no distant metastasis
- Stage I – the cancer has grown into tissue below the top skin layer, but has not spread to nearby blood vessels, lymph vessels, or nerves; it has not spread to nearby lymph nodes; and has no distant metastasis
- Stage IIA – the cancer has grown into tissue below the top skin layer, into nearby blood vessels, lymph vessels, or nerves, and/or it is considered high grade (3); it has not spread to nearby lymph nodes; and has no distant metastasis, OR: the cancer has grown into the corpus spongiosum, but has not spread to nearby lymph nodes; and has no distant metastasis
- Stage IIB – the cancer has grown into the corpus cavernosum, but has not spread to nearby lymph nodes; and has no distant metastasis
- Stage IIIA – the cancer has grown into tissue below the top skin layer and may have grown into the corpus spongiosum, cavernosum, or both; it has spread to one or two nearby inguinal lymph nodes on the same side of the body; and has no distant metastasis
- Stage IIIB – the cancer has grown into tissue below the top skin layer and may have grown into the corpus spongiosum, cavernosum, or both; it has spread to three or more nearby inguinal lymph nodes on the same side of the body, or to inguinal lymph nodes on both sides of the body; and has no distant metastasis

- Stage IV – the cancer has grown into the scrotum, prostate, or pubic bone, and may or may not have spread to nearby lymph nodes; and has no distant metastasis, OR: the cancer may or may not have grown into deeper layers of the penis or nearby structures, has spread to nearby lymph nodes in the pelvis, or has grown outside of a lymph node into surrounding tissue; and has no distant metastasis, OR: the cancer may or may not have grown into deeper layers of the penis or nearby structures, may or may not have spread to nearby lymph nodes, but has definitely metastasized to distant sites

Treatment

Early squamous cell carcinomas and premalignant epidermal lesions are often ignored, even though they can be easily treated. Treatment delays occur because of embarrassment, denial, fear, guilt, ignorance, or failure to detect lesions under a phimotic foreskin. If detected early, carcinoma of the penis is treated by local surgical excision, radiation, laser surgery, or cryosurgery. All of these methods can be curative. If the cancer has metastasized, it may not be curable, but chemotherapy can be used to place it into remission and control the disease. *Penile preserving therapy* is used to reduce physical and psychological morbidities, plus long-term problems related to treatment. Locally advanced, regionally spread, and metastasized disease will require therapy throughout the patient's lifetime. If a penile cancerous tissue is surgically removed, this can cause decreased sexual performance ability. Rarely, it causes decreased urinary stream and problems emptying the bladder. Radiotherapy is often used preoperatively and postoperatively. In some cases, chemotherapy (paclitaxel, ifosfamide, cisplatin) is indicated.

Prevention and Early Detection

The prevention of carcinoma of the penis is easily accessible, via the HPV vaccination, which is available now for young boys. This vaccine can greatly decrease the incidence of penile cancer. Stopping the smoking of tobacco products and preventing sexually transmitted infections, plus early detection of penile cancer by regular self-examinations are also essential.

Prognosis

For localized penile cancer, the five-year relative survival rate is 80%. For regionalized disease, with the cancer having spread to nearby structures or lymph nodes, the five-year relative survival rate is 50%. For distant metastases, such as the lungs, liver, or bones, the five-year relative survival rate is only 9%. The overall combined five-year relative survival rates for all stages are 65%. If untreated, progression of the disease can cause death within two years.

Significant Point

The HPV is detectable in 30–50% of all penile carcinomas. In an uncircumcised man, if the foreskin area is not cleaned regularly, HPV or the HIV can congregate, and may be picked up by immune cells. In the United States, penile cancer is curable in 80–90% of cases. The two general surgeries include partial penectomy, in which enough penile length is maintained to allow for normal urination, or complete removal of the penis, if the disease has become advanced. There is also a plastic surgery procedure that can create a new penis, using muscles from other parts of the body.

Clinical Case

1. When is penile cancer usually diagnosed?
2. Which type of cancer makes up the majority of cases of penile cancer?

3. Are there any methods of preventing penile cancer?

A 64-year-old man had been diagnosed with moderate to poorly differentiated squamous cell carcinoma of the penis. He underwent four cycles of chemotherapy (paclitaxel, ifosfamide, cisplatin), followed by partial penectomy with lymph node dissection. There was bilateral inguinal lymph metastases with extranodal extension, plus a positive right obturator pelvic lymph node metastasis. Adjuvant EBRT was administered along with weekly cisplatin. Within two years, there was increasing hypermetabolic right pelvic adenopathy, plus new bone metastasis in the right anterior acetabulum. The patient was started on pembrolizumab, and then had a wide resection hemipelvectomy with acetabular reconstruction and total hip arthroplasty. Imaging done three months later revealed complete resolution of the lymph node metastasis, and no further metastatic disease. Over three years of follow-up, there was still no evidence of metastatic disease.

Answers:

1. **About 80% of cases of penile cancer are diagnosed in men over age 55, and about 66% are diagnosed in those over age 65.**
2. **About 95% of cases of penile cancer are squamous cell carcinoma. It affects the skin or mucosal membranes, and when it spreads, the inguinal lymph nodes are usually affected.**
3. **The prevention of carcinoma of the penis is easily accessible via the HPV vaccination, which is available now for young boys. This vaccine can greatly decrease the incidence of penile cancer. Stopping the smoking of tobacco products and preventing sexually transmitted infections, plus early detection of penile cancer are also essential.**

Key Terms

Active surveillance
Beam radiation therapy
Benign prostatic hyperplasia
Beta human chorionic gonadotropin
Bipolar resectoscope
Boswellia
Bowen's disease
Brachytherapy
Buschke–Lowenstein tumor
Cellules
Conformal radiation therapy
Coudé tip
Electrovaporization
Erythroplasia of Queyrat
Filiforms
Foley catheter

Followers
Gamma radiation
Gynecomastia
Holmium laser enucleation of the prostate
Lichen planus
Median furrow
Percussible
Polyploidization
Port cannula
Prostate Health Index
Rete testis
Robotic surgery
Salvage radiation
Uroflowmetry
Vasovagal syncope

Bibliography

1 American Cancer Society. (2021). *Key statistics for prostate cancer*. American Cancer Society, Inc. https://www.cancer.org/cancer/prostate-cancer/about/key-statistics.html. Accessed 2021.

2 American Cancer Society. (2021). *Initial treatment of prostate cancer, by stage*. American Cancer Society, Inc. https://www.cancer.org/cancer/prostate-cancer/treating/by-stage.html. Accessed 2021.

3 American Cancer Society. (2021). *Testicular cancer – causes, risk factors, and prevention*. American Cancer Society, Inc. https://www.cancer.org/cancer/testicular-cancer/causes-risks-prevention.html. Accessed 2021.

4 American Cancer Society. (2021). *Penile cancer stages*. American Cancer Society, Inc. https://www.cancer.org/cancer/penile-cancer/detection-diagnosis-staging/staging.html. Accessed 2021.

5 American Cancer Society. (2021). *Survival rates for penile cancer*. American Cancer Society, Inc. https://www.cancer.org/cancer/penile-cancer/detection-diagnosis-staging/survival-rates.html. Accessed 2021.

6 American Cancer Society Journals – Cancer. (2017). *Future of testicular germ cell tumor incidence in the United States: Forecast through 2026*. John Wiley & Sons, Inc. https://acsjournals.onlinelibrary.wiley.com/doi/full/10.1002/cncr.30597. Volume 123, Issue 12, pp. 2320–2328. Accessed 2021.

7 American Urological Association. (2020). *Management of benign prostatic hyperplasia/lower urinary tract symptoms*. American Urological Association. https://www.auanet.org/guidelines/guidelines/benign-prostatic-hyperplasia-(bph)-guideline. Accessed 2021.

8 American Urological Association. (2020). *Medical student curriculum: Prostate cancer screening and management*. American Urological Association. https://www.auanet.org/education/auauniversity/for-medical-students/medical-students-curriculum/medical-student-curriculum/prostate-cancer/psa. Accessed 2021.

9 BeatCancer.org – Center for Advancement in Cancer Education. (2017). *How to prevent testicular cancer*. BeatCancer.org. https://beatcancer.org/blog-posts/how-to-prevent-testicular-cancer. Accessed 2021.

10 British Journal of Urology International. (2007). *Holmium laser enucleation of the prostate (HoLEP)*. John Wiley & Sons, Inc. https://bjui-journals.onlinelibrary.wiley.com/doi/10.1111/j.1464-410X.2007.07341.x. Volume 101, Issue 1, pp. 131–142. Accessed 2021.

11 Centers for Disease Control and Prevention. (2020). *Prostate cancer statistics*. U.S. Department of Health & Human Services/USA.gov. https://www.cdc.gov/cancer/prostate/statistics/index.htm. Accessed 2021.

12 Chodak, G. (2013). *Winning the Battle against Prostate Cancer: Get the Treatment That's Right for You*, 2nd Edition. New York: Demos Health.

13 Clinical Cases in Advanced Prostate Cancer – Episode 1. (2020). *Case 1: MRI/TRUS fusion biopsy for nonmetastatic CRPC*. Targeted Oncology. https://www.targetedonc.com/view/case-1-mri-trus-fusion-biopsy-for-nonmetastatic-crpc. Accessed 2021.

14 Cohen, J.S. (2018). *Prostate Cancer Breakthroughs: The New Options You Need to Know About*. New York: Square One Publishers.

15 Cross, S. (2020). *Prostate Cancer: Diagnosis, Treatment and Recovery*. Foster Academics.

16 Culkin, D.J. (2014). *Management of Penile Cancer*. New York: Springer.

17 DoveMed. (2018). *Invasive squamous cell carcinoma of penis*. DoveMed. https://www.dovemed.com/diseases-conditions/invasive-squamous-cell-carcinoma-penis. Accessed 2021.

18 Duffy, R. (2018). *Testicular Cancer: The Essential Guide*. St. Ives: BxPlans.Ltd.

19 Foulkes, W.D. and Cooney, K.A. (2010). *Male Reproductive Cancers: Epidemiology, Pathology and Genetics (Cancer Genetics)*. New York: Springer.

20 Gaglani, V. (2019). *Life after Prostate Cancer and Other Medical Conditions: A Step-by-Step*

Guide to Stop Urinary Leakage in Ten Weeks. Baltimore: Osmosis Publications.

21 Gracia, C. and Woodruff, T.K. (2012). *Oncofertility Medical Practice: Clinical Issues and Implementation.* New York: Springer. Accessed 2021.

22 Hayes, P. (2019). *Prostate Cancer: Assessment and Treatment.* New York: Hayle Medical.

23 Healio – Hematology/Oncology – Genitourinary Cancer. (2012). *A 46-year-old male with advanced nonseminomatous testicular cancer, renal and lung impairment.* Healio. https://www.healio.com/news/hematology -oncology/20120331/a-46-year-old-male- with-advanced-nonseminomatous-testicular- cancer-renal-and-lung-impairment. HemOnc today Issue: March 10, 2012. Accessed 2021.

24 Healthy Male. (2014). *Testicular Cancer,* 5th Edition. Melbourne (Australia): Healthy Male.

25 Johns Hopkins Medicine – Health Conditions and Diseases. (2021). *Testicular cancer tumor markers.* The Johns Hopkins University, The Johns Hopkins Hospital, and Johns Hopkins Health System. https://www. hopkinsmedicine.org/health/conditions-and- diseases/testicular-cancer/testicular-cancer- tumor-markers. Accessed 2021.

26 Majzoub, A. and Agarwal, A. (2017). *The Complete Guide to Male Fertility Preservation.* New York: Springer.

27 Medical News Today. (2021). *What is benign prostatic hyperplasia?* Healthline Media UK Ltd. https://www.medicalnewstoday.com/ articles/314998. Accessed 2021.

28 Mulhall, J.P., Applegarth, L.D., Oates, R.D., and Schlegel, P.N. (2013). *Fertility Preservation in Male Cancer Patients.* Cambridge: Cambridge University Press.

29 Mulhall, J.P., Incrocci, L., Goldstein, I., and Rosen, R. (2011). *Cancer and Sexual Health (Current Clinical Urology).* Totowa: Humana Press.

30 Muneer, A. and Horenblas, S. (2017). *Textbook of Penile Cancer,* 2nd Edition. New York: Springer.

31 Muneer, A., Arya, M., and Horenblas, S. (2011). *Textbook of Penile Cancer.* New York: Springer.

32 National Center for Advancing Translational Sciences/Genetic and Rare Diseases Information Center. (2021). *Testicular seminoma.* Genetic and Rare Diseases Information Center. https://rarediseases.info. nih.gov/diseases/4792/testicular-seminoma. Accessed 2021.

33 National Library of Medicine – National Center for Biotechnology Information. (2014). *Basal cell carcinoma of the penis: A case report and review of the literature.* National Library of Medicine. https://pubmed.ncbi.nlm.nih. gov/25298901. Accessed 2021.

34 Nursing Made Incredibly Easy! (2011). *The ABCs of male reproductive cancer.* Wolters Kluwer Health, Inc. https://journals.lww.com/ nursingmadeincrediblyeasy/fulltext/2011/07000/ the_abcs_of_male_reproductive_cancer.7.aspx. Volume 9, Issue 4, pp. 28–38. Accessed 2021.

35 Olshan, A.F. and Mattison, D.R. (2012). *Male-Mediated Developmental Toxicity: Reproductive Biology.* New York: Springer.

36 Onik, G. (2005). *The Male Lumpectomy: A Rational New Approach to Treating Prostate Cancer.* Bloomington: AuthorHouse.

37 Orwig, K.E. and Hermann, B.P. (2011). *Male Germline Stem Cells: Developmental and Regenerative Potential (Stem Cell Biology and Regenerative Medicine).* Totowa: Humana Press.

38 Panda, A., Gulani, V., and Ponsky, L. (2020). *Reading MRI of the Prostate: A Practical Guide.* New York: Springer.

39 PathologyOutlines.com. (2020). *Testis & epididymis – Germ cell tumors – Seminoma.* PathologyOutlines.com. https://www. pathologyoutlines.com/topic/testisseminomas. html. Accessed 2021.

40 Prime Health Channel. (2013). *Seminoma (cancer).* Prime Health Channel. https://www. primehealthchannel.com/seminoma.html. Accessed 2021.

41 Prostate Conditions Education Council. (2021). *About prostate conditions: Early detection & prevention.* Prostate Conditions Education Council. https://www. prostateconditions.org/about-prostate-conditions/early-detection-prevention. Accessed 2021.

42 Radiopaedia. (2021). *Testicular seminoma.* Radiopaedia.org. https://radiopaedia.org/articles/testicular-seminoma-1. Accessed 2021.

43 Radiopaedia. (2021). *Non-seminomatous germ tell tumors.* Radiopaedia.org. https://radiopaedia.org/articles/non-seminomatous-germ-cell-tumours-2?lang=gb#nav_epidemiology. Accessed 2021.

44 Scholz, M. (2018). *The Key to Prostate Cancer: 30 Experts Explain 15 Stages of Prostate Cancer.* Marina del Ray: Prostate Oncology Specialists.

45 ScienceDirect – Gene. (2018). *Epigenetics and testicular germ cell tumors.* Elsevier B.V. https://www.sciencedirect.com/science/article/pii/S0378111918303160. Volume 661, 30 June 2018, pp. 22–33. Accessed 2021.

46 Sikka, S.C. and Hellstrom, W.J.G. (2017). *Bioenvironmental Issues Affecting Men's Reproductive and Sexual Health.* Cambridge: Academic Press.

47 Spiess, P.E. (2016). *Penile Cancer: Diagnosis and Treatment (Current Clinical Urology)*, 2nd Edition. Totowa: Humana Press.

48 Stein, G.S. and Luebbers, K.P. (2019). *Cancer: Prevention, Early Detection, Treatment and Recovery*, 2nd Edition. Hoboken: Wiley-Blackwell. Figure 1 from Page. 371.

49 Turkington, C. and Pound, C. (2005). *Encyclopedia of Men's Reproductive Cancer (Facts on File Library of Health and Living).* New York: Facts on File, Inc.

50 University of Washington – Department of Radiology. (2021). *Testicular choriocarcinoma (pure).* University of Washington. https://rad.washington.edu/body-teaching-files/22143. Accessed 2021.

51 Walsh, P.C. and Farrar Worthington, J. (2018). *Dr. Patrick Walsh's Guide to Surviving Prostate Cancer*, 3rd Edition. New York: Grand Central Life & Style.

52 Wassersug, R.J., Walker, L.M., Robinson, J.W. et. al. (2014). *Androgen Deprivation Therapy: An Essential Guide for Prostate Cancer Patients and Their Loved Ones.* New York: Demos Health. Accessed 2021.

53 Wiley Online Library – International Journal of Urology. (2019). *Clinical Investigation – Robot-assisted single-port radical prostatectomy: A phase 1 clinical study.* John Wiley & Sons, Inc. https://onlinelibrary.wiley.com/doi/full/10.1111/iju.14044. Volume 26, Issue 9, pp. 878–883. Accessed 2021.

54 Wiley Online Library – Clinical and Experimental Dermatology. (2017). *Recurrent penile squamous cell carcinoma in an elderly circumcised man.* John Wiley & Sons, Inc. https://onlinelibrary.wiley.com/doi/abs/10.1111/ced.13051. Volume 42, Issue 3, pp. 360–362. Accessed 2021.

55 World Cancer Research Fund/American Institute for Cancer Research/Continuous Update Project. (2021). Prostate cancer statistics: Prostate cancer is the second most common cancer in men worldwide. World Cancer Research Fund International. https://www.wcrf.org/dietandcancer/prostate-cancer-statistics. Accessed 2021.

9

Female Reproductive Tumors

Benign Breast Tumors

Benign breast tumors are masses that may be of any size. A benign tumor may be discovered during breast self-examination, incidentally, or by a physician during physical examination. Benign masses may be painless or painful. There are sometimes other features such as discharge from the nipple, or skin changes.

Epidemiology

Statistics on prevalence and incidence of benign breast tumors are not well documented. Fibrocystic changes affect 50–60% of all women in the United States. Fibrocystic changes of the breast are most common in women that had early menarche, the first live birth when they were 30 years or older, or in women that have never given birth. They usually develop in women between ages 20 and 50. Fibroadenomas usually develop when a woman is in her reproductive years, occurring most frequently between ages 18 and 35. Generally, 7–13% of women are affected. A variant called *juvenile fibroadenoma* occurs in teenagers and continues to grow over time – this is different from fibroadenomas in older women. **Phyllodes tumor** is most common in middle-aged women, but make up less than 1% of all breast neoplasms. *Intraductal papilloma* is most common between ages 30 and 50, though overall this is a rare tumor that grows in a dilated duct, often close to the nipple, causing discharge. Intraductal papillomas make up about 2% of all benign breast lesions. **Mammary duct ectasia** is most common during pregnancy and lactation, or after menopause, though actual epidemiological statistics are limited. *Fat necrosis* occurs between the ages of 14 and 80 years, with an average age of 50, though documentation of

Global Epidemiology of Cancer: Diagnosis and Treatment, First Edition. Jahangir Moini,
Nicholas G. Avgeropoulos, and Craig Badolato.
© 2022 John Wiley & Sons Ltd. Published 2022 by John Wiley & Sons Ltd.

the number of cases is limited. For some reason, African American women that are relatively young have the highest rates of *fibroadenomas*. Otherwise, the various types of benign breast tumors affect women of all racial and ethnic groups nearly evenly.

Global statistics on the prevalence and incidence of benign breast tumors are lacking. However, a 2003 study in Germany revealed that there were 23.3 cases out of every 100,000 women. Generally, most benign breast tumors occur in women between ages 18 and 50. There is no significant racial or ethnic predilection for these tumors, except for younger black women having a higher number of fibroadenomas.

Etiology and Risk Factors

Approximately 90% of breast masses are benign. They are usually caused by fibrocystic changes or fibroadenomas. Fibrocystic changes were previously referred to as *fibrocystic disease*. This refers to breast cysts, **mastalgia**, and nondescript masses that are usually in the upper, outer area of the breast. These different findings may occur as a single manifestation or together. Continued stimulation by estrogen and progesterone may cause fibrocystic changes. Fibrocystic changes are also related to genetic background, age, number of children, history of lactation, consumption of caffeine, and the use of exogenous hormones. Rupture of a cyst releases secretory material into nearby breast tissues, resulting in chronic inflammation and scarring fibrosis. Fibrous tissue increases until menopause. *Usual ductal hyperplasia* is the presence of more than two cell layers above the basement membrane, within the ductal space. There is distention of the ducts and lobules by luminal and myoepithelial cells. Risk factors for fibroadenomas include puberty and early adulthood.

Clinical Manifestations

With fibrocystic changes, there may be a dense and nodular texture of the breast, or it can feel uncomfortable and rather heavy compared with the other breast. Sometimes, a burning pain is felt. Symptoms usually resolve after menopause. Fibrocystic changes are responsible for the most commonly documented breast symptoms. Fibroadenomas are usually smooth and rounded masses that are mobile and painless. *Intraductal papillomas* manifest spontaneous or induced nipple discharge that can be bloody, watery, or serous. Rarely, nipple retraction occurs. *Mammary duct ectasia* may cause nipple retraction or subareolar induration. There is spontaneous discharge from multiple ducts that appears bloody, thick, and sticky. The areolar area may have burning pain or swelling. After rupture, there is a palpable mass.

Pathology

Fibroadenomas are often solitary and well circumscribed, being 1–5 cm in diameter. They usually decrease in size over time, in older women. Simple fibroadenomas are not believed to increase risks for breast cancer. However, complex fibroadenomas may increase the risks to a small degree. Fibroadenomas grow slowly, and are composed of varying amounts of epithelial and connective tissues, probably under the influence of estrogen. *Phyllodes tumors* are fibroepithelial, with significant proliferation of connective tissue stroma and large size. They are multinodular; 2–20 cm in diameter, and late in their progression may cause trophic cutaneous ulcerations. They grow slowly at first, and 10–25% become malignant. *Intraductal papillomas* are usually small, friable, and yellow–red in color. Most of these papillomas are about 5 mm in size and attached to the wall of the duct by a short, thin stalk. *Mammary duct ectasia* occurs as the main lactiferous ducts become dilated. They fill with cellular debris. There is a secondary inflammatory reaction, and sometimes, rupture of the ducts. *Fat necrosis* is yellow or gray necrotic foci.

Diagnosis

For diagnosis, patient history should take into account the length of time that the mass has been present, if it is constant or intermittent, or if there is pain. Any previous masses and outcomes must be discussed. Nipple discharge must be assessed to determine whether it only responds to breast manipulation or occurs spontaneously. Discharge must also be assessed concerning its appearance – clear, bloody, or milky. Symptoms of advanced cancer such as bone pain, malaise, and weight loss must be ruled out. Previous medical history should assess risk factors for breast cancer. These include history of radiation therapy to the chest area before age 30, and previous breast cancer diagnoses. Family history should document breast cancer in a first-degree relative and if positive, whether a mother, sister, or daughter carried the BRCA1 or BRCA2 gene mutations, predisposing them for breast cancer.

Physical examination of the breast also takes into account surrounding tissues, with inspection for skin changes. These may occur above the mass, or include nipple retraction and discharge. Skin changes may include rash, redness, exaggerated skin markings, and orange peel skin due to edema. The mass must be palpated for size, tenderness, hardness, or softness, and mobility or fixture to the chest wall or skin. The axillary, infraclavicular, and supraclavicular areas are also palpated for adenopathy and masses. Findings that are of the most concern include the following:

- Bloody or spontaneous nipple discharge
- A mass fixed to the chest wall or skin
- Fixed or matted axillary lymph nodes
- Skin dimpling
- A stony, hard, irregular mass
- Thickened and reddened skin

In a woman with a history of similar findings, during reproductive age, any painful, rubbery, or tender mass is suggestive of fibrocystic changes. There is considerable overlap between the features of benign and malignant lesions. Risk factors can be present or absent. Therefore, most patients must be tested with accuracy so that breast cancer can be ruled out.

Differentiating between cysts and solid masses is important, because cysts are usually not cancerous. Ultrasound is usually done. Cystic lesions may be aspirated if they are causing symptoms. Solid masses are first assessed via mammography, and then with imaging-guided biopsy. Often, any type of mass is evaluated with needle aspiration. If fluid is not obtained, or if aspiration does not eliminate the mass, mammography is done, followed by imaging-guided biopsy. Aspirated cystic fluid is only sent for cytological study if it is extremely bloody, turbid, if only a small amount of fluid can be obtained, and if a mass is still present after aspiration. The patient is examined again in 1–2 months. A cyst is considered benign if it is no longer palpable. If a cyst recurs, **reaspiration** is performed. Obtained fluid is sent for cytology no matter how it appears. A third recurrence or continued presence of a mass after the first aspiration – even with negative cytology – indicates that a biopsy is necessary.

Treatment

Benign breast tumors are treated based on the causative component. Symptoms of fibrocystic changes can be relieved by acetaminophen, non-steroidal anti-inflammatory drugs (NSAIDs), and by wearing athletic bras, since these reduce trauma to the breasts. Also, taking a supplement called *evening primrose oil* (linoleic acid) may help relieve breast pain for some patients. Fibroadenomas are usually surgically removed if they grow or are symptomatic. If they are less than 3 cm in diameter, fibroadenomas can be **cryoablated** after the patient is given a local anesthetic. Unfortunately, these tumors often recur. If a patient has a fibroadenoma that is not removed, she should be followed-up periodically to assess any changes. After a patient has had several benign fibroadenomas, she may not want to have additional tumors removed. For juvenile fibroadenomas, surgical excision is indicated because they usually enlarge.

Phyllodes tumors are locally excised unless they have become voluminous or malignant. In this case, a simple mastectomy is performed. *Intraductal papillomas* are treated by excision of the involved duct or ducts. *Mammary duct ectasia* is treated with antibiotics and anti-inflammatory medications. *Fat necrosis* is either observed for any worsening, or can be locally excised. Medications that can be used for breast pain caused by benign breast tumors include danazol, bromocriptine, tamoxifen, iodine, and progesterone.

Prevention and Early Detection

There is no significant way to prevent benign breast tumors, though there are some steps that can be taken to improve overall health, and reduce the likelihood of developing benign or malignant tumors. These include self-examination, regular mammograms, regular exercising to maintain a healthy weight, eating a nutritious diet, avoiding smoking, drinking alcohol only in moderation, considering the use of hormone replacement therapy if needed, and switching to a non-hormonal contraceptive. Early detection of benign breast tumors is the goal, since it has the potential to assess tumors that have the ability to cause significant symptoms, or that have a higher likelihood of becoming malignant over time.

Prognosis

Most women with benign breast tumors do not develop breast cancer. If there are increased risks, based on the type of benign tumor, more frequent cancer screenings may be indicated. Anytime there are changes in the appearance or feel of the breasts, a physician must be notified so that they can be assessed. Overall, the prognosis for benign breast tumors is good.

Breast Cancer

Breast cancer is a malignant neoplastic disease of breast tissue. It is a common malignancy in women and is very rare in men. Breast cancers are often found as asymptomatic masses during examination or screening mammography. Metastasis occurs through the lymphatic system to the axillary lymph nodes and to the bones, lungs, brain, and liver. There is evidence that primary carcinomas of the breast may exist in multiple sites and that tumor cells may enter the bloodstream directly without passing through the lymph nodes.

Epidemiology

In the United States, breast cancer is the second leading cause of cancer deaths in women, though it is the *leading* cause of death in Hispanic women. Approximately 276,500 cases of invasive breast cancer were diagnosed in 2020, with about 42,200 cases being fatal. There were over 48,500 new cases of in situ breast cancer in the same year. Incidence rates are highest in non-Hispanic white women (130.8 per 100,000), followed by African American women (126.7 per 100,000). However, African American women have the highest breast cancer *death rate*, at 28.4 deaths per 100,000, which is more than double that of Asian American or Pacific Islander women, in whom there are 11.5 deaths per 100,000. Women near age 70 have the highest rates of breast cancer diagnoses (1 in 24 women), followed by those near age 60 (1 in 28). The lowest rates of breast cancer diagnoses are in women near age 30 (1 in 204). Breast cancer is rare in men, but it may occur often in older people. Cases of female breast cancer far exceed cases of male breast cancer, with male cases making up of 1% of total cases. In men, there were approximately 2,620 new cases of invasive breast cancer, with about 520 deaths, in 2020 in the United States.

According to the World Health Organization in 2021, breast cancer has now overtaken lung cancer as the most commonly diagnosed cancer throughout the world. Based on statistics from 2018, there are more than 2.09 million new global cases of invasive breast cancer annually. Incidence ranges between 25.9 cases per 100,000 women in South Central Asia to 94.2 cases per 100,000 in Australia and New Zealand.

Approximately 66% of invasive breast cancer occurs in women aged 55 or older. Global cases of male breast cancer are about 0.61 of every 100,000 men. Caucasians are the most likely group to be diagnosed with breast cancer, in women and men, followed by people of African descent. According to the World Cancer Research Fund in 2020, the countries with the highest rates of breast cancer in women included Belgium, Luxembourg, Netherlands, metropolitan France, New Caledonia, Lebanon, Australia, the United Kingdom, Italy, New Zealand, Ireland, Sweden, Finland, Denmark, Switzerland, Montenegro, Malta, Norway, Hungary, Germany, Iceland, the United States, Canada, Cyprus, and Samoa (see Figure 9.1).

Etiology and Risk Factors

Breast cancer may develop from cells with multiple genetic aberrations that are influenced by hormonal exposures and inherited susceptibility genes. About 12% of breast cancers occur due to inheritance of a susceptible gene or genes. Risks are higher after age 60. The risk of dying from breast cancer is about 10% by five years following diagnosis. The most important risk factor is aging, with the majority of diagnoses occurring after age 50, peaking at 70–80 years. If a woman has a first-degree relative – a sister, mother, or daughter with breast cancer, the risk is doubled or tripled. Breast cancer in more distant relatives only slightly raises the risk. Between 5% and 10% of all women with breast cancer have a mutation in either breast cancer gene *BRCA1* or *BRCA2*. Lifetime risk of the disease when a BRCA gene is present is 50–85%. With a BRCA1 mutation, the risk of breast cancer developing by age 80 is about 72%. With a BRCA2 mutation, this same risk is about 69%. Also, women with BRCA1 mutations have a 20–40% risk of developing ovarian cancer, but BRCA2 mutations are not as commonly linked with ovarian cancer. If a woman has no family history of breast cancer in at least two first-degree relatives, she is not likely to carry a BRCA mutation, and screening for the mutation is not required. The most common group that carries a BRCA mutation consists of *Ashkenazi Jews*. If a BRCA is present, the woman needs close surveillance, preventive medications (raloxifene or tamoxifen), or a double mastectomy. It should be noted, however, that as many as 75% of women have no identifiable risk factors for breast cancer.

Regarding personal history of breast cancer, previous in situ or invasive breast cancer

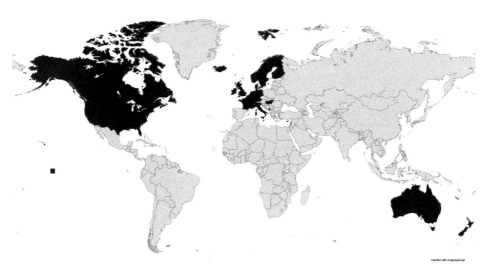

Figure 9.1 Countries with the highest rates of breast cancer.

increases risks, and the risk of developing cancer, after a single mastectomy, in the contralateral breast is 0.5–1% per year of follow-up. Risks are also increased by early menarche, late menopause, or a late first pregnancy. Women with a first pregnancy after age 30 have a higher risk of breast cancer than a woman that has never given birth. Risks are slightly increased if a woman has had a breast lesion that required a biopsy. Women are not at high risk if they have more than one breast mass, with no high-risk patterns seen in histology. Invasive breast cancer can develop from benign lesions, including complex fibroadenoma, florid or moderate hyperplasia that lacks atypia, papilloma, and sclerosing adenosis. If a woman has atypical ductal or lobular hyperplasia, risks for breast cancer are 4–5 times higher. If she has a family history of invasive breast cancer in a first-degree relative, and has atypical ductal or lobular hyperplasia herself, the risks are 10 times higher. An increased risk of breast cancer is related to increased breast density, as visualized during mammography.

Lobular carcinoma in situ (LCIS) increases the risk of invasive carcinoma in either breast by 25 times. With LCIS, invasive carcinoma develops in 1–2% of patients every year. The use of oral contraceptives increases breast cancer risks by about 5 more cases per 100,000 women than is seen in women that do not use oral contraceptives. The risk mostly increases during the use of the contraceptives, and reduces within 10 years after stopping them. After three years of use, postmenopausal estrogen plus progestin, through hormonal therapy, increases the risk of breast cancer slightly. This is an approximate 24% increase in relative risks. Without progestin, estrogen therapy does not appear to increase the risk of developing breast cancer. Risks are lowered if selective estrogen-receptor (ER) modulators such as raloxifene are used.

Risks of breast cancer are also increased by exposure to radiation therapy before age 30. When mantle-field radiation therapy is used to treat Hodgkin's lymphoma, risks of breast cancer are about four times higher over the next 20–30 years. Diet may be related to breast cancers, though evidence for this is controversial. While improving diet is not a certain factor for risk reduction, obese postmenopausal women have a higher risk of breast cancer. If obese women menstruate later than average, risks may be reduced. There is a higher risk of breast cancer in people that smoke or drink alcohol excessively. Women should stop smoking and reduce alcohol consumption. The American Cancer Society recommends that women consume no more than one alcoholic drink per day. Risks for female breast cancer are calculated by using the following:

- *Breast Cancer Risk Assessment Tool* (BCRAT) – which assesses personal history, previous radiation therapy, BRCA mutations, genetic cancer syndromes, age, race or ethnicity, previous benign breast tumors, age of first menstrual period, age of first childbirth, number of first-degree relatives with breast cancer
- *Gail model* – which assesses women based on age of first menstrual period, number of previous biopsies, number of first-degree relatives with breast cancer, history of atypical hyperplasia, and patient age
- *Claus model* – uses family history for up to two first- or second-degree relatives, or both; short- and longer-term risks are calculated, but atypia seen during breast biopsy is not included
- *Tyrer-Cuzick model* – uses a variety of risk factors, including mammographic density

Clinical Manifestations

Breast cancers are often discovered during regular self-examinations or clinical breast examination with mammography, though they sometimes cause breast pain or enlargement, or thickening of breast tissues. Nearly half of affected patients have a palpable breast mass when they are clinically examined. During physical examination, the breasts may be asymmetrical, or there may be a *dominant mass*, which is very different from surrounding tissues. Diffuse fibrotic changes are most common in the upper outer quadrant of a breast, but can be present in any quadrant. These changes usually signify a benign tumor. If one breast has slightly firmer thickening than the other, this may indicate breast cancer. When breast cancer is more advanced, there may be one or more of the following present:

- Exaggerated normal skin markings – from edema, due to invasion or dermal lymphatic vessels (referred to as orange peel skin)
- A mass that is fixated to the chest wall or overlying skin
- Satellite nodules or skin ulcers

Tumor spread is signified by matted or fixed axillary lymph nodes, supraclavicular lymphadenopathy, or infraclavicular lymphadenopathy. *Inflammatory breast cancer* involves orange peel skin, reddening, and enlargement. A mass is often not present, but nipple discharge is common. This type of breast cancer is highly aggressive.

Pathology

The majority of breast cancers are epithelial tumors, arising from cells that line ducts or lobules. Less often, they are nonepithelial cancers of the supporting stroma – classified as angiosarcomas, phyllodes tumors, or primary stromal sarcomas. Breast cancers are classified as *carcinoma in situ* or *invasive cancer*. Carcinoma in situ is diagnosed when there is cancer cell proliferation in the ducts or lobules, but no invasion into the stromal tissue. *Ductal carcinoma in situ* (DCIS) makes up about 85% of these tumors, and is usually found during mammography. A small or wide breast area may be affected. If the area is wide, microscopic invasive foci may eventually develop. LCIS is often multifocal as well as bilateral. The *classic type* is not malignant, yet increases the likelihood for invasive carcinoma in either breast. It is not palpable, and usually detected by a biopsy, being rarely seen during mammography. The *pleomorphic type* is more similar to DCIS, and must be excised to negative margins.

Invasive carcinoma is usually adenocarcinoma. Approximately 80% of these tumors are called *infiltrating ductal* tumors, while the remainder is *infiltrating lobular* tumors) – see Figure 9.2. There are also rare types known as *medullary, metaplastic, mucinous,* and *tubular* carcinomas. The mucinous subtype usually develops in older women, and grows slowly and the outlook is much better. *Inflammatory breast cancer* grows quickly and is often fatal. Cancer cells block lymphatic vessels within the skin of the breast, causing an appearance of inflammation. The skin resembles an orange peel, referred to as *peau d'orange* and is thicker than normal. Inflammatory breast cancer often spreads to the armpit lymph nodes, which then feel hard. There is often no breast mass since the cancer is dispersed throughout the breast tissue. *Paget disease of the nipple* is a type of DCIS that extends over the nipple and areola skin, as an eczematous or psoriaform lesion. Paget cells are present within the epidermis.

Breast cancer is locally invasive. It spreads through the bloodstream, regional lymph nodes, or both. Metastatic breast cancer can affect nearly every body organ, but mostly, the lungs, liver, bones, skin, and brain. With skin metastases, they usually occur close to the site of breast surgery. Metastases to the scalp are rare. Recurrence of breast cancer is varied, often predictable by tumor markers. When a woman is negative for tumor markers, metastatic breast cancer can occur within three years. If a patient has an ER-positive (ER +) tumor, metastatic breast cancer may occur within more than 10 years after the first diagnosis and treatment.

Estrogen and progesterone receptors are present in some breast cancers. They are nuclear hormone receptors, promoting replication of DNA and cell division when appropriate hormones bind to them. Therefore, for tumors with the receptors, drugs that block them may be successful. Approximately 66% of postmenopausal breast cancer patients have an ER + tumor. In premenopausal patients, incidence of ER-positive tumors is lower. Human epidermal growth factor receptor 2 (HER2, also known as

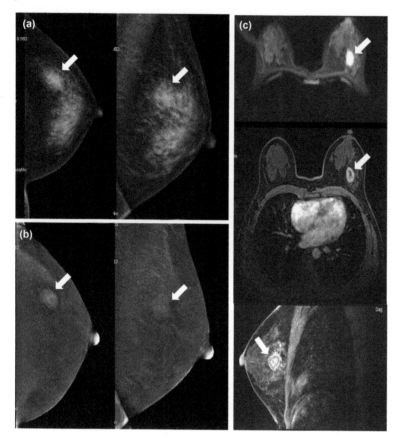

Figure 9.2 (a) Digital mammography image showing focal asymmetry (white arrows); (b) contrast-enhanced images showing enhancement of the mass (white arrows) with surrounding edema; (c) contrast-enhanced magnetic resonance imaging (MRI) views of the mass, which was diagnosed in pathology as invasive ductal carcinoma. *Source*: Figure 1 from Wiley Online Library – Cancer Medicine [58].

HER2/neu or ErbB2) is another cellular receptor. If present, it is linked to a worsened outlook regardless of cancer staging. The HER2 receptors are overexpressed in about 20% of patients with breast cancer.

Diagnosis

If physical breast examination or mammography detects a breast abnormality, testing is needed to differentiate a benign lesion from cancer. Earlier diagnosis improves outlook, so accurately diagnosing breast cancer must be conclusive. When advanced cancer is suspected after physical examination, a biopsy is performed first. If advanced cancer is not suspected, ultrasound is usually performed first to differentiate cancer from benign tumor. Any lesion that may be cancer must be biopsied. A pre-biopsy bilateral mammogram can help identify other areas for biopsy, and gives a baseline for future assessments. Mammogram results must not alter any decision to perform a biopsy if the decision was made from physical findings.

The preferred form of biopsy is percutaneous core needle biopsy. It can be done with imaging guidance or freehand – simply by using palpation. For improved accuracy, a stereotactic biopsy is common, as well as ultrasound-guided biopsy (see Figure 9.3). A stereotactic biopsy is a needle biopsy guided by mammography, in two planes. A computer, producing a three-dimensional

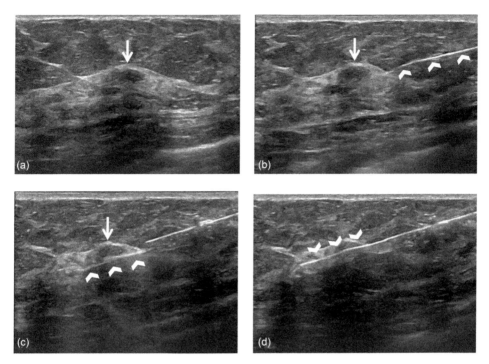

Figure 9.3 (a) Pre-biopsy ultrasound image of a hypoechoic mass (arrow); (b) biopsy needle (arrowheads) directed toward the mass; (c) the needle is through the mass (arrowheads); (D) the cannula has covered the core trough and the specimen is secured. *Source*: Figure 1 from Wiley Online Library – Journal of Ultrasound in Medicine – Early View [59].

image, analyzes the biopsy. A lesion that is excessively posterior makes a core biopsy impossible, so a surgical biopsy can be done. To identify the biopsy site, a guidewire is inserted, by using imaging for accuracy. Any skin removed with a tissue biopsy must be examined since it can reveal cancer cells in the dermal lymphatic vessels. The specimen is X-rayed for comparison with the pre-biopsy mammogram, to judge whether the entire lesion has been successfully excised. When an original lesion had microcalcifications, mammography is performed again once the breast has lost tenderness. This is usually 6–12 weeks after biopsy, and assesses any residual microcalcifications. Mammography is performed prior to any radiation therapy being done.

Once breast cancer is diagnosed, professionals from different disciplines, including a breast surgical oncologist, medical oncologist, radiation oncologist, and cancer experts, plan testing and treatments. A portion of a positive specimen from biopsy is analyzed for the HER2 protein, and for estrogen and progesterone receptors. Blood and saliva cells are tested for inherited gene mutations that predispose to breast cancer, if there is any of the following:

- Family history – of multiple cases of early-onset breast cancer
- Ovarian cancer in the patient – with family history of breast or ovarian cancer
- Breast and ovarian cancer – occurring in the same patient
- Ashkenazi Jewish heritage
- Family history of one case of male breast cancer
- Age below 45 when breast cancer developed
- No estrogen or progesterone receptors, or overexpression of HER2 protein – this is known as *triple negative breast cancer*

Certain experts for all patients with breast cancer recommend genetic testing. The patient is referred to a genetic counselor, to create a detailed family history, choose appropriate tests, and interpret results. To assess metastatic disease, a chest X-ray, CBC, serum calcium measurement, and liver tests are done. An oncologist should determine whether there is a need for measuring serum carcinoembryonic antigen (CEA) or the cancer antigens (CA) 15-3 or 27-29. Indications for a bone scan include bone pain, elevated serum alkaline phosphatase, or stage III or IV breast cancer. An abdominal computed tomography (CT) scan is needed if there are abnormal liver test results, abnormal abdominal or pelvic examinations, or stage III or IV breast cancer. A chest CT scan is needed if there is shortness of breath or any other pulmonary symptom, and stage III or IV breast cancer. An MRI may be used to plan surgery since it can determine the size of the tumor, the number of tumors, and any chest wall involvement. An MRI is often reserved for women at very high risk, while ultrasound is usually used for those at moderate risk.

Tumor grading is based on the histology of the biopsied tissue. The grade describes how the abnormal cells and tissue appear microscopically. Staging utilizes the tumor, node, and metastasis classification. Since clinical examination and imaging are not highly sensitive for lymph node involvement, staging is refined as part of surgery, since regional lymph nodes can be assessed. If the patient has axillary lymph nodes that feel abnormal upon palpation, pre-surgical ultrasound-guided fine needle aspiration or core biopsy may be performed. If the biopsy results are positive, axillary lymph node dissection is usually done during surgery. Neoadjuvant chemotherapy can result in sentinel lymph node biopsy being possible if it changes lymph node status from N1 to N0. When biopsy results are negative, the less aggressive sentinel lymph node biopsy can be performed.

Staging of the tumor may follow either the *anatomic* staging model or the *prognostic* staging model. The anatomic staging model is based on tumor anatomy (see Table 9.1). It is used in areas of the world where biomarkers are not regularly obtainable. The prognostic staging model is based on tumor anatomy plus status of biomarkers. It is used most often in the United States.

During any treatment for breast cancer, the patient should avoid becoming pregnant. If the patient wishes to preserve fertility, she should be

Table 9.1 The anatomic staging model for breast cancer.

Stage	Tumor classification	Regional lymph node/distant metastasis
0	Tis (in situ)	N0/M0
IA	T1 (with or without micrometastases)	N0/M0
IB	T0 to T1 (with or without micrometastases)	N1 (with micrometastases)/M0
IIA	T0, T1 (with or without micrometastases), T2	N1 (without micrometastases)/M0, N0/M0
IIB	T2, T3	N1/M0, N0/M0
IIIA	T1 (with or without micrometastases), T2, T3	N2/M0, N1/M0
IIIB	T4	N0/M0, N1/M0, N2/M0
IIIC	Any T	N3/M0
IV	Any T	Any N/M1

referred to a reproductive endocrinologist immediately. Fertility preservation can occur via assisted reproductive techniques (ART) or with ovarian suppression. The ARTs involve ovarian stimulation, plus oocyte and embryo cryopreservation. Use of ART may cause adverse effects in patients that have ER + tumors. Ovarian suppression, such as that utilizing leuprolide, minimizes destruction of the ova by the chemotherapy used. The type of fertility preservation used is based on the diagnosed type of breast cancer, anticipated treatments, and the patient's preference.

Biomarkers have greatly affected the diagnosis of breast cancer. They help determine risks for developing the disease and guide screening as well as monitoring. The BRCA1 and BRCA2 mutations identify patients at an increased risk. They may improve screening methods and chemoprevention. The mutations can easily be found in DNA from a blood or saliva sample. When breast cancer is diagnosed, biomarkers help determine the type that is present, affecting treatment choices and prognosis. The performance of *immunohistochemistry* (IHC) *staining* determines expression of estrogen and progesterone hormone receptors, as well as the HER2 status of the patient. This status is also determined by the use of *fluorescence in situ hybridization* (FISH) to examine the expression of the encoding RNA. Androgen receptor status is also often assessed via IHC staining. Assessment of circulating tumor cells (CTCs) has become an excellent tool to evaluate breast cancer development. When less than five CTCs are present in a 7.5 mL sample, the patient has a better prognosis. The important factor is to delineate and characterize the cells found in the bloodstream of a cancer patient. The cells are separated from other cell types in the blood by using anti-epithelial cell adhesion molecule (anti-EpCAM) antibodies, and classified further.

Treatment

For most breast cancers, treatments involve surgery, radiation therapy, and systemic therapy, based on the actual tumors and characteristics of the patient. Surgical recommendations are evolving, including earlier referrals to plastic surgeons or reconstructive surgeons for **oncoplastic surgery**. This technique removes the cancer while reconstructing the breast. Mastectomy is the removal of the entire breast, while breast-conserving surgery preserves as much breast tissue as possible. Surgery of either type is combined with radiation therapy. There are five types of mastectomy, as follows:

- Radical mastectomy – also removes the axially lymph nodes and pectoral muscles – this type is reserved for cases in which the pectoral muscles have been invaded by the cancer; this procedure has become nearly obsolete because of the development of better treatment methods
- Modified radical mastectomy – removes some axillary lymph nodes but not the pectoral muscles

Simple mastectomy – spares the pectoral muscles and axillary lymph nodes

- Skin-sparing mastectomy – does not remove the pectoral muscles or axillary lymph nodes, and leaves enough skin to cover the surgical wound to make breast reconstruction much easier
- Nipple-sparing mastectomy – is the same as skin-sparing mastectomy, but the nipple and areola are also spared

Breast-conserving surgery is based on the determination of tumor size and the required margins that must be removed, based on a size comparison between the tumor and entire breast volume. To describe the extent of breast tissue that must be removed, the terms *lumpectomy, quadrantectomy*, and *wide excision* are used. If the cancer is invasive, survival and recurrence rates are not widely different between mastectomy and breast-conserving surgery with radiation therapy – as long as the entire tumor is removable.

The patient's preference is very important, guided by the multidisciplinary team's expert opinions. Breast-conserving surgery with radiation therapy offers the advantage of less extensive surgery, so that the patient can keep the breast as intact as possible. Cosmetic results are considered excellent in 15% of patients. Cosmetic appearance is compromised by the requirement for total tumor removal plus tumor-free margins. A plastic surgeon can perform oncoplastic surgery, which is helpful for sagging breasts, yet this procedure also allows for adequate resection margins. Preoperative chemotherapy is sometimes used to shrink the tumor. This means that some patients who may need a mastectomy can instead have breast-conserving surgery.

The axillary lymph nodes are usually evaluated regardless of the chosen surgical method. *Axillary lymph node dissection* (ALND) is extensive, with as many axillary nodes being removed as possible. Adverse effects commonly occur – primarily lymphedema. Therefore, *sentinel lymph node biopsy* (SLNB) is usually performed first unless a biopsy of lymph nodes has already detected cancer. The risk of lymphedema is lower with SLNB, which has more than 95% sensitivity for axillary lymph node involvement. This makes it an overall better choice than ALND. During SLNB, blue dye with or without radioactive colloid is injected in the tissues around the breast. If only the blue dye is used, direct inspection and a gamma probe are used to locate the lymph nodes that the dye drains into. When radioactive colloid is used, the gamma probe is sufficient to determine this. Since these lymph nodes are the first to receive tracers, they are the most likely to also receive metastatic cells. Therefore, they are called *sentinel nodes.*

If any of them contain cancer cells, ALND may be needed. This is based on tumor stage, hormone-receptor status, and the number of involved nodes. Frozen section analysis during mastectomy with SLNB may be performed. The surgeon should get the patient's approval to perform ALND if the nodes are found to be positive for cancer. Other surgeons wait for standard pathology results, performing ALND as a follow-up procedure when needed. With lumpectomy, frozen section analysis is not usually done.

After axillary node removal (regardless of the method used) and radiation therapy, impaired lymphatic drainage of the ipsilateral arm is common. This may cause extreme swelling because of lymphedema. The amount of swelling is basically proportional to the number of nodes removed. After ALND, the lifetime risk of lymphedema is approximately 25%, and after SLNB, there is a 6% lifetime risk. To reduce risks, IV infusions are usually avoided on the affected side. It is important that the patient wear compression garments and preventing infections in the affected limb. Sometimes, patients are advised to avoid ipsilateral venipuncture or blood pressure measurement. Lymphedema requires treatment by a specially trained therapist. Once or twice daily massage may help drain fluid toward functional lymphatic basins. Low-stretch bandaging is applied immediately afterward. The patient should exercise every day as instructed. After lymphedema reduces over 1–4 weeks, the patient continues daily exercise and overnight bandaging for as long as the lymphedema is present.

After breast surgery, reconstruction may be *prosthetic* or *autologous.* In prosthetic reconstruction, a silicone or saline implant is placed, sometimes after a tissue expander is used. In autologous reconstruction, there can be a muscle flap transfer or a muscle-free flap transfer. A muscle flap transfer utilizes the latissimus dorsi, gluteus maximus, or lower rectus abdominis muscles. Breast reconstruction can be performed during a first mastectomy or breast-conserving surgery, or it can be performed later. Scheduling of surgery is based on the patient's choices and the need for adjuvant radiation or other therapies. Administration of radiation therapy first reduces the types of reconstructive surgery that will be possible. Therefore, a plastic surgeon must be consulted early in the treatment planning process.

The advantages of breast reconstruction after mastectomy include improved mental health. Disadvantages include complications from surgery, and possible effects of implants over time. A plastic surgeon should also be consulted when lower breast or upper inner quadrant lumpectomy will be performed. The best candidates for oncoplastic surgery are patients with sagging breasts. Symmetry may be improved by a *contralateral mastopexy*. For some women with breast cancer, such as those with a related genetic mutation that makes them "high risk," *contralateral prophylactic mastectomy* is an option. Invasive cancer is just as likely to develop in either breast when a woman has a LCIS in one breast. Therefore, the only way to stop breast cancer in this case is bilateral mastectomy. Women that are of high risk of invasive breast cancer often choose this option. Advantages include decreased anxiety, decreased risk of contralateral breast cancer (primarily when there is a family history of breast or ovarian cancer), improved survival (in patients with an inherited gene mutation or when cancer diagnosis occurs below age 50), and a reduced need for excessive follow-up imaging procedures. Disadvantages include a nearly doubled increase in surgical complications. Instead of contralateral prophylactic mastectomy, close surveillance is a good alternative.

After mastectomy, radiation therapy is required if the primary tumor is 5 cm or larger, and any axillary lymph nodes are involved. Radiation greatly reduces local recurrences on the chest wall and in regional lymph nodes. It also improves overall survival. If the patient is older than 70 and has early ER + breast cancer, there may be no benefit from addition radiation therapy to lumpectomy plus tamoxifen. Radiation does not greatly decrease rates of mastectomy for local recurrence, development of distant metastases, and also does not increase survival rates. Adverse effects of radiation such as skin changes and fatigue are usually mild and transient. Late adverse effects are not common, but include brachial plexopathy, lymphedema, radiation pneumonitis, rib damage, cardiac toxicity, and secondary cancers. Newer radiation therapies target the radiation to the cancer with more precision, sparing the remainder of the breast from adverse effects.

For patients with LCIS, daily oral tamoxifen is often used. Raloxifene or an aromatase inhibitor is sometimes substituted for tamoxifen in postmenopausal women. With invasive breast cancer, chemotherapy is usually started quickly after surgery. If systemic chemotherapy is not needed, hormone therapy is usually started quickly after surgery, accompanied by radiation therapy, and continues for years. Recurrence in nearly all patients is prevented, and for some, survival is prolonged. Some oncologists believe these therapies are not needed for tumors of 0.5–1 cm in size without lymph node involvement – especially for postmenopausal patients – due to the already excellent prognosis. For tumors larger than 5 cm, adjuvant systemic therapy may be initiated prior to surgery. Regardless of the stage of the cancer, the relative risk reduction for recurrence and death, with chemotherapy or hormone therapy, is the same. The absolute benefit is increased for patients that have a greater risk of recurrence or death. For example, a 20% relative risk reduction causes a 10% recurrence rate to lower to 8%, while a 50% recurrence rate lowers to 40%. Adjuvant chemotherapy reduces annual relative risk of death by 25–35% for premenopausal patients. In postmenopausal patients, the reduction is 9–19%, and the absolute benefit for 10-year survival is much less.

With ER tumors, postmenopausal patients receive the greatest benefit from adjuvant chemotherapy. With ER + tumors, predictive genomic testing is becoming more common, to assess risks in primary breast cancer patients, and to determine if combination chemotherapy or hormone therapy on its own would be best. Prognostic tests often include the 21-gene recurrence score assay (based on Oncotype Dx), the Amsterdam 7-gene profile (MammaPrint), and the 50-gene risk of recurrence score (the PAM50 assay). Most American women with breast cancer have the ER +/PR +/HER- form, with negative axillary lymph nodes. Low or intermediate scores on the 21-gene recurrence score assay will predict similar survival rates with chemotherapy + hormone therapy, and with only hormone therapy. This means that for this group of patients, neoadjuvant chemotherapy may not be needed.

Combination chemotherapy is more effective than only using one drug. A dose-dense regimen, in which the time between doses is shorter than in standard regimens, is started, lasting for 4–6 months. A common regimen is called ACT (which combines doxorubicin [Adriamycin], cyclophosphamide [Cytoxan], and paclitaxel [Taxol]). All regimens cause various adverse effects, which generally include nausea, vomiting, fatigue, mucositis, alopecia, cardiotoxicity, myelosuppression, and thrombocytopenia. To reduce risks of fever and infection from chemotherapy, growth factors are often used, which stimulate the bone marrow. These include filgrastim and pegfilgrastim. Most chemotherapy regimens cause few long-term adverse effects. Deaths from infection or bleeding only occur in 0.2% of cases. Since there is no advantage over standard therapy, high-dose chemotherapy + bone marrow or stem cell transplantation should not be used.

When a tumor overexpresses HER2 (called HER2 +), anti-HER2 drugs such as pertuzumab or trastuzumab are indicated. These are humanized monoclonal antibodies. Adding trastuzumab to chemotherapy greatly improves results. This drug is usually given for one year, though the best duration of its use is not known. When the lymph nodes are also involved, pertuzumab is added, improving disease-free survival. However, both trastuzumab and pertuzumab can cause decreased cardiac ejection fraction, a serious adverse effect. Benefits from hormone therapy with raloxifene, tamoxifen, or aromatase inhibitors (AIs) are based on estrogen and progesterone receptor expression. Benefits are best when the tumor has expressed estrogen and progesterone receptors. Benefit is slightly less when there are only ERs, and minimal when there are only progesterone receptors. If neither receptor is present, there is no benefit in using raloxifene, tamoxifen, or AIs. Hormone therapy can replace chemotherapy in patients with ER tumors, especially if the patients are of low risk.

Tamoxifen competitively binds with ERs, and adjuvant use of this drug over five years lowers annual risks of death by approximately 25% in female patients of all ages regardless of axillary lymph node disease. Treatment over two years is not as effective. If the tumors have ERs, 10-year-long treatment prolongs survival and reduces recurrence risks compared with 5-year-long treatment. Tamoxifen can cause or worsen symptoms of menopause, yet lowers incidence of contralateral breast cancer. It also lowers serum cholesterol. Tamoxifen increases the bone density of postmenopausal women. It can reduce risks of fractures as well as ischemic heart disease. Unfortunately, tamoxifen greatly increases risks for endometrial cancer, with incidence being 1% in postmenopausal use after five years. If this group of patients experiences any spotting or bleeding, there must be an evaluation of endometrial cancer. However, improved survival rates greatly outweigh any increased risk of death from endometrial cancer. There is also an increased risk of thromboembolism.

In postmenopausal women, AIs such as anastrozole, exemestane, and letrozole block peripheral estrogen production. These drugs are more effective than tamoxifen. Today, they are preferred for postmenopsual patients with early-stage hormone-receptor-positive breast cancer. After tamoxifen treatments are completed, letrozole may be used in postmenopsual women. The best duration of therapy with AIs is not proven. In a recent trial, treatment that was extended to 10 years gave a lower rate of breast cancer recurrence, and better rates of disease-free survival. There was no change in overall survival however, and with extended treatment, a higher rate of osteoporosis and fractures. Raloxifene is not used for treatment, but is indicated for prevention.

An immediate assessment is needed if there is any indication of metastases. Treatment can increase median survival by six months or more. Though chemotherapy is relatively toxic, it can relieve symptoms and improve quality of life, so treatment decisions are highly individualized. Chosen therapies are based on four factors: the tumor's hormone-receptor status, length of the disease-free interval between remission to signs of metastases, the number of metastatic sites and which organs are affected, and whether the patient is pre- or postmenopausal. For symptomatic metastatic disease, systemic chemotherapy or hormone therapy is usually indicated. At first, systemic therapy is given for multiple metastatic sites outside the CNS. If there are no symptoms of metastasis, treatment is not proven to greatly increase survival, yet often reduces the quality of life.

Any patient with ER-positive tumors, disease-free intervals of over two years, and with disease that is not soon to be life-threatening, hormone therapy is preferred. Tamoxifen is often used initially for premenopausal women. Alternatives include ovarian ablation via surgery, use of a luteinizing-releasing hormone agonist such as buserelin, goserelin, or leuprolide, and radiation therapy. Sometimes, ovarian ablation is combined with an aromatase inhibitor or tamoxifen. For postmenopausal women, AIs are becoming the primary hormone therapy. If the cancer responds initially, yet progresses over months or years, other hormonal therapies may be used sequentially until they become no longer effective. These include progestins and the antiestrogen called *fulvestrant*.

Chemotherapy drugs with the highest effects include capecitabine, doxorubicin of various formulations, gemcitabine, vinorelbine, and the taxanes called docetaxel and paclitaxel. Drug combinations have better response rates than single drugs. However, toxicity is increased, and survival is not improved. As a result, single drugs may be used in a sequence instead of concurrently. For tumors overexpressing HER2, and anti-HER2 drugs such as pertuzumab or trastuzumab are used, to treat and control visceral metastatic sites. Trastuzumab may be used alone, or combined with hormone therapy, chemotherapy, or pertuzumab. Trastuzumab with chemotherapy and pertuzumab impedes growth of HER2 + metastatic breast cancer, while increasing survival more than when trastuzumab is used with chemotherapy. Tyrosine kinase inhibitors include lapatinib and neratinib. They are becoming more popular for use with HER2 + tumors. For symptomatic bone lesions or local skin recurrences that are not likely to be well treated with surgery, only radiation therapy may be used. It is the most effective therapy for brain metastases, and can provide long-term control. For stable metastatic breast cancer, palliative mastectomy may be an option. Intravenous bisphosphonates such as pamidronate and zoledronate reduce bone pain and bone loss. They also prevent or delay skeletal complications from bone metastases. Approximately 10% of patients with bone metastases will develop hypercalcemia. This is also treated with IV bisphosphonates.

Near the end of a breast cancer patient's life, further treatments are unlikely to prolong survival. Palliation often becomes the most important goal. Cancer pain can be controlled with opioid analgesics, and symptoms such as breathing difficulty, nausea, and constipation must also be treated. The patient should be offered psychological and spiritual counseling. For those with metastatic breast cancer, there should be counseling about updating wills, and preparing advance directives that indicate which types of care are wanted in case the patient loses the ability to make such decisions.

Prevention and Early Detection

Prevention of breast cancer basically involves lifestyle modification, chemoprevention, and surgical prevention. Lifestyle modification involves changes in behavior – adequate physical activity and exercise to avoid obesity, a healthy diet, smoking cessation, and alcohol reduction. Chemoprevention has involved two classes of drugs: the selective estrogen-receptor modulators (SERMs) and the AIs. The SERMs include raloxifene and tamoxifen, while the AIs include arimidex and exemestane. Tamoxifen decreases the incidence of breast cancer by 49%, and raloxifene is just as effective, but for postmenopausal women. Unfortunately, adverse effects that include endometrial cancer, blood clot formation, and strokes limit the use of SERMs. The AIs are only used for postmenopausal women, but have had greater success than the SERMs, with less severe adverse effects such as muscle pain, joint pain, and osteoporosis. Surgical prevention involves removal of non-affected organs as a preventive measure against breast cancer. It is considered for high-risk patients, and includes prophylactic/risk-reducing mastectomy and salpingo-oophorectomy. The prophylactic mastectomy can reduce the risk of breast cancer development by 95%, and the prophylactic salpingo-oophorectomy can reduce risks by about 50%.

Screening for the early detection of breast cancer is essential for all women. Monthly self-breast examination is required for the evidence of change that could indicate a malignant mass. There is disagreement as to patient age for the first screening procedure (mammography), and how often it should be performed. Screening is with digital and three-dimensional mammography, clinical breast examination, and MRI if the patient is of high risk. With mammography, both breasts receive low-dose X-rays in oblique and craniocaudal views. Mammography is most accurate for older women. This is because fibroglandular breast tissue is usually replaced with fatty tissue due to aging. This fatty tissue is easier to distinguish from abnormal tissue. In women with dense breast tissue, mammography is not as sensitive. In certain states, patients must be informed that they have dense breast tissue when it is discovered during mammography.

For women with an average risk of breast cancer, screening mammography generally begins at age 40, 45, or 50. It is repeated annually or every two years until age 75, or when the life expectancy of the patient is less than 10 years. Each patient should be educated about her individual risk of breast cancer, and asked about preferred testing methods. A woman is considered to be at average risk if her lifetime breast cancer risk is lower than 15%. Mammography accuracy, risks, and costs must all be discussed. This is partly because there is an 85–90% false-positive rate for breast cancer during screening mammography. False-negative results may be higher than 15%. Often, benign cysts or fibroadenomas cause false-positives. Accuracy is based on the type of procedure and the mammographer's experience.

Breast tomosynthesis, performed with digital mammography, slightly increases rates of cancer detection, and lowers the rate of repeated imaging. It is useful for women with dense breast tissue, but exposes patients to nearly two times the radiation as standard mammography. Radiation exposure has cumulative effects upon cancer risk. Costs include the imaging procedure, plus the diagnostic tests required for evaluation of false-positive results.

Prognosis

Over time, the prognosis for breast cancer is based on tumor staging. The number and location of affected lymph nodes determines the patient's *nodal status*. It is related with disease-free and overall survival more than any other prognostic factor. According to the National Cancer Institute's Surveillance, Epidemiology, and End Results (SEER) Program, the patient's five-year survival rate is based on cancer stage as follows:

- 98.8% – Localized – confined to the primary site
- 85.5% – Regional – confined to the regional lymph nodes
- 54.4% – Unknown – when these determinations are not clear
- 27.4% – Metastasized to distant sites (see Figure 9.4)

A worsened prognosis is given for a variety of factors. It is worse if the patient is diagnosed during the 20s or 30s, than when diagnosed during middle age. Larger breast tumors are more often lymph node-positive. However, regardless of nodal status, larger breast tumors have a worsened prognosis. Patients with poorly differentiated tumors also have a worsened prognosis. For patients with ER + tumors, the prognosis is improved, and hormone therapy is often beneficial. Those with progesterone receptors on tumors may also have an improved prognosis. It

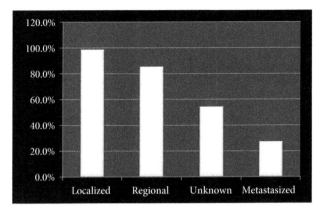

Figure 9.4 Five-year survival rates for breast cancer, based on stage.

is uncertain whether having both estrogen and progesterone receptors on a tumor gives a better prognosis than having only one of these receptors.

More aggressive tumor cells often are present when the HER2 gene is amplified and HER2 is overexpressed. The overexpression of HER2 worsens prognosis on its own, and is linked to high histologic grade ER tumors, as well as increased proliferation, and larger tumor size. Patients with the BRCA1 mutation have a worse prognosis than patients with sporadic tumors. This may be because they have a larger proportion of high-grade hormone-receptor-negative cancers. With the BRCA1 or BRCA2 mutations, the risk of another cancer in the remaining breast tissue may be increased to as high as 40%.

Significant Point

Regular mammography can lower the risk of dying from breast cancer. The Centers for Disease Control and Prevention (CDC) offer free and low-cost mammography for qualifying women. Women may qualify if they have no insurance, or their insurance does not cover screening mammograms. Other qualifications include a yearly income at or below 250% of the federal poverty level, being 40–64 years of age, and being in the high-risk group of patients.

Clinical Case

1. Which type of tumors are most commonly seen in breast cancer?
2. What is the importance of HER-2 in relation to breast cancer?
3. Which chemotherapy regimen is extremely common for breast cancer patients?

A 46-year-old woman had her first screening mammogram, which revealed a dense lesion in her left breast. She had previously felt the lesion during self-examination, as well as a lump in her left armpit. Ultrasound revealed a suspicious mass of 15 mm in diameter in the breast, and an axillary mass of 35 mm in diameter. The patient was referred to a surgical oncologist. Ultrasound-guided core biopsies were performed. The lesions were grade III infiltrating ductal carcinomas, estrogen and progesterone receptor negative, and HER-2 positive. A positron emission tomography (PET) scan revealed tumors isolated in the breast and axilla. There were no satellite lesions, and the right breast was normal. It was determined that the patient was an ideal candidate for adjuvant chemotherapy, given systemically. A group of diverse professionals discussed the case and agreed the treatment course would be systemic chemotherapy followed by surgery and postoperative radiation therapy. The chemotherapy resolved all palpable disease. The patient was given the choice of breast-conserving lumpectomy or mastectomy, and she chose mastectomy. An SLNB was also performed. There was no residual carcinoma in the breast or lymph nodes. Radiation therapy was completed, and breast reconstruction was scheduled. The patient survived without recurrence.

Answers:

1. **The majority of breast cancers are epithelial tumors, arising from cells that line ducts or lobules. Less often, they are nonepithelial cancers of the supporting stroma – classified as angiosarcomas, phyllodes tumors, or primary stromal sarcomas.**
2. **Human epidermal growth factor receptor 2 (HER2, also known as HER2/neu or ErbB2) is a cellular receptor. If present in a breast cancer patient, it is linked to a worsened outlook, regardless of cancer staging. The HER2 receptors are overexpressed in about 20% of patients with breast cancer.**
3. **Combination chemotherapy for breast cancer patients that is very common is called ACT, which combines Adriamycin with Cytoxan, and Taxol.**

Benign Ovarian Masses

Benign ovarian masses may be functional cysts or tumors. The majority of these masses are asymptomatic, and treatment is based on whether the patient intends to have children or not, or is already postmenopausal. The two types of functional cysts are *follicular*, developing from graafian follicles, and *corpus luteum* cysts that can hemorrhage into the cyst cavity. This distends the ovarian capsule, or ruptures into the peritoneum. The majority of functional cysts are smaller than 1.5 cm in diameter, but they rarely can be larger than 5 cm. These cysts usually resolve without treatment in days to weeks, and they are not common after menopause. Benign ovarian cysts are the fourth leading diagnosis in patients hospitalized for gynecological reasons.

Polycystic ovary syndrome is usually of clinical definition and is not based on ovarian cysts being present. The ovaries usually contain many follicular cysts of 2–6 mm in size. Sometimes, there are larger cysts, up to 10 cm in size, with **atretic cells**. Benign ovarian tumors are usually slow-growing, and rarely become malignant. *Benign cystic teratomas* consist mostly of **ectodermal** tissue, but are derived from all three germ cell layers. *Fibromas* are slow-growing tumors, usually less than 7 cm in diameter. *Cystadenomas* are usually mucinous or serous.

Epidemiology

The prevalence of benign ovarian cysts ranges between 8% and 18% of premenopausal and postmenopausal women. Benign cysts make up 70% of all ovarian cysts, functional cysts make up 24%, and malignant cysts make up only 6% (see Figure 9.5) In the United States, 5–10% of women undergo surgical exploration for ovarian cysts, which usually are not malignant. The overall incidence of malignancy is 1 in 1,000 in premenopausal women, and 3 in 1,000 by the age of 50. Benign ovarian *tumors* occur in 30% of women with regular menses and 50% of women with irregular menses. They mostly occur in premenopausal women and are uncommon in premenarchal and postmenopausal women. Benign neoplastic cystic tumors of germ cell origin are most common in younger women, accounting for 15–20% of all ovarian neoplasms. Benign ovarian cysts and tumors are most common during a woman's reproductive years, and mostly when these years begin and when they end – at puberty and menopause. They also occur in fetal development and childhood, but

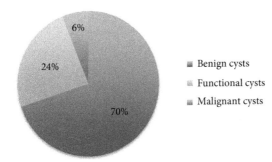

Figure 9.5 Percentages of different types of ovarian cysts.

much less often. Global epidemiology of benign ovarian masses is not well documented, but generally believed to be very similar to the statistics from the United States.

Etiology and Risk Factors

Benign ovarian enlargement in an ovulating woman is often caused by follicular and corpus luteum cysts, which are functional since they develop from variations of normal physiology. Both types of cysts are usually unilateral. The causes of endometrial polyps are usually related to estrogen stimulation. They may result from obesity, hypertension, anovulatory cycles, and use of tamoxifen.

Clinical Manifestations

The majority of functional cysts and benign ovarian tumors are asymptomatic. However, menstrual abnormalities are reported. Pain or signs of peritonitis may occur from hemorrhagic corpus luteum cysts – especially if they rupture. Rarely, severe abdominal pain is caused by **adnexal torsion** of a mass or cyst that is usually larger than 4 cm. Some patients become nauseous, develop a fever, or experience urinary urgency. Fibromas may be accompanied by ascites, or less often by pleural effusion. Follicular cysts cause bloating, heavy or irregular menses, and swelling and tenderness of the breasts. They can vary in size and symptoms between episodes, and often recur. Symptoms of corpus luteum cysts include slight pelvic pain, amenorrhea, and delayed menstruation. Bleeding that is irregular or heavier than normal may follow this. A rupture only happens occasionally, but can cause massive bleeding and extreme pain. This may indicate a need for immediate surgery. In nonpregnant women, these cysts usually regress spontaneously. With *ovarian torsion*, the patient develops acute and severe unilateral abdominal or pelvic pain.

Pathology

Benign ovarian cysts form when a follicle or follicles are stimulated, with no dominant follicle developing and becoming mature. There are about 120 follicles per month that are stimulated, but normally, only one ovulates a mature ovum. Follicles normally respond to hormonal signals from the pituitary gland during the early follicular phase of the menstrual cycle. Follicle-stimulating hormone (FSH) from the pituitary matures ovarian follicles. As they enlarge, granulosa cells inside them multiply, secreting estradiol. When a dominant follicle forms, increased levels of estradiol are secreted from it, stimulating a surge in luteinizing hormone (LH) from the pituitary. During the follicular phase, a small ovarian cyst is normal. The surge of LH stimulates the follicle, and it ruptures, releasing the ova and changing the granulosa cells of the dominant follicle into the corpus luteum. Normally, the corpus luteum becomes vascularized and secretes progesterone, which stops the development of other follicles, in both ovaries, during this cycle. LH, enzymes, and prostaglandins trigger follicular rupture and release of the ovum.

Follicular cysts may develop when the dominant follicle does not rupture, or nondominant follicles do not regress. The hypothalamus may not receive or send a strong message that increases FSH, resulting in a dominant follicle simply not developing or maturing. The hypothalamus monitors estradiol and progesterone in the blood. When FSH is low, estradiol does not increase to an amount needed to stimulate LH. When progesterone is not produced, the hypothalamus releases GnRH, increasing the FSH level. The FSH continually stimulates follicles to mature. Granulosa cells increase in size, and it is believed that estradiol increases. This is an abnormal cycle that continually stimulates the size of follicles, causing follicular cysts to develop. After a few cycles, when hormone levels become regular and progesterone levels are restored, the cysts are usually absorbed, or they regress. Most cysts are filled with fluid. The risk of malignancy is higher when an ovarian cyst is relatively solid.

Granulosa cells that remain after ovulation usually form corpus luteum cysts. They are extremely vascularized and limited in size. Abnormal or hemorrhagic cysts may develop from hormonal imbalances with low LH and progesterone levels. The corpus luteum then does not develop sufficiently. Sometimes, large cysts rupture, resulting in hemorrhage. Corpus luteum cysts are less common than follicular cysts, but they usually cause more systems, especially after rupturing. These cysts are normal during the first trimester of pregnancy, until the placenta is formed.

Dermoid cysts are actually teratomas of the ovaries. They contain components of all three germ layers, and are quite common. Dermoid cysts may contain mature tissues such as hair, skin, muscle fibers, sebaceous and sweat glands, bone, and cartilage. They are usually asymptomatic and only found incidentally during pelvic examination. However, since dermoid cysts have a potential to become malignant, they must be carefully evaluated for surgical removal. Complications of various ovarian cysts and tumors include *torsion of the ovary*, which can occur at any age. Large cysts can cause an ovary to twist on its ligaments. This event stops the blood supply and results in extreme pain. Though rare, ovarian torsion is a gynecologic emergency.

Diagnosis

Benign ovarian masses are usually found incidentally, but can be indicated by signs and symptoms. A pregnancy test is given so that an ectopic pregnancy may be excluded. Diagnosis is usually confirmed by **transvaginal ultrasound**. Masses that have radiographic features of cancer must be assessed by a specialist, and excised. These features include cystic or solid components, multiocular features, irregular shapes, and surface **excrescences**. Tumor marker tests are performed when a mass must be excised, or if ovarian cancer is thought to be present. There are commercially available tests for five tumor markers that help determine whether surgery is needed. These tumor markers include *apolipoprotein A-1, beta-2 microglobulin, cancer antigen* (CA) *125-II, prealbumin*, and *transferrin*. The best use of tumor markers is to monitor treatment responses however, and they are not highly sensitive to screening. They are also not highly specific or predictive.

Treatment

Often, functional ovarian cysts less than 5 cm in diameter resolve on their own. This can be documented by using serial ultrasound. If the patient is asymptomatic, within reproductive age, and has simple, thin-walled cystic adnexal masses of 5–8 cm that are usually follicular and lack signs of cancer, repeated ultrasound is effective. Benign tumors, however, require treatment. Any mass with radiographic features of cancer is excised via laparotomy or via a laparoscopic procedure. The goal is to preserve the ovaries, often via cystectomy. However, oophorectomy is performed if any of the following are present:

- Cystadenomas
- Cystic teratomas larger than 10 cm
- Cysts that cannot be surgically removed without also removing the ovary
- Fibromas that cannot be removed via cystectomy
- Cysts larger than 5 cm that are found in postmenopausal women

Follicular cysts can be treated with oral contraceptives since they block the hypothalamic–pituitary–gonadal (HPG) axis, which helps to normalize the ovary. For corpus luteum cysts that become large, painful, or hemorrhagic, oral contraceptives help suppress ovarian function, preventing additional cysts from forming. Dermoid cysts may be surgically removed but require careful evaluation since they can become malignant. Ovarian torsion is also treated surgically.

Prevention and Early Detection

There is no way to prevent benign ovarian masses from developing. However, regular pelvic examinations help in the early detection of changes in the ovaries. Women should be instructed about noticing any changes in their monthly cycles. These include unusual symptoms, especially if they persist for more than a few cycles.

Prognosis

Prognosis of benign ovarian masses is variable, based on the type and size of the mass, any complications, and the age of the patient. Most small ovarian masses have a good prognosis because they self-resolve. For ovarian torsion, prognosis is mixed. If surgery is done promptly, the tissues will usually remain viable, and pregnancy is still possible. Prognosis of surgically removed cysts depends on the histology.

Clinical Case

1. What is the description and the characteristics of dermoid cysts?
2. When is oophorectomy performed in regard to ovarian cysts?
3. What is the pathology involved in the development of ovarian cysts?

A 35-year-old woman was taken by her husband to the emergency department because of acute right lower quadrant and right flank pain, accompanied by nausea. The patient also had a fever and urinary urgency. After physical examination revealed tenderness in the patient's abdomen, a CT scan was ordered, which revealed a 5 cm right ovarian mass that strongly appeared to be a dermoid cyst. A laparoscopic right ovarian cystectomy was performed, with no complications. Postoperative diagnosis was consistent with a dermoid cyst, and gross inspection was consistent with a pathological diagnosis of a mature teratoma. There were no signs of malignancy, and the patient was discharged two days later.

Answers:

1. **Dermoid cysts are actually teratomas of the ovaries. They contain components of all three germ layers, and are quite common. Dermoid cysts may contain mature tissues such as hair, skin, muscle fibers, sebaceous and sweat glands, bone, and cartilage. They are usually asymptomatic and only found incidentally during pelvic examination. However, since dermoid cysts have a potential to become malignant, they must be carefully evaluated for surgical removal.**
2. **Oophorectomy is performed if there are cystadenomas, cystic teratomas larger than 10 cm, cysts that cannot be surgically removed without also removing the ovary, fibromas that cannot be removed via cystectomy, or if there are cysts larger than 5 cm and the patient is postmenopausal.**
3. **Benign ovarian cysts form when a follicle or follicles are stimulated, with no dominant follicle developing and becoming mature. During the follicular phase, a small ovarian cyst is normal. Follicular cysts may develop when the dominant follicle does not rupture, or nondominant follicles do not regress. With continuous stimulation of follicle size, follicular cysts develop. Corpus luteum cysts usually form from granulosa cells that remain after ovulation.**

Ovarian Cancer

Ovarian cancer is a serious form of cancer because it is often advanced upon diagnosis, and therefore, highly fatal. In fact, ovarian cancer is the most lethal type of gynecologic cancer. Symptoms are often nonspecific even when it has become advanced. Types of ovarian cancer include: clear cell carcinomas, endometrioid carcinomas, mucinous carcinomas, serous cystadenocarcinomas, transitional cell carcinomas, dysgerminomas, embryonal carcinomas, immature teratomas, and polyembryomas. Ovarian germ cell cancer is predisposed by **XY gonadal dysgenesis**. The various types of ovarian cancers are further summarized in Table 9.2.

Epidemiology

Overall, the various forms of ovarian cancer comprise the second most common gynecological cancer in the United States. Approximately 1 of 70 women develop some form of ovarian cancer, which is the fifth leading cause of female cancer-related deaths, totaling about 22,000 new cases annually, and causing 14,000 deaths. Incidence is the highest in developed countries such as the United States. Older women are mostly affected, especially those that are perimenopausal or postmenopausal. In the United States, rates of ovarian cancer are the highest in Caucasians (13.1 cases out of every 100,000 women), followed by Native Americans (10.2 cases), Hispanic Americans (9.4 cases), African Americans (9 cases), and Asians/Pacific Islanders (8.4 cases).

Ovarian cancer is the 18th most common cancer worldwide, and the 8th most common female cancer. According to the World Ovarian Cancer Atlas in 2020, an average of 7 women per 100,000 develop the disease annually, with 3 cases out of 100,000 being fatal. The area of the world with the highest incidence is Asia (154,000 cases), followed by Europe (68,000),

Table 9.2 Types of ovarian cancers.

Site of origination	Types
Epithelium	Brenner tumor
	Clear cell carcinoma
	Endometrioid carcinoma
	Mucinous carcinoma
	Serous cystadenocarcinoma (the most common)
	Transitional cell carcinoma
	Unclassified carcinoma
Primary germ cells	Choriocarcinoma
	Dysgerminoma
	Embryonal carcinoma
	Endodermal sinus tumor
	Immature teratoma
	Polyembryoma
Sex cord and stromal cells	Granulosa-theca cell tumor
	Sertoli–Leydig cell tumor
Metastases	Breast cancer
	Cancer of the gastrointestinal tract

North America (28,000), Latin America and Caribbean (24,000), Africa (22,000), and the Oceanic areas (2,200). The actual countries with the largest number of ovarian cancer cases are China, India, the United States, Russian Federation, Indonesia, Japan, Germany, Brazil, United Kingdom, Poland, the Philippines, Italy, Mexico, Ukraine, and Pakistan (see Figure 9.6).

Etiology and Risk Factors

The causes of ovarian cancer are linked to genetic mutations. In 14–18% of patients with high-grade serous tumors, there are identified germline alterations of the BRCA1 and BRCA2 genes. About 3% have somatic BRCA mutations or inactivation because of methylation. In about 50% of high-grade patients, there is a deficiency of homologous recombination, in which is involved repair of DNA damage and replication. Women with BRCA1 mutations have a 20–40% risk of ovarian cancers, and the BRCA2 mutations carry a lower risk. These mutations are most common in Ashkenazi Jews.

Risk factors for the various forms of ovarian cancer are increased by: history of the disease in a first-degree relative, never having had children or delays in childbearing, early menarche, delayed menopause, and a personal or family history of endometrial, breast, or colon cancer. Using oral contraceptives decreases risks.

Clinical Manifestations

Usually, early ovarian cancer is asymptomatic. There may be an incidental discovery of an adnexal mass that is usually fixed, irregular, and solid. Diffuse nodularity is often found during pelvic and rectovaginal examinations. Sometimes there is severe abdominal pain because of ovarian mass torsion. When ovarian cancer is advanced, there are usually nonspecific symptoms. These include bloating, dyspepsia, early satiety, backache, and gas pains. Over time, anemia, pelvic pain, abdominal swelling from ovarian enlargement or ascites, and **cachexia** usually develop. Germ cell tumors and stromal tumors may cause functional effects such as feminization, hyperthyroidism, and virilization.

Pathology

Serous tumors that are high grade may be subclassified as epithelial ovarian, fallopian tube, and peritoneal carcinomas. They behave

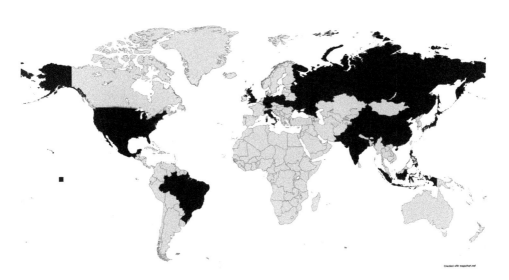

Figure 9.6 Countries with the highest rates of ovarian cancer.

similarly and require treatment. The majority of ovarian tumors develop from epithelial cells. Germ cell tumors usually occur in women under the age of 30. The high-grade and low-grade serous tumors are epithelial ovarian carcinomas, with the high-grade form making up over 70% of all epithelial carcinomas. Low-grade serous ovarian cancers usually appear as if they are benign, with slow cell growth, insubstantial cell and nucleus changes, and cell uniformity. The other types of epithelial ovarian carcinomas include the endometrioid, clear cell, and mucinous types. The pathology of ovarian cancer involves spreading by direct extension, peritoneal seeding, lymphatic dissemination to the pelvis and around the aorta, and uncommonly, via hematogenous spread to the liver or lungs.

The epithelial subtype of ovarian carcinomas is most common, usually originating from the distal portion of the fallopian tubes or because of endometriosis. Therefore, not all ovarian cancers originate within the ovaries. The high-grade epithelial ovarian cancers are extremely aggressive and grow quickly. They are genetically unstable and poorly differentiated. There is less overall survival, and they are usually discovered at later stages, with extensive metastasis. Precursor lesions often develop in the fallopian tubes. The tumors have TP53 mutations or gene loss. Lesions located at the distal fallopian tubes are either related to, or may be precursors of, high-grade serous ovarian cancer.

Endometrioid ovarian cancers are believed to develop from the uterine endometrium as well as from endometriosis that reaches the ovaries via retrograde flow, through the fallopian tubes. The clear cell subtype is likely to be high grade when found, with a very poor outlook. Like endometrioid tumors, the clear cell carcinomas have microsatellite instability. The mucinous subtype usually grows slowly and is unilateral. They are often large when they are discovered. Histology includes extremely well-differentiated cells, with low cellular division activity and nuclei that appear normal.

The nonepithelial subtype includes germ cell and sex cord stromal tumors. Germ cell tumors are exemplified by **dysgerminomas**, while sex cord stromal tumors include granulosa, Sertoli–Leydig cell tumors, sarcomas, and lipoid tumors. Only a small percentage of nonepithelial tumors become malignant. These tumors often are successfully treated in comparison with epithelial ovarian tumors.

Diagnosis

For suspected early ovarian cancer, ultrasound is used for diagnosis. For suspected advanced cancer, CT or MRI is used. Ovarian cancer is suspected if any of the following are present:

- Changes in bowel habits
- Unexplained abdominal pain, adnexal masses, or abdominal bloating
- Unintended weight loss

Ovarian masses are most likely to be cancer in older patients. In young woman, benign functional cysts may be similar to functional germ cell tumors or stromal tumors. Ovarian cancer is usually indicated by a pelvic mass accompanied with ascites. However, this sometimes indicates **Meigs syndrome**, which combines a right hydrothorax with a benign fibroma accompanied by ascites.

Biopsies are not usually recommended, except for patients that are not candidates for surgery. Needle biopsies are used for masses, and needle aspiration is used for ascitic fluid. Staging of ovarian cancer during surgery is summarized in Table 9.3.

When early-stage ovarian cancer is suspected, laparoscopy or robotic-assisted laparoscopic surgery may be done. Without these techniques, an abdominal midline incision

Table 9.3 Surgical staging for ovarian cancer (as well as fallopian tube and peritoneal cancer).

Stage	Description
I	Tumor only in the ovaries or fallopian tubes
IA	Tumor in one ovary (intact capsule) or fallopian tube surface; no malignant cells in peritoneal washings or ascitic fluid
IB	Tumor in one or both ovaries (intact capsule) or fallopian tubes; no tumor on external surface of ovary or fallopian tube; no malignant cells in peritoneal washings or ascitic fluid
IC	Tumor in one or both ovaries or fallopian tubes plus any of the following: IC1 (surgical spill), IC2 (capsule ruptured prior to surgery, or tumor on surface of ovary or fallopian tube), IC3 (malignant cells in peritoneal washings or ascitic fluid)
II	Tumor in one or both ovaries or fallopian tubes, with pelvic extension below pelvic brim, or primary peritoneal cancer
IIA	Extension, implants, or both, on uterus, fallopian tubes, ovaries, or all
IIB	Extension, implants, or both, on other pelvic intraperitoneal tissues
III	Tumor in one or both ovaries or fallopian tubes, or primary peritoneal cancer with microscopically confirmed peritoneal metastases outside pelvis, and/or metastasis to retroperitoneal lymph nodes
IIIA	Positive retroperitoneal lymph nodes, with or without microscopic peritoneal metastases extending beyond pelvis: IIIA1 (positive retroperitoneal lymph nodes only that are proven by histology), IIIA1I (metastasis is 10 mm or smaller in the largest dimension), IIIA1II (metastasis is larger than 10 mm in the largest dimension, IIIA2 (microscopic extrapelvic peritoneal involvement, with or without positive retroperitoneal lymph nodes)
IIIB	Macroscopic peritoneal metastases extending beyond pelvis of 2 cm or less in the largest dimension, with or without positive retroperitoneal lymph nodes
IIIC	Macroscopic peritoneal metastases extending beyond pelvis of larger than 2 cm in the largest dimension, with or without metastasis to retroperitoneal lymph nodes; this includes extension to the capsule of liver and spleen without any parenchymal involvement
IV	Distant metastases
IVA	Pleural effusion and positive cytology
IVB	Liver or splenic parenchymal metastasis, and/or metastases to extra-abdominal organs, including lymph nodes outside abdominal cavity or inguinal lymph nodes, and/or transmural disease of the intestine

must be made, allowing access to the upper abdomen. There is inspection and palpation of peritoneal surfaces, abdominal and pelvic viscera, and *hemidiaphragms*. Pelvic washings, **abdominal gutters**, and diaphragmatic recesses are taken, plus multiple biopsies of the peritoneum of the abdomen and the central and lateral pelvis are done. The **infracolic omentum** is removed for early-stage cancer. The para-aortic and pelvic lymph nodes are sampled. A significant tumor marker, such as cancer antigen 125, is helpful.

Treatment

For most ovarian cancers, hysterectomy and bilateral salpingo-oophorectomy are usually indicated. This is true except for younger women with stage I nonepithelial or low-grade unilateral epithelial ovarian cancer. When the unaffected ovary and the uterus are left intact, fertility can be preserved. The preferred first treatment for stage III or IV ovarian cancer is primary surgical cytoreduction, followed by systemic chemotherapy. Neoadjuvant chemotherapy is used if the patient is not a surgical candidate, due to the cancer's location and volume, or because of comorbid conditions. Surgery is either not indicated or can be deferred if any of the following are present:

- Diffuse mesenteric disease
- Evidence of parenchymal or pleural lung disease
- Lymphadenopathy in the porta hepatis
- Multiple liver metastases
- Suprarenal para-aortic lymph nodes

For these patients, neoadjuvant chemotherapy, such as carboplatin plus paclitaxel, is used. Surgery may be possible after initial chemotherapy. During hysterectomy and bilateral salpingo-oophorectomy, all visibly affected tissue is removed if possible. For epithelial ovarian cancers, there is less response to chemotherapies, due to their genetic makeup, and a slower rate of cellular division. First-line chemotherapies for high-grade epithelial, fallopian, and peritoneal carcinoma combine carboplatin or cisplatin with paclitaxel. It can be IV or by intraperitoneal instillation. High-grade epithelial ovarian carcinoma usually responds well. Chemotherapies for nonepithelial ovarian carcinomas include bleomycin, cisplatin, and etoposide.

For epithelial ovarian cancers, immune therapy is a new area of focus. Certain immune cells are linked to increased progression-free survival. They can be induced via chemotherapy to increase sensitivity to, recognition of, and attack upon tumor cells. This makes chemotherapies more effective. When cytotoxic T cells invade ovarian tumors, disease progression is delayed, and overall survival is improved.

Prevention and Early Detection

There is no preventive screening test for ovarian cancer. Women with BRCA mutations or other known hereditary risks are followed closely. The CA 125 marker has up to 99.9% specificity for ovarian cancer, but only 71% sensitivity. It has a

low positive predictive value. Therefore, CA 125 is not used to screen asymptomatic women of average risk. Using CA 125 plus ultrasound can detect certain cases of ovarian cancer, but outcomes are not improved, even in the high-risk subgroup. Hereditary cancer syndromes must be considered for all patients with ovarian, fallopian tube, or peritoneal cancers. A genetic risk evaluation is performed. Detailed personal and family histories of all types of cancers are obtained to identify patients most likely to have a hereditary cancer syndrome, such as those involving BRCA mutations, or **Lynch syndrome**.

Women are screened for BRCA abnormalities if their family history reveals any of these factors:

- Diagnosis of breast and ovarian cancer in one first-degree relative, if one of the cancers was diagnosed before age 50
- Diagnosis of ovarian cancer in a first-degree relative before age 40
- One case of breast cancer and one case of ovarian cancer in first- or second-degree relatives of the same lineage, if breast cancer was diagnosed before age 40, or if ovarian cancer was diagnosed before age 50
- Two cases of ovarian cancer in first- and second-degree relatives of the same lineage
- Two cases of breast cancer and one case of ovarian cancer in first- or second-degree relatives of the same lineage
- Two cases of breast cancer in first- or second-degree relatives of the same lineage, if both cases were diagnosed before age 50
- Two cases of breast cancer in first- or second-degree relatives of the same lineage, if one case was diagnosed before age 40

Prognosis

The outlook for ovarian cancer ranges from good to poor based on staging. For stage I, 90% of patients survive for five years. For stage II, this is 74%, and for stage III, it is 50%. Stage IV ovarian cancer patients have only 18% survival over five years (see Figure 9.7). The prognosis is worsened if the tumor grade is higher, or if surgery is

Figure 9.7 Five-year survival rates for ovarian cancer.

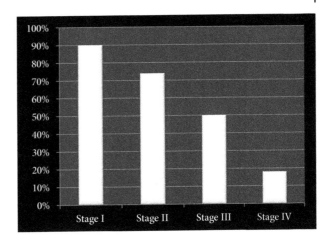

unable to remove all visibly diseased tissue. Then, prognosis is best when involved tissue can be reduced to less than 1 cm in diameter, or to a microscopically residual amount in cytoreductive surgery. Recurrence is about 70% for stage III and IV ovarian cancer.

Significant Point

Most ovarian cancers begin in the cells lining the ovaries, and fallopian tubes. About 50% of women that are diagnosed are 63 years old or more. Risks can be lowered by having a full-term pregnancy during peak childbearing years, breastfeeding, and by taking oral contraceptives. The best ways to detect ovarian cancer early is to get recommended screenings such as pelvic exams, transvaginal ultrasound, and a CA 125 blood test.

Clinical Case

1. How common is ovarian cancer?
2. What are the nonspecific symptoms of advanced ovarian cancer?
3. What is the description of stage IIIc ovarian cancer?

A 64-year-old woman went to her physician because of abdominal distention, fatigue, nausea, and vomiting. Physical examination revealed ascites. A CT scan showed a bulky adnexal mass. Paracentesis confirmed the mass to be an adenocarcinoma, consistent with a diagnosis of primary ovarian cancer. The patient's hemoglobin level was 9.5 g/dL. Esophagogastroduodenoscopy revealed a benign ulcer at the gastroesophageal junction, and a colonoscopy found extensive diverticular disease. Ovarian cancer was diagnosed as stage IIIc, and the patient underwent debulking surgery. At this time, the patient received two units of transfused blood. Follow-up chemotherapy was with carboplatin + paclitaxel. Her hemoglobin level at discharge was 10.8 g/dL. Within 10 days, a follow-up appointment showed the hemoglobin to be at 8.5 g/dL. This signified quickly worsening anemia, indicating the need for additional blood transfusions. It was suspected that the patient's anemia could be caused by blood loss related to ovarian cancer, the ulcer or diverticulosis, impaired erythropoiesis because of vitamin or mineral deficiency, or chemotherapy.

Answers:

1. **Overall, the various forms of ovarian cancer comprise the second most common gynecological cancer in the**

United States. Approximately 1 or 70 women develop some form of ovarian cancer, which is the fifth leading cause of female cancer-related deaths. Incidence is the highest in developed countries such as the United States. Ovarian cancer is the 18th most common cancer worldwide, and the 8th most common female cancer.

2. The nonspecific symptoms of advanced ovarian cancer include bloating, dyspepsia, early satiety, backache, and gas pains. Over time, anemia, pelvic pain, abdominal swelling from ovarian enlargement or ascites, and cachexia usually develop.

3. Stage IIIc ovarian cancer is described as follows: macroscopic peritoneal metastases extending beyond the pelvis, larger than 2 cm in largest dimension, with or without metastasis to retroperitoneal lymph nodes; this include extension to capsule of liver and spleen without any parenchymal involvement.

Uterine Fibroids

Uterine fibroids are benign tumors that originate from smooth muscles. They are also referred to as *leiomyomas* and *myomas*. Uterine fibroids may cause pain and pressure in the pelvis and pregnancy complications. However, they usually remain small and insignificant, causing no symptoms. They are the most common benign tumors of the uterus.

Epidemiology

Uterine fibroids are the most common form of pelvic tumor, affecting approximately 70% of women, everywhere in the world. Prevalence increases in women aged 30–50, but decreases with menopause. Based on various populations and diagnostic methods,

incidence of uterine fibroids ranges from 217 to 3,745 cases per 100,000 women. About 50% of African American and Asian American women, and 25% of Caucasian women, will develop symptomatic uterine fibroids. Global statistics on uterine fibroids are not well documented.

Etiology and Risk Factors

The cause of uterine fibroids is unknown. However, their size is related to estrogen, progesterone, angiogenesis, **apoptosis**, and **growth factors**. Fibroids have tissue changes. They are sensitive to estrogen and progesterone, and have increased amounts of ERs. These lesions do not appear before menarche. Development is often linked with exposure to estrogen. In pregnant women, they may enlarge quickly, but often decrease in size after pregnancy ends. Risk factors for uterine fibroids include family history, having no children, obesity, polycystic ovary syndrome, diabetes mellitus, the African or Asian races, and hypertension.

Clinical Manifestations

Many uterine fibroids are small and asymptomatic. However, complications from these lesions are the primary reason for gynecologic hospitalizations. They can cause abnormal bleeding from the uterus, such as **menometrorrhagia** or **menorrhagia**. Submucosal bleeding can sometimes be severe, resulting in anemia. An enlarged fibroid and a pedunculated fibroid twisted can cause severe pressure and pain. Urinary frequency or urgency may be caused by bladder compression. Constipation and other intestinal symptoms can be caused by intestinal compression. Chances for a woman becoming infertile can be increased. When a woman is pregnant and fibroids are present, there may be premature contractions, abnormal fetal presentation, or the requirement for a cesarean delivery. Recurrent spontaneous abortions and postpartum hemorrhage can also happen.

Pathology

Uterine fibroids are more common in women with a high body mass index. Most are *subserosal*, followed in occurrence by **intramural** and *submucosal* fibroids. Subserosal fibroids are under the outer uterine surface. Intramural fibroids are within the uterine wall. Submucosal fibroids are under the lining of the uterus. Sometimes fibroids develop in the broad ligaments and are called **intraligamentous fibroids**. They may also develop in the cervix or fallopian tubes. Some fibroids are *pedunculated*, meaning that they grow on a stalk.

Fibroids usually occur in multiple numbers, and each one develops from a single smooth muscle cell – meaning that they are monoclonal in origin. Figure 9.8 shows the various locations of uterine fibroids. Fibroids usually enlarge during a woman's reproductive years since they respond to estrogen. After menopause, they decrease in size. Fibroids can outgrow their supplies of blood and degenerate in various ways, becoming hyaline, calcific, **myxomatous**, cystic, fatty, necrotic, and usually only during pregnancy, reddened. Transformation into sarcomas only occurs in less than 1% of patients.

Diagnosis

Diagnosis of uterine fibroids often is made when bimanual pelvic examination finds an enlarged uterus that is irregular and mobile during palpation. Imaging studies confirm diagnosis and are usually required if the fibroids are new, have grown, are causing symptoms, or must be differentiated from ovarian masses and other abnormalities. Usually, transvaginal imaging or **sonohysterography** is done. In sonohysterography, saline is instilled inside the uterus, allowing the technician to better locate the fibroid. If these procedures are inconclusive, MRI is usually done since it offers the most accurate imaging. Hysteroscopy can visualize submucosal uterine fibroids, and allow for biopsy or resection of smaller lesions.

Treatment

There is no required treatment for asymptomatic uterine fibroids. The patient is re-evaluated every 6–12 months. When fibroids become symptomatic, suppression of ovarian hormones to stop the bleeding usually does not provide enough relief. Even so, medications to achieve this are used first before any surgery is

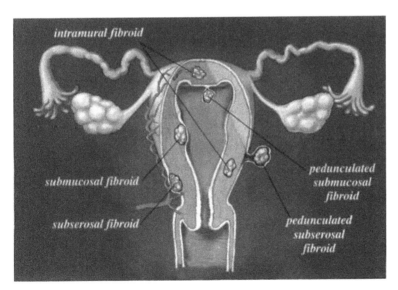

Figure 9.8 Locations of uterine fibroids. *Source*: AORN Journal – Clinical [9].

considered. The gonadotropin-releasing hormone (GnRH) agonists may shrink fibroid tissues, often stopping menses and allowing the patient's blood counts to increase. Since fibroids decrease in size after menopause, expectant management may be done for perimenopausal women.

Medications for uterine fibroids, besides the GnRH agonists, include antiprogestins, exogenous progestins, danazol, nonsteroidal antiinflammatory drugs (NSAIDs), SERMs, and tranexamic acid. The GnRH agonists are usually preferred, and are able to reduce bleeding and size of the fibroids. These agonists can be given intramuscularly (leuprolide), subcutaneously (goserelin), as subdermal pellets, and as nasal spray (nafarelin). These agonists reduce estrogen production, and are best used before surgery, to reduce the volume of the fibroids as well as uterus. This makes surgery better tolerated and also reduces blood loss. The GnRH agonists are usually not used for a long period of time, since there can be rebound fibroid growth that reaches the pretreatment size within six months. Bone demineralization is another factor of long-term GnRH use. When these drugs are required for a long time, supplemental estrogen, known as *add-back therapy* is given, which sometimes involves low doses of a combination estrogen–progestin.

The estrogen stimulation of uterine fibroid growth is partially suppressed by exogenous progestins. They are able to decrease uterine bleeding, but their ability to shrink fibroids is not as significant as that of the GnRH agonists. To limit heavy bleeding during the menstrual cycle, oral medroxyprogesterone or megestrol acetate can be used. The use of these drugs can be once per day for 10–14 days, or as continuous therapy, taken every day of the month. Their use often provides contraception as well as reducing bleeding. Depot medroxyprogesterone acetate can be injected intramuscularly every three months, with similar effectiveness. However, before this is done, oral progestins should be tried to see if the patient can tolerate effects such as depression, irregular bleeding, and weight gain. Another factor to consider is that progestins sometimes cause uterine fibroids to grow. Another option is to use an intrauterine device (IUD) that releases levonorgestrel, reducing uterine bleeding.

For mifepristone and other antiprogestins, taken daily for 3–6 months, doses are lower than the 200-mg used for termination of pregnancy. The smaller doses require special pharmaceutical mixing and are not always available. Using SERMs can reduce fibroid growth. These agents may or may not be able to relieve other symptoms that are present. The androgenic agonist called *danazol* can suppress fibroid growth but has many adverse effects. These include acne, weight gain, edema, hirsutism, voice deepening, hair loss, flushing, sweating, and vaginal dryness. For pain, NSAIDs are used, though they are not believed to decrease bleeding. The antifibrinolytic drug called *tranexamic acid* reduces bleeding by as much as 40%. It is administered every eight hours for up to five days, and is becoming more popular as a treatment.

Surgical treatment of uterine fibroids involves a variety of signs and symptoms. These include the following:

- A quickly enlarging pelvic mass
- An enlarged uterus, with mass abdominal effects that cause urinary or intestinal symptoms, or compress organs and cause dyspareunia, hydronephrosis, or urinary frequency
- Infertility (when the patient desires to become pregnant)
- Recurrent uterine bleeding that is refractory to medications
- Recurrent spontaneous abortions (when pregnancy is desired)
- Severe or persistent pressure or pain, such that may require opioids for control, or when it is intolerable
- When childbearing is completed and no other children are desired
- If the patient wants definitive treatment

Myomectomy is usually performed hysteroscopically or laparoscopically. The surgical instrument has a wide-angle scope and an electrical wire loop used for excision. Robotic techniques may or may not be used. **Hysterectomy** can be performed laparoscopically, via laparotomy, or vaginally. Indications for both myomectomy and hysterectomy are similar. The patient must be completely informed about possible problems and sequelae, comparing the two techniques. There can sometimes be adhesions, pain, or bleeding. After a myomectomy, there is occasional uterine rupture during a subsequent pregnancy.

The reasons that hysterectomy may be favored over myomectomy include the following:

- It is the definitive treatment for uterine fibroids, since myomectomy can result in new fibroids starting to grow – about 25% of patients have a hysterectomy 4–8 years after a myomectomy
- Multiple myomectomy may be extremely difficult compared with hysterectomy
- Less invasive treatments have failed
- Myomectomy may be complicated by other conditions such as endometriosis and extensive adhesions
- Hysterectomy can decrease risks for cervical intraepithelial neoplasia, endometrial hyperplasia, endometriosis, and in patients with a BRCA mutation, ovarian cancer

There are newer procedures able to relieve symptoms that require more evaluation concerning efficacy and restoring of fertility. These include cryotherapy, high-intensity focused sonography, **radiofrequency ablation**, MR-guided focused ultrasound surgery, and uterine artery embolization, which attempts to preserve normal uterine tissue while causing infarction of fibroids. The patient can recover more quickly from uterine artery embolization than from myomectomy or hysterectomy. However, complications are more frequent, as well as the need for further treatment. Complications include bleeding and uterine ischemia. Uterine artery embolization fails in 20–23% of patients, ultimately requiring a hysterectomy.

Treatment choices for uterine fibroids are highly individualized. The factors that help women decide include being asymptomatic, requiring no treatment. For postmenopausal women, expectant management is used first since symptoms often remit with a decrease in fibroid size after menopause. If pregnancy is desired, symptomatic fibroids are treated with uterine artery embolization, high-focused intensity focused sonography, or myomectomy. When other treatments are insufficient and the symptoms are severe – especially if pregnancy is not desired – GnRH agonist therapy may be tried, often followed by hysterectomy.

Prevention and Early Detection

Protective factors against uterine fibroids include **parturition** and for some reason, cigarette smoking. Otherwise, uterine fibroids cannot be prevented. The best method of early detection for uterine fibroids is regular gynecological examinations, and alerting the physician to any signs and symptoms as soon as they develop.

Prognosis

The prognosis for uterine fibroids are generally good, since only about 1 of every 1,000 lesions is malignant or become malignant, usually as a leiomyosarcoma. A sign of malignancy is growth of fibroids after menopause.

Significant Point

Uterine fibroids are the most common uterine tumors. Though benign, they may have similar symptoms to those of uterine sarcoma. They are most common in African American women. Uterine fibroids are the leading cause of hysterectomies.

Clinical Case

1. How common are symptomatic uterine fibroids in African American women?
2. What are the risk factors for uterine fibroids?
3. What does uterine fibroid embolization attempt to preserve?

A 44-year-old African American woman was suffering from uterine fibroids that caused heavy menstrual bleeding, prolonged periods, and the passing of blood clots. The condition progressed to cause extreme anemia, and the woman was hospitalized. Blood transfusions were required, and a hysterectomy was suggested, which gave the patient a lot of anxiety due to her high-level job and fears of losing it. A specialist informed the patient about uterine fibroid embolization, which could be performed in less time, with less cost, and with a faster rehabilitation time. The procedure was performed, and the patient's symptoms began to improve. After four months of follow-up, the patient's menstrual flow was under control, and no more clots were being passed. After two years, the patient's health was completely back to normal.

Answers:

1. **About 50% of African American women will develop symptomatic uterine fibroids. The same percentage is found in Asian American women, yet for some reason, only 25% of Caucasian women develop them.**
2. **Risk factors for uterine fibroids include family history, having no children, obesity, polycystic ovary syndrome, diabetes mellitus, the African or Asian races, and hypertension.**
3. **Uterine fibroid embolization attempts to preserve normal uterine tissue while causing infarction of fibroids.**

The patient can recover more quickly from this procedure than from myomectomy or hysterectomy, but complications are more frequent (bleeding and uterine ischemia), as well as the need for further treatment. The procedure fails in 20–23% of patients, ultimately requiring a hysterectomy.

Endometrial Cancer

Endometrial cancer is commonly referred to as *uterine cancer*, and it arises in the glandular epithelium of the uterine lining. It is the most prevalent gynecological malignancy, most often occurring in the fifth or sixth decade of life. The disease is diagnosed via biopsy and staged surgically. Endometrial cancer occurs most often in developed countries that have high-fat diets. It is believed that the disease will become more prevalent because of the increase in metabolic syndrome worldwide.

Epidemiology

Endometrial cancer is the fourth most common cancer in women in the United States. Women are at an overall 3% lifetime risk of endometrial cancer. According to the American Association for Cancer Research, more than 65,620 new cases are diagnosed, and nearly 12,600 deaths occur every year. Incidence and deaths are increasing continually. Postmenopausal women are mostly affected by endometrial cancer, with a mean patient age of 61 years at diagnosis. About 92% of all cases occur in women aged 50 or older. Caucasian women are affected the most, followed by African American women. However, mortality rates are the highest in African American women, possibly because of less access to adequate treatment. The prevalence is approximately 500,000 women in the United States.

Globally, endometrial cancer is the sixth most common female cancer, and is more common in developed countries, affecting 1.6% of the population. The incidence in developed countries is 13 of every 100,000 women. In developing countries, it only affects 0.6% of the population. Northern and Eastern Europe, plus North America, have the highest rates of endometrial cancer, while Africa and Western Asia have the lowest rates. Cases of global endometrial cancer are increasing. Women between 50 and 65 are most often affected, with more than 75% of cases occurring after menopause. The worldwide median age is 63. The countries with the highest rates of endometrial cancer are Belarus, Samoa, Macedonia, Lithuania, Canada, Greece, Ukraine, the United States, Slovakia, Croatia, Serbia, Jamaica, Poland, Singapore, and the Czech Republic.

Etiology and Risk Factors

Although the cause of endometrial cancer is not clear. In a small number (5%) of patients, inherited gene mutations are linked to endometrial cancer. About 50% of the inherited cases occur in families that have hereditary nonpolyposis colorectal cancer (HNPCC, also called *Lynch syndrome*). Patients with HNPCC have a high risk of secondary colorectal or ovarian cancers.

Primary risk factors include age over 50 diabetes mellitus, obesity, and **unopposed estrogen**. Additional risk factors include a personal or family history of breast or ovarian cancer, family history of HNPCC, gallbladder disease, hypertension, previous pelvic radiation therapy, and the use of tamoxifen for five years or more. There is a possible risk factor of having a first-degree relative that had endometrial cancer. Unopposed estrogen may be linked to anovulation, early *menarche*, and estrogen therapy without progesterone, late menopause, never having given birth, obesity, and polycystic ovary syndrome.

Clinical Manifestations

Over 90% of women with endometrial cancer experience abnormal vaginal bleeding. This may include postmenopausal bleeding or premenopausal metrorrhagia that recurs. About 33% of women with postmenopausal bleeding are diagnosed with endometrial cancer. This is the cardinal symptom. Lower abdominal and lower back pain may also be present. A large, boggy uterus is often a sign of advanced disease.

Pathology

Endometrial hyperplasia usually precedes endometrial cancer, which is classified as low-grade, either *type 1* or *type 2*. Type 1 endometrial cancer is more common, making up 90% of all cases. The tumors are usually responsive to estrogen and progesterone, and observed in women that are of younger age, obese, or are perimenopausal. The most common histology is endometrioid adenocarcinoma, grade 1 and grade 2. There may be microsatellite instability, and mutations of the following genes may be implicated: *catenin beta 1, Kirsten rat sarcoma* (KRAS), and *phosphatase and tensin homolog* (PTEN). Inactivation of PTEN is present in 83% of these tumors. *Mucinous carcinomas* are usually low-grade tumors with a good prognosis, and often result from KRAS mutations. Most type 1 tumors are well differentiated.

The type 2 endometrial carcinomas are usually high grade, and make up only 10% of all cases. They are more aggressive and include grade 3 endometrioid carcinomas or tumors with non-endometrioid histologies. These include clear cell, serous, mixed cell, and undifferentiated carcinomas as well as carcinosarcomas. There is atrophy of the endometrium and estrogen dependency. The type 2 tumors mostly occur in older women, and 10–30% of cases have *tumor protein 53 mutations*. *Endometrioid adenocarcinomas* make up 85% of endometrial cancers. The *uterine papillary serous carcinomas* make up only 10% and the *clear cell carcinomas* make up less than 5% (see Figure 9.9). These uncommon tumors are more aggressive and of higher risk. They are linked to a greater incidence of extrauterine disease when diagnosed.

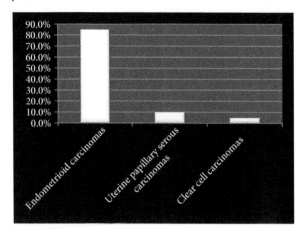

Figure 9.9 Subtypes of type 2 endometrial carcinomas.

Diagnosis

Diagnosis of endometrial cancer is based on biopsy and surgical staging. The cancer is suggested by abnormal bleeding (in premenopausal or postmenopausal women). A routine Pap test shows endometrial cells (in postmenopausal women), or a Pap test shows atypical endometrial cells (in any women). Once cancer is suspected, an outpatient endometrial biopsy is performed, which is over 90% accurate. Especially for women over 40 years of age, endometrial sampling is recommended when there is abnormal bleeding. If results are not conclusive or there is complex hyperplasia with atypia, outpatient *fractional dilation and curettage* (D&C) with hysteroscopy is performed. Transvaginal ultrasound is an alternative, but histologic diagnosis is required. Routine preoperative MRI, CT, or PET scan are not recommended.

Pelvis and abdominal CT checks for extrauterine or metastatic cancer. This is done for patients that have an abdominal mass or hepatomegaly, abnormal liver function tests. The papillary tumors, upon diagnosis, are present outside of the uterus in 40–70% of cases.

Surgical staging is based on histologic differentiation, and the extent of spread. This includes depth of invasion, cervical involvement, and extrauterine metastases. Staging includes abdominopelvic exploration and total hysterectomy. For a patient with high-risk features, pelvic and para-aortic lymphadenectomy is performed. Staging is via laparotomy, laparoscopy, or robotic-assisted surgery. If the cancer is only within the uterus, **sentinel lymph node mapping** may be done instead of pelvic and para-aortic lymphadenectomy. Table 9.4 summarizes the Federation of Gynecology and Obstetrics (FIGO) stating of endometrial carcinoma.

Except for Stage IVB, grading (G) shows percentage of tumor with a nonsquamous or **nonmorular** solid growth pattern:

- G1 – 5% or less
- G2 – 6–50%
- G3 – over 50%

Nuclear grading is more important for serous adenocarcinomas, clear cell adenocarcinomas, and squamous cell carcinomas. The nuclear grade of the glandular component is used for adenocarcinomas with squamous differentiation.

Sentinel lymph node (SLN) mapping is considered for staging if the cancer appears to be only within the uterus (stage I cancer). This SLN mapping is the standard of cancer for many cancers that are high risk, including carcinosarcomas, clear cell carcinoma, and papillary serous carcinoma. In various studies, SLN mapping with indocyanine green (ICG) has been proven highly accurate to diagnose endometrial cancer

Table 9.4 Federation of Gynecology and Obstetrics (FIGO) staging of endometrial carcinoma.

Stage	Definition
I	Only in the uterine corpus
IA	Only in endometrium, involving less than 50% of myometrium
IB	Invasion of 50% or more of the myometrium
II	Invasion of cervical stroma; no extension outside uterus
III	Local and/or regional spread
IIIA	Invasion of serosa, adnexa, or both (direct extension or metastasis)
IIIB	Metastases or direct spread to vagina, parametria, or both
IIIC	Metastases to pelvic or para-aortic lymph nodes, or both
IIIC1	Metastases to pelvic lymph nodes
IIIC2	Metastases to para-aortic lymph nodes, and/or pelvic lymph nodes
IV	Involvement of bladder and/or intestinal mucosa and/or distant metastases
IVA	Invasion of bladder, intestinal mucosa, or both
IVB	Distant metastases to inguinal lymph nodes, lungs, liver, bones, plus intraperitoneal disease

metastases, and it may replace complete lymphadenectomy. Cervical injection with ICG provides a higher detection rate than hysteroscopic injection. The anatomic nodal distribution is similar. Usually, dye is injected in the cervix superficially and deep in locations described as "3 o'clock" and "9 o'clock." The dye penetrates the uterine lymphatic trunks that meet in the parametria, and appears in the broad ligament that leads to the pelvic lymph SLNs and sometimes the para-aortic SLNs. No lymphadenectomy is indicated if the SNLs are identified bilaterally. If one or both sides have no identified sentinel nodes, complete lymphadenectomy is required on that side. The surgeon decides if dissection of the para-aortic nodes is required.

Treatment

Endometrial cancer should be removed *en block*. This requires either a total hysterectomy or bilateral salpingo-oophorectomy. Morcellation or intraperitoneal tumor fragmentation should not be performed. Surgery may be by the laparoscopic, open, robotic, or vaginal routes. If the tumor is only within the uterus, minimally invasive surgery is preferred. There are similar outcomes for laparoscopic surgery and laparotomy. For young women with stage IA or IB endometrioid adenocarcinoma, ovarian preservation is often safe, and recommended to preserve ovarian function. Complete lymphadenectomy is needed on the side in which an SLN is not identified.

Stage II or III endometrial cancer must be treated with pelvic radiation therapy, with or without chemotherapy. For stage III cancer, treatment is individualized, with surgery being an option. Patients undergoing combined surgery and radiation therapy generally have a better prognosis. Total hysterectomy and bilateral salpingo-oophorectomy are avoided if the patient has bulky parametrial disease. Stage IV cancer usually involves surgery combined with radiation and chemotherapy. Hormone therapy is sometimes used. In 20–25% of patients, tumors respond to hormone therapy with a progestin. Carboplatin plus paclitaxel is an example of a highly effective cytotoxic drug combination. These drugs are mostly given to women with metastatic or recurrent tumors. Doxorubicin may also be used. Carboplatin plus paclitaxel is the standard treatment for advanced cancer. Recent studies support use of lenvatinib and pembrolizumab, with an objective response rate of 39.6% for this combination.

More targeted therapies may be highly beneficial for recurrent cancer. These include a combination of everolimus with letrozole, providing a clinical benefit rate of 40%, and an objective response rate of 32%. For recurrent uterine papillary serous carcinoma, trastuzumab was added to the standard carboplatin plus paclitaxel regimen. Progression-free survival was increased from 8 months to 12 months. Patients with complex endometrial hyperplasia and atypia have up to a 50% risk of concurrent endometrial cancer. Progestins or definitive surgery are used for endometrial hyperplasia. Progestin alone is an option if the patient is young, has grade 1 tumors, no myometrial invasion, and wants to preserve fertility. Within three months of initiating therapy, 46–80% of patients have a complete response. After three months, reevaluation requires D & C. The use of a levonorgestrel-releasing IUD is becoming more popular for patients with complex atypical hyperplasia or grade I endometrial cancer. Surgery is recommended if the cancer is still present after 6–9 months of treatment, or if the patient has completed having children. Fertility-sparing treatment is contraindicated for high-grade endometrial cancers. For young women with stage IA or IB endometrioid adenocarcinomas, ovarian preservation is approved. Patients benefit from counseling about the importance of overall health, including adequate exercise, diet, and weight loss. Avoiding obesity and hypertension is extremely beneficial.

For high-risk patients, multimodality therapy is usually recommended, including hysterectomy, bilateral salpingo-oophorectomy with pelvic and para-aortic lymphadenectomy, plus omental and peritoneal biopsies. For gross extrauterine disease, cytoreduction can reduce the tumor bulk to achieve no gross residual disease. Adjuvant therapy for papillary serous and clear cell carcinomas is based on the stage. For stage IA with no myometrial invasion and no residual disease in hysterectomy specimens, observation and close follow-up is approved. For other stage IA or IB, or stage II cancers, vaginal brachytherapy is often done, followed by systemic carboplatin + paclitaxel. For more advanced cancer, carboplatin + paclitaxel is the standard of care. Adjuvant therapy for carcinosarcoma is also stage-based, and is the same for stage I cancers. For all other stages, the preferred treatment is systemic ifosfamide + paclitaxel.

Administration of progesterone counteracts the effects of estrogen regarding the neoplasia of endometrial cells. Progesterone also downregulates ER expression, and leads to cell death in the endometrial glands and stroma via transforming growth factor beta. Therefore, use of progesterone has been focused on while treating endometrial cancer. For the papillary serous carcinomas, targeted therapy is focused on their specific gene pathway alterations. Metformin has been found to have antitumor effects against endometrial adenocarcinomas. It lowers the risk of all types of cancers. In diabetic patients, metformin improves outcomes of endometrial cancer, with fewer recurrences and longer overall survival. Metformin also appears to have synergistic effects when combined with progesterone analogs.

Significant Point

The use of oral contraceptives can decrease risks for endometrial cancer by 80%, up to about 10 years after being taken. A progestin-containing IUD helps to prevent endometrial abnormalities in women taking tamoxifen as an agent to prevent breast cancer.

Prevention and Early Detection

While there is no clear method of preventing endometrial cancer, there are ways to reduce risks. Protective factors that decrease the risk of endometrial cancer include pregnancy, breastfeeding, hormonal contraceptives, physical activity, and weight loss. The protective effects of cigarette smoking are opposed by the more significant adverse effects. New ways of preventing endometrial cancer are being studied in clinical trials, including ketogenic diets, brachytherapy, and many different medications. Screening methods to detect endometrial cancer early are extremely effective, although Pap tests are not helpful in early stage. Transvaginal ultrasound measures the thickness of the endometrium, providing screening for postmenopausal women and high-risk premenopausal women. If the endometrium is thicker than 5 mm, endometrial biopsy is performed to rule out cancer. A thin tube is placed through the cervix to collect endometrial tissue. Early detection of endometrial cancer provides excellent treatment outcomes in most cases.

Prognosis

Higher-grade endometrial cancers have a worsened prognosis, as do cases in which the patient is older, or there is more extensive spread. Average five-year survival rates for stage I or II cancer is 70–95%. With stage III or IV cancer, average five-year survival rates are 10–60%. Generally, 63% of patients have no cancer within five or more years after treatment. The prognosis is poorer for the type 2 endometrial cancers. The papillary serous carcinomas have a five-year overall survival of only 27–55%. They make up 39% of all deaths from uterine cancers.

Significant Point

Most endometrial cancers are adenocarcinomas, and endometrioid cancer is the most common type of adenocarcinoma. Endometrioid cancers begin in gland cells and resemble the normal uterine endometrium. The other variants of endometrioid cancers include adenocanthoma, adenosquamous cancer, ciliated carcinoma, secretory carcinoma, and villoglandular adenocarcinoma.

Clinical Case

1. Which group of women are most often affected by endometrial cancer?
2. Which subtype of endometrial cancer is most common?
3. What are the treatments for malignant and invasive endometrial cancer?

A 60-year-old woman presented to the emergency department because of continual abnormal uterine bleeding. She stated that she had never entered menopause. Her other complaints were weight loss, shortness of breath, urinary frequency, fatigue, and night sweats. Physical examination revealed an enlarged uterus and left lower quadrant abdominal tenderness. The patient also had a white purulent discharge with blood. Endometrial biopsy, tissue culture, and blood culture were collected. Results showed anemia and leukocytosis. Urinary analysis suggested a urinary tract infection. The patient was hospitalized and underwent a hysterectomy. The diagnosis was of a malignant and invasive endometrial tumor.

Answers:

1. **In the United States, postmenopausal women are mostly affected by endometrial cancer, with a mean patient age of 61 years at diagnosis. About 92% of all cases occur in women aged 50 or older. Globally, women between 50 and 65 are most often affected, with more than 75% of cases occurring after menopause. The worldwide median age is 63.**
2. **Type 1 endometrial cancer is the most common subtype, making up 90% of all cases. The most common histology is endometrioid adenocarcinoma, grade 1 and grade 2. The type 2 endometrial carcinomas are usually high grade, and make up only 10% of all cases.**

3. **Endometrial cancer should be removed en block. This requires either a total hysterectomy or bilateral salpingo-oophorectomy. If the tumor is only within the uterus, minimally invasive surgery is preferred. Stage II or III endometrial cancer must be treated with pelvic radiation therapy, with or without chemotherapy. Stage IV cancer usually involves surgery combined with radiation and chemotherapy. Hormone therapy is sometimes used.**

Uterine Sarcoma

Uterine sarcoma is malignant cancer that develops from the uterine corpus, causing abnormal bleeding, pelvic pain, or a pelvic mass. These tumors evolve from **mesenchymal** tissues that include myometrial smooth muscle, nearby connective tissues, or the endometrial stroma. Most uterine sarcomas are diagnosed histologically, following hysterectomy or myomectomy.

Epidemiology
Uterine sarcomas are rare and make up 3–8% of all types of uterine cancers. They also make up 3% of all genital tract cancers. According to the American Cancer Society, there are more than 65,600 cases of uterine cancer diagnosed in the United States annually, and about 12,600 of these are fatal. More than 90% of cases occur in the endometrium. Average age at diagnosis is in the early 50s. There is a lack of epidemiological data because of low occurrence rates. African American women, for some reason, have the highest number of cases of uterine sarcoma, with nearly two times higher rates than that of Caucasian or Asian women.

Statistics on the global prevalence of uterine sarcoma are not well documented, and it is estimated that less than 1% of the world female population is affected. Incidence rates are estimated to be approximately 0.4 out of every 100,000 women, globally. Most patients are in their 50s when diagnosed. Individual data from different countries throughout the world are lacking.

Etiology and Risk Factors
Uterine sarcoma is of uncertain cause. Risk factors for uterine sarcomas include previous pelvic radiation (within 5–25 years) and the use of tamoxifen. Excess estrogen exposure over time is also a risk factor. Women who previously had retinoblastoma, due to an abnormal copy of the RB gene, have an increased risk of uterine leiomyosarcomas.

Clinical Manifestations
The majority of uterine sarcomas cause abnormal vaginal bleeding. Less often, there is pelvic pain or pressure, abdominal fullness, a vaginal mass, frequent urination, or a pelvic mass that can be palpated. There may be significant vaginal discharge that has a foul odor. Patients may complain of gastrointestinal as well as genitourinary abnormalities.

Pathology
The most common pathological subtypes of uterine sarcomas include leiomyosarcomas (63% of all cases) and endometrial stromal sarcomas (21%). There are also undifferentiated uterine sarcomas, adenosarcomas, and rhabdomyosarcomas. Carcinosarcomas are now classified and treated as high-grade epithelial tumors, while previously, they were classified as uterine sarcomas. The growth of high-grade sarcomas is usually hematogenous and often metastasizes to the lungs.

Diagnosis
Diagnosis of uterine sarcoma is based on symptoms that indicate the need for transvaginal ultrasound, endometrial biopsy, or D&C. These tests only offer limited sensitivity. After

hysterectomy or myomectomy, endometrial stromal sarcoma or uterine leiomyosarcoma may be diagnosed incidentally. If a sarcoma is identified before surgery, a CT or MRI is usually performed. If diagnosed after surgical resection, imaging is indicated, and additional explorative surgery may be discussed. The surgical staging for the uterine sarcomas called leiomyosarcoma and endometrial stromal sarcoma is described in Table 9.5.

Table 9.6 summarizes the surgical staging of the uterine adenosarcomas.

Treatment

Treatment of uterine sarcomas involves total abdominal hysterectomy and bilateral salpingo-oophorectomy. There should be en block removal of the tumors, and Morcellation must not be performed. For a specimen broken up during surgery, imaging is indicated, and surgical re-exploration should be discussed. Chemotherapy is recommended. For early-stage uterine leiomyosarcoma, if the patient wants to preserve hormonal function, the ovaries may be preserved.

Intraoperative results prompt any additional surgical resection. For leiomyosarcoma or endometrial stromal sarcoma, lymphadenectomy is not done since there is evidence that risks for lymph node metastases are less than 2%. If the sarcoma is inoperable, pelvic radiation therapy with or without brachytherapy, systemic therapy or both are recommended. Adjuvant radiation is usually used and delays local recurrence yet does not improve the survival rate.

Chemotherapy is usually used when sarcomas advanced or recur, chosen by tumor type. Combination chemotherapies that are recommended include: docetaxel + gemcitabine (best used for leiomyosarcoma), doxorubicin + dacarbazine, doxorubicin + ifosfamide, gemcitabine + dacarbazine, and gemcitabine + vinorelbine. Unfortunately, overall response to chemotherapy is poor. Therefore, hormonal therapy may be used for hormone-receptor-positive uterine leiomyosarcoma, or for endometrial stromal sarcomas. Hormone therapies include: AIs, GnRH agonists, medroxyprogesterone acetate, and megestrol acetate.

Table 9.5 Surgical staging of uterine sarcomas: leiomyosarcoma and endometrial stromal sarcoma.

Stage	Description
I	Only within the uterus
IA	Tumor 5 cm or less in largest dimension
IB	Tumor larger than 5 cm
II	Tumor extends beyond uterus, but within pelvis
IIA	Tumor involves the adnexa
IIB	Tumor involves other pelvic tissues
III	Tumor infiltrates abdominal tissues
IIIA	Tumor is only in one site
IIIB	Tumor is in one or more sites
IIIC	There is regional lymph node metastasis
IVA	Tumor invades bladder or rectum
IVB	There is distant metastases

Table 9.6 Surgical staging of uterine adenosarcomas

Stage	Description
I	Tumor only within the uterus
IA	Tumor in the endometrium and/or endocervix
IB	Tumor invades less than 50% of myometrium
IC	Tumor invades more than 50% of myometrium
II	Tumor extends beyond uterus, but is within pelvis
IIA	Tumor involves the adnexa
IIB	Tumor involves other pelvic tissues
III	Tumor infiltrates abdominal tissues
IIIA	Tumor is within one site
IIIB	Tumor is in one or more sites
IIIC	There are metastases to the regional lymph nodes
IVA	Tumor invades the bladder or rectum
IVB	There are distant metastases

Prevention and Early Detection

Uterine sarcoma is usually not preventable, but early detection can be very helpful. It is important to understand the signs and symptoms of uterine sarcoma and see a physician quickly if they develop. Unfortunately, many uterine sarcomas are already advanced by the time manifestations develop. There are no current tests or examinations to detect uterine sarcomas in asymptomatic women. Pap tests are not extremely effective in finding uterine sarcomas, though they are good for finding early cervical carcinomas.

Prognosis

Compared with endometrial cancer of similar stages, the prognosis for uterine sarcoma is generally worse. Survival is usually poor if the cancer has spread beyond the uterus. The five-year survival rates for uterine sarcoma have been reported as stage I (51%), stage II (13%), stage III (10%), and stage IV (3%). The cancer usually recurs locally, in the abdomen, or the lungs.

Significant Point

Uterine leiomyosarcomas begin in the myometrium and are the most common subtype of uterine sarcomas. They can grow and spread quickly. Endometrial stromal sarcomas begin in the supporting stroma of the uterine endometrium, and are relatively rare. Undifferentiated uterine sarcomas begin in either the myometrium or endometrium, growing and spreading quickly.

Clinical Case

1. What are the most common pathological subtypes of uterine sarcomas?
2. Based on the advanced disease described in this scenario, what stage would this patient's condition be listed as?

3. What are the five-year survival rates for uterine sarcomas?

A 71-year-old woman was diagnosed with a uterine leiomyosarcoma after experiencing recurrent vaginal bleeding. The tumor extruded into the vagina. An MRI revealed that the tumor had enlarged enough to actually invert the patient's uterus. The patient's bleeding and anemia were worsening, so a laparotomy procedure was performed to achieve a total hysterectomy and bilateral salpingo-oophorectomy. Microscopically, the tumor had both sarcoma and carcinoma features. The patient then received five courses of chemotherapy, with docetaxel + gemcitabine. Later, this was followed on an outpatient basis with doxorubicin for four weeks. In less than a year, metastatic tumors appeared in the patient's right lung that resulted in pleural effusion and respiratory distress. Her condition deteriorated quickly and death occurred within a few months.

Answers:

1. **The most common pathological subtypes of uterine sarcomas include leiomyosarcomas (63% of all cases) and endometrial stromal sarcomas (21%). The growth of high-grade sarcomas is usually hematogenous and often metastasizes to the lungs.**
2. **Because there were distant metastases of the uterine leiomyosarcoma to the right lung, this patient's condition would be listed as Stage IVB – the most serious stage possible for this type of tumor.**
3. **The five-year survival rates for uterine sarcoma have been reported as stage I (51%), stage II (13%), stage III (10%), and stage IV (3%).**

Choriocarcinoma

Choriocarcinoma is a rare tumor that is part of a group of tumors referred to as *gestational*

trophoblastic disease (GTD), which affect the uterus (see Figure 9.10). However, GTD tumors begin in cells that would normally form the placenta during pregnancy – hence the term "gestational." Choriocarcinoma is a malignant form of GTD, but most GTD tumors are benign, including **hydatidiform mole**, invasive mole, placental-site trophoblastic tumor, and epithelioid trophoblastic tumor. The term *choriocarcinoma* is based on the word **chorion** of a fetus.

Epidemiology

Choriocarcinoma occurs in about 1 of every 12 women (8%) after a **molar pregnancy**. Only about 1 in every 590 pregnancies is a molar pregnancy. These statistics mean that only about 1 in every 50,000 pregnancies will result in a choriocarcinoma. Most patients are within 25 and 35 years of age at diagnosis. Women of Asian, Native American, and African American descent have an increased risk. Though little global data are available, rates of choriocarcinomas are the highest in Southeast Asia (9.2 cases per 40,000 pregnancies) and Japan (3.3 per 40,000).

Etiology and Risk Factors

About 50% of choriocarcinomas begin as molar pregnancies. About 25% develop in women who have a spontaneous or intentional abortion, or a tubal pregnancy, with the fetus developing in the fallopian tubes instead of the uterus. Another 25% of choriocarcinomas occur after normal pregnancy and delivery. Risk factors include previous hydatidiform mole, older maternal age, long-term oral contraceptive use, and women of the blood group A, with the father of the baby also having blood group A.

Clinical Manifestations

Choriocarcinoma may cause extremely painful cramps or dysmenorrhea. A choriocarcinoma that forms in the vagina can cause bleeding. If it spreads to the abdomen, there may be pain and/or pressure. If the tumor has reached the lungs or brain, it can cause coughing, difficulty breathing, chest pain, nausea, headache, and dizziness.

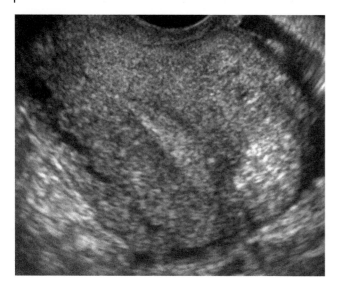

Figure 9.10 Via transvaginal ultrasound, an epithelioid trophoblastic choriocarcinoma is present within the uterus. *Source*: AORN Journal – Clinical [9].

Pathology

Choriocarcinoma begins in the **trophoblast cells**, which would normally surround an embryo. Early on, these cells form villi, which are tiny finger-like projections. The villi grow into the uterine lining. Over time, the trophoblast layer forms the placenta, which protects and provides nourishment to a developing fetus. Choriocarcinomas can develop months to years after a pregnancy. They appear as bulky dark masses in the uterus, with significant central hemorrhage and varying necrosis. The tumor may have sheets of **trimorphic** malignant trophoblasts, with intermediate trophoblasts and cytotrophoblasts surrounded by **syncytiotrophoblasts**. There is extreme cytologic atypia and many mitotic figures. Lymphovascular invasion is common. In cytology, there are large atypical cells with abundant cytoplasm, plus intracellular globules, and small atypical cells that have hyperchromatic nuclei and high nucleus/cytoplasm ratios. The tumor cells are positive for human chorionic gonadotropin (hCG).

Diagnosis

Diagnosis of choriocarcinoma starts with a pelvic examination, measuring hCG, and imaging tests such as CT, MRI, ultrasound, or X-ray. A red, hemorrhagic mass may be seen in the uterus, of various sizes. The stage of the tumor will be determined, based on size and spread. Laboratory testing may also include weekly hCG tests for stage II, III disease, and I over 3 consecutive weeks, and then once per month for 12 months. Patients with stage IV disease are followed similarly, over 24 months. All of the tumor cells stain positively for cytokeratin AE1/AE3, with more than 90% positive for Ki67.

Treatment

When a tumor is low risk, chemotherapy is the primary treatment. If it is high-risk, surgery, chemotherapy, and radiation may all be required. For some patients, a hysterectomy is required, followed by radiation. Most women (more than 90%) are curable unless the disease has reached the liver or brain. For brain metastases, radiation therapy is indicated. The non-gestational choriocarcinomas may be less responsive to chemotherapy.

Prevention and Early Detection

In one study, systemic methotrexate was used to prevent choriocarcinoma from developing after persistent trophoblastic disease had developed following a hydatidiform mole. Otherwise, the main prevention is the early detection of hydatidiform mole, so that early removal and management can be performed.

Prognosis

Prognosis can be very good without spread or metastasis. Upon diagnosis however, lung metastases are seen in over 90% of patients. Metastases to the liver and brain are less common. With treatment, patients have 80% survival over five years. If death occurs, it is usually due to liver and brain metastases. The non-gestational choriocarcinomas may have a less favorable prognosis. A prognostic score is calculated based on age 40 years or higher, related pregnancy and its characteristics, the number of months since gestation, hCG levels prior to treatment, the largest tumor size (if multiple tumors are present), the location and number of metastases, and any prior failed chemotherapy. Prognostic scores are calculated as low risk (six or less) or high risk (seven or more) based on the Staging and Risk Factor Scoring System for Gestational Trophoblastic Disease.

Significant Point

Choriocarcinoma is a malignant and highly aggressive tumor that originates from placental tissues. It can quickly spread to the lungs and other organs. It usually occurs after a molar pregnancy, and is 1,000 times more likely in these cases, compared with other forms of pregnancy. Fortunately, the tumor can be easily seen during imaging studies such as ultrasound.

Cervical Polyps

Cervical polyps are outgrowths of columnar epithelial tissue of the endocervical canal. They are common benign mass. Cervical polyps affect about 2–5% of women, globally. Most cervical polyps originate in the endocervical canal, and are often red, purple, or gray. Endocervical polyps may form because of chronic inflammation, and rarely become malignant. They can be shaped like a thin stem, a bulb, or may even resemble a finger, ranging in size from a few millimeters to several centimeters.

Epidemiology

After endometrial polyps, cervical polyps are the second most common type of gynecological polyps seen. Cervical polyps are estimated to affect 2–5% of the global female population. The incidence of cervical polyps is not well documented, but they are most common in women older than age 20 when they have given birth to two or more children. Malignancies occur in 0.2–1.5% of all cases of cervical polyps and is very rare – usually in postmenopausal women. There is no racial predilection for cervical polyps. Statistics on the global occurrence of cervical polyps are not well documented.

Etiology and Risk Factors

The actual cause of cervical polyps is unknown, but they may be related to cervical infections, chronic inflammation, an abnormal response to estrogen, or clogged blood vessels close to the cervix. Risk factors may include being premenopausal (this is under debate), having multiple children, having a sexually transmitted infection, and previous history of cervical polyps.

Clinical Manifestations

The majority of cervical polyps are asymptomatic, but endocervical polyps can bleed, either between menstrual periods or after intercourse. If they become infected, they can cause leukorrhea, a purulent vaginal discharge. Endocervical polyps are usually shiny, red to pink, less than 1 cm in diameter, and may be friable.

Pathology

Most cervical polyps do not recur. Histologically, they show vascular connective tissue, and stromal cells covered by the papillary cell proliferation. The cells contain columnar, squamous, or squamocolumnar epithelium. The polyps form from glandular epithelial hyperplasia, but the tip of each polyp is usually squamous metaplasia. Histological patterns include typical mucosa, inflammatory, vascular, fibrous, pseudo-decidual, mixed cervical/endometrial, and pseudosarcomatous. Endocervical polyps are more common than ectocervical polyps. Endocervical polyps have a loose, edematous stroma, and large dilated or small thick-walled vasculature. The stromal cells often have mixed acute or chronic inflammation, benign microglandular hyperplasia, and erosion. These features are usually seen on the surface of larger polyps that protrude through the cervical os, based on the amount of irritation that is present.

Diagnosis

The diagnosis of cervical polyps requires examination with a speculum, which will allow visualization of polypoid lesions within the cervix. They are often discovered during routine pelvic examinations or Pap tests. They may sometimes be discovered during colposcopy or ultrasound procedures. A biopsy is usually taken so that cancer can be ruled out. Triple smear or vaginal-cervical-endocervical smear is often used, as is transvaginal ultrasound to evaluate related endometrial pathologies. When indicated, an endometrial sample is taken.

Treatment

Cervical polyps that bleed or cause discharge should be surgically excised, which can be done in a physician's office by grasping the base of each polyp with forceps and twisting it off. This is known as *polypectomy*, and does not require anesthetics. Bleeding after a polyp is removed is rare, but chemical cauterizing agents can be used. Cervical cytology is then performed. After treatment, if bleeding or discharge continues, and endometrial biopsy is performed so that cancer can be excluded. Cramping also sometimes follows the procedure, which can be relieved by OTC acetaminophen or ibuprofen. For large polyps, actual surgery may be needed, using a local or general anesthetic.

Prevention and Early Detection

There is no prevention for cervical polyps, but routine pelvic examinations and Pap tests detect them early, allowing for treatment to occur before any symptoms manifest.

Prognosis

The prognosis for cervical polyps is excellent. Nearly all of them are benign and do not recur.

Significant Point

Cervical polyps are finger-like growths on the cervical canal, and rarely cause any symptoms. They are usually discovered during regular pelvic examinations. Usually, only one polyp is present, but two or three may be present. Though nearly all cervical polyps are benign, they must be examined for signs of cancer after being removed. They are most common in premenopausal women.

Cervical Cancer

Cervical cancer is a neoplasm of the uterine cervix that can be detected in the early, curable stage by Pap test. About 90% of cervical tumors are squamous cell carcinoma. It is caused mostly by the human papillomavirus (HPV) infection. The initial symptom of cervical cancer is usually vaginal bleeding that occurs irregularly, and often happens after intercourse.

Epidemiology

Cervical cancer is the third most common gynecological cancer, and the eighth most common cancer in American women. It affects more than 14,000 women in the United States annually, and is fatal in about 4,300 cases. Incidence rates of cervical cancer were reduced by over 50% from the mid-1970s to the mid-2000s partly because of increased screening. Decreasing incidence in younger women is believed to be due to the use of the HPV vaccine. Deaths from cervical cancer in the United States have also been reduced. The mean age at diagnosis is 50, but cases have occurred in women as young as 20. Hispanic American and African American women have slightly higher rates of cervical cancer.

Cervical cancer is the fourth most common malignancy diagnosed in women throughout the world. It is also the most common type of cancer in women that have HIV, who are six times as likely to develop cervical cancer eventually. According to the World Health Organization, over 300,000 women died in 2018 from cervical cancer. It is most fatal in low- and middle-income countries, which lack sufficient public health services, plus the fact that screening and treatment have not been widely established. About 60% of the deaths from cervical cancer occur in low- and middle-income countries. Globally, the average age at diagnosis of cervical cancer was 53 years, within an average range of 44–68 years. The countries with the highest rates of cervical cancer include Swaziland, Malawi, Zambia, Zimbabwe, Tanzania, Burundi, Uganda, Lesotho, Madagascar, and Comoros. Except for Madagascar and Comoros, which are off the coast of Africa, all of these countries are within the continent of Africa.

Etiology and Risk Factors

The exact cause is unknown, but factors that may be associated with the development of cervical cancer are coitus at an early age, relations with many sexual partners, genital herpesvirus infections (cytomegalovirus), HPV, and poor obstetric and gynecological care. Cervical cancer develops from cervical intraepithelial neoplasia, which is related to an infection with the HPV virus types 16, 18, 31, 33, 35, or 39. Other risk factors for cervical cancer include immunodeficiency and cigarette smoking.

Clinical Manifestations

Early cervical cancer is often asymptomatic. Symptoms usually start with irregular vaginal bleeding, usually after intercourse but also happening spontaneously in between periods. In advanced lesions may cause a dark, foul-smelling vaginal discharge, leaking from bladder or rectal fistulas. Anorexia, weight loss, pelvic pain, back pain, and leg swelling are also observed.

Pathology

Cervical intraepithelial neoplasia has three grades. Grade 1 is mild cervical dysplasia. Grade 2 is moderate dysplasia, and grade 3 is severe dysplasia with carcinoma in situ. This final stage is not likely to regress on its own. Squamous cell carcinomas make up 90% of all cervical cancers, and the rest are nearly always adenocarcinomas. Sarcomas and small cell neuroendocrine tumors only occur rarely. Invasive cervical cancer, via direct extension into nearby tissues or through the lymphatic system, spreads to the pelvic and para-aortic lymph nodes, in most cases. Rarely, spreading is hematogenous. If the cancer reaches the pelvic or para-aortic lymph nodes, it worsens prognosis, and the radiation therapy field will be affected.

Diagnosis

For diagnosis of cervical cancer, each patient has been exposed to another person that had HPV. Diagnosis combines a Pap test, biopsy and staging. The cancer may be suspected during routing gynecological examinations. It should be considered when there are visible **acetowhite** lesions on the cervix, abnormal Pap test results, or abnormal vaginal bleeding. The acetowhite changes indicate high-grade cervical intraepithelial neoplasia (see Figure 9.11). When no obvious cancer is revealed by cytology, colposcopy is used to find areas that should be

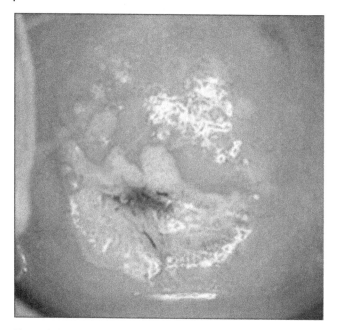

Figure 9.11 Acetowhite changes on the cervix, indicating high-grade cervical intraepithelial neoplasia. *Source*: Courtesy: Mr. John Tidy, Royal Hallamshire Hospital, Sheffield. AORN Journal – Clinical [9].

biopsied. Diagnosis is usually confirmed by colposcopy-directed biopsy with endocervical curettage. If this cannot be done, cone biopsy is required, in which a cone of tissue is removed with a loop electrical excision procedure (LEEP), scalpel, or laser.

As of 2018, the staging for cervical cancer was revised from the 2009 staging system, which only allowed for clinical examination and a few tests. The new system allows for cross-section imaging and pathology results as supplemental procedures for all stages. Cross-section imaging methods include CT, ultrasound, MRI, PET, PET-CT, and MRI-PET. However, imaging and pathology results are sometimes not available in lower-income and middle-income countries, where cervical cancer occurs more often. Therefore, these procedures are considered optional in these countries. Other updates to the 2018 staging system include the following:

- Horizontal tumor spread is no longer a part of stage IA1 or IA2 cancers.
- Lymph node status is now included. Positive pelvic lymph nodes are stage IIIC1, and positive para-aortic lymph nodes are stage IIIC2. If there are micrometastases in the lymph nodes, this is considered positive for cancer. If these isolated tumor cells do not indicate that the stage should be III, they are still documented. If the lymph nodes are classified positive during imaging, an "r" is added to the stage, such as IIIC1r or IIIC2r. If the lymph nodes are classified positive from pathology results, a "p" is added, such as IIIC1p or IIIC2p.
- Stage I is now subdivided into three subgroups based on tumor size. IB1 is less than 2 cm in diameter, IB2 is 2–4 cm, and IB3 is 4 cm or larger. Previously there were two subgroups.

If the cancer is staged at IA2 or higher, CT or MRI of the abdomen and pelvis is usually performed for better determination of tumor size, nodal metastases, parametrial involvement, and invasion into the vagina. To assess for spread beyond the cervix, PET-CT is being used more often today. When this, standard CT, or MRI are not available, cystoscopy, sigmoidoscopy, or IV urography are staging options. If imaging shows that pelvic or para-aortic lymph nodes are larger than 2 cm, there may be a need for surgical exploration, often using a retroperitoneal approach. The only reason for this is to remove enlarged lymph nodes, allowing radiation therapy to be more accurately targeted, for better effect.

Treatment

Treatments of cervical cancer include surgery or curative radiation therapy – if there is no spread to the parametrium or beyond. Also, chemoradiation can be used if there is spread to the parametrium or beyond. Chemoradiation is also used if hysterectomy is indicated but the patient is not a good candidate for it. Chemoradiation provides similar results as hysterectomy. For metastatic and recurrent cancers, chemotherapy is used.

For Stage IA1, in which there is no lymphovascular space invasion (LVSI), conization or simple hysterectomy is performed. This **microinvasive** cervical cancer has less than a 1% risk of lymph node metastases. It may be conservatively managed with conization via LEEP, scalpel, or laser. The procedure preserves fertility while obtaining (when possible) a non-fragmented sample with a 3 mm margin. If the patient does not intend to have children or if the margins are positive after conization, a simple hysterectomy is performed. If the margins are positive, there should be consideration of SLN mapping. If the patient wants to have children, repeated conization may be done. Other recommended treatments for Stage IA1 that does include LVSI, which are also indicated for Stage IA2, include external pelvic radiation therapy + brachytherapy, and modified radical hysterectomy + pelvic lymphadenectomy, with or without SLN mapping.

For Stages IB1, IB2, and IIA1 cervical cancers, open radical hysterectomy + bilateral pelvic lymphadenectomy, with or without SLN mapping, is usually performed. The uterus and cervix are surgically resected, along with parts of the cardinal and uterosacral ligaments, the pelvic lymph nodes, and the upper 1–2 cm of the vagina. Minimally invasive surgery (MIS) has provided a poorer survival rate and a higher recurrence rate than total abdominal radical hysterectomy (TARH). There are four types of radical hysterectomy procedures, plus some subtypes that also consider nerve preservation and paracervical lymphadenectomy. Because of comorbid conditions, some patients are not ideal surgical candidates. Therefore, external pelvic radiation + brachytherapy, with or without concurrent platinum-based chemotherapy, is used. Another option is radical hysterectomy + bilateral pelvic lymphadenectomy, with or without para-aortic lymphadenectomy, sometimes accompanied by adjuvant radiation therapy. During radical hysterectomy, if extracervical spread is found, the procedure must be stopped. Postoperative radiation therapy + chemotherapy is recommended to stop any local recurrence.

For Stages, IB3, IIA2, IIB, III, and IVA, external pelvic radiation therapy + brachytherapy + platinum-based chemotherapy is used. Surgical staging helps determine whether the para-aortic lymph nodes are involved, indicating the use of extended-field radiation therapy. This is especially true if the patient has positive pelvic lymph nodes, found during imaging. A laparoscopic retroperitoneal approach is indicated. If cancer is only within the cervix, pelvic lymph nodes, or both, treatment is usually with external beam radiation therapy that is followed by brachytherapy to the cervix, which uses local radioactive implants. These usually contain **cesium**. Acute radiation proctitis and cystitis may develop. Later complications may include intestinal obstruction, vaginal stenosis, or the formation of rectovaginal or vesicovaginal fistulas. Chemotherapy with carboplatin or cisplatin usually accompanies radiation therapy, which can sensitize the tumor to the radiation. Stage IVA cancers are usually treated with radiation therapy first, but pelvic exenteration – the excision of all pelvic organs – may be considered. After radiation therapy, if the cancer is still present but only within the central pelvis, exenteration is done. It is curative for up to 40% of patients. Exenteration may include continent or incontinent **urostomy**, low anterior rectal anastomosis with an end-descending colostomy or without colostomy, omental carpet to close the pelvic floor (known as a *J-flap*), and the use of gracilis or rectus abdominis myocutaneous flaps for vaginal reconstruction.

For Stage IVB and recurrent cervical cancer, chemotherapy is the main form of treatment, with response rates at about 48%. For patients with recurrent, persistent, or metastatic cancers, the addition of bevacizumab to either cisplatin/paclitaxel or topotecan/paclitaxel gave an improvement of 3.7 months in median overall survival. For metastases outside the radiation field, there is a better response to chemotherapy than with previously irradiated tumors or pelvic metastases. For recurrent, progressive, or metastatic cervical cancers, there should be consideration of testing for mismatch repair (MMR) expression, microsatellite instability (MSI), neurotrophic tyrosine kinase (NTRK) gene fusion, and programmed cell death-ligand 1 (PD-L1) expression. The results from these tests help predict how PD-LI inhibitors and other immunotherapies will affect the cancer.

For patients with IA1 with LVSI, IB1, IB2, or IIA1 cervical cancer, SLN mapping may be done instead of full pelvic lymphadenectomy. This is because only 15–20% of these patients have positive lymph nodes. Therefore, SLN mapping decreases the number of full pelvic lymphadenectomies, which can cause effects such as lymphedema and nerve damage. As discussed previously, SLN mapping involves injection of dyes into the cervix, which can be monitored during surgery. Ultrastaging of SLNs can detect micrometastasis and isolated tumor cells, signifying low-volume disease. Regardless of mapping, grossly suspicious lymph nodes are removed. If no mapping occurs on a hemipelvis, a side-specific lymphadenectomy is performed. Only macrometastases and micrometastases are considered for the classification of IIIC cases. Isolated tumor cells are considered pN0 and do not change the stage. Detection rates are best for tumors smaller than 2 cm.

A **radical trachelectomy** may be performed for IA1 with LVSI, IA2, IB1, certain IB2 cases, and for patients who still want to have children. There are abdominal, laparoscopic, robotic-assisted, and vaginal approaches available. The cervix, parametria adjacent to the cervix, the upper 2 cm of the vagina, and the pelvic lymph nodes are removed. The remaining uterus is reattached to the upper vagina so that fertility can be preserved. The best candidates for this procedure are those with cancer that is Stage IA1/grade 2 or 3 with LVSI, Stage IA2, Stage IB1, or with histologic subtypes such as squamous cell carcinoma, adenocarcinoma, or adenosquamous carcinoma. Before surgery, an MRI is used to exclude invasion of the upper cervix and lower uterus. Recurrence and death rates are similar with this procedure to those of radical hysterectomy. If the patient wants to have children, any delivery will have to be cesarean. Following radical trachelectomy, fertility rates are between 50% and 70%. Recurrence rates are 5–10%.

Prevention and Early Detection

To aid in the prevention of cervical cancer, the Papanicolaou test and HPV test are used for screening, to achieve the earliest possible detection. As of 2020, the American Cancer Society set forth new screening guidelines. These include the following:

- Screening begins at age 25, instead of at age 21
- If HPV testing is available, it is started at age 25, instead of at 30 years, and performed every 5 years; cytology via Pap tests is not needed
- If primary HPV testing is not available, a Pap test is done every three years, or co-testing with Pap and HPV tests are done every five years
- When primary HPV testing becomes available, Pap tests and co-testing are phased out
- For women over age 65, the same is true: testing is stopped if results have been normal for the previous 10 years; testing is continued if they have not been normal for the previous 10 years

Screening is not indicated if a woman had a hysterectomy for a disorder other than cancer, and she has had no abnormal Pap test results. HPV testing is preferred for follow-up of atypical squamous cells of undetermined significance (ASCUS), an inconclusive finding in Pap tests. If the woman does not have HPV, screening continues at the normal intervals. If she does have HPV, a colposcopy is performed.

Preventive HPV vaccines are available. The first is the bivalent vaccine. It protects against HPV subtypes 16 and 18, which cause the majority of cervical cancers. The second is the quadrivalent vaccine. It protects against subtypes 6, 11, 16, and 18. The final vaccine is the 9-valent vaccine, which offers the widest protection. It protects against subtypes 6, 11, 16, 18, 31, 33, 45, 52, and 58 (which cause approximately 15% of cervical cancers). Also, subtypes 6 and 11 cause more than 90% of genital warts that are visible. The HPV vaccines are preventive, but are not used to treat cervical cancer. If the patient is 15–26 years old, or is immunocompromised, 3 doses are given, at zero, 1–2, and 6 months. For patients under age 15, two doses are given, 6–12 months apart. The HPV vaccine is recommended for boys as well as girls, and should be given before they become sexually active. They are recommended to be vaccinated starting at age 11–12, but vaccination can be as early as 9 years of age.

Prognosis

For squamous cell carcinomas, distant metastases usually occur if the cancer is advanced or recurrent. The five-year survival rates are 80–90% for Stage I, 60–75% for Stage II, 30–40% for Stage III, and 0–15% for Stage IV. Almost 80% of recurrences occur within two years. Prognosis is worsened if there is deep cervical stromal invasion, a large tumor size and volume, lymph node involvement, LVSI, a nonsquamous histology, or parametrial invasion.

Significant Point

Cervical cancer is, fortunately, not as commonly diagnosed as pre-cancerous conditions. With increased use of the Pap test over decades, cervical cancer death rates have dropped significantly. Also, the HPV test has improved cervical cancer screening by detecting the human papillomavirus, which is linked to nearly all cervical cancers. The HPV vaccination has been proven to reduce the incidence of cervical cancer – especially for teenagers who receive it prior to becoming sexually active.

Clinical Case

1. Which factors are associated with the development of cervical cancer?
2. Which type of tumor is the most common cervical cancer?
3. What are the American Cancer Society's new screening guidelines for cervical cancer?

A 45-year-old woman went to her physician because of abnormal vaginal bleeding, abdominal pain, constipation, poor appetite, and anemia. After evaluation, she was found to have a large cervical mass. A biopsy was taken, confirming an invasive cervical carcinoma. A CT scan showed the cancer to be 8.6 cm in diameter, which was staged as IIB. The patient was positive for HPV. A hysterectomy was performed, followed by weekly IV cisplatin plus daily pelvic radiation therapy. The patient recovered well, and was soon able to return to normal activities. She was counseled about a healthy lifestyle, and the need to return for annual Pap tests to ensure that the cancer would not recur.

Answers:

1. **The factors that may be associated with the development of cervical cancer are coitus at an early age, relations with many sexual partners, genital herpesvirus infections (cytomegalovirus), HPV, and poor obstetric and gynecological care. Cervical cancer develops from cervical intraepithelial neoplasia, which is related to an infection with the HPV virus types 16, 18, 31, 33, 35, or 39. Other risk factors include immunodeficiency and cigarette smoking.**
2. **Squamous cell carcinomas make up 90% of all cervical cancers, and the rest are nearly always adenocarcinomas. Sarcomas and small cell neuroendocrine tumors only occur rarely.**
3. **The Papanicolaou test and HPV test are used to screen for cervical cancer, and the new screening guidelines are as follows: screening begins at age 25 instead of 21, if HPV testing is available it is started at age 25 and performed every 5 years, if HPV testing is not available a Pap test is done every 3 years, if both tests are available they are done every 5 years, when primary HPV testing becomes available the Pap tests and co-testing are phased out. For women over age 65, testing is stopped if results have been normal for the previous 10 years, or continued if they have not been normal for the same time period.**

Vaginal and Vulvar Cancer

Vaginal cancer, as a primary cancer, is rare, making up less than 1% of all gynecological cancers in the United States. Metastases to the vagina or local extension from nearby gynecological structures are more common than primary vaginal tumors. Vaginal cancer is usually squamous cell carcinoma, occurring in older women most often. It is usually signified by abnormal bleeding and diagnosed by biopsy. Treatment requires hysterectomy, vaginectomy, and lymph node dissection if the cancer is small and localized. The majority of other vaginal cancers require radiation therapy.

Vulvar cancer is usually a squamous cell skin cancer, and is most common in older women. In most cases, there is a palpable lesion, and it is diagnosed via biopsy. Treatment usually includes excision with lymph node dissection or SLN mapping. Vulvar cancer is the fourth most common gynecological cancer in American women, making up 5% of female genital tract cancers.

Epidemiology

There are about 8,200 cases of vaginal cancer diagnosed annually in the United States, and just over 1,500 deaths. This means that there are about 0.7 cases per 100,000 women, with about 0.2 per 100,000 being fatal. Most vaginal cancers occur in women older than age 60, with the average age at diagnosis being 60–65. The rare form called clear cell adenocarcinoma of the vagina, from in utero diethylstilbestrol exposure, has a mean age at diagnosis of 19. A form called **sarcoma botryoides** has a peak incidence of age 3. African American women have the highest rates (0.9 per 100,000), followed by Hispanic American (0.7 per 100,000), Caucasian (0.6 per 100,000), and Asian Americans or Pacific Islanders (0.5 per 100,000). Information for Native Americans or Alaskan Natives has not been well documented. Global data are not well documented as well.

There are about 6,200 new cases of vulvar cancer annually in the United States, and nearly 1,400 cases are fatal. This means there are approximately 2.7 cases per 100,000 women, with about 0.7 being fatal. The average age at diagnosis is about 70 years, and incidence increases with aging. For some reason, incidence also appears to be increasing in young women.

Caucasian women have the highest rates (2.8 per 100,000 women), followed by African Americans (1.9 per 100,000), Hispanic Americans (1.6 per 100,000), Native Americans or Alaskan Natives, and Asian Americans or Pacific Islanders (each of these groups has 0.9 cases per 100,000). Global data are not well documented.

Etiology and Risk Factors

The exact cause of vaginal cancer is uncertain. Risk factors for vaginal cancer include the HPV infection, cervical cancer, and vulvar cancer. Most vaginal cancers are related to HPV. Rarely, exposure to diethylstilbestrol in utero predisposes a woman to clear cell adenocarcinoma of the vagina. The exact cause of vulvar cancer is also not certain. Risk factors for vulvar cancer include vulvar intraepithelial neoplasia, chronic granulomatous disease, heavy cigarette smoking, HPV infection, lichen sclerosus, squamous carcinoma of the cervix or vagina, and squamous hyperplasia.

Clinical Manifestations

The majority of patients with vaginal cancer have abnormal vaginal bleeding that may be intermenstrual, **postcoital**, or postmenopsual. There may be dyspareunia or a watery vaginal discharge. Some patients are asymptomatic, with lesions found during routine pelvic examinations or when a Pap test is evaluated. Advanced disease is signified by rectovaginal or vesicovaginal fistulas.

Vulvar cancers are usually palpable lesions, often noticed by a woman during bathing, or by a clinician during a pelvic examination. Often, there has been a long previous history of itching. Many patients are not diagnosed until vulvar cancer has become advanced. Lesions may be necrotic or ulcerated. They sometimes cause bleeding or a watery vaginal discharge. If the cancer is a melanoma, it may appear bluish-black, papillary, or pigmented.

Pathology

About 95% of primary vaginal cancers are squamous cell carcinomas. There are also primary and secondary adenocarcinomas, clear cell adenocarcinomas in younger women, secondary squamous cell carcinomas in older women, and melanomas. The most common type of vaginal sarcoma is *sarcoma botryoides*, also called *embryonal rhabdomyosarcoma*. The majority of vaginal cancers occur in the upper third of the posterior vaginal wall. Pathological spread can be via direct extension, through the inguinal lymph nodes, through the pelvic lymph nodes, or hematogenously. Direct extension occurs into the local paravaginal tissues, bladder, or rectum. Lower vaginal lesions spread through the inguinal lymph nodes. Upper vaginal lesions spread through the pelvic lymph nodes.

Approximately 90% of vulvar cancers are squamous cell carcinomas, and only 5% are melanomas. The other subtypes include adenocarcinomas, adenoid cystic carcinomas, adenosquamous carcinomas, and transitional cell carcinomas. All subtypes may originate within the **Bartholin glands**. Additionally, there are sarcomas and basal cell carcinomas that have underlying adenocarcinomas. The spreading of vulvar cancer may be by direct extension, hematogenously, to the inguinal lymph nodes, or from the inguinal lymph nodes to the pelvic and para-aortic lymph nodes. Direct extension may reach into the urethra, bladder, perineum, vagina, anus, or rectum.

Diagnosis

For diagnosis, a punch biopsy is usually sufficient, though wide local excision is sometimes needed. Vaginal cancers are staged clinically, via physical examination, cystoscopy, proctoscopy, chest X-ray to assess pulmonary metastases, and usually, CT to assess abdominal or pelvic metastases. Survival rates are based on the stage of the cancer. Outlook will be worse for large or poorly differentiated primary tumors.

Vulvar cancer can be diagnosed when a woman develops a vulvar lesion, but is at a low risk of sexually transmitted diseases, or does not respond to treatment for an STD. Vulvar cancer can mimic sexually transmitted chancroid as well as basal cell carcinoma, Bartholin gland cysts, Condyloma acuminatum infection, or vulvar Paget disease, which is a pale, eczematoid lesion. For must vulvar cancers, dermal punch biopsy with a local anesthetic is diagnostic. Sometimes, wide local excision is necessary to differentiate cancer from vulvar intraepithelial neoplasia. Non-obvious lesions may be found by staining the vulva with toluidine blue, or via colposcopy. Staging is based on tumor size and location, plus regional lymph node spread, via dissection. This is performed as part of initial surgery.

Treatment

Stage I tumors in the upper third of the vagina are treated with radical hysterectomy, upper vaginectomy, and pelvic lymph node dissection. Radiation therapy may be used after surgery. The majority of other primary vaginal tumors are treated with radiation therapy. This usually combines external beam radiation therapy with brachytherapy. If radiation therapy is contraindicated due to vesicovaginal or rectovaginal fistulas, pelvic exenteration is performed.

For vulvar cancer, a wide 2 cm or larger margin, radical excision of the local tumor is done if the tumor is only within the vulva, and has no extension to nearby perineal structures. If stromal invasion is 1 mm or larger, lymph node dissection may be done. This is unnecessary if stromal invasion is less than 1 mm. Radical vulvectomy is usually only done for Bartholin gland adenocarcinoma. If the tumor extends to perineal structures such as the urethra, vagina, or anus, a modified radical vulvectomy is done, regardless of tumor size. For some patients with squamous cell vulvar carcinoma, SLNB may be done instead of lymph node dissection. For mapping, a dye is injected intradermally around and in front of the leading edge of the tumor. If cancer has spread to the lymph nodes of the groin, SLN mapping is not needed. If the lesion is lateralized and 2 cm or less, unilateral wide local excision + unilateral SLN dissection is indicated. Bilateral SLN dissection is needed for lesions near the midline, as well as for the majority of lesions larger than 2 cm. For stage III disease,

lymph node dissection followed by chemoradiation is usually done before radical excision. Cisplatin is preferred as the chemotherapy agent, though fluorouracil may be used. Without these procedures, more radical or exenterative surgery will be required. For stage IV disease, treatment combines pelvic exenteration, radiation, and systemic chemotherapy.

Prevention and Early Detection

Except for avoiding HPV infection, there is no proven method of preventing vaginal cancer. Early detection of small, localized lesions can provide a better outlook, but many vaginal cancers do not cause any symptoms until they have already grown and spread. Pre-cancerous vaginal intraepithelial neoplasia does not usually cause any symptoms. Routine pelvic examinations and cervical cancer screening sometimes discover cases of neoplasia and early invasive vaginal cancer.

Vulvar cancer can also not be prevented, but avoiding HPV infection greatly reduces the chances of developing the disease. Routine pelvic examinations greatly improve the chances of early detection and successful treatment. There is no standard screening method currently available.

Prognosis

The prognosis for vaginal cancer is intermediate to poor. For localized vaginal cancer, the five-year survival rate is 66%. If the cancer is regional, the rate is 55%, and if distant, only 21% over five years. With all stages combined, vaginal cancer has a 49% survival rate over five years. For vulvar cancer, overall five-year survival rates depend on the stage, with risk of lymph node spreading being proportional to tumor size and invasion depth. If the cancer is a melanoma, these often metastasize, based mostly on invasion depth, but also on the size of the tumor. The five-year relative survival rate for localized vulvar cancer is good, at 86%. However, if regional, this is only 53%, and if distant, 19%. With all stages combined, vulvar cancer has a 71% survival rate over five years.

Clinical Case

1. What are the risk factors for vaginal cancer?
2. Which type of tumor is the most common vaginal cancer?
3. What is the prognosis for vaginal cancer?

A 66-year-old woman was taken to the emergency department because of continual vaginal bleeding. She denied history of multiple sex partners, but was uncertain about having HPV or not. Family history revealed that her brother had stage IV colon cancer at 68 years of age. The patient also had a 5 cm nodule in her left breast. There was a 3 cm mass on the lower third of her vagina. She had not seen a gynecologist for many years, so there were no relatively current Pap test or mammogram reports available. The vaginal mass was biopsied and diagnosed as a poorly differentiated, invasive squamous cell carcinoma. Core biopsy of the left breast nodule revealed the same characteristics as the vaginal mass. Hysterectomy, resection of both masses, and lymph node dissection were performed. Both masses were confirmed to be squamous cell carcinomas. Final diagnosis was a Stage IVB primary vaginal carcinoma, with metastasis to the left breast. After surgery, the patient was treated with carboplatin, and later, pelvic external beam radiation therapy, brachytherapy, and breast irradiation. The patient was monitored every three months for two years, and remained cancer-free.

Answers:

1. **Risk factors for vaginal cancer include the HPV infection, cervical cancer, and vulvar cancer. Most vaginal cancers are related to HPV. Rarely, exposure to diethylstilbestrol in utero predisposes a woman to clear cell adenocarcinoma of the vagina.**
2. **About 95% of primary vaginal cancers are squamous cell carcinomas. There are also primary and secondary adenocarcinomas, clear cell adenocarcinomas in younger women, secondary squamous cell carcinomas in older women, and melanomas.**
3. **The prognosis for vaginal cancer is intermediate to poor. For localized vaginal cancer, the five-year survival rate is 66%. If the cancer is regional, the rate is 55%, and if distant, only 21% over five years. With all stages combined, vaginal cancer has a 49% survival rate over five years.**

Key Terms

Abdominal gutters
Adnexal torsion
Apoptosis
Atretic cells
Bartholin glands
Breast tomosynthesis
Cachexia
Cesium
Choriocarcinoma
Chorion
Cryoablated
Dysgerminomas

Ectodermal
Excrescences
Growth factors
Hydatidiform mole
Hysterectomy
Infracolic omentum
Intraligamentous fibroids
Intramural
Invasive carcinoma
Lobular carcinoma in situ
Lynch syndrome
Mammary duct ectasia

Mastalgia
Meigs syndrome
Menometrorrhagia
Menorrhagia
Mesenchymal
Microinvasive
Molar pregnancy
Myomectomy
Myxomatous
Nonmorular
Parturition
Phyllodes tumor
Polycystic ovary syndrome
Postcoital
Radical trachelectomy

Radiofrequency ablation
Reaspiration
Sarcoma botryoides
Sentinel lymph node mapping
Sonohysterography
Syncytiotrophoblasts
Transvaginal ultrasound
Trimorphic
Trophoblast cells
Unopposed estrogen
Urostomy
Uterine sarcoma
Vaginal cancer
Vulvar cancer
XY gonadal dysgenesis

Bibliography

1 Albuquerque, K., Beriwal, S., Viswanathan, A.N., and Erickson, B. (2019). *Radiation Therapy Techniques for Gynecological Cancers: A Comprehensive Practical Guide. (Practical Guides in Radiation Oncology)*. New York: Springer.

2 Al-Mudhaffar, S.A. and Al-Qadi, S.X. (2015). *Characterization of Progesterone and Its Receptors in Ovarian Tumors "Benign and Malignant" (Progesterone and Ovarian Tumors)*. Scotts Valley: CreateSpace Independent Publishing Platform.

3 American Association for Cancer Research. (2020). *Endometrial Cancer*. American Association for Cancer Research. https://www.aacr.org/patients-caregivers/cancer/endometrial-cancer. Accessed 2021.

4 American Cancer Society. (2021). *Uterine Sarcoma*. American Cancer Society, Inc. https://www.cancer.org/cancer/uterine-sarcoma.html. Accessed 2021.

5 American Cancer Society. (2021). *What Is Gestational Trophoblastic Disease?* American Cancer Society, Inc. https://www.cancer.org/cancer/gestational-trophoblastic-disease/about/what-is-gtd.html. Accessed 2021.

6 American Cancer Society. (2020). *Key Statistics for Uterine Sarcoma*. American Cancer Society, Inc. https://www.cancer.org/cancer/uterine-sarcoma/about/key-statistics.html. Accessed 2021.

7 American Cancer Society. (2018). *Vaginal Cancer – Early Detection, Diagnosis, and Staging – Can Vaginal Cancer Be Found Early?* American Cancer Society, Inc. https://www.cancer.org/cancer/vaginal-cancer/detection-diagnosis-staging/detection.html. Accessed 2021.

8 American Cancer Society Journals – Cancer. (2003). *Incidence of ovarian cancer by race and ethnicity in the United* States, *1992–1997*. John Wiley & Sons, Inc. https://acsjournals.onlinelibrary.wiley.com/doi/full/10.1002/cncr.11349. 97 (S10): 2676–2685. Accessed 2021.

9 AORN Journal – Clinical. (2001). *Uterine Artery Embolization*. John Wiley & Sons, Inc. https://aornjournal.onlinelibrary.wiley.com/doi/abs/10.1016/s0001-2092%2806%2961807-3. 73 (4): 788–807 Accessed 2021.

10 Augustin, H.G., Iruela-Arispe, M.L., Rogers, P.A.W., and Smith, S.K. (2012). *Vascular*

Morphogenesis in the Female Reproductive System. Basel: Birkhauser.

11 Aydiner, A., Igci, A., and Soran, A. (2019). *Breast Disease: Diagnosis and Pathology*, Volume 1, 2nd Edition. New York: Springer.

12 Benigno, B.B. and Manning-Geist, B. (2016). *The Ultimate Guide to Ovarian Cancer: Everything You Need to Know about Diagnosis, Treatment, and Research*, 2nd Edition. Atlanta: Sherryben Publishing House.

13 Benoit, M., Williams-Brown, M.Y., and Edwards, C.L. (2017). *Gynecologic Oncology Handbook: An Evidence-Based Clinical Guide*, 2nd Edition. New York: DemosMedical.

14 Bristow, R.E., Karlan, B.Y., and Chi, D.S. (2015). *Surgery for Ovarian Cancer*, 3rd Edition. Boca Raton: CRC Press.

15 British Medical Journal Best Practice. (2021). *Uterine fibroids*. BMJ Best Practice. https://bestpractice.bmj.com/topics/en-gb/567. Accessed 2021.

16 Cancer Research U.K. (2021). *About persistent trophoblastic disease and choriocarcinoma*. Cancer Research U.K. https://www.cancerresearchuk.org/about-cancer/gestational-trophoblastic-disease-gtd/persistent-trophoblastic-disease-ptd-choriocarcinoma/about. Accessed 2021.

17 CancerWall.com – Cancers, Tumors, Swellings Information & Research. (2021). *What is Choriocarcinoma?* CancerWall.com. https://cancerwall.com/choriocarcinoma-symptoms-prognosis-treatment-diagnosis. Accessed 2021.

18 Coukos, G., Berchuck, A., and Ozols, R. (2008). *Ovarian Cancer: State of the Art and Future Directions in Translational Research (Advances in Experimental Medicine and Biology, Volume 622)*. New York: Springer.

19 Dizon, D.S. and Abu-Rustum, N.R. (2008). *Gynecologic Tumor Board-Clinical Cases in Diagnosis & Management of Cancer of the Female Reproductive System*. Burlington: Jones & Bartlett Learning.

20 Drugs.com. (2020). *What are Cervical Polyps?* Drugs.com https://www.drugs.com/health-guide/cervical-polyps.html. Accessed 2021.

21 Drunpanthel, F. (2021). *Symptoms of Cervical Cancer: Abnormal Vaginal Bleeding, Pelvic Pain, Dyspareunia, Loss of Appetite, Weight Loss, Fatigue, Vaginal Discharge, Urinary Symptoms, General Feelings of Illness, Nausea and Vomiting*. New York: Drunpanthel.

22 Elsevier – Maturitas. (2012). *Incidence of uterine leiomyosarcoma and endometrial stromal sarcoma in Nordic countries: Results from NORDCAN and NOCCA databases*. Elsevier B.V. https://www.sciencedirect.com/science/article/abs/pii/S0378512212000515. 72 (1): 56–60. Accessed 2021.

23 ePainAssist.com. (2021). *What is Gestational Choriocarcinoma: Causes, Symptoms, Treatment, Life Expectancy, Prognosis*. PainAssist Inc (ePainAssist). https://www.epainassist.com/pregnancy-and-parenting/gestational-choriocarcinoma. Accessed 2021.

24 Goldblum, J.R., Lamps, L.W., McKenney, J.K., and Myers, J.L. (2017). *Rosai and Ackerman's Surgical Pathology*, 11th Edition. Amsterdam: Elsevier.

25 Hirschmann, K. (2010). *Cervical Cancer (Diseases & Disorders)*. New York: Lucent Books.

26 Hunt, K.K., Robb, G.L., Strom, E.A., Ueno, N.T., Buzdar, A.U., and Freedman, R.S. (2007). *Breast Cancer (M.D. Anderson Cancer Care Series)*, 2nd Edition. New York: Springer.

27 Icon Health Publications. (2004). *Cervical Polyps – A 3-in-1 Medical Reference: Medical Dictionary, Bibliography & Annotated Research Guide*. San Diego: Icon Health Publications.

28 Imiline, Y. (2021). *Signs of Cervical Cancer*. New York: Imiline.

29 International Agency for Research on Cancer. (2014). *WHO Classification of Tumours of the Female Reproductive Organs*, 4th Edition. Geneva: World Health Organization.

30 Jenkins, D. and Bosch, X. (2019). *Human Papillomavirus: Proving and Using a Viral Cause for Cancer*. Cambridge: Academic Press.

31 Johnson, T. and Schwartz, M. (2012). *Gestational Trophoblastic Neoplasia: A Guide for Women Dealing with Tumors of the*

Placenta, Such as Choriocarcinoma, Molar Pregnancy and Other Forms of GTN. New York: Your Health Press.

32 Lee, S.H. (2021). *From Pap Smears to HPV Vaccines: Evolution of the Cervical Cancer Prevention Industry.* Hauppauge: Nova Science Publishing Inc.

33 Mayo Clinic. (2021). *Patient Care & Health Information – Diseases & Conditions – Uterine fibroids.* Mayo Foundation for Medical Education and Research (MFMER). https://www.mayoclinic.org/diseases-conditions/uterine-fibroids/symptoms-causes/syc-20354288. Accessed 2021.

34 Metwally, M. and Li, T.C. (2020). *Modern Management of Uterine Fibroids.* Cambridge: Cambridge University Press.

35 Mirza, M.R. (2020). *Management of Endometrial Cancer.* New York: Springer.

36 Mitidieri, M., Danese, S., and Picardo, E. (2021). *Uterine Fibroids: From Diagnosis to Treatment (Obstetrics and Gynecology Advances).* Hauppauge: Nova Science Publishing Inc.

37 Muggia, F. and Oliva, E. (2009). *Uterine Cancer: Screening, Diagnosis, and Treatment.* Totowa: Humana Press.

38 National Cancer Institute – Surveillance, Epidemiology, and End Results Program. (2020). *Cancer Stat Facts: Female Breast Cancer.* U.S. Department of Health and Human Services – National Institutes of Health – National Cancer Institute – USA.gov. https://seer.cancer.gov/statfacts/html/breast.html. Accessed 2021.

39 National Cancer Institute. (2021). *Endometrial Cancer Prevention (PDQ) – Patient Version.* U.S. Department of Health and Human Services – National Institutes of Health – National Cancer Institute – USA.gov. https://www.cancer.gov/types/uterine/patient/endometrial-prevention-pdq. Accessed 2021.

40 National Cancer Institute. (2021). *Clinical Trials Search Results.* U.S. Department of Health and Human Services – National Institutes of Health – National Cancer Institute – USA.gov. https://www.cancer.gov/about-cancer/treatment/clinical-trials/search/r?loc=0&pn=41&t=C7558. Accessed 2021.

41 National Comprehensive Cancer Network. (2018). *NCCN Guidelines for Patients: Uterine Cancer (Endometrial Cancer, Uterine Sarcoma).* Plymouth Meeting: National Comprehensive Cancer Network (NCCN).

42 National Library of Medicine – National Center for Biotechnology Information. (2017). *Epidemiology of uterine fibroids: A systematic review.* National Library of Medicine. https://pubmed.ncbi.nlm.nih.gov/28296146. Accessed 2021.

43 National Library of Medicine – National Center for Biotechnology Information. (2018). *Relative Effects of Age, Race, and Stage on Mortality in Gestational Choriocarcinoma.* National Library of Medicine. https://pubmed.ncbi.nlm.nih.gov/29232272. Accessed 2021.

44 PathologyOutlines.com. (2021). *Placenta – Gestational trophoblastic disease – Neoplasms – Choriocarcinoma.* PathologyOutlines.com, Inc. https://www.pathologyoutlines.com/topic/placentachoriocarcinoma.html. Accessed 2021.

45 Petrozza, J.C. (2020). *Uterine Fibroids.* Boca Raton: CRC Press.

46 Pritchett Mims, M., Miller-Chism, C., and Sosa, I.R. (2019). *Handbook of Benign Hematology.* New York: DemosMedical.

47 Rajaram, S., Chitrathara, K., and Maheshwari, A. (2015). *Uterine Cancer: Diagnosis and Treatment.* New York: Springer.

48 Rosenblatt, A. and De Campos Guidi, H.G. (2009). *Human Papillomavirus: A Practical Guide for Urologists.* New York: Springer.

49 Rowe, J.J. and Downs-Kelly, E. (2021). *Mesenchymal Tumors of the Breast and Their Mimics: A Diagnostic Approach.* New York: Springer.

50 StatPearls. (2021). *Cervical Polyps.* StatPearls. https://www.statpearls.com/articlelibrary/viewarticle/19243. Accessed 2021.

51 Sugino, N. (2018). *Uterine Fibroids and Adenomyosis (Comprehensive Gynecology and Obstetrics).* New York: Springer.

52 Syrjanen, K. and Syrjanen, S. (2000). *Papillomavirus Infections in Human Pathology.* Hoboken: Wiley.

53 Tabar, L., Tot, T., and Dean, P.B. (2011). *Breast Cancer: Early Detection with Mammography – Crushed Stone-like Calcifications: The Most Frequent Malignant Type.* Stuttgart: Thieme.

54 Veronesi, U., Goldhirsch, A., Veronesi, P., Gentilini, O.D., and Leonardi, M.C. (2017). *Breast Cancer: Innovations in Research and Management.* New York: Springer.

55 WebMD – Cancer Center. (2019). *What is Choriocarcinoma?* WebMD LLC. https://www.webmd.com/cancer/what-is-choriocarcinoma. Accessed 2021.

56 WebMD – Women's Health – Guide. (2021). *What Are Cervical Polyps?* WebMD LLC. https://www.webmd.com/women/guide/cervical-polyps. Accessed 2021.

57 Wiley InterScience – Ultrasound Obstet Gynecol. (2010). *Sonographic appearance of gestational trophoblastic disease evolving into epithelioid trophoblastic tumor.* John Wiley & Sons, Inc. https://obgyn.onlinelibrary.wiley.com/doi/pdf/10.1002/uog.7560. 36: 249–251. Accessed 2021.

58 Wiley Online Library – Cancer Medicine. (2020). *Contrast-enhanced spectral mammography: A potential exclusion diagnosis modality in dense breast patients.* John Wiley & Sons, Inc. https://onlinelibrary.wiley.com/doi/full/10.1002/cam4.2877. 9 (8): 2653–2659. Accessed 2021.

59 Wiley Online Library – Journal of Ultrasound in Medicine – Early View. (2020). *Ultrasound-Guided Breast Biopsies – Basic and New Techniques.* John Wiley & Sons, Inc. https://onlinelibrary.wiley.com/doi/full/10.1002/jum.15517. Accessed 2021.

60 Wiley Online Library – Trends in Urology, Gynaecology & Sexual Health. (2010). *Gynaecological Malignancies – Diagnosis and management of primary cervical carcinoma.* John Wiley & Sons, Inc. https://onlinelibrary.wiley.com/doi/10.1002/tre.151. 15 (3):24–30. Accessed 2021.

61 World Cancer Research Fund – American Institute for Cancer Research. (2018). *Breast cancer statistics – Breast cancer is the most common cancer in women worldwide.* WCRF International – Continuous Update Project. https://www.wcrf.org/dietandcancer/breast-cancer-statistics. Accessed 2021.

62 World Cancer Research Fund – American Institute for Cancer Research. (2018). *Endometrial cancer statistics – Endometrial cancer is the 15th most common cancer worldwide.* WCRF International – Continuous Update Project. https://www.wcrf.org/dietandcancer/endometrial-cancer-statistics. Accessed 2021.

63 World Health Organization. (2021). *Breast cancer now most common form of cancer: WHO taking action.* World Health Organization. https://www.who.int/news/item/03-02-2021-breast-cancer-now-most-common-form-of-cancer-who-taking-action. Accessed 2021.

64 World Health Organization – Human Reproduction Programme. (2019). *Sexual and reproductive health – Cervical cancer.* World Health Organization. https://www.who.int/reproductivehealth/topics/cancers/en. Accessed 2021.

65 World Ovarian Cancer Coalition. (2020). *World Ovarian Cancer Coalition Atlas 2020 – Global trends in incidence, mortality, and survival.* World Ovarian Cancer Coalition. https://worldovariancancercoalition.org/wp-content/uploads/2020/10/2020-World-Ovarian-Cancer-Atlas_FINAL.pdf. Accessed 2021.

10

Skin Tumors

OUTLINE

Moles
Dermatofibromas
Infantile Hemangiomas
Lipoma and Liposarcoma
Keloids
Melanoma
Basal Cell Carcinoma
Squamous Cell Carcinoma
Bowen Disease
Merkel Cell Skin Cancer
Kaposi Sarcoma
Key Terms
Bibliography

Moles

Moles are skin growths that usually appear in childhood or adolescence. Most moles are close to the color of the surrounding skin, but they can also be much darker than the skin. They are clinically also referred to as macules, nodules, or papules, and are made up of groupings of melanocytes or nevus cells. It is important to monitor moles for alterations in their appearance such as developing more than one color simultaneously, having irregular borders, and symptoms such as bleeding, itching, or ulceration. These changes may suggest atypia or the development of melanoma. Atypical moles are also called *benign melanocytic nevi*. They have borders that are irregular and poorly defined. The colors are usually brown or tan, and macular or papular features are present. Atypical moles increase the risk of developing melanoma.

Epidemiology

Though present in nearly every human, the lifetime risk of a mole becoming malignant is about 1 in every 3,000–10,000 people. People with 50 or more benign moles have an increased risk of developing melanoma. Prevalence of atypical moles in the United States is 4% of people with lighter skin, though an estimated 7.5% of the general population has them. Common and atypical moles generally decrease in number with aging, starting when people are in their 20s. However, atypical moles can continue to appear throughout life. Prevalence is slightly higher in males than in females, but this has been linked to higher ultraviolet radiation exposure in men because more of them work in occupations that require them to be outside of buildings. Prevalence of atypical moles is the lowest in dark-skinned people, at only 13% of the fair-skinned rate.

Global Epidemiology of Cancer: Diagnosis and Treatment, First Edition. Jahangir Moini, Nicholas G. Avgeropoulos, and Craig Badolato.
© 2022 John Wiley & Sons Ltd. Published 2022 by John Wiley & Sons Ltd.

Global prevalence of atypical moles is in the range of 2–18%, with a higher incidence in European countries of 7–24%, predominantly in fair-skinned people. More cases of atypical moles occur in adults, and pediatric incidence is low. Throughout the world, men have atypical moles slightly more often than women. While there is no actual racial or ethnic predilection, skin color is generally the most important factor. However, there are exceptions, such as in Japan, where skin color is lighter, yet this population has a low incidence of atypical moles. Overall, there is a lack of studies on the actual number of global cases of atypical moles, however.

Etiology and Risk Factors

While normal moles have no specific cause and develop naturally, atypical moles may be inherited in an autosomal dominant fashion. They can also form sporadically with no family history. **Familial mole-melanoma syndrome** involves multiple atypical moles and melanoma developing in two or more first-degree relatives. These individuals are at a 25-times higher risk of eventually developing melanoma. Risk factors for atypical moles include puberty, pregnancy, fair skin, genetics, and have excessive sun exposure.

Clinical Manifestations

Most moles are less than 6 mm in diameter and usually light brown to dark brown in color. They can be flat or elevated, and described as nodular macules or papules. Atypical moles, however, are often 6 mm or larger in diameter and mostly round in shape, but with non-distinct borders and slight asymmetry. They differ in appearance from melanomas, which have more color irregularities, including red, blue, black, off-white, and depigmented. Some melanomas look like scars.

Table 10.1 compares characteristics that are different between typical and atypical moles.

Pathology

There are five different pathological classifications of moles, which are also singularly referred to as a **nevus**, and when there are multiple moles, as **nevi**. The classifications are as follows:

- Blue nevus – bluish gray to bluish-black in color, often flat but can be slightly elevated macules or thin papules, 2–4 mm in diameter, though there have been sizes up to 2 cm in diameter; there are deeply pigmented dendritic melanocytes, plus scattered melanophages in the dermal layer of the skin as well as adipose tissues; there may be alveolar and pigmented dendritic cellular patterns; the

Table 10.1 Characteristics of typical and atypical moles.

Typical moles	Atypical moles
Appear in childhood or adolescence	Continue to appear in adulthood
Flesh-colored to yellow–brown to black	Tan to dark brown with a pink background, with a light or dark target appearance, with the rim being flatter than the center; the pigment may be "blurry" at the edges, or have notches
Can appear anywhere on the body	Usually appear on areas of skin exposed to the sun, but can also occur on "covered" areas, such as the scalp, breasts, or buttocks
Range from 1 to 10 mm in size, but usually are less than 6 mm	Range from 5 to 12 mm in size
Usually less than 10 moles in total	One to several dozen moles in total
Symmetrical shape with regular borders	Symmetrical or asymmetrical, with borders that can be regular or irregular

blue color is due to the depth and density of pigment within the skin

- Halo nevus – can be of any color or elevation, but surrounded by a 2–6 mm ring of depigmented skin; their histology is like the other classifications, but there is inflammation and loss of melanocytes in the "halo skin"
- Junctional nevus – can range from very light in color to almost black, they are usually flat but can be somewhat elevated, and 1–10 mm in diameter; there are nests of melanocytes at the epidermodermal junction
- Compound nevus – light to dark brown in color, slightly or extremely elevated, 3–6 mm in diameter; there are "nests" of melanocytes located at the epidermodermal, and the dermal layer
- Intradermal nevus – can range from the same color as the surrounding skin to brown in color, and can be smooth or have protruding hairs, or even warts; they are elevated, with a 3–6 mm diameter; melanocytes and nevus cells are almost totally confined to the dermal layer

During adolescence, there is often an increase in the number of moles on the body, with existing moles increasing in diameter or darkening in color. Nevus cells may be replaced with fibrous tissue or fat. Moles often change in consistency, becoming softer, spongy, firmer, and can lose pigment with aging. Atypical moles are different in appearance and histology. They have a disordered structure, and the melanocytes are atypical. Most melanomas arise *de novo*, which means they form from normal skin and are not connected to a mole. Some patients have one or a small number of atypical moles, but others can have many of them.

Diagnosis

Due to the commonality of benign moles and the rareness of melanoma, they are usually not removed on a prophylactic basis. Even so, biopsy and histological study is concert when a mole has concerning features. These are known as the ABCDEs of melanoma, as follows:

- Asymmetry – the appearance is not symmetrical
- Borders – they are irregular and not oval or round
- Color – there are variations of color in the mole, some of which may be unusual, or the suspect mole is much different or darker than other moles on the patient's body
- Diameter – the mole is larger than 6 mm in diameter
- Evolution – a mole has suddenly appeared in a patient older than 30 years of age, or a mole has started to have visible changes

Biopsy is also considered if a mole starts to hurt, itch, ulcerate, or bleed. The specimen must be deep to allow for accurate diagnosis under a microscope. The entire lesion should be biopsied if possible – especially when suspicion of cancer is significant. Wide primary excision is not the first procedure, however, even when a mole is extremely abnormal in appearance. There are many abnormal moles that are not actually melanomas. Even when they are, the correct margins for biopsy and recommendations for sampling nearby lymph nodes are based on histopathology. An excisional biopsy does not reduce the change for metastasis when the mole is malignant. It also avoids excessively extensive surgery for a benign mole.

Atypical moles must be differentiated from melanomas by using the ABCDEs of melanoma. Though diagnosis can be established by clinical findings, visual differences between atypical moles and melanomas may sometimes be difficult to see. The most abnormal-appearing moles should be biopsied to establish diagnosis and determine how much atypia is present. The complete depth and width of the mole should be biopsied – excisional biopsy is often best. Examination is done every year or more often for patients with many atypical moles, or with personal or family history of melanoma. A hand-held **dermoscope** may be used so that extremely small structures can be seen. Dermoscopy can reveal high-risk features such as irregular globules or dots, an abnormal pigment network, a blue-white veil, or a reverse network. An abnormal pigment network contains intersecting brown lines in a reticular pattern that resembles a mesh-like grid. A blue-white veil is a focal, relatively non-structured zone with an overlying white "haze" that resembles ground glass, occurring in raised or palpable area of a mole. A reverse network is also called a *negative pigment network*. It is a milky, laced network that develops between the brown areas of a mole.

Treatment

For cosmetic purposes, moles can be surgically removed by shaving or excision. In shave excision, a scalpel is used to shave off the mole. In excision biopsy, the mole is cut out of the skin and stitches are used if necessary to close the wound. In serial excision, multiple surgical sessions are used to remove larger moles in small stages. With cryotherapy, the mole is frozen with liquid nitrogen, causing it to be gradually shed as the skin continually regenerates. If the mole does not fall off, a physician can easily remove it later. With electrocautery, the mole is burned off and removed from the skin via an electrically heated wire. The upper skin layers that contain the mole are also burned off. All moles that are removed should be histologically examined. For any mole from which a hair grows, it should be sufficiently excised and not shaved because the hair will simply regrow. The prophylactic removal of all atypical moles does not mean that melanoma will be prevented, so it is not recommended. Even so, these moles can be removed if any of the following exist:

- The mole has high-risk features found during dermoscopy
- The mole is located in any area that makes monitoring for changes difficult or impossible
- The patient has a high-risk history, with personal or family history of melanoma
- The patient cannot ensure that close follow-up will occur

Nonsurgical treatments include chemical peels that use glycolic acid or azelaic acid, lasers, and **dermabrasion**, which is a skin-resurfacing procedure that uses a quickly rotating device to remove the outer layer of the skin. The new skin that replaces it is usually smooth and of a more cosmetically appealing appearance.

Prevention and Early Detection

Prevention of atypical moles involves avoiding excessive sun exposure and the use of sun-protecting agents. It is also important to take enough vitamin D as a supplement. Patients should be instructed about the proper methods to examine their skin for changes in moles, and how to recognize the characteristic features of melanomas. New or changing moles can be discovered by full-body photography, and regular follow-up examinations should occur. For any patient with a history of melanoma or other types of skin cancers, first-degree relatives must also be examined. If there is a family history of melanomas, individuals have a higher-than-average risk of developing them. Such individuals should have examinations of their skin, including the scalp skin, to assess risks of developing melanoma, and follow-up examinations are required. Early detection of atypical moles is very important, along with close monitoring for any changes that may indicate the development of melanoma. Vigilant self-examination and reviewing any possibly atypical moles with a physician should occur every 4–6 months for high-risk individuals, and every 6–12 months for those not at high risk. Regular clinical photography of suspect moles should be done to assist in detecting changes.

Prognosis

The prognosis for atypical moles is varied. Studies have reported a 0.5–46% rate of progression to melanoma. Different forms of diagnostic criteria explain this large range.

Significant Point

Patients with 50 or more moles on their bodies must be taught how to self-monitor for warning signs of malignancy. Skin surveillance must become part of their primary care. Protection from ultraviolet radiation is important, and requires avoiding excessive sun exposure and indoor tanning.

Clinical Case

1. What are the chances of a mole becoming malignant?
2. What are the five pathological classifications of moles?
3. What are the treatment options for atypical moles?

A 41-year-old woman had previously been diagnosed with nodular melanoma. She visited her dermatologist because of a dome-shaped nodule in the gluteal region. It was bluish-black in color and had a diameter of 1.2 cm. It was clinically diagnosed as a blue nevus. The nodule had recently enlarged slightly, so a complete resection was performed. In histology, it was found to have an increasing pattern of extension into the dermis as well as subcutaneous adipose tissue. There was an alveolar pattern and a pigmented dendritic cell pattern. This was consistent with a cellular blue nevus. Due to the patient's history of nodular melanoma, immunohistochemistry and molecular analysis were performed. These procedures, fortunately, confirmed the diagnosis of a benign, cellular blue nevus.

Answers:

1. **The lifetime risk of a mole becoming malignant is about 1 in every 3,000–10,000 people. People with 50 or more benign moles have an increased risk of developing melanoma.**
2. **The five pathological classifications of moles are: blue nevus, halo nevus, junctional nevus, compound nevus, and intradermal nevus.**
3. **Treatment options for atypical moles include shave excision and excision biopsy, serial excision, cryotherapy, electrocautery, chemical peels, lasers, and dermabrasion.**

Dermatofibromas

Dermatofibromas are also known as *benign fibrous histiocytomas* and *cutaneous fibrous histiocytomas*. They are red to brown in color, and are small, firm nodules or papules made up of fibroblastic tissue, usually on the thighs or legs. However, they can occur anywhere on the body, with the upper arms and upper back being the next most common sites. Over years, some dermatofibromas change color. They remain on the body for life unless surgically removed.

Epidemiology

Dermatofibromas, since they are benign, have not been widely studied as to their prevalence or incidence. Based on a few small-scale studies, they are estimated to affect the global population at a percentage between 0.5% and 2%, though in two more recent studies, estimates were between 14% and 18%. Dermatofibromas are common in adults between the ages of 40 and 48, though they have been seen in adults as young as 18 and as old as 86. They appear more often in women than men, in an estimated ratio between 2 : 1 and 5 : 1. They are rare in children, but have appeared between the ages of 12 and 17. There is no racial or ethnic predilection, as they occur in people from all countries, and dermatofibromas have been documented as occurring on all continents of the world.

Etiology and Risk Factors

Dermatofibromas may be genetically related. Sometimes, they develop on the skin after an insect bite, an injection, or an injury from a sharp plant such as a rose bush. Risk factors for multiple dermatofibromas include poor immune system function, immunosuppression, and autoimmune conditions.

Clinical Manifestations

Dermatofibromas are usually between 0.5 and 1.5 cm in diameter, and are firm. They sometimes "dimple" inward if they are gently squeezed. This is known as the *pinch sign*. In some people, dermatofibromas feel like there is a hard structure below the skin. The majority of dermatofibromas are asymptomatic, but for some individuals, if a minor trauma occurs to them, they may itch or ulcerate. Due to being raised, they can be traumatized during shaving. Sometimes, these lesions are painful or tender. The color ranges from pink to light brown in Caucasians, and dark brown to black in darker-skinned people. Sometimes, the center of a dermatofibroma is paler in color than the rest of the lesion.

Pathology

It is unknown if dermatofibromas are part of a reactive process or are neoplasms. Their pathological makeup includes proliferating fibroblasts as well as histiocytes. Under a microscope, there are whirling fascicles of spindle cell proliferation and excessive collagen deposition in the dermal layer. Pathological variants include: aneurysmal, atypical, cellular, cholesterotic, epithelioid, lipidized ankle-type, and palisading. Dermatofibromas are attached to the surface of the skin, and are mobile structures above the subcutaneous tissues. Rarely, dozens of dermatofibromas may develop over a few months, usually in immunosuppressed individuals. The subtype known as *atrophic dermatofibroma* usually occurs on the shoulders, followed by the lower legs and back. Dermatofibromas of all types do not lead to skin cancer.

Diagnosis

The diagnosis of dermatofibromas is usually clinical, often assisted by dermoscopy. They may be biopsied so that any melanocytic proliferation can be excluded. This proliferation can lead to a mole, **solar lentigo**, melanoma, and other skin cancers. Diagnostic excision or skin biopsy is performed if there is recent enlargement, asymmetrical structures or colors, or ulceration. Diagnostic confirmation is via immunohistochemical staining. Dermatofibromas can be misdiagnosed as **dermatofibrosarcoma protuberans** or *desmoplastic melanoma*.

Treatment

While asymptomatic dermatofibromas are not treated, those that cause any trouble to the patient can be surgically excised. However, recurrence is common since dermatofibromas often extend beyond the clinical margin. Surgical removal requires a deep cut because dermatofibromas extend below the skin surface, and a noticeable scar is usually present after surgery. Only rarely are treatments such as cryotherapy, laser treatments, or shave biopsies successful in permanently removing dermatofibromas.

Prevention and Early Detection

There is no known way to prevent dermatofibromas because they are of unknown cause. Because dermatofibromas are easily seen, they are usually detected early. When they are in locations that are hard to see, they are often found early because they frequently rub up against clothing.

Prognosis

The prognosis of dermatofibromas is excellent because they do not become cancerous.

Infantile Hemangiomas

Infantile hemangiomas are the most common tumors that occur in infants, and appear as raised hyperplastic vascular lesions during the first year of life. They are red or purple to blue in color. Most infantile hemangiomas spontaneously decrease in size, but those that obstruct the eyes, the airway, or other important body structures must be treated.

Epidemiology

Globally, including in the United States, infantile hemangiomas affect 10–25% of infants within the first 12 months of life. They are present *at birth* in 10–20% of affected infants. However, true incidence is unknown due to lack of documentation, but infantile hemangiomas are estimated to affect about 5% of infants of all ages throughout the world. They occur slightly more often in females, Caucasians, and those that are born prematurely or that have a low birthweight.

Etiology and Risk Factors

The cause of infantile hemangiomas is not known, but estrogen signaling in proliferation is believed to be involved. Local soft-tissue hypoxia and increased levels of circulating estrogen after birth may be implicated. Risk factors for infantile hemangiomas include the female gender, the Caucasian race, premature birth, and low birth weight.

Clinical Manifestations

Sometimes, deeper infantile hemangiomas do not appear until a few months after birth. Their size and extent of vascularity increase quickly, usually reaching a peak of development in about 12 months. When superficial, these lesions are often bright red in color, but when they are deeper, they appear almost blue. Minor trauma can cause them to bleed or ulcerate, and ulcerated lesions can become painful. In some areas of the body, the lesions may interfere with normal functioning. Those located on the face or in the oropharynx can interfere with sight or breathing. If located near the anus or urethral meatus, they can affect defecation or urination. A *periocular hemangioma* is considered an emergency in infants and should be removed soon to avoid possible permanent visual abnormalities. When there is a lumbosacral hemangioma, this can indicate a neurologic or genitourinary abnormality.

Beginning at 12–18 months of age, the lesions start to slowly resolve, with decreases in vascularity and size. Usually, infantile hemangiomas resolve by about 10% with each year of age. They are usually completely resolved by the age of 10 years, though they often leave behind a discoloration that is yellowish or resembles multiple tiny blood vessels. The texture of the lesion site may be wrinkled, or have a loose structure of adipose tissue. These changes are almost always proportional to the lesion's largest size and extent of vascularity.

Pathology

The pathological classifications of infantile hemangiomas include superficial, deep, or cavernous appearances, and those that are known as **strawberry hemangiomas** (see Figure 10.1). All types of hemangiomas have the same pathophysiology and type of development.

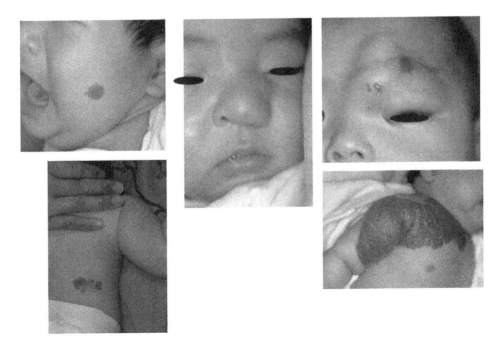

Figure 10.1 Strawberry hemangiomas. (a) Cheek; (b) nose; (c) forehead and eyebrow; (d) back; (e) shoulder and neck. *Source*: https://onlinelibrary.wiley.com/doi/10.1111/j.1346-8138.2010.00927.x. Journal of Dermatology [20].

Diagnosis

Infantile hemangiomas are diagnosed clinically. Their size can be evaluated via an MRI if they are believed to affect a vital body structure. Most infantile hemangiomas can be diagnosed by history and physical examination. Based on the location of the tumor, confirmation is by Doppler ultrasound, MRI, cytology, and histopathology. Tissue can be obtained via excisional biopsy, fine-needle aspiration, or skin biopsy. Another diagnostic factor is that these hemangiomas show mostly volumetric growth over the first 4–8 weeks of life. After that, growth slows over 6–9 months, but 80% of the growth has occurred by 3 months of age.

Treatment

There are many different treatment methods for infantile hemangiomas. Surgery is usually avoided unless essential. Treatments are individualized based on the lesion size, location, and severity. When a superficial or uncomplicated hemangioma requires treatment, topical or intralesional corticosteroids may be used, as well as topical beta-blockers such as propranolol. If the hemangioma is complicated or of high risk, oral propranolol may be administered. Complicated or high-risk hemangiomas are those that threaten life or essential functions such as vision, affect a large part of the face, are distributed over the jaw area, or are lumbosacral, multiple, or ulcerated. The ulcerated hemangiomas require generalized wound care. Topical treatments for these hemangiomas help to prevent bleeding, pain, and scarring. Infections can be prevented, and colonization of pathogens can be stopped by using compresses, barrier creams or dressings, and topical metronidazole or mupirocin. Barrier dressings usually involve a polyurethane film dressing or gauze that has been impregnated with petrolatum. Since most hemangiomas resolve on their own, observation is usually used before any treatment is given.

Surgery or other invasive procedures are reserved for hemangiomas that are life-threatening or compromise the function of any vital organ. However, they usually leave more scarring than what remains after a hemangioma resolves naturally. Physicians often discuss hemangiomas with the parents of affected infants and show them photographs of how they resolve over time. They can also photograph the lesions at every visit to document that they are resolving, helping to encourage parents as needed.

Prevention and Early Detection

There is no known method of preventing infantile hemangiomas. Since they usually completely resolve on their own, early detection plays no role in their development or resolution.

Prognosis

The prognosis for most infantile hemangiomas is very good, since they completely resolve during childhood. Though the vascular component resolves, about half of all affected children still have skin changes in the area where the tumor was located. For those that resolve by 6 years of age, 38% of cases have a scar, **telangiectasia**, or **anetodermic** skin. About 80% of lesions that resolve by 6 years of age leave severe skin abnormalities.

Significant Point

Infantile hemangiomas are benign tumors that form from an overgrowth of blood vessels. They are sometimes referred to as "strawberry marks" because of their color and surface appearance. They can occur anywhere on the body, but most often appear on the face and neck, often forming a nodule or having a plaque-like appearance.

Clinical Case

1. How common are infantile hemangiomas?
2. When do these hemangiomas start to resolve?

3. Though prognosis is generally good, what skin changes usually remain?

A 9-week-old boy is brought by his mother to their pediatrician to assess a bluish mass of his right eyelid and orbit. The mass has increased in size over the past month, but the baby had no other health problems. The mass inferiorly displaced his right eye and caused severe ptosis of the right eyelid. It was a large orbital lesion, and a diagnosis of a non-periocular infantile hemangioma was made. The baby was assessed for cardiac abnormalities, which were not present, and then treated over the next year with propranolol, which was successful in resolving the hemangioma completely.

Answers:

1. **Globally, infantile hemangiomas affect 10–25% of infants within the first 12 months of life. They are present at birth in 10–20% of affected infants. They are estimated to affect about 5% of infants of all ages throughout the world.**

2. **Beginning at 12–18 months of age, infantile hemangiomas start to slowly resolve, with decreases in vascularity and size. Usually, they resolve by about 10% with each year of age, and are usually completely resolved by the age of 10 years. They often leave behind discolorations and skin texture changes.**

3. **Though the vascular component of infantile hemangiomas resolves, about half of all affected children still have skin changes in the area where the tumor was located. For those that resolve by 6 years of age, 38% of cases have a scar, telangiectasia, or anetodermic skin. About 80% of lesions that resolve by 6 years of age leave severe skin abnormalities.**

Lipoma and Liposarcoma

A **lipoma** of skin is a common, benign tumor that is usually solitary. However, some people develop multiple lipomas. They are soft when palpated, can be moved back and forth, and lie within the subcutaneous skin layer. They are nodules of adipocytes. The skin above them appears normal. Most often, lipomas develop on the upper arms, neck, chest, abdomen, or upper legs. When multiple, lipomas may be familial or related to genetic disorders. Liposarcomas are cancerous tumors that are made up of cells that resemble those of adipose tissue.

Epidemiology

Approximately 2% of the general global population, including that of the United States, has a lipoma, and they may affect about 1 of every 1,000 people. Lipomas occur in people of all ages, but are most common between the years of 40 and 60. Skin lipomas are rare in children, but may appear in relation to **Bannayan–Zonana syndrome**. Lipomas occur almost equally in men and women, except for multiple lipomas (lipomatosis), which has a male predilection. There is no racial or ethnic predilection, and they occur in all people throughout the world. Liposarcomas are most common in adults above age 40, and after malignant fibrous histiocytomas, they are the second most common of all soft-tissue sarcomas. However, there are only about 2.5 cases per 1 million people, globally.

Etiology and Risk Factors

Lipomas may develop on their own or as part of a hereditary condition such as familial multiple lipomatosis. In rare cases, minor traumatic injuries have triggered the growth of lipomas, but this is not proven. Risk factors include family history, obesity, and lack of exercise. Liposarcomas arise from fat cells in soft tissues.

Clinical Manifestations

Lipomas are usually asymptomatic, but may be tender or painful. Over time, some lipomas become relatively firm. Lipomas are usually only 1–3 cm in diameter, but rarely, they reach 10–20 cm across, with weights as much as 4–5 kg. Liposarcomas most often appear inside the thighs or in the retroperitoneum. They are usually large and bulky, with many smaller satellites extending outward.

Pathology

There are many pathological subtypes of lipomas. These include: adenolipomas, angiolipomas, chondroid lipomas, subcutaneous lipomas, and liposarcomas. All of these subtypes are benign except liposarcomas that account for 1% of cases of lipomas. Liposarcomas are larger than 5 cm, with calcification, fast growth, and invasion into nearby tissues or through the fascia into muscle tissues. Under a microscope, liposarcomas appear similar to fat cells. However, lipoblasts are present. These cells have a large quantity of clear multivacuolated cytoplasm, with an eccentric dark-staining nucleus indented with vacuoles. Cell features include spindle, round, and myxoid structures.

Diagnosis

The diagnosis of lipomas is usually clinical, though quickly growing lesions should be biopsied. A physical examination is the simplest method of diagnosis. In rare cases, imaging studies may be needed – usually MRI, since this method can distinguish a lipoma from a cancerous liposarcoma. Other imaging methods include traditional X-rays and ultrasound. Diagnosis of liposarcomas is via biopsy or surgical excision.

Treatment

For cosmetic purposes or lipomas become troubling due to their location, they can be surgically excised. Simple surgical excision is most commonly used, and only 1–2% of lipomas recur. A new method of treatment that is being developed is the injection of compounds that trigger lipolysis, such as phosphatidylcholine or steroids. Other new methods include cauterization, **electrosurgery**, and **harmonic scalpel**. If a liposarcoma is diagnosed, surgery is required, and then, radiation therapy.

Prevention and Early Detection

There is no known method to prevent lipomas from developing. Early detection of a fast-growing lipoma is the best way of avoiding the tumor from evolving into a liposarcoma.

Prognosis

Subcutaneous lipomas have an excellent prognosis, but those growing within the internal organs have a worsened prognosis due to their ability to cause bleeding, obstructions, and ulceration. Malignant transformation into liposarcoma is very rare. Deeper lipomas recur more often than superficial lipomas. Prognosis for liposarcoma varies based on the site of origin, cell type, tumor size and depth, and how close the tumor is to lymph nodes. The five-year survival rates range between 56% and 100%.

Clinical Case

1. How common are liposarcomas?
2. What do the lipoblasts of a liposarcoma contain?
3. What are the five-year survival rates for liposarcomas?

A 54-year-old woman went to her physician because of nausea and abdominal distention. A CT scan revealed a subepithelial mass on the upper gastric corpus, with low density, filling most of the left side of the patient's abdomen. Abdominal ultrasonography revealed a 15 cm tumor. Partial hyperechoic lesions suggested hemorrhage inside the tumor. Aspiration needles were used to biopsy the mass. Cytopathological examination revealed spindle, myxoid, and round lipoblasts. A high-grade liposarcoma was diagnosed, but the patient declined any aggressive treatment for the tumor. Therefore, radiation therapy was scheduled.

Answers:

1. **Liposarcomas are seen in adults above age 40, and after malignant fibrous histiocytomas, are the second most common of all soft-tissue sarcomas. Even so, there are only about 2.5 cases per 1 million people, globally.**
2. **The lipoblasts of a liposarcoma have a large quantity of clear multivacuolated cytoplasm, with an eccentric dark-staining nucleus indented with vacuoles.**
3. **The five-year survival rates for liposarcomas range between 56% and 100%.**

Keloids

Keloids are relatively smooth overgrowths and thickened of collagenous scar tissue at the site of skin injury, particularly a wound or a surgical incision. The new tissue is elevated, rounded, and firm. Keloids extend beyond the original wound margin.

Epidemiology

The actual prevalence and incidence of keloids is not known. Keloids can develop in people of all ages, but are least common in children under 10 years of age. According to the American Academy of Dermatology Association, keloids have been documented as most common in younger people between the ages of 10 and 30. There is no male or female predilection, though they occur slightly more often in younger females in comparison with younger males. Keloids are more common in people with darker skin. However, it can occur in all skin types. The only epidemiological studies of keloids have shown that they are least common in England, with only 0.09% of the population affected, and most common in the African country of Zaire, where 16% of the population is affected. Keloids are also more common in people from Asian or Latino heritage in comparison with Caucasians.

Etiology and Risk Factors

Trauma is the major causative factor for keloids, though the tendency for them to form is believed to be hereditary. An individual is more likely to develop keloids if one or both parents had them. There is no single causative gene, but susceptibility loci have been discovered, mostly in chromosome 15. Risk factors include **pseudofolliculitis barbae**, tattoos, burns, acne, chickenpox, ear piercing, skin scratches, surgical incisions, and vaccinations.

Clinical Manifestations

Keloids appear smooth, firm, shiny, and are usually oval. However, they can be webbed or contracted. Their color is often pinkish, though they can be hyperpigmented. Keloids can cause pain, itching, and significant disfigurement. They may or may not resolve over time. If located over a joint, they can impair mobility.

Pathology

Keloids are fibrotic tumors, in which there are atypical fibroblasts with extremely large deposits of collagen, elastin, fibronectin, and proteoglycans. Collagen forms nodules within the deep dermal areas of the tumors.

Diagnosis

The diagnosis of keloids is clinical, and is simple, based on physical examination only.

Treatment

Unfortunately, treatment of keloids is often not effective. Sometimes, they can be flattened by corticosteroid injections given on a monthly basis. Triamcinolone acetonide is often the corticosteroid of choice. Debulking of keloids by pulsed dye laser or surgical excision can result in the recurrence of even larger keloids. Excision has better results when corticosteroids are injected into the site before and after the procedure. Other methods include solid carbon dioxide, liquid nitrogen, and silicon gel, radiation therapy, interferon, and 5-fluorouracil. Recent techniques include imiquimod or other topical immunomodulators, which prevent the development or recurrence of keloids.

Prevention and Early Detection

The only method of preventing keloids is in people with a known predisposition is by avoiding unneeded trauma or surgery. This includes avoiding ear piercing or having moles removed for cosmetic reasons. Prevention is also based on treating infections or acne as early as possible. Early detection is easy, simply by physical examination, but does not prevent keloids from becoming larger.

Prognosis

Patients should be told that keloid scarring is very difficult to treat, and the prognosis is usually uncertain. There is no preferred treatment strategy, and each patient's response to treatment is variable and unpredictable.

Significant Point

Keloids are collections of overgrown scar tissue that resemble shiny and raised skin. They form within months after an injury and are more common in dark-skinned people. Causes of keloids include cuts, surgery, and acne, but sometimes they form for no obvious reason.

Melanoma

A **melanoma** is a malignant tumor that arises from melanocytes in a pigmented area such as skin, eyes, mucous membranes, and brain. Even though melanoma makes up only 4% of all skin cancers in the United States, it causes about 80% of all deaths from skin cancer.

Epidemiology

Melanoma is the fifth most common type of cancer in men and the seventh most common type in women. There has been an increase in melanoma cases affecting younger women between 20 and 24 years. Only 0.6% of melanoma cases occur below the age of 20 years. The median age

at diagnosis is approximately 60 years in the United States. About 7% of those diagnosed are older than 85. For some reason, men over age 60 are also experiencing an increase in melanoma cases. Caucasians with lighter skin are the individuals most affected by melanoma. The lowest numbers of cases occur in African Americans and other dark-skinned people. Though the Southern states generally have hotter climates, and Northern states have the cooler climates. However, the highest rates of new melanoma cases occur in the Northern states. Human behaviors regarding sun exposure are the biggest factor, with many Northerners spending increased time indoors, yet when they do go outside they seldom use any protection against ultraviolet radiation. People in the Southern states generally use sun protection much more regularly. According to the CDC in 2016, the 10 U.S. states with the highest rates of melanoma are shown in Figure 10.2.

Globally, there are over 160,000 new cases of melanoma annually, and 48,000 of these are fatal. Cases have been increasing worldwide in developed countries, likely due to more sun exposure as part of recreation. The incidence rates in all populations have increased 5%, meaning that they double every 10–20 years. The highest incidence is in Australia and New Zealand, with as many as 60 cases per 100,000 people annually. The lowest rates of melanoma occur in Africa and Asia. Ages have ranged between 15 and 85 years. In Australia, New Zealand, and most of Europe, men are affected more often than women. For some reason, in the Northern and Western portions of Europe, women are more affected.

Etiology and Risk Factors

Approximately 80% of melanomas develop from normal skin, and 20% from melanocytic moles. It is uncertain whether some moles are actually precancerous, or if melanoma development on a mole might happen only from the effects of melanocytes. Sun exposure, particularly repeated blistering sunburns and repeated tanning with ultraviolet A (UVA) are important risk factors.

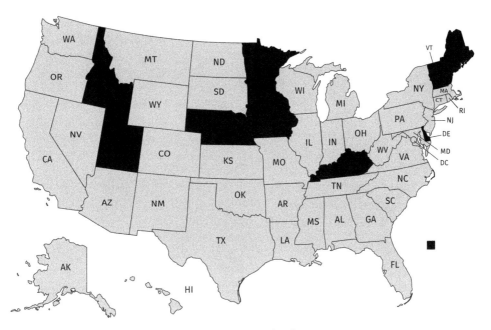

Figure 10.2 The 10 U.S. states with the highest rates of melanoma.

Atypical moles, particularly larger than 5 cm, congenital melanocytic maligna, and atypical mole syndrome may also cause malignant melanoma. Overall, family history of melanoma is linked to a two times higher risk of developing melanoma. Other risk factors for developing melanoma include lack of skin pigmentation or increased numbers of melanocytic nevi. *Fitzpatrick's classification* is used to assess estimates of relative risk factors for developing melanoma, as follows:

- Type I – white skin, red or blonde hair, blue eyes, freckles, always burns but does not tan
- Type II – fair skin, red or blonde hair, blue/brown/or green eyes, usually burns, only tans slightly
- Type III – darker but still white skin, eyes and hair of any color, sometimes burns, tans gradually
- Type IV – light brown skin or Mediterranean Caucasian skin, burns rarely, tans easily
- Type V – dark brown skin as in East Asia, burns very rarely, and can darkly tan easily
- Type VI – black skin, never burns, and tans easily

Skin type I has about two times higher risk for melanoma than skin type IV. There is also a 2 times higher risk for fair skin versus dark skin, and about 1.5 times higher risk for people with blue eyes than brown eyes. There is also a 3.5 times higher risk for red-haired versus brown or black-haired people, and about a 2 times higher risk if a person has a large number of freckles. Risk factors are also higher for people with *atypical or dysplastic nevus syndrome (DNS)*, which consists of more than 30 atypical or dysplastic moles. For people with 100–120 common moles, there is also increased risk for melanoma – of about 7 times higher – compared with people who have less than 15 common moles. When any atypical moles are present, the risk for melanoma is about four times higher. This increases to over six times higher if a person has more than five atypical moles. Cumulative risks in people affected by a familial type of atypical or dysplastic nevi syndrome are about 49% between ages 10 and 50, but about 82% in people 72 years or older.

Clinical Manifestations

The lesion of melanoma is similar to an atypical mole – basically a flattened, pigmented macule. Over time, it becomes more irregular in its shape, and its colors may include brown, black, red, gray, and depigmented areas. The changes usually occur over several months or years. Regression is signified by the depigmented areas.

Pathology

The two primary pathological forms of melanoma are described as *thick* or *thin* melanomas. The thicker melanomas, larger than 4 mm in diameter, are either stabilized in the number of cases or are increasing in most countries throughout the world. Thinner melanomas are increasing in the United States, Central Europe, and Australia, however. Along with the factor that the global mortality rates from melanoma are relatively stable, there may be a subtype of pathologically aggressive melanoma that can be fatal even if it is found early and is of a thinner diameter. For large cutaneous melanocytic moles, mutations may be present that are not the same as those of common moles in adults. The malignant transformation usually occurs during childhood. The *histoclinical* subtypes of melanomas are divided into four primary types, as follows:

- *Superficial spreading melanoma (SSM)* – the most common subtype, making up about 70% of melanomas; it starts growing on the middle skin layer but then penetrates deeper; this subtype is most common when a person under age 40 develops melanoma. It occurs mostly on women's legs and men's torsos. Histologically, atypical melanocytes invade the dermis and epidermis.
- *Nodular melanoma (NM)* – grows quickly, causing nearly 50% of all melanoma related deaths; it appears like a mole, insect bite, or pimple that is often round and black but can be other colors; only about 15% of all melanoma cases are nodular. It may occur on any parts of the body as a dark papule or a plaque.
- *Lentigo maligna melanoma (LMM)* – this accounts for 5% of melanomas. They grow deeper into the skin and are considered invasive and mostly appear on the upper body areas of elderly people. LMM occur on the face or other parts of chronic sun exposure as a flat, tan, brown, or black spots.

- *Acral-lentiginous melanoma (ALM)* – this type accounts for 5% of melanomas. A black or brown discoloration on the sole of the foot or palm of the hand that grows in size over time; it is the most common melanoma in dark-skinned people, and is the only subtype not associated with sun exposure; this type can also occur under the nails and in the oral mucosa; it usually appears in people between 60 and 70 years of age. For people with a large number of moles, sun exposure is needed only to begin the development of melanoma, with other factors enabling the progression to cancer. However, in people with a low number of moles, significant sun exposure is required to cause melanocytes to transform into melanomas. Growth rate, tumor thickness, and the time required for the tumor to develop are predictors of aggressiveness.

Diagnosis

Melanomas can be distinguished from benign lesions by using polarized light and immersion contact dermoscopy (see Figure 10.3). However, biopsy and histological evaluation are also needed. Patients should be instructed how to examine their bodies to detect changes in existing moles, and which features are suggestive of melanomas. Any mole that has recently enlarged, changed shape, or has developed signs of inflammation around it must be clinically evaluated. Ulceration, itching, or tenderness must also be evaluated. Recent darkening, enlargement, bleeding, or ulceration usually means that melanoma is present and has already invaded deeper skin layers.

When biopsied, the full depth of the dermis must be evaluated as well as areas slightly past the lesion's edges. Even a lesion of only slight suspicion should be biopsied. An earlier diagnosis can be made from lesions with mixed colors, visible or palpable irregular elevations, and borders with notches or angled indentations. Biopsy should be excisional for most of these lesions, except if they are located in areas that can be sensitive or cosmetically important. For these, broad shave biopsy is performed. For wider lesions, such as **lentigo maligna**, shave

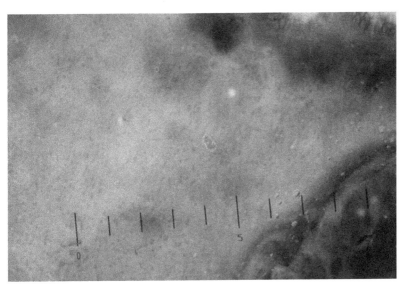

Figure 10.3 Melanoma viewed with immersion contact dermoscopy, revealing many dotted vessels in the depigmented area. *Source*: Figure 5 from https://onlinelibrary.wiley.com/doi/full/10.1111/1346-8138.13686. Journal of Dermatology [21].

biopsies from various areas can improve the accuracy of the diagnosis. Step sections allow the determination of the maximum thickness of the lesion. Radical surgery should only occur once the histologic diagnosis is made. Melanomas, especially when metastatic, may be tested for gene mutations. Differential diagnoses include basal cell carcinoma, **seborrheic keratoses**, squamous cell carcinoma, atypical moles, blue nevi, dermatofibromas, common moles, hematomas, **pyogenic granulomas, venous lakes**, and warts that have focal thromboses. Staging is similar to the tumor–node–metastasis (TNM) system, as follows:

- Stage 0 – in situ or intraepithelial melanoma
- Stage I – localized primary melanoma
  - IA – up to 0.8 mm in thickness with no ulceration
  - IB – less than 0.8 mm and up to 1 mm, with ulceration
- Stage II – localized primary melanoma
  - IIA – 1.01–2 mm with ulceration
  - IIB – 2.01–4 mm with ulceration
  - IIC – larger than 4 mm with ulceration
- Stage III – metastasis to regional lymph nodes
- Stage IV – distant metastasis

Staging is extremely influential regarding prognosis. Better staging can be done since the development of **sentinel lymph node biopsy** (SNLB). Staging is based on *Breslow depth*, which is how deeply the tumor cells have invaded, as well as histology. Ulceration means that the melanoma is of higher risk, even if they are less than 0.8 mm of Breslow depth. Additional staging methods include complete blood count, lactate dehydrogenase testing, liver tests, chest X-rays, CT scan, and PET. Staging procedures are done by a combination of dermatologists, general surgeons, oncologists, dermatopathologists, and plastic surgeons.

Treatment

Wide local surgical excision is the treatment of choice, for a lesion that is less than 0.8 mm in thickness and 1 cm diameter. For a tumor of this size that has ulceration, SNLB is considered. For thicker lesions, the margins may be larger and surgery more radical, along with SNLB. Lentigo maligna and lentigo maligna melanoma are usually treated with wide local excision, and sometimes, skin grafts. Intensive radiation is not as effective. Melanoma in situ is also best treated via surgical excision. If the patient is not a candidate for surgery or declines it, *imiquimod* and cryotherapy can be used. Nodular or spreading melanomas usually require wide local excision.

For metastatic melanoma, oncologists consider all immunotherapy, molecular targeted therapy, and radiation therapy. Since metastatic melanoma is usually inoperable, surgical resection is rare, though localized and regional metastases can be removed to reverse the disease and lengthen survival. Immunotherapy is helpful. Molecular targeted therapy includes use of the BRAF inhibitors *dabrafenib, encorafenib,* and *vemurafenib*, decreasing or stopping tumor cell proliferation. Since cytotoxic chemotherapy does not usually lengthen survival, it is usually only used when there are no other treatment options. For inoperable metastatic melanoma, adjuvant therapy includes recombinant biologic response modifiers. For brain metastases, radiation therapy may be used palliatively, though results are poor. New treatments under study include vaccine therapy and infusion of lymphokines-activated killer cells or antibodies (reserved for advanced melanoma).

Prevention and Early Detection

The prevention of melanoma is focused on limiting exposure to ultraviolet radiation. People are advised to mostly stay in the shade when outdoors, minimize outdoor activities when the rays of the sun are strongest (10:00 am-3:00 pm), and avoid sunbathing as well as tanning beds. Protective clothing should be worn, including wide-brimmed hats, long-sleeved shirts, and long pants. Sunscreen with a sun protection factor (SPF) of 30 or higher should be used, and it should have broad-spectrum ultraviolet A as well as ultraviolet B protection. Sunscreen must be reapplied every two hours and also after sweating or swimming. Early detection is helpful for starting treatment more quickly and improving prognosis. An early melanoma may be difficult to distinguish from a benign, pigmented lesion. Determination between them is based on the color distribution and the shape of the lesion. Highly aggressive melanomas grow quickly and have a high Breslow depth upon presentation. Even early detection may not change the outcome after surgery is performed. Screening usually finds less aggressive tumors earlier than the more aggressive types, so the impact upon survival is minimal.

Prognosis

A cure for melanoma highly depends on early diagnosis and treatment. The five-year survival rate when the lesion is very superficial and found early is high. However, melanoma can spread quickly, and be fatal without only a few months. When the tumor originates from the skin and has not metastasized, survival is based on tumor thickness upon diagnosis. Example five-year survival times are: Stage IA – 97% and Stage IIC – 53%. Example 10-year survival times are: Stage IA – 93% and Stage IIC – 39%. Anorectal melanomas and other mucosal melanomas have a poor prognosis even if they seem very limited upon diagnosis. After metastasis to the lymph nodes, five-year survival is between 25% and 70%, based on how many lymph nodes are involved and the level of ulceration present. After metastasis to distant sites, five-year survival is approximately 10%. The level of lymphocytic infiltration indicates a reaction by the immune system, and may be related to the extent of invasion, affecting prognosis. A cure is most possible when lymphocytic infiltration is only in very superficial lesions.

Significant Point

A gene expression test called *DecisionDx®-Melanoma* is available, to aid in determining whether a stage I or II melanoma is likely to metastasize. It is still not widely used, but in the future may help to determine whether immunotherapies would be helpful for individual patients.

Clinical Case

1. What age group is most affected by melanoma?
2. What are the risk factors for melanoma?
3. What are the characteristics of superficial spreading melanoma?

A 75-year-old woman went to her dermatologist for evaluation of a pigmented lesion on the medial aspect of her left ankle. There was painless inguinal swelling about 10 × 15 cm in size. The patient was referred for surgery, which involved wide local excision of the lesion with skin grafting, along with inguinal lymph node excision and biopsy. The lymph node had an appearance of cystic degeneration with hemorrhagic fluid aspirated from it, suggesting a superficial spreading melanoma with a maximum size of 2.5 cm. Lymphatic tumor emboli were detected but there were no other signs of metastasis. The melanoma was determined to be Stage II. Post-operative radiation therapy was also performed. The patient has had no relapse over five years of follow-up.

Answers:

1. **Only 0.6% of melanoma cases occur below the age of 20 years. The median age at diagnosis is approximately 60 years in the United States. About 7% of those diagnosed are older than 85. There has been an increase in melanoma cases affecting younger women between 20 and 24 years. For some reason, men over age 60 are also experiencing an increase in melanoma cases. Globally, ages have ranged between 15 and 85 years.**
2. **Sun exposure, particularly repeated blistering sunburns and repeated tanning with UVA are important risk factors. Atypical moles, especially if larger than 5 cm, congenital melanocytic maligna, and atypical**

mole syndrome may also cause malignant melanoma. Family history is linked to a two times higher risk. Other risk factors include lack of skin pigmentation or increased numbers of melanocytic nevi. People at the highest risk are those with white skin, red or blonde hair, blue eyes, freckles, and those that always burn but do not tan.

3. **Superficial spreading melanoma is the most common subtype, making up about 70% of melanomas. It starts growing on the middle skin layer but then penetrates deeper. It occurs mostly on women's legs and men's torsos. Histologically, atypical melanocytes invade the dermis and epidermis.**

Basal Cell Carcinoma

Basal cell carcinoma of the skin is a superficial cancer. It forms from keratinocytes near the basal skin layer. These cells are sometimes referred to as *basaloid keratinocytes*. The lesion grows slowly and appears as a nodule or papule, and is derived from epidermal cells. Though localized growth can cause extreme skin destruction, metastasis is rare. Other names for this cancer are *basiloma* and *rodent ulcer*.

Epidemiology

Basal cell carcinoma is the most common type of skin cancer globally, and in general, cases appear to be increasing in incidence by about 10% per year. In the United States, there are more than 4.3 million new cases every year. Over 245,000 basal cell carcinomas have been linked annually to the use of indoor tanning beds. People who use these devices have a 29% increased risk of developing basal cell carcinoma. Any history of indoor tanning increases risks for the disease by 69% before age 40. Most basal cell carcinomas occur in older adults, primarily between ages 50 and 80, with a median age at diagnosis being 65 years. The disease affects men two times as often as women, and this may be related to the fact that more men work in outdoor jobs. Most cases occur in light-skinned people that receive excessive sun exposure. This cancer is very rare in dark-skinned people.

Global prevalence and incidence are difficult to determine accurately because basal cell carcinoma is so common that it is not reported to cancer registries. The non-melanoma skin cancers, which include basal cell carcinoma, are the fifth most commonly occurring cancer in men and women throughout the world. Most people affected are above age 50. The only statistics found came in 2002 from Australia, in which there were 1,041 cases per 100,000 men, and 745 cases per 100,000 women; as well as in 2014, with 899 cases per 100,000 men, and 656 cases per 100,000 women.

Etiology and Risk Factors

Aside from ultraviolet light exposure, basal cell carcinomas are also linked to genetic syndromes, and can form in a **nevus sebaceous**. This cancer, along with melanoma can be related to an inherited DNA repair defect, and may develop after **xeroderma pigmentosum** that carries a 2,000 times increased risk of developing cancer at some point. Multiple basal cell carcinomas may be linked to *Gorlin syndrome*, which is also called *basal cell nevus syndrome*, an autosomal dominant disorder. Early onset of multiple basal cell carcinomas may be caused by **Bazex syndrome**, which is a rare form of **genodermatosis**. Other genetic syndromes linked to basal cell carcinoma include **Rombo syndrome**, *generalized follicular basaloid hamartoma syndrome*, and **Happle–Tinschert syndrome**. Additional risk factors for basal cell carcinoma include the human papillomavirus, chronic arsenic exposure, AIDS, *and ultraviolet A radiation therapy*, and photosensitizing drugs.

Clinical Manifestations

Basal cell carcinomas start as shiny papules. Over months to years, there is a pearl-like, shiny border with prominent telangiectases on the surface. In the center, there is an ulcer or a **dell**. Crusting or bleeding often continues as the tumor enlarges. Often, these carcinomas crust and then heal, so the patient and even the physician may not be suitably aware of exactly what the lesion is. There is no obvious premalignant stage. Usually, basal cell carcinomas progress very slowly, with peripheral extension. Sometimes there are spontaneous size changes, and many superficial tumors resemble scars. About 80% of these carcinomas develop on the face and neck.

There are many different signs and symptoms as well as biologic behaviors of basal carcinomas, which are of four general types, as follows (also see Figure 10.4):

- *Nodular* – this subtype makes up 60% of all basal cell carcinomas – small in size, firm, shiny, nearly translucent to pink in color with telangiectases; usually appearing on the face, often with crusting and ulceration (see Figure 10.5)
- *Superficial* – makes up 30% of all basal cell carcinomas – marginated, pink or red in color with thin papules or plaques; most common on the trunk and highly resemble localized dermatitis or psoriasis
- *Morpheaform* –8% of all basal cell carcinomas– flat, indurated, and scar-like; they have vague borders and may be flesh-colored or light red
- *Pigmented* – makes up 2%, the nodular and superficial subtypes can produce pigment and are sometimes referred to as *other basal cell carcinomas*

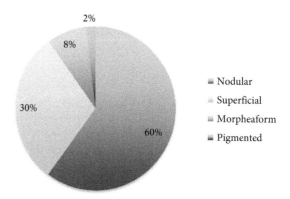

Figure 10.4 Percentages of various basal cell carcinomas.

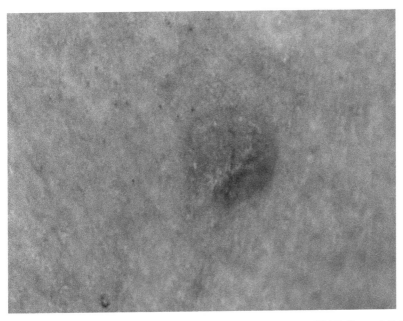

Figure 10.5 A nodular basal cell carcinoma. *Source*: Burns et al. (2013), Figure 141.3 from Page 3634. With permission of John Wiley & Sons.

Pathology

The stage of a basal cell carcinoma is not as important as for melanoma, since these cancers are nearly always cured before they spread. These cancers are related to the pilo-sebaceous structures and are believed to originate from **pluripotent cells** in the basal layer of the epidermis. The tumor protein 53 (TP53) is also involved in the development of basal cell carcinoma.

Basal cell carcinoma cells resemble cells of the basal epidermal layer as well as matrix cells of the appendages. They have a small quantity of cytoplasm, and their compact nuclei are close together and stain darkly. The cytoplasm, however, only slightly stains. Cell margins are indistinct, and adjacent cells are connected by bridge-like structures. Desmosomes and **tonofibrils** are present. Cells within the marginal palisade have little differentiation or organization. Mitotic figures are often frequent. A large number of cells within a basal cell carcinoma die quickly, and some cells become amyloid and **acantholytic**. With tumor progression, the masses extend into the dermis, and can separate from all other masses. The infiltrate of mast cells and Langerhans cells is linked to the aggressive nature of the tumor. Histological patterns are widely varied, and include superficial, nodular, infiltrative, micronodular, and pigmented subtypes. Advanced and metastatic basal cell carcinomas are only seen in 1–2% of cases, due to a long period of avoiding treatment. If the tumor progresses to cause severe damage, it can be fatal.

Diagnosis

The diagnosis of a basal cell carcinoma requires a biopsy and histologic examination. Diagnosis also includes medical history, physical examination, dermoscopy with cross-polarized light, high-frequency ultrasonography, and optical coherence tomography with infrared light. Methods of biopsy include shave biopsy, punch biopsy, excisional biopsy to remove the entire tumor, and incisional biopsy to remove part of the tumor. If the lymph nodes have been affected, they may be assessed via fine-needle aspiration or surgical lymph node biopsy. Imaging tests are usually not needed, but for very deep tumor invasion, MRI or CT may be performed.

Differential diagnoses include: various types of moles, **molluscum contagiosum**, sebaceous hyperplasia, **keratoacanthoma**, Bowen disease, squamous cell carcinoma, eczema, psoriasis, **chondrodermatitis nodularis helicis**, melanoma, and viral warts.

Treatment

The treatment of basal cell carcinoma requires a specialist. Treatments are based on the histologic subtype, location, size, and clinical appearance of the tumor. Methods include curettage with **electrodesiccation**, cryosurgery, surgical excision, topical 5-fluorouracil or imiquimod, photodynamic therapy, carbon dioxide or pulsed dye lasers, and **brachytherapy**. Curettage with electrodesiccation can achieve five-year cure rates of as much as 92% for many primary basal cell carcinomas. Mohs microscopic surgery is often used for large tumors, recurring or incompletely treated tumors. Surgical excision can achieve complete clearance, and recurrence rates are only 5% over five years.

Prevention and Early Detection

The prevention of basal cell carcinoma is focused on limiting exposure to ultraviolet radiation. People are advised to mostly stay in the shade when outdoors, minimize outdoor activities when the rays of the sun are strongest (10:00 am–3:00 pm), and avoid sunbathing as well as tanning beds. Protective clothing should be worn, including wide-brimmed hats, long-sleeved shirts, and long pants. Sunscreen with a sun protection factor (SPF) of 30 or higher should be used, and it should have *broad-spectrum ultraviolet A as well as ultraviolet B protection*. Sunscreen must be reapplied every two hours and also after sweating or swimming.

Early detection of basal cell carcinoma may be achieved by teaching patients how to correctly perform skin self-examinations, at least once per month. Like other skin cancers, any changes of skin lesions must be evaluated clinically. Also, regular skin examinations in the medical office are very important for patients that have a high risk of skin cancer. These include individuals with a weakened immune system, Gorlin syndrome, or xeroderma pigmentosum.

Prognosis

The prognosis for basal cell carcinoma is generally good. Deaths from these cancers are rare, but can occur if the disease invades or affects vital orifices such as the mouth, eyes, ears, dura mater, or bones. Nearly 25% of all patients will develop a new basal cell carcinoma within five years after an initial one had been treated. Therefore, patients with such history must have an annual skin examination.

Significant Point

Basal cell carcinomas are abnormal, uncontrolled lesions arising from the skin's basal cells, which line the deepest layer of the epidermis. They often appear as open sores of various colors, shiny bumps, or scars. They are usually caused by exposure to the sun, and nearly never spread beyond the original tumor site. However, if not treated properly, they can cause disfigurement.

Clinical Case

1. What are the epidemiological statistics about basal cell carcinoma?
2. What are the four general types of basal cell carcinoma?
3. What is the prevention of basal cell carcinoma centered on?

An 85-year-old man that previously had melanoma and squamous cell carcinoma is taken to visit a dermatologist because of a 6 × 6 mm pearly lesion on his forehead. Examination and biopsy revealed the lesion was a basal cell carcinoma. Options for treatment included wide localized excision,

Mohs micrographic surgery, and superficial radiation therapy. The patient chose radiation for treatment. The procedure focused on the area of the lesion as well as a 10-mm border around it. Tumor depth was estimated to be less than 5 mm The patient received several radiation treatments over two weeks. There were no side effects except for slight redness and erythema after the final session. During follow-up, the patient had a very good cosmetic result with very little visible scarring.

Answers:

1. **Basal cell carcinoma is the most common type of skin cancer globally, and cases appear to be increasing in incidence by about 10% per year. In the United States, there are more than 4.3 million new cases every year. Most cases occur in adults between 50 and 80, with men affected 2 times as often as women. Global prevalence and incidence are difficult to determine accurately because basal cell carcinoma is so common that it is not reported to cancer registries.**
2. **The four general types of basal cell carcinomas include the nodular, superficial, morpheaform, and other types. The nodular subtype makes up 60% of all basal cell carcinomas, and the superficial subtype makes up 30%. The morpheaform subtype is seen in 8% of all cases, and the "other" type, sometimes called "pigmented," is very rare.**
3. **The prevention of basal cell carcinoma is centered on limiting exposure to ultraviolet radiation. People should minimize outdoor activities when the rays of the sun are strongest, from 10 a.m.–4 p.m., and avoid sunbathing as well as tanning beds. Protective clothing and sunscreen should be worn.**

Squamous Cell Carcinoma

Squamous cell carcinoma is a malignancy forming from epidermal keratinocytes that invaded into the dermal layer. It is most common in areas of the body that are most often exposed to the sun. There can be localized tissue destruction, and if advanced, metastases. The cancer can develop within an actinic keratosis, in a burn scar, within oral leukoplakia, or in normal tissue. Generally, squamous cell carcinomas have low rates of local, regional, or distant spreading. The high-risk subtype indicates carcinomas that are the most likely to spread.

Epidemiology

Squamous cell carcinoma is the second most common type of skin cancer. There are more than 1 million cases in the United States every year, with 2,500 being fatal. Epidemiology has changed over about six decades due to decreases in occupational carcinogen exposures and increases in recreational sun exposure and population aging. Incidence is high in the United States compared with much of the world, with 290 cases out of every 100,000 people. Cases increase with age and peak incidence is at approximately 60 years. Males are affected in a 2 : 1 ratio compared with females. Caucasians are most likely to be affected, especially in those with lighter skin.

Globally, squamous cell carcinoma has been increasing in incidence since 1960. Accurate figures are not available because, like basal cell carcinoma, this type of cancer is basically not reported – both because of its commonality and low death rates. However, statistics from Australia show the highest number of cases: 387 out of every 100,000 people. Figures from England describe annual incidence to be about 23 cases out of every 100,000. In Wales, incidence is between 15 and 19 out of every 100,000; in Scotland, it is over 37 cases out of every 100,000. The highest European incidence rate recorded was in Switzerland, with nearly 30 cases out of every 100,000 people. Cases of squamous cell carcinoma increase with age, with about 27 cases out of every 100,000 people aged 85 or older. Cases are three times higher in this age group than in people aged 65–84, and seven times higher than people under age 64. Like basal cell carcinoma, this type of cancer is more prevalent in men than in women, and is usually seen on the face and neck. The disease mostly affects Caucasian populations, though it is also seen in people of all racial and ethnic groups.

Etiology and Risk Factors

The causes of squamous cell carcinoma include mutations of the tumor protein 53 (TP53) gene. These mutations are seen in 90% of cases. Methylation occurs, which influences the likelihood of cellular damage. Chromosomal abnormalities include losses at chromosomes 3p, 8q, 9p, 11p, 13q, 17p, and 18p. Risk factors for squamous cell carcinoma include excessive ultraviolet radiation exposure, immunosuppression, use of azathioprine or cyclosporin, chronic lymphocytic leukemia and HIV. Rarely, squamous cell carcinoma is a complication of chronic ulceration and radiation therapy. The cancer is also linked to **hidradenitis suppurativa**, lymphedema, dystrophic epidermolysis bullosa, and **Hailey–Hailey disease**.

Clinical Manifestations

There are many variations in the appearance of squamous cell carcinoma. All non-healing lesions on skin that are exposed to the sun should be carefully evaluated. The tumor may start as a reddened papule or plaque. The surface can be crusted or scaly. It may become hyperkeratotic or nodular, and the raised surface may resemble a wart (see Figure 10.6). In some patients, squamous cell carcinomas are tender when touched. Sometimes, most of the lesion is actually below the level of surrounding skin tissue. Over time, the tumor will ulcerate and invade deeper tissues. Late-stage disease is the most likely to metastasize to surrounding skin, nearby organs, or lymph nodes.

Pathology

Invasive squamous cell carcinoma starts when atypical keratinocytes enter the basement membrane of the epidermis and then invade the dermis. Differentiation from precursors is structural, based on descending strands of malignant keratinocytes or even single atypical keratinocytes being present. *Pseudoepitheliomatous hyperplasia* may also occur at an ulcer margin or in various dermal inflammatory or neoplastic developments. Grading of squamous cell carcinoma is

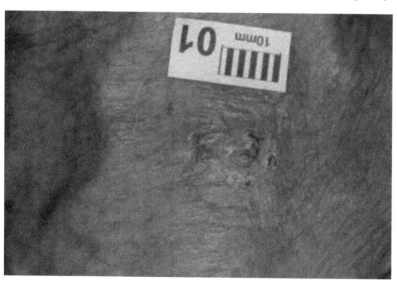

Figure 10.6 Squamous cell carcinoma showing hyperkeratosis with a raised nodule. *Source:* Burns et al. (2013), Figure 142.6 from Page 3646. With permission of John Wiley & Sons.

based on the *worst component* found in them, despite the extent of tissue that contains the component. Diagnosis of poorly differentiated tumors and the spindle cell variant requires identifying an in situ tumor, plus the expression of cytokeratin markers in immunohistochemistry. Histological specimens are described in terms of tumor type, differentiation grade, thickness, invasion level, presence of perineural invasion, lymphovascular invasion, margins of the excision, and pathological stage.

Diagnosis

To diagnose a squamous cell carcinoma, a biopsy is required. Accurate diagnosis takes into account the presence of tenderness and induration, as well as a raised "shoulder" extending past the area of disordered scaling. Approximately 33% of lingual or mucosal squamous cell carcinomas have already metastasized prior to diagnosis. Differential diagnoses include pyodermas gangrenosum, venous stasis ulcer, keratoacanthoma, verruca vulgaris, actinic keratosis, basal cell carcinoma, seborrheic keratosis, nummular dermatitis, and psoriasis.

Treatment

Treatment for squamous cell carcinoma includes curettage with electrodessication, cryosurgery, surgical excision, topical chemotherapy with 5-fluorouracil or imiquimod, photodynamic therapy, and radiation therapy. Late-stage squamous cell carcinoma may require extensive surgery. The patient must be closely monitored because the risk of metastasis is so high. If located on the lips or another mucocutaneous area, the tumor must be surgically excised, but achieving a cure is not common. Large tumors and recurrent tumors are aggressively treated with Mohs microscopically controlled surgery. The tissue borders are progressively excised until no more tumor cells are seen. Radiation therapy and chemotherapy may be used adjunctively. For tumors with perineural invasion, radiation therapy is usually used after surgery. When a metastasis can be identified and is isolated, radiation therapy is usually effective. However, widespread metastases do not respond well to chemotherapy. New options for inoperable, advanced squamous cell carcinoma or for metastatic disease are the programmed death receptor 1 (PD-1) inhibitors such as cemiplimab and pembrolizumab.

Prevention and Early Detection

Preventive measures for squamous cell carcinoma include avoiding sunlight exposure, reducing outdoor activities between 10 a.m. and 3 p.m., avoiding sunbathing and tanning beds, wearing protective clothing, and using adequate sunscreen correctly. Early detection is the key to diagnosing and treating squamous cell carcinoma. Like basal cell carcinoma, squamous cell carcinoma can be detected by proper self-examinations of the skin, and then consultation with a physician.

Prognosis

Generally, prognosis for small squamous cell carcinomas that are surgically removed early in their development is excellent. Regional and distant metastases are not common, but do occur, often from a tumor that is poorly differentiated. When these carcinomas are more aggressive, they are usually larger than 2 cm in diameter and have an invasion depth of more than 2 mm The overall 5-year survival rate for metastatic squamous cell carcinomas, even when treated, is only 34%.

Significant Point

Squamous cell carcinoma is more aggressive than basal cell carcinoma. However, the spread of this cancer is usually slow, and most cases are diagnosed before it has progressed beyond the upper skin layer. Most squamous cell carcinomas can be cured if they are treated early. After treatment, it is important to have regular follow-up skin examinations.

Clinical Case

1. What are the risk factors for squamous cell carcinoma?
2. What are the features of the classic subtype of squamous cell carcinoma?
3. What are the prognostic factors concerning squamous cell carcinoma?

An 86-year-old man was evaluated for a neck mass near his right ear that had grown rapidly over 2 months. He had previously had a squamous cell carcinoma a year before, in the same area. It had been surgically excised, and a skin graft was performed. A CT scan revealed that the tumor had attached to the carotid artery as well as surrounding it. Therefore, the patient was referred to a vascular surgeon, who determined that the carotid artery involvement made the surgery a high-risk factor for the patient having a stroke. The only way to remove the tumor would be to remove and replace the carotid artery. The surgery was scheduled, and the surgeon performed an extended radical neck resection with flap repair. The carotid artery was replaced with a vein graft from the patient's thigh. After the successful operation, an ultrasound confirmed that the vein graft was successful. The patient recovered, and was scheduled for adjuvant radiation and chemotherapy. The final diagnosis of the tumor was a classic squamous cell carcinoma.

Answers:

1. **Risk factors for squamous cell carcinoma include immunosuppression, use of azathioprine or cyclosporin, excessive ultraviolet radiation exposure, chronic lymphocytic leukemia or other blood malignancies, and HIV. Rarely, this cancer is a complication of chronic ulceration and radiation therapy. It is also linked to hidradenitis suppurativa, lymphedema,** morpheaform, dystrophic epidermolysis bullosa, and Hailey–Hailey disease.
2. **The classic squamous cell carcinoma is the most common subtype. Its cells may be large and polygonal with vesicular nuclei, prominent nucleoli, and abundant cytoplasm, with keratinization and intercellular bridges – or pleomorphic cells that are poorly differentiated.**
3. **Generally, prognosis for small squamous cell carcinomas that are surgically removed early in their development is excellent. The overall 5-year survival rate for metastatic squamous cell carcinomas, however, is only 34% - even when they are treated.**

Bowen Disease

Bowen disease is also called *intraepidermal squamous cell carcinoma.* Is usually occurs in skin areas exposed to the sun, but can occur anywhere on the body. This means that Bowen disease is an in situ form of cancer. The plaques are persistent and not elevated. They appear red and can be scaly or crusted. In most cases, the lesions grow progressively, though spontaneous, and partial regression may occur. Other terms used to describe Bowen disease are *Bowenoid keratosis* and *squamous cell carcinoma in situ.*

Epidemiology

The prevalence of Bowen disease is about 15 of every 100,000 people in North America, based on a range of 15–28 per 100,000. There may be a higher incidence because of increased sun exposure. Bowen disease occurs in adults of all ages, but is most common over the age of 60, and rare in those under 30. However, unlike other skin cancers, Bowen disease occurs 70–85% of the time in women. It is most common in Caucasians.

Global statistics on prevalence and incidence are not well documented, but in the United Kingdom, most cases of Bowen disease occur in people over 60, with Caucasians most often affected. Areas of the world with high sunlight exposure are more likely to have increased cases of Bowen disease.

Etiology and Risk Factors

Some patients also have other ultraviolet radiation-related skin cancers as well as Bowen disease. In various studies, approximately 40% of cases had a previous or subsequent skin cancer–usually basal cell carcinoma. Bowen disease is also associated with internal malignancies. There is a link between the disease and ingestion of arsenic – even decades before. For example, agricultural workers have higher cases of Bowen disease, and may be exposed to arsenic salts that are present in pesticides, fungicides, and weed killing agents. Though not highly prevalent in Westernized countries, arsenic has contaminated water supplies in Argentina, Bangladesh, and Taiwan. Human papillomavirus type 16 and 18 DNA has been found in anogenital Bowen disease. HPV16 is also present in 60% of periungual and palmoplantar lesions. Risk factors for Bowen disease include immunosuppression (HIV), chronic lymphocytic leukemia, radiation exposure, skin injuries, and chronic inflammatory conditions including **lupus vulgaris** and chronic lupus erythematosus.

Clinical Manifestations

Bowen disease may manifest as single or multiple lesions, though multiple lesions are present in only 10–20% of cases. Lesions can be occurred on the lower legs (see Figure 10.7). They are reddish brown in color, with crusting or scaling. The scale is white or yellowish in color, and can easily be pulled away to reveal a wet, red, and sometimes granular surface without any visible blood. Margins are well demarcated. There is a slight raised portion while the surface is overall usually flat, thought it can become hyperkeratotic. There is only a small level of induration. The lesions

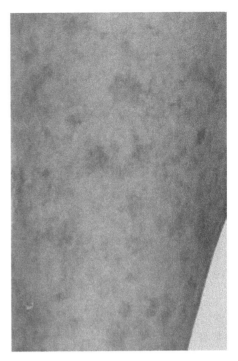

Figure 10.7 Multiple areas of Bowen disease on the lower leg. *Source*: Burns et al. (2013), Figure 142.23 from Page 3655. With permission of John Wiley & Sons.

often resemble a local, thin plaque – such as those of dermatitis, psoriasis, or a dermatophyte infection. Ulcerations usually signify that an invasive carcinoma has developed, but this may occur years after the initial intraepidermal manifestations. With multiple lesions, there can be wide spreading or they can remain close together and become confluent, with extension. Complications of Bowen disease include nonmelanoma skin cancers and lip cancers. On the perianal skin, there is an increased risk of invasion, recurrence, and cervical or vulval dysplasia. If the disease affects the nail areas, there is also a higher risk of invasion and recurrence.

Pathology

The pathology of Bowen disease involves full-thickness dysplasia in the epidermal layer, plus disordered differentiation, and loss of polarity in the epithelia. Usually, the intraepidermal areas of the **cutaneous adnexae** are affected. The keratinocytes have varying pleomorphism, and acanthosis as well as parakeratosis are usually evident. There is enlargement and hyperchromasia of the cell nuclei. The cells become prematurely keratinized. When a PAS stain is used, clear cell changes may be seen because of increased quantities of intracytoplasmic glycogen. Mitotic figure can be frequent. The cells may be multinucleate and have a giant form. The junction between the dermis and epidermis remains intact.

In the papillary dermis, there is an inflammatory cell infiltrate that is very dense. Vascular **ectasia** may be extreme. The infiltrate can be band-like and resemble **lichenoid dermatoses**. Variants of Bowen disease include: atrophic, psoriaform, and verrucous. However, mixtures of these patterns may exist in just one lesion. In *Bowenoid papulosis*, there are varying degrees of epidermal dysplasia, from mild to full-thickness features. HPV-related changes can be slight or extreme. They include hypergranulosis and coarse granules of **keratohyalin** that have encircling halos.

Diagnosis

The diagnosis of Bowen disease is via biopsy, which will reveal full-thickness dysplasia in the epidermal layer, but no involvement of the dermal layer. Dermoscopy reveals vascular structures that are characteristic of the disease. The differential diagnoses include basal cell carcinoma, seborrheic keratosis, **discoid dermatitis**, squamous cell carcinoma, and psoriasis. Bowen disease must also be differentiated from lichen simplex. Bowenoid papulosis mimics Bowen disease but is usually found on the genital skin in younger people that are sexually active. It is diagnosed because of the appearance of single or multiple small papules of a red, brown, or flesh color. The surfaces are flat to verrucous. The lesions can coalesce into larger plaques.

Treatment

The treatment of Bowen disease is based on the characteristics of the lesions. Options include topical chemotherapeutic agents, curettage with electrodesiccation, electrocautery, surgical excision, and cryosurgery. When the disease does not improve after topical corticosteroids, this suggests a diagnosis of Bowen disease. Without treatment, the disease can metastasize. For recurrent perianal Bowen disease, surgery with wide excision may be required. Sometimes, finger amputation is needed.

Prevention and Early Detection

The prevention of Bowen disease is the same as for other skin cancers: avoiding excessive sun exposure, minimizing outdoor activities between 10 a.m. and 3 p.m., avoiding sunbathing and tanning beds, wearing protective clothing, and using adequate sunscreen correctly. Early detection is important to guide diagnosis and treatment, and if signs of cancerous transformation are detected – such as a fleshy nodule or a lump in a skin lesion – they may be more successfully treated. Patients should be taught how to look for these changes and also to note if there is any tenderness, easy bleeding, ulceration, or induration.

Prognosis

The prognosis of Bowen disease, in most cases, is excellent since the risk of malignant transformation is low. Most patients that receive treatment will recover completely. Prognosis is improved when the patient follows the requirements for reducing sun exposure and wearing sunscreen when outdoors.

Significant Point

Bowen disease only affects the epidermis, and treatment is usually successful. Even so, it is a pre-cancerous condition. It was first described in 1912 and is considered an early noninvasive form of intraepidermal squamous cell carcinoma. The most important step to lower risks of this disease is to limit or avoid excessive exposure to the ultraviolet radiation.

Clinical Case

1. Is Bowen disease more common in women or men?
2. Which factors may be potential causes of Bowen disease?
3. What are the potential complications of Bowen disease?

A 57-year-old woman had been diagnosed with Bowen disease because of a lesion on her forehead. It was about 5 cm in diameter. Fluorouracil, cryotherapy, and photodynamic therapy were not successful. The patient was then treated with radiation therapy, which reduced the size of the lesion. Over one year of follow-up, the lesion was completely resolved, and the patient was very happy that the cosmetic appearance of her forehead looked just as it had prior to the lesion developing.

Answers:

1. **Unlike other skin cancers, Bowen disease occurs 70–85% of the time in women, usually over the age of 60.**
2. **Causative factors include ultraviolet radiation exposure, previous skin cancers, internal malignancies, ingestion of arsenic, and the human papillomavirus type 16 and 18.**
3. **Potential complications of Bowen disease include non-melanoma skin cancers and lip cancers, invasion, recurrence, cervical or vulval dysplasia, and the development of metastatic squamous cell carcinoma.**

Merkel Cell Skin Cancer

Merkel cell skin cancer is also known as *Merkel cell carcinoma, neuroendocrine skin carcinoma, primary small cell skin carcinoma, trabecular cell carcinoma*, and *anaplastic skin cancer*. It is a rare and aggressive carcinoma that is most common in older Caucasians. Merkel cell skin cancer often undergoes lymphatic spreading.

Epidemiology

Merkel cell skin cancer is increasing in prevalence and incidence in the United States. There are over 2,000 cases per year. Annual incidence has increased over the previous 25 years from 0.15 cases per 100,000 people to 0.44 cases per 100,000. Merkel cell skin cancer is most often diagnosed at approximately age 75. It also affects younger people that are immunosuppressed. The disease is just slightly more common in men compared with women. Like most skin cancers, it is most common in Caucasians. Globally, prevalence and incidence statistics are difficult to obtain but appear to be the same. Merkel cell skin is most commonly found in areas with increased sun exposure. Australia and New Zealand are the countries with the highest incidence.

Etiology and Risk Factors

The cause of Merkel cell skin cancer is not fully understood. The disease begins in the Merkel cells at the base of the epidermis. These cells are connected to the nerve endings responsible for the sense of touch. Risk factors include cumulative ultraviolet light exposure, the Merkel cell polyomavirus, and personal history of cancers such as chronic lymphocytic leukemia, melanoma, and multiple myeloma. Additional risk factors include immunosuppression, older age, and lighter skin color.

Clinical Manifestations

The lesions of Merkel cell skin cancer are usually shiny and firm. They may be flesh-colored or have a bluish-red color, and nodularity is common. They grow quickly, but do not cause any pain or tenderness. Merkel cell skin cancer is most common on sun-exposed areas, but can occur anywhere on the body. The face, head, and neck are the most common sites where this cancer develops. Even with treatment, this cancer often metastasizes via the lymphatics, reaching the lymph nodes, brain, bones, liver, or lungs.

Pathology

There is emerging evidence that Merkel cell skin cancer utilizes specific oncogenetic pathways. Up to 80% of cases are associated with the Merkel cell polyomavirus, mediated by ultraviolet light exposure. The cells show a varying mixture of nodules, sheets, nests, and trabeculae. The tumors are usually small round blue cell neoplasms with a high nucleus to cytoplasm ratio, round or oval nuclei, finely dispersed chromatin, indistinct nucleoli, obvious mitoses, and apoptotic bodies. There are variations in nuclear molding and crush artifacts. Most cases have a pure neuroendocrine morphology, known as *pure Merkel cell carcinoma*. A smaller number of cases are *combined Merkel cell carcinoma*, with squamous or sarcomatoid differentiation, or a close connection with in situ or invasive squamous cell carcinoma.

Diagnosis

The diagnosis of Merkel cell skin cancer is via skin and SNLB. Staging is based on tumor size, imaging, and the results of a SNLB. Serology tests are also performed to assess the presence of the Merkel polyomavirus. A baseline oncoproteins antibody test within 2–3 months of first evidence of the disease is suggested for all patients. Patients that do not produce antibodies have a higher risk for recurrence. Those that produce **oncoprotein antibodies** have a decreased need for follow-up imaging. Antibodies that recognize the oncoproteins are present in the blood of 50% of newly diagnosed patients. These proteins are hardly ever present in anyone that has not had Merkel cell skin cancer.

Treatment

Treatment of Merkel cell skin cancer is based on staging. It usually involves wide localized excision, which is often followed by lymph node dissection, radiation therapy, or both. For metastatic or recurrent tumors, systemic therapy may be required. This usually involves conventional chemotherapeutic agents, or a PD-1 inhibitor such as avelumab. Leukocyte growth factors such as *sargramostim* are sometimes required to reduce the likelihood of infections after chemotherapy. Additional treatment options include immunotherapy, Mohs micrographic surgery, as well as complementary and alternative therapies. Immunotherapies include the immune checkpoint inhibitors *pembrolizumab, avelumab, nivolumab,* and *ipilimumab.* Complementary and alternative therapies include optimizing fruit and vegetable intake and nutritional supplements.

Prevention and Early Detection

Prevention of Merkel cell skin cancer is based on protection from sun exposure between 10 a.m. and 3 p.m., avoiding sunbathing and tanning beds, wearing protective clothing, and using adequate sunscreen. Early detection requires regular self-examinations and immediately reporting any skin changes to a physician.

Prognosis

The prognosis of Merkel cell skin cancer is poor because most patients have metastases upon diagnosis. Unfortunately, about 80% of all Merkel cell skin cancers recur in the first two years following diagnosis and treatment. Most deaths from the disease occur in the first three years after diagnosis. The five-year relative survival rates for Merkel cell skin cancer are as follows: 76% if localized, 53% if regional, and only 19% if distant metastasis has occurred.

Significant Point

Merkel cell skin cancer is a rare and aggressive carcinoma, with a high risk of recurrence and metastases. Merkel cells are located deep in the epidermis, and are connected to nerves. The tumors are not as distinctive as other types of skin cancer, but the rapid speed at which they grow often prompts patients and physicians to have them biopsied.

Clinical Case

1. Which people are most likely to develop Merkel cell skin cancer?
2. Aside from sun exposure, what are the other risk factors for Merkel cell skin cancer?
3. What is the outlook for Merkel cell skin cancer?

A 66-year-old man went to his physician because of a superficial plaque on his left leg. The area was biopsied, and a diagnosis of Merkel cell skin cancer was made. The patient underwent a wide surgical excision and SNLB, which was negative. Radiation therapy was directed just at the localized lesion area. Two years later, the patient had a recurrence of the same cancer, close to but not exactly in the same area. Another wide surgical excision was performed with adjuvant radiation therapy. PET scans were ordered every three months to monitor the patient. A year later, another lesion was found in a similar area, diagnosed again as Merkel cell skin cancer. The patient had another wide local excision, radiation therapy, and chemotherapy. After three years of follow-up, there has been no recurrence.

Answers:

1. **Merkel cell skin cancer is most common in older adults, often diagnosed around age 75, in younger people that are immunosuppressed, and is seen slightly more often in men than in women – especially in Caucasians. Sun-exposed regions such as Australia and New Zealand have the highest incidence.**
2. **Risk factors include the Merkel cell polyomavirus, personal history of chronic lymphocytic leukemia, melanoma, and multiple myeloma as well as immunosuppression, older age, and lighter skin color.**
3. **The outlook is poor because most patients have metastases upon diagnosis. About 80% of all cases recur in the first two years following diagnosis and treatment. Most deaths occur in the first three years after diagnosis. The five-year relative survival rates are: 76% if localized, 53% if regional, and only 19% if distant metastasis has occurred.**

Kaposi Sarcoma

Kaposi sarcoma is a vascular tumor of a multicentric nature. It may be of endemic or iatrogenic forms. The endemic form is also referred to as the classic form, and is associated with autoimmune deficiency syndrome (AIDS). The iatrogenic form may occur after organ transplantation due to immunosuppression. Kaposi sarcoma is also called *multiple idiopathic hemorrhagic sarcoma*.

Epidemiology

Kaposi sarcoma was rare in the United States before the AIDS epidemic, with only about two new cases out of every one million people annually. Once the epidemic hit, cases peaked at about 47 per 1 million annually, in the early 1990s. Today, there are only about six cases per one million annually, mostly in HIV-infected individuals. Also, about 1 in 200 transplant patients develops the disease, usually when they already had *Kaposi sarcoma associated herpesvirus (KSHV)* prior to transplantation. The classic form of Kaposi sarcoma is most common in men older than age 60, of Eastern European, Italian, or Jewish ancestry. It is only rarely seen in children. Overall, Kaposi sarcoma is much more common in men than in women. The disease is most common in African Americans than in other groups.

In Africa and parts of the world where KSHV and HIV infection rates are significant, endemic and AIDS-associated Kaposi sarcomas occur in men, women, and children.

Etiology and Risk Factors

Kaposi sarcoma is caused by herpesvirus type 8 (HHV-8), and originates in the endothelial cells as a response to infection. The likelihood of developing this disease is greatly increased by immunosuppression. Epidemic Kaposi sarcoma is the most common cancer associated with AIDS. Risk factors include Jewish or Mediterranean descent, equatorial African descent, the male gender, HHV-8, KSHV, immune deficiency, homosexual intercourse, or sexual activity with multiple partners, and sharing intravenous needles.

Clinical Manifestations

The classic form of Kaposi sarcoma is indolent, and there are usually only a small number of lesions on the skin of the legs. Visceral involvement occurs in less than 10% of cases. Skin lesions are asymptomatic and of a pink, purple, or red color. They appear as macules, but may coalesce over time into bluish violet to black nodules and plaques (see Figure 10.8). Edema may be present, and sometimes the nodules **fungate** or penetrate into soft tissues and bones. However, epidemic Kaposi sarcoma is much more aggressive than the classic form of the disease. Many skin lesions are usually present, often on the face and trunk. There is usually gastrointestinal, lymph node, and mucosal involvement. Mucosal lesions are dark macules, plaques, or tumors. Visceral involvement is common in the oral cavity, GI tract, and lungs. Symptoms vary based on the affected organs. The GI lesions are usually asymptomatic but can bleed and even hemorrhage.

In some cases, Kaposi sarcoma is the initial manifestation of AIDS. Also, endemic Kaposi sarcoma occurs in Africa even without HIV infection being present. The *prepubertal lymphadenopathic subtype* mostly affects children. There are primary tumors of the lymph nodes, and skin lesions may or may not be present. This subtype is usually fulminant and fatal. The *adult subtype* of endemic Kaposi sarcoma is like the classic form of the disease. *Iatrogenic Kaposi sarcoma* usually develops a few years after organ transplantation, with a variably fulminant course, based on the level of immunosuppression.

Pathology

The tumor cells of Kaposi sarcoma have a spindle shape. Their appearance is similar to that of fibroblasts, myofibroblasts, and smooth muscle cells. Endothelial cells infected with HHV-8 have changes in lymphatic differentiation. They manufacture cytokines, which creates a favorable environment for angiogenesis. There are three pathological stages, as follows:

- *Patch stage* – dilated vascular channels dissect through the dermal collagen; the promontory sign is an uncommon feature, in which the

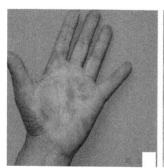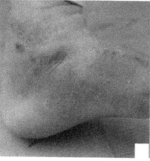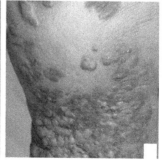

Figure 10.8 Kaposi sarcoma on (a) palm; (b) foot; (c) trunk. *Source*: https://onlinelibrary.wiley.com/doi/10.1111/jdv.12349. Journal of the European Academy of Dermatology and Venereology [22].

tumor's vascular channels surround and entrap the native blood vessels; this may be very slight when the lesions are early in their development

- *Plaque stage* – there are more extensive and compressed, thin vascular channels that infiltrate the deeper dermis; infiltrative proliferation occurs of the spindled endothelial cells, which may look similar to fibroblasts; these cells often infiltrate and destroy the eccrine coils
- *Tumor (nodular) stage* – there are discrete nodules made up of intersecting fascicles consisting of uniform spindle cells; between them are intervening blood-filled spaces; longitudinal section reveals slit-like spaces, but cross section reveals **sieve-like spaces**; there may be intracytoplasmic hyaline globules

In all pathological stages, mitoses are common, but there is usually only slight pleomorphism. In rare, poorly differentiated cases, pleomorphism is severe. This must be confirmed using the HHV-8 immunostain to exclude angiosarcoma. There are usually extravasated erythrocytes and hemosiderin, and often, plasma cells are present.

Diagnosis

The diagnosis of Kaposi sarcoma is confirmed via punch biopsy. If the patient has AIDS or immunosuppression, visceral spreading must be evaluated via chest and abdominal CT scan. If this is negative but there are GI or pulmonary symptoms, bronchoscopy or GI endoscopy may be required. The differential diagnoses include angiosarcoma, severe vascular stasis, hobnail hemangioma, spindle cell hemangioma, and Kaposiform hemangioendothelioma.

Treatment

There are many identical treatments used for both classic and endemic forms of Kaposi sarcoma. No treatment is often needed for indolent lesions. One to several superficial lesions can be surgically excised, removed by cryotherapy or electrocoagulation, or interferon alfa or intralesional vinblastine can be applied. Topical

imiquimod is another choice. If the patient has many lesions, diffuse tumor involvement, and lymph node disease, radiation therapy and chemotherapy are indicated. Recurrence often happens, and a complete cure is rare. Endemic Kaposi sarcoma treatments are often palliative.

For AIDS-related Kaposi sarcoma, highly active antiretroviral therapy (HAART) is often effective. This may be since the patient's CD4 + count will improve and the viral load of HIV will decrease. Also, protease inhibitors used in this regimen may be able to block angiogenesis. For AIDS patients with indolent localized disease, CD4 + counts above 150 per microliter, and HIV RNA of less than 500 copies per milliliter, intralesional vinblastine may be also used. For more indolent lesions, pomalidomide is an option. If there is more extensive or visceral disease, pegylated liposomal doxorubicin can be given every 2–3 weeks. An alternative first-line agent is paclitaxel, which can also be given if pegylated liposomal doxorubicin fails. Potentially adjunctive therapies include desferrioxamine, interleukin-12, and oral retinoids. Treatment for most AIDS patients does not actually lengthen their lives. This is because infections are so prevalent and severe.

For iatrogenic Kaposi sarcoma, immunosuppressants should be stopped. For organ transplant patients, reducing these agents often reduces the extent of Kaposi sarcoma lesions. If the patient's doses cannot be reduced, the local and systemic treatments used for other types of Kaposi sarcoma should be administered. Another agent that can improve iatrogenic disease is *sirolimus*.

Prevention and Early Detection

There is no known way to completely prevent Kaposi sarcoma. Therefore, avoiding known risk factors is suggested. There are no recommended routine screening tests to detect this disease in individuals that are not at increased risk. For HIV-infected people, there should be regular examination by experienced physicians to recognize the presence of the disease early.

Prognosis

Classic Kaposi sarcoma is usually not fatal. Prognosis is based on the clinical variant, disease stage, and immune status. Generally, the five-year relative survival rate for Kaposi sarcoma is based on staging. This is 81% if localized, 62% if regional, and 41% with distant metastasis. These percentages only apply to the stage of cancer upon initial diagnosis, and do not apply later if the disease grows, spreads, or recurs after treatment.

Clinical Case

1. What are the causes and risk factors for Kaposi sarcoma?
2. What are the three stages of Kaposi sarcoma?
3. Which treatment options are available for Kaposi sarcoma?

A 55-year-old man went to his physician because of skin lesions on his legs and in his mouth. The lesions were dark in color. Punch biopsies revealed the lesions to be Kaposi sarcoma, and CT scans were taken of his chest and abdomen. Testing showed that the man was HIV-negative, but that he had immune system impairment. Histopathology showed spindle cells that formed slit-like spaces, with some of them containing red blood cells. He was treated with paclitaxel, and his condition improved. After six months, the patient's lesions were greatly reduced in size and he had no other complications.

Answers:

1. **Kaposi sarcoma is caused by herpesvirus type 8 (HHV-8), and originates in the endothelial cells as a response to infection. The likelihood of developing this disease is greatly increased by immunosuppression. Risk factors** include Jewish or Mediterranean descent, equatorial African descent, the male gender, HHV-8, KSHV, immune deficiency, homosexual intercourse or sexual activity with multiple partners, and sharing intravenous needles.

2. **The three stages of Kaposi sarcoma are the patch, plaque, and tumor (nodular) stages. Dilated vascular channels dissecting through the dermal collagen define the patch stage. In the plaque stage, there are more extensive and compressed, thin vascular channels that infiltrate the deeper dermis. In the tumor (nodular) stage, there are discrete nodules made up of intersecting fascicles consisting of uniform spindle cells.**

3. **Treatment options for Kaposi sarcoma include observation (for indolent lesions), surgical excision, cryotherapy, electrocoagulation, interferon alfa, intralesional vinblastine, topical imiquimod, radiation therapy, chemotherapy, palliative treatments, HAART, protease inhibitors, pomalidomide, pegylated liposomal doxorubicin, paclitaxel, desferrioxamine, interleukin-12, oral retinoids, and sirolimus.**

Significant Point

Kaposi sarcoma is caused by human herpesvirus 8 (HHV-8). In AIDS patients, it usually appears as a quickly progressing tumor affecting the skin, lymph nodes, GI tract, lungs, liver, or spleen. Fortunately, incidence is decreasing due to HAART.

Key Terms

Acantholytic
Anetodermic
Bannayan–Zonana syndrome
Basal cell carcinoma
Bazex syndrome
Bowen disease
Brachytherapy
Chondrodermatitis nodularis helicis
Cutaneous adnexae
Dell
Dermabrasion
Dermatofibromas
Dermatofibrosarcoma protuberans
Dermoscope
Discoid dermatitis
Ectasia
Electrodesiccation
Electrosurgery
Familial mode-melanoma syndrome
Freckles
Fungate
Genodermatosis
Hailey–Hailey disease
Happle–Tinschert syndrome
Harmonic scalpel
Hidradenitis suppurativa
Infantile hemangiomas
Kaposi sarcoma

Keloids
Keratoacanthoma
Keratohyalin
Lentigo maligna
Lichenoid dermatoses
Lipoma
Lupus vulgaris
Melanoma
Merkel cell skin cancer
Molluscum contagiosum
Nevi
Nevus
Nevus sebaceous
Oncoprotein antibodies
Pluripotent cells
Pseudofolliculitis barbae
Pyogenic granulomas
Rombo syndrome
Seborrheic keratoses
Sentinel lymph node biopsy
Sieve-like spaces
Solar lentigo
Squamous cell carcinoma
Strawberry hemangiomas
Telangiectasia
Tonofibrils
Venous lakes
Xeroderma pigmentosum

Bibliography

1 Alhumidi, A. (2013). *Immunohistochemistry of Epithelial Skin Tumors*. Riga (Latvia): Lap Lambert Academic Publishing.

2 American Academy of Dermatology Association (AAD). (2021). *Keloids: Who Gets and Causes*. https://www.aad.org/public/diseases/a-z/keloids-causes Accessed 2021.

3 Baykal, C. and Yazganoglu, K.D. (2014). *Clinical Atlas of Skin Tumors*. New York: Springer.

4 Baumann, K., Halata, Z., and Moll, I. (2013). *The Merkel Cell: Structure-Development-Function-Cancerogenesis*. New York: Springer.

5 Burg, G., Kutzner, H., Kempf, W., Feit, J., and Smoller, B.R. (2018). *Atlas of Dermatopathology: Tumors, Nevi, and Cysts*. Hoboken: Wiley-Blackwell.

6 Centers for Disease Control and Prevention. (2016). *States With the Highest Rate of Skin Cancer – Rankings*. QuoteWizard. https://quotewizard.com/news/posts/skin-cancer-rates-by-state. Accessed 2021.

7 Cerroni, L. (2020). *Skin Lymphoma: The Illustrated Guide*, 5th Edition. Hoboken: Wiley-Blackwell.

8 Cognetta, Jr., A.B. and Mendenhall, W.M. (2013). *Radiation Therapy for Skin Cancer.* New York: Springer.

9 Elder, D.E. and Murphy, G.F. (2010). *Melanocytic Tumors of the Skin (AFIP Atlas of Tumor Pathology Series 4).* Arlington: American Registry of Pathology.

10 Elder, D.E. (2018). *World Health Organization Classification of Skin Tumors (Medicine),* 4th. Geneva: World Health Organization.

11 Franchi, A. (2019). *Pearls and Pitfalls in Head and Neck Pathology.* Cambridge: Cambridge University Press.

12 Griffiths, C.E.M., Barker, J., Bleiker, T., Chalmers, R., and Creamer, D. (2016). *Rook's Textbook of Dermatology,* 9th Edition. Hoboken: Wiley. Figure 141.3 from Page 3634.

13 Griffiths, C.E.M., Barker, J., Bleiker, T., Chalmers, R., and Creamer, D. (2016). *Rook's Textbook of Dermatology,* 9th Edition. Hoboken: Wiley. Figure 142.6 from Page 3646.

14 Griffiths, C.E.M., Barker, J., Bleiker, T., Chalmers, R., and Creamer, D. (2016). *Rook's Textbook of Dermatology,* 9th Edition. Hoboken: Wiley. Figure 142.23 from Page 3655.

15 Hanlon, A. (2018). *A Practical Guide to Skin Cancer.* New York: Springer.

16 Hassan, I., Ahmad, P.S., and Handa, S. (2013). *Clinical Synopsis and Color Atlas of Skin Tumors.* New Delhi: Jaypee Brothers Medical Publishers Pvt Ltd.

17 Huang, J.T. and Coughlin, C.C. (2017). *Skin Tumors and Reactions to Cancer Therapy in Children.* New York: Springer.

18 Ibekwe, P. (2012). *Prevalence of HHV8 in AIDS Patients with Kaposi's Sarcoma.* Riga (Latvia): Lap Lambert Academic Publishing.

19 Ishikawa, K. (2012). *Adnexal Tumors of the Skin: An Atlas.* New York: Springer.

20 Journal of Dermatology, The. (2010). *Strawberry hemangiomas in different locations.* https://onlinelibrary.wiley.com/doi/10.1111/j.1346-8138.2010.00927.x. 37 (11): 969–955. Accessed 2021.

21 Journal of Dermatology, The. (2017). *Melanoma viewed with immersion contact dermoscopy, revealing many dotted vessels in the depigmented area.* https://onlinelibrary.wiley.com/doi/full/10.1111/1346-8138.13686. 44 (5): 525–532. Figure 5. Accessed 2021.

22 Journal of the European Academy of Dermatology and Venereology. (2014). *Kaposi sarcoma on palm, foot, and trunk.* https://onlinelibrary.wiley.com/doi/10.1111/jdv.12349. 28 (11): 1545–1552. Accessed 2021.

23 Kazakov, D.V., McKee, P., Michal, M., and Kacerovska, D. (2012). *Cutaneous Adnexal Tumors.* Philadelphia: Lippincott, Williams, and Wilkins.

24 Longo, C. (2019). *Diagnosing the Less Common Skin Tumors: Clinical Appearance and Dermoscopy Correlation.* Boca Raton: CRC Press.

25 Lowther, C.M. (2009). *An Atlas of Histology of Basal Cell Carcinoma (For Physicians Learning Mohs Surgery).* Nikki & Lowther Scientific Publishing.

26 Lund, H.Z., and Armed Forces Institute of Pathology (U.S.). (2012). *Tumors of the Skin.* United States Armed Forces Institute of Pathology.

27 Massi, G. and LeBoit, P.E. (2014). *Histological Diagnosis of Nevi and Melanoma,* 2nd Edition. Springer.

28 Mattassi, R., Loose, D.A., and Vaghi, M. (2015). *Hemangiomas and Vascular Malformations – An Atlas of Diagnosis and Treatment,* 2nd Edition. Springer.

29 Morgan, M., Hamill, J.R., and Spencer, J.M. (2010). *Atlas of Mohs and Frozen Section Cutaneous Pathology.* Springer.

30 Patterson, J.W. (2006). *Nonmelanocytic Tumors of the Skin (Atlas of Tumor Pathology Series 4).* American Registry of Pathology.

31 Plaza, J.A. and Prieto, V.G. (2016). *Applied Immunohistochemistry in the Evaluation of Skin Neoplasms.* Springer.

32 Rathod, G. and Parmar, P. (2014). *Tumors of Skin – A Histopathological Study.* Lap Lambert Academic Publishing.

33 Reichrath, J. (2020). *Sunlight, Vitamin D and Skin Cancer (Advances in Experimental Medicine and Biology,* 3rd Edition. Springer.

34 Requena, L. and Sangueza, O. (2018). *Cutaneous Adnexal Neoplasms*. Springer.

35 Riffat, F., Palme, C.E., and Veness, M. (2015). *Non-Melanoma Skin Cancer of the Head and Neck (Cancer Clinics)*. Springer.

36 Robins, P. and Perez, M. (2015). *Understanding Melanoma – What You Need to Know*, 5th Edition. The Skin Cancer Foundation.

37 Rongioletti, F., Margaritescu, I., and Smoller, B.R. (2015). *Rare Malignant Skin Tumors*. Springer.

38 Rosendahl, C. and Marozava, A. (2019). *Dermatoscopy and Skin Cancer: A Handbook for Hunters of Skin Cancer and Melanoma*. Scion Publishing Ltd.

39 Sand, M. (2016). *MicroRNAs in Malignant Tumors of the Skin – First Steps of Tiny Players in the Skin to a New World of Genomic Medicine (Research)*. Springer.

40 Sangueza, O.P. and Requena, L. (2003). *Pathology of Vascular Skin Lesions: Clinicopathologic Correlations*. Humana Press.

41 Thompson, J.F., Morton, D.L., and Kroon, B.B.R. (2020). *Textbook of Melanoma: Pathology, Diagnosis and Management*. CRC Press.

42 Warnakulasuriya, S. and Khan, Z. (2017). *Squamous Cell Carcinoma: Molecular Therapeutic Targets*. Springer.

43 Zalaudek, I., Argenziano, G., and Giacomel, J. (2016). *Dermatoscopy of Non-Pigmented Skin Tumors: Pink-Think-Blink*. CRC Press.

11

Bone Tumors

Benign Bone Tumors

Benign bone tumors include many different types of neoplasia. These include the following: benign giant cell tumors of bone, chondroblastomas, chondromyxoid fibromas, enchondromas, nonossifying fibromas, osteoblastomas, osteochondromas, and osteoid osteomas. Nonossifying fibromas are also known as *fibroxanthomas* and, when very small, *fibrous cortical defects*. Osteochondromas are also known as *osteocartilaginous exostoses*, and are the most common benign bone tumors.

Epidemiology

Benign giant cell tumors of bone usually affect individuals in their 20s or 30s. Chondroblastomas are rare, occurring mostly in people between age 10 and 20, which is the same age group as for osteochondromas. Chondromyxoid fibromas are very rare, usually occurring before age 30. Enchondromas occur in all ages, but mostly between ages 10 and 40. Nonossifying fibromas are common in children. Osteoblastomas are much more common in males, usually developing between ages 10 and 35. Osteoid osteomas usually occur in males in their teens and 20s. There is no racial or ethnic predilection for benign bone tumors.

Etiology and Risk Factors

Benign giant cell tumors of bone are generally of unknown cause or risk factors. With enchondromas, overgrowth of cartilage lining at the ends of bones is implicated, as is persistent growth of original embryonic cartilage. The risk factors for osteochondromas include younger age (children and teenagers) and the male gender, as well as having family members with these tumors.

Clinical Manifestations

Benign giant cell tumors of bone, because of continued growth, can cause pain. Enchondromas are usually asymptomatic, as are nonossifying fibromas when they are small. Lesions that affect more than 50% of the bone diameter make pathologic fractures more likely. Osteoblastomas cause sustained pain that is relatively less responsive or OTC pain relievers than other tumors. These tumors also cause spinal nerve compression, as well as swelling and tenderness in the general tumor location. Osteochondromas usually cause painless and hard immobile masses, lower than normal height for the patient's age, differences in the size of one arm or leg, irritation or pressure with exertion, and soreness of surrounding muscles. Some patients have no symptoms at all with osteochondromas. Osteoid osteomas may cause pain that is usually worse at night, indicating increased nocturnal inflammation from the effects of prostaglandins, especially prostaglandin E_2 (PGE_2) from proliferating osteoblasts.

Pathology

Benign giant cell tumors of bone develop in the epiphyses and distal epiphyseal–metaphyseal region. They are locally aggressive, continually enlarging. The tumors destroy and erode bones and may extend into soft tissue. After treatment, these tumors have a high rate of recurrence. Chondroblastomas form in the epiphysis, and can continually grow, destroying bones and joints. Chondromyxoid fibromas form near the end of long bones – usually in the proximal tibia and iliac wing. Enchondromas usually form in the medullary bone metaphyseal–diaphyseal area. They are like periosteal chondromas that occur on the surface of bones.

Nonossifying fibromas are fibrous lesions. The small subtype known as fibrous cortical defects occur during development, as areas of bone that would normally ossify fill with fibrous tissue. Most often, fibrous cortical defects are in the *metaphyses* of the distal femur, distal tibia, and proximal tibia. They may continually enlarge, becoming **multioculated**. However, most lesions eventually become ossified and are remodeled, leaving areas that are dense and sclerotic.

Osteoblastomas are consisting of tissue that is similar in histology to osteoid osteoma. Sometimes, osteoblastomas are considered to be large osteoid osteomas of more than 2 cm in diameter. Most

often, osteoblastomas develop in the posterior spine, legs, hands, and feet. They grow slowly and destroy normal bone, without significant bony reactions. There is a variation called *aggressive osteoblastoma* that is histologically and radiographically like osteosarcoma. However, malignant transformation of osteoblastomas is rare. Osteochondromas usually occur near the ends of long bones, but may arise in any bone. They may be single or multiple, with multiple osteochondromas often running in families. In less than 1% of cases, single osteochondromas develop into secondary malignant chondrosarcomas. However, with multiple osteochondromas, this occurs in about 10% of cases. Multiple hereditary osteochondromas involve more tumors, which more often develop into chondrosarcomas. Multiple hereditary osteochondromas were formerly known as *multiple hereditary exostoses type 1 and 2*. Bone fractures only occur in rare cases of osteochondromas. Osteoid osteomas are most common in long bones, but can occur in any bone – often in the appendicular skeleton, and are usually less than 2 cm in diameter. About half of all cases are in the femur or tibia, mostly in the cortex, and less often in the medullary cavity. A thick portion of reactive cortical bone is usually present, and may be the only identifying feature in imaging studies.

Diagnosis

Benign giant cell tumors of bone appear in imaging as expanding, lytic lesions. They have a margin lacking a **sclerotic rim**, at the end point of the tumor and the beginning of normal, trabecular bone. A biopsy is required for diagnosis. A chest CT is performed early to assess any metastasis to the lungs. Chondroblastomas appear in imaging as sclerotic marginated cyst-like lesions with areas of **punctate** calcification. An MRI can aid in diagnosis, by revealing large amounts of edema around the tumor. Chondromyxoid fibromas usually appear in imaging as eccentric, highly circumscribed, lytic lesions. Their location prompts diagnosis.

Enchondromas are often found incidentally during imaging for other reasons. On X-ray, the tumor may appear lobulated and calcified. Some have less calcification, and X-rays or CT may show stippling of the calcified portions. If the tumor is near the cortex, there is slight endosteal scalloping. Because most enchondromas have increased uptake in bone scans, cancer is often considered, but is not actually present. MRI and CT may be diagnostic, but if not, a tumor that is causing pain is diagnosed via open biopsy. Bone tumor pain and joint pain can be differentiated by injecting the joint with bupivacaine or another long-lasting anesthetic. If the pain continues, it may be due to the tumor. Nonossifying fibromas appear as well-defined lucent cortical lesions in X-rays. They are usually found incidentally, often after trauma, and are usually single lesions less than 2 cm in diameter. There is an oblong appearance and well-defined sclerotic borders within the cortex. They may also be multioculated.

Osteoblastomas are visualized via X-rays, CT, and MRI (see Figure 11.1). Open biopsies are usually done for accurate diagnosis. Osteochondromas appear in imaging as bony prominences with cartilage caps that are usually less than 2 cm in diameter. The caps develop from the bone surfaces, and there is no underlying cortex below them. An MRI may help to differentiate between thick cartilage caps, bursa, or surrounding masses of soft tissue. At the base of the exostosis, there is no actual underlying cortex, and the medullary canal is continuous with the base of the exostosis. Sometimes, a painful bursa forms over the cartilage cap.

Osteoid osteomas, when they occur in growing children, result in an inflammatory response and hyperemia. If this is close to the open growth plate, there may be resulting overgrowth and discrepancies in limb length. In physical examination, there may be regional muscle atrophy, since pain causes the child to avoid using the muscle. In imaging, osteoid osteomas appear as small radiolucent areas surrounded by larger sclerotic areas. When a tumor is suspected, a whole-body technetium-99 m bone scan is performed. The tumor appears as an area of increased uptake, as do many other bone lesions. An excellent way to distinguish osteoid osteomas is CT with fine image sequences, or MRI (see Figure 11.2). Plain X-rays or fine cut CT scans may reveal a "bull's eye" appearance of the actual nidus of the tumor, which is surrounded by reactive bone.

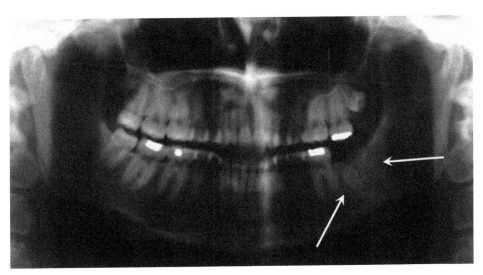

Figure 11.1 Osteoblastoma of the mandible, with arrows indicating the tumor. *Source*: Wiley Online Library– Journal of the Sciences and Specialties of the Head and Neck [66].

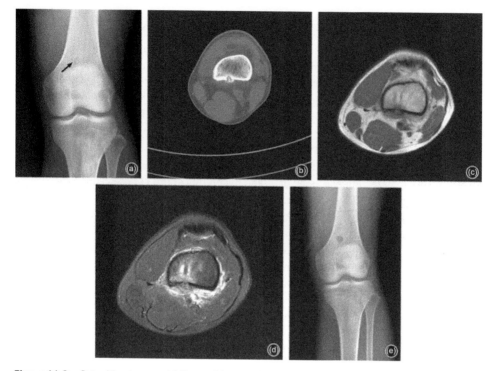

Figure 11.2 Osteoid osteomas. (a) X-ray with arrow indicating the nidus; (b) CT scan of high intensity lesion; (c) T1-weighted MRI showing low-intensity nidus; (d) T2-weighted MRI showing increased intensity in nidus; (e) X-ray done four months after surgery showing small local bone loss. *Source*: Figure 1, Wiley Online Library – Orthopaedic Surgery [67].

Treatment

Benign giant cell tumors of bone are treated with radical curettage, then packing with methyl methacrylate or bone graft. An adjuvant is often used, including thermal heat via the hardening of *polymethyl methacrylate*, thermal heat via an argon beam, chemical treatment with phenol, or cryotherapy using liquid nitrogen. If the tumor is very large and is destroying the joint, complete excision with joint reconstruction may be indicated. Denosumab, a monoclonal antibody, can be used if the tumor is large and essentially inoperable. This agent is a receptor activator of nuclear factor kappa-B ligand (RANKL) inhibitor. Chondroblastomas must be surgically excised by curettage. The cavity must then be bone grafted. The local recurrence rate is 10–20%. Recurrent chondroblastomas are often resolved by repeated bone curettage and grafting. Chondromyxoid fibromas are treated, after biopsy, with surgical excision or curettage. An adjuvant such as an argon beam, liquid nitrogen, or phenol may be used, and bone grafting is often indicated. Enchondromas do not require treatments or biopsy if they are asymptomatic. Additional imaging may be done to exclude progression to chondrosarcoma, which only occurs rarely. The imaging is done at six months and one year, or when symptoms develop. Multiple enchondromas (**Ollier disease**) and multiple enchondromatosis that involves soft-tissue hemangiomas (**Maffucci syndrome**) greatly increase risks of chondrosarcoma developing. Nonossifying fibromas, if small, do not require treatment and follow-up needs only be limited. If they are causing pain or are about 50% of the bone diameter in size, curettage and bone grafting may be needed to lower the risk of pathologic fractures.

Osteoblastomas are treated with surgery that often includes curettage and bone grafting.

Local recurrence, after treatment with intralesional curettage, may be in 10–20% of cases. If the lesion appears to be more aggressive, it is treated with surgical en bloc resection, and bony reconstruction. Osteochondromas are excised if they compress large nerves or vessels, if they disturb growth, appear destructive in imaging, or cause pain – mostly when they impinge muscles to create an inflamed bursa. Excision is also done if there is a soft-tissue mass, or a cartilaginous cap that has thickened to become larger than 2 cm, which suggests the development of malignant chondrosarcoma. In adults, enlargement of an osteochondroma should prompt consideration of chondrosarcoma, indicated biopsy or excision. The pain of osteoid osteomas may be relieved by aspirin and other NSAIDs that target prostaglandins. Ablation of the small radiolucent area, using percutaneous radiofrequency energy, usually provides permanent relief. Interventional musculoskeletal radiologists most often perform this procedure, with percutaneous techniques along with anesthesia. Less frequently, surgical curettage or excision is done. If the osteoid osteoma is close to a nerve or skin (hands, feet, or spine), surgical excision or curettage may be preferred, since damage can be caused by the radiofrequency ablation heat.

Prevention and Early Detection

Benign giant cell tumors of bone have no known method of prevention, though they can be detected early if bone pain has manifested. Chondroblastomas are the same, as are chondromyxoid fibromas. Enchondromas are not preventable, and though early detection improves treatment and outlook, there is a lack of screening tests available. Nonossifying fibromas are not preventable, and there are no standard methods for their early detection. Osteoblastomas can also not be prevented, but are sometimes discovered early in their development via MRI. Osteochondromas have not been found to be preventable, and may be detected early because, if multiple, there will be more obvious signs than with a single osteochondroma. As with the other benign bone tumors, osteoid osteomas are not preventable. There is no approved screening method for their early detection.

Prognosis

Benign giant cell tumors of the bone have varying prognoses based on the patient's age, tumor's size and location, and treatment method. They can recur, so patients must have regular follow-up visits for years after treatment, utilizing various X-ray procedures. Chondroblastomas have 5-year and 10-year relapse-free survival rates of 86.6%. Recurrence can occur as long as 51 months after initial treatment, and all local recurrences have occurred in patients over age 16. With surgery, most cases of chondromyxoid fibromas have a good prognosis. However, there is a 10–20% chance of recurrence, so follow-up care is very important. Enchondromas have a good prognosis in 82.6% of patients, and malignant transformation is not extremely common. Long-term outlook for nonossifying fibromas is very good, and most patients resume normal activities within 3–6 months after surgery. Long-term prognosis is equally good, since the tumors resolve once skeletal maturity is reached. Osteoblastomas usually have an excellent prognosis, based on tumor activity, response to treatment, age, overall health, and tolerance for the various types of treatment. Recurrence can occur, and continuous follow-up care is essential. Osteochondromas have varied

---

Significant Point

Fortunately, most bone tumors are benign and usually not life-threatening. The most common types include nonossifying fibroma, osteochondroma, giant cell tumor of bone, and enchondromas. Many benign tumors only require observation. Some are treated effectively with medication, and some disappear over time – especially in children. However, some benign bone tumors spread or become malignant, and can even recur after being surgically removed.

prognoses, based on patient health, extent of progression, and how early treatment began. Prognosis is usually excellent if treatment was started early in the disease course. Osteoid osteomas usually have a good prognosis since they are not life-threatening and usually only require analgesics and anti-inflammatory medications. If surgery is needed, the patient usually returns to normal activities and only requires follow-up care.

Multiple Myeloma

Multiple myeloma is the most common of the primary malignant bone tumors. However, it is commonly considered to be a bone marrow cell tumor, rather than an actual tumor of the bone itself. It is of hematopoietic origin, and occurs mostly in adults. Usually, its development and progression are multicentric. The bone marrow is often so diffusely involved that the disease is easily diagnosed by bone marrow aspiration. Different from metastatic bone tumors, radionuclide bone scans may be unable to reveal lesions. Therefore, skeletal surveys are performed, which usually show extremely circumscribed, lytic lesions that appear to be "punched out," or sometimes have diffuse demineralization. In rare cases, multiple myeloma lesions appear sclerotic or as diffuse osteopenia – especially within a vertebral body. A *plasmacytoma* is a single, isolated lesion that does not have systemic involvement of the bone marrow. Some bony lesions respond to radiation therapy quite well. Multiple myeloma was discussed in detail in Chapter 7.

Osteosarcoma

Osteosarcoma is also known as *osteogenic sarcoma*, and after multiple myeloma, is the second most common primary bone tumor. There is immature bone known as *malignant osteoid* produced from the tumor bone cells. These bulky tumors always contain osteoid and callus (osteoblastic sarcoma). The osteoid and callus are produced by atypical anaplastic stromal cells, which

are not normal or embryonal. The tumors may also contain cartilage (chondroblastic sarcoma) or fibrinoid (fibroblastic sarcoma) tissues. Osteoid is deposited in thick collections between the trabecular of callus. As normal compact bone is destroyed, it is replaced with dense callus and osteoid masses. The bone tissue that is produced never matures to become compact bone. Osteosarcoma is most common around the knee, in the distal femur, but also sometimes in the proximal tibia (see Figure 11.3). It may occur in other long bones – especially the metaphyseal–diaphyseal location. Metastasis is usually to the other bones and lungs. Osteosarcoma is signified in most cases by pain and swelling.

Epidemiology

According to the American Cancer Society, there are about 1,000 cases of osteosarcoma diagnosed annually in the United States, and about half of them occur in children and adolescents. In fact, most osteosarcomas occur between the ages of 10 and 30, with adolescents having the most cases. Between 56% and 60% of all bone malignancies in children and adolescents under age 20 are osteosarcomas. They are not common in children under 5 years of age, and incidence peaks at age 15. About 1 of every 10 osteosarcomas occurs in people over age 60, which is equivalent to 28% of bone tumors in this group. There is a slight male predilection with these tumors, of 1.4:1, which has sometimes been reported as 3:2. Osteosarcomas mostly affect African American adolescents, followed by Hispanic Americans and Caucasians. The rates of childhood and adolescent osteosarcomas are approximately as follows, in the United States:

- African American – 6.8 per million children and adolescents, annually
- Hispanic American – 6.5 per million
- Caucasians – 4.6 per million (also see Figure 11.4)

Global statistics on osteosarcomas are lacking. There is limited information from the United Kingdom, listing about 2.6 cases out of every million people annually. This totals about 160 new cases per year. In Ireland, there about 11 new cases diagnosed annually.

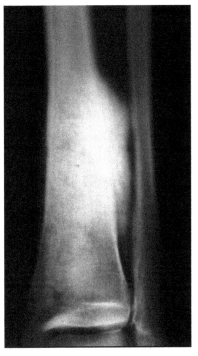
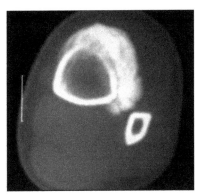

Figure 11.3 Left: anteroposterior X-ray showing a densely mineralized osteosarcoma at the distal metadiaphysis of the tibia. Right: a CT scan showing the lesion on the bone surface, with slight breakthrough of the anterolateral cortex and over 50% circumferential involvement. *Source*: American Cancer Society (ACS) Journals – Cancer [10].

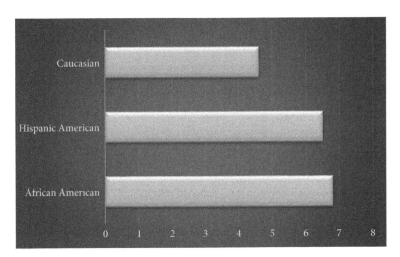

Figure 11.4 Rates of various children and adolescents with osteosarcomas, per million.

Etiology and Risk Factors

Osteosarcomas appear to be related to both environmental and genetic factors. These tumors have complex genetic abnormalities. In most cases, these involve *tumor protein 53 (TP53)*, *cyclin-dependent kinase inhibitor 2A and B (CDKN2A/B)*, *proto-oncogene MDM2*, *retinoblastoma (RB)*, and similar genes. External radiation therapy is implicated; however, higher incidence of osteosarcomas exists in people that survived childhood cancers, mostly with genetic syndromes such as hereditary retinoblastoma. A high risk for osteosarcoma is related to germline abnormalities in *TP53, checkpoint kinase 2 (CHEK2; Li-Fraumeni syndrome)*, or *RB1*. With the RB1 gene mutation, a child has up to 500 times higher risks of developing an osteosarcoma. Osteosarcomas are also associated with the *SRC* proto-oncogene. Risk factors for osteosarcomas include age, increased height, race, gender, bone diseases, and inherited cancer syndromes.

Clinical Manifestations

The main complaint of patients is pain, a secondary symptom is swelling due to the soft-tissue mass, and sometimes, pathologic fractures, which most often are attributed to a sports injury. The symptoms are located around the knee and distal femur, fibula, or proximal tibia. Pain worsens, usually at night, and requires medications.

Pathology

Osteosarcomas usually develop as intramedullary metaphyseal bone lesions that originate from the mesenchyme. They are less common on the surfaces of long bones. They may occur in the leg bones, humerus, pelvis, and jaw. Histological subtypes of osteosarcomas include osteogenic, conventional, Paget disease-associated, parosteal, periosteal, radiation-associated, small cell, and telangiectatic subtypes.

The majority of osteosarcomas form in the medullary canal and spread centrifugally. They invade the cortex and periosteum, developing a soft-tissue mass. However, the parosteal and periosteal osteosarcomas form in the cortex. The parosteal form is most common in adults, often located in the femur, and usually is more indolent. The periosteal subtype occurs in all ages, progressing in a way that is between the effects of the parosteal and other subtypes of osteosarcomas. The most common subtype of osteosarcoma is the classic form, which is referred to as *osteoblastic, chondroblastic,* or *fibroblastic.*

Osteosarcomas can be subclassified into a round-cell type or short, spindle-cell type. In the round-cell type, there are either round or oval-shaped cells with a nuclear diameter ranging from 57 to 15 μm. Most nuclei are uniform in shape and size, with slight variations. They contain fine, hyperchromatic, or coarse chromatin. Nucleoli may be inconspicuous, prominent, or absent. The round-cell type may have tumor cells that are very small, small, or medium (see Figure 11.5).

Diagnosis

Diagnosis begins with plain X-rays or the primary area. There is often a sunburst sign that indicates horizontal, new bone spicules around the tumor, due to it breaking through the cortex. A Codman triangle is also common. This occurs from periosteal new bone formation at the tumor margin. Lytic or sclerotic features signify osteosarcoma, but accurate diagnosis requires a biopsy. A CT scan shows cortical destructions, and the soft-tissue component is best shown in MRI, along with skip metastases and intramedullary spread. Chest X-rays and CT scans can also detect lung metastases. Bone scans are used to detect bone metastases.

Biopsy should be performed by a surgeon experienced with these tumors. Based on location and imaging results, open biopsy or core needle biopsy may be done. Any soft-tissue mass is biopsied, since it usually contains a viable tumor, which is usually of a high grade upon diagnosis. Most osteosarcomas metastasize to the lungs, followed by metastasis to other bones. Skip metastases are seen in up to 2% of cases, as are synchronous regional bone metastases, either in the primary bone, or transarticularly. These must be identified before any surgery. Metastatic disease is present in 20% of cases upon first diagnosis of an osteosarcoma. This means that a CT scan should be done to assess any pulmonary or bone metastases. A PET-CT scan is being used more often because of higher sensitivity.

Treatment

Treatment of osteosarcoma combines chemotherapy with surgery. Adjuvant chemotherapy

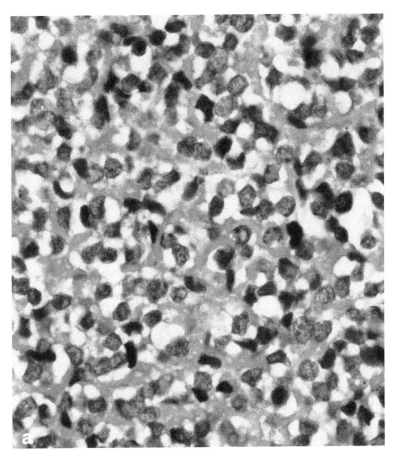

Figure 11.5 Lace-like osteoid and multinuclear giant cells of an osteosarcoma, in large areas of round cells that have medium-sized nuclei. *Source*: American Cancer Society (ACS) Journals – Cancer [12].

can increase survival from less than 20% of patients to more than 65% of patients, over five years. Neoadjuvant chemotherapy is started before surgery. The desired response is for more than 95% tumor necrosis to be seen during a histological study of a resected specimen. Some amount of response to chemotherapy is indicated by decreased size of the tumor in X-rays, reduction of pain, and decreased serum alkaline phosphatase. Several courses of chemotherapy are given over several months, after which limb-sparing surgery and reconstruction can be performed. Sometimes, for a fungating tumor, surgical amputation is required before chemotherapy can be started. Early micrometastatic disease that is believed to exist must be treated, even if it does not appear during imaging studies to determine the stage of the disease.

During limb-sparing surgery, the tumor undergoes en bloc resection, which includes all nearby reactive tissue, plus a rim of surrounding normal tissue. The tumor is not cut apart so that microscopic spillage of tumor cells will not occur. Chemotherapy is usually continued afterward. If there is about 95% complete tumor necrosis from the preoperative chemotherapy, over 90% of patients will survive for at least five years. If there is limited metastasis to the lungs, this may occasionally be treated with thoracotomy and *metastatectomy*, plus *wedge resection* of the lung lesion. When complete surgical resection is not possible, radiation therapy may be used. For the low-grade parosteal osteosarcomas, chemotherapy is not needed prior to surgical resection. These tumors must undergo en bloc resection, and chemotherapy is not needed if the resected specimen proves that the tumor is well differentiated. Usually, periosteal osteosarcomas are treated like the conventional form, with chemotherapy + surgical en bloc resection. For children and adolescents, **rotationplasty** may be performed, with major areas of the thigh, tumor, and knee being resected, as the sciatic nerve supply to the leg and foot is preserved. The proximal tibia is internally fixed to the remaining proximal femur after it is rotated 180°. The foot is positioned as needed so that the ankle joint functions as a knee joint and the foot acts as the tibial stump, as in a below-knee amputation. When amputation is required, the patient is closely monitored with **roentgenograms** and CT scans.

Cisplatin + doxorubicin can provide cure rates higher than 50% when the disease is localized. However, a three-drug regimen is even more effective, usually involving the addition of methotrexate. The current standard regimen is called MAP, which consists of high-dose <u>m</u>ethotrexate, <u>A</u>driamycin (doxorubicin), and <u>P</u>latinol (cisplatin). However, there are toxicities and treatment complications with MAP. Therefore, some treatment regimens use carboplatin + doxorubicin + ifosfamide, with similar results. Though surgery is extremely important for survival, about 80% of patients with metastatic disease would die without the use of systemic chemotherapy.

Radiation therapy for primary osteosarcomas is used for unresectable tumors or sometimes, as perioperative treatment or palliation. When the tumor is non-resectable or when wide surgical margins are not achievable, high doses of ionizing radiation increase localized control of the disease. Proton irradiation is also becoming more common, especially for younger patients, since it allows lower doses to reach non-targeted tissues. This reduces adverse effects and risks for secondary cancers. Surgical margins of less than 1.5 cm, along with poor responses to pre-surgical chemotherapy are factors more often linked to localized recurrences. Patients with better tissue responses have a five-year EFS above 75%, if there is 90% or higher tumor necrosis after

surgery. The rate is only 50–60% in patients with less than 90% tumor necrosis after surgery.

Patients that remain disease-free are closely followed for recurrences, with X-rays of the primary site, plus chest CT scans to assess lung metastases. Intervals between visits increase over time. Children are eventually transitioned to long-term follow-up clinics, usually after five years, since recurrence past this point are extremely rare. For secondary neoplasms, clinical monitoring is also needed since some patients have an inherited cancer predisposition syndrome. Late complications of treatments include doxorubicin-related cardiotoxicity (up to decades after therapy is completed). The drug called *dexrazoxane* can decrease cardiotoxicity without negative outcomes. Other toxicities from therapy include cisplatin-related hearing loss, and kidney damage from cisplatin and ifosfamide. Also, cyclophosphamide and ifosfamide can impact fertility. Complications of limb-sparing surgery include uneven leg lengths and fractures of prosthetic implants.

Prevention and Early Detection

There are no known ways to prevent osteosarcomas, but maintaining a healthy weight and avoiding smoking can improve overall health. Reducing exposure to all forms of radiation may also be preventive. There are no widely recommended screening tests for osteosarcoma for people that are not at an increased risk. With certain bone diseases or inherited cancer syndromes, increased monitoring for osteosarcoma may be recommended. This type of cancer does not usually run in families.

Prognosis

For osteosarcomas, a worsened prognosis exists if there is metastasis at diagnosis, primary disease in the axial skeleton, or if the tissues respond poorly to treatments. For non-metastatic osteosarcomas, the outcome of surgery plus chemotherapy is 60–70% survival over five years. For metastatic osteosarcomas, this survival rate is less than 40%. Long-term survival can be achieved with pulmonary metastases if they can all be surgically resected.

Clinical Case

1. How common are osteosarcomas in younger people?
2. What are the characteristic signs of osteosarcomas seen in imaging?
3. What are the good prognostic signs following preoperative chemotherapy and surgery?

A 16-year-old boy was playing soccer and suffered a fracture of the right femur. Upon evaluation, the boy's mother told the physician that her son had complained of pain in the femur for a few days prior to the fracture. Treatments included surgical resection of the tumor and three months of chemotherapy. Fortunately, the tumor necrosis rate was over 90% after surgery. There was no spread of the tumor, which was diagnosed as an osteoblastic osteosarcoma, and after one year of follow-up, the boy had no recurrence.

Answers:

1. **Osteosarcoma is the second most common primary bone tumor after multiple myeloma. It is most common around the knee, in the distal femur, and sometimes in the proximal tibia. About half of all diagnosed cases occur in children and adolescents.**

Most occur between the ages of 10 and 30, with adolescents having the most cases. Between 56% and 60% of all bone malignancies in children and adolescents under age 20 are osteosarcomas.

2. In imaging, there is often a sunburst sign that indicates horizontal, new bone spicules around the tumor, due to it breaking through the cortex. A Codman triangle is also common. This occurs from periosteal new bone formation at the tumor margin. Lytic or sclerotic features signify osteosarcoma, but accurate diagnosis requires a biopsy.

3. If there is about 95% complete tumor necrosis from the preoperative chemotherapy, over 90% of patients will survive for at least five years. Patients with better tissue responses have a five-year EFS above 75%, if there is 90% or higher tumor necrosis after surgery.

Chondrosarcoma

Chondrosarcoma is a malignant cartilage tumor. They are chondrogenic. Chondrosarcomas are very different from osteosarcomas on a clinical level, and in their treatment and prognosis. About 90% of chondrosarcomas are primary tumors, and chondrosarcomas make up about 20% of all bone tumors. They can also form as part of pre-existing conditions such as multiple osteochondromas and multiple enchondromatosis, which may be part of Maffucci syndrome or Ollier disease. Chondrosarcomas usually develop in the legs, arms, pelvis, scapula, and ribs.

Epidemiology

Chondrosarcoma is the most common malignant cartilage tumor. It is also the third most common bone sarcoma. Incidence of chondrosarcomas ranges between 0.1 and 0.3 cases per every 100,000 people. There are about 600 cases annually in the United States. Chondrosarcomas mostly occur in older adults, and make up more than 40% of primary bone sarcomas in adults of all ages. The average age of diagnosis is 51 years, within a range of 20–70 years in most cases. In children and adolescents, chondrosarcomas only make up 6% of all primary bone sarcomas. Males are slightly more affected than females, with peaks during the fifth and seventh decades. In younger people, there are usually higher rates of malignancy and metastases. Chondrosarcomas are more common in the United States and other Westernized countries. However, there are no clear racial or ethnic differences in occurrence. Because of the rarity of these tumors, there are no significant global data available.

Etiology and Risk Factors

Chondrosarcomas may be caused by genetic mutations. Pre-existing chondral lesions such as osteochondromas, can cause secondary chondrosarcomas to form, which are usually quite treatable. Risk factors include aging, and conditions that are signified by increased amounts of enchondromas in the body, such as Ollier disease and Mafucci syndrome.

Clinical Manifestations

There is an insidious onset to symptoms of chondrosarcomas. Patients often go to their physicians because of localized pain and swelling. The pain starts as a dull ache that occurs intermittently. It slowly worsens and occurs constantly, sometimes being severe enough to awaken the patient from sleep.

Pathology

Chondrosarcomas are common in flat bones such as the pelvis or scapula. They also develop in other bones and various areas of them, but usually in long bones such as the femur and humerus. Sometimes, chondrosarcomas have soft-tissue components that affect softer tissues than bone. The pathological subtypes of chondrosarcomas include: *chondrogenic, dedifferentiated, mesenchymal,* and *primary central,* which may be low-, intermediate-, or high-grade. The primary composition of chondrosarcomas consists of cartilaginous elements.

Chondrosarcomas are relatively large tumors with poor definition. They infiltrate the trabeculae of spongy bone. Cartilage-forming cells are produced, but ossification does not occur. Chondrosarcomas may form in the metaphysis or diaphysis of a long bone such as the femur. There are large lobules of hyaline cartilage, separated by fibrous tissue bands and anaplastic cells. Chondrosarcomas usually implant in surrounding tissues.

Diagnosis

In X-rays, chondrosarcomas often have punctate calcifications. They commonly cause cortical bone destruction, plus a loss of normal bone trabeculae (see Figure 11.6). X-rays must be carefully evaluated to assist with diagnosis. A CT scan is also used for imaging. A soft-tissue mass may appear on MRI. Bone scans often reveal these tumors as well. Tissue diagnosis is required, and can determine the tumor grade and likelihood of metastasis. Needle biopsies often are unable to extract enough tissue for diagnosis. Via imaging, and sometimes histology, it may be hard to identify low-grade chondrosarcomas because they are like enchondromas. Chondrosarcomas may cause elevation of serum glucose levels. Biopsy is performed at the time of surgery since seeding of tumor cells can occur if it is done before surgical resection. Accurate diagnosis relies on enough tumor tissue being obtained.

Treatment

The low-grade chondrosarcomas, of grade 1, must often undergo wide curettage, along with some type of adjuvant therapy. These include an argon beam, freezing with liquid nitrogen, and heating with methyl methacrylate, phenol, or via radiofrequencies. Surgical en bloc resection is sometimes preferred for low-grade chondrosarcomas to reduce recurrence risks. Higher-grade chondrosarcomas undergo surgical en bloc resection. If this surgery will impair function significantly, amputation is sometimes necessary. To avoid implantation of the tumor, great care is required to avoid any spillage of tumor cells into

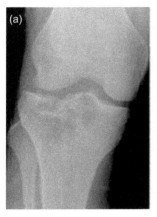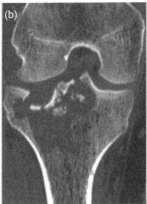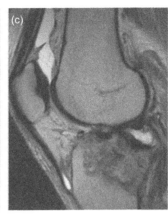

Figure 11.6 Chondrosarcoma of the tibia with a pathological fracture, osteolytic destruction, and a small soft-tissue component. (a) X-ray; (b) Coronal CT scan; (c) Sagittal T2-weighted MRI.
Source: Wiley Online Library – Diagnostic Cytopathology [68].

the soft tissues, as part of biopsy or surgery. If these cells spill, the chondrosarcoma will recur. If they do not, a cure is based on the grade of the tumor. Low-grade tumors are usually curable.

Since the tumors have a small amount of vascularity, chemotherapy and radiation are not extremely effective. For the dedifferentiated form of chondrosarcoma, doxorubicin + cisplatin may be effective. For the mesenchymal form, the *vincristine, Adriamycin, and cyclophosphamide (VAC)/ifosfamide and etoposide (IE)* regimen is preferred. This involves vincristine + Adriamycin (doxorubicin) + cyclophosphamide, alternating with ifosfamide + etoposide. There are many clinical trials ongoing for chondrosarcomas, including those that assess the use of the *isocitrate dehydrogenase 1 and 2 (IDH1 and IDH2)* inhibitors, and the *vascular endothelial growth factor (VEGF)* inhibitors such as pazopanib.

Prevention and Early Detection
There is no known prevention for chondrosarcomas. People with rare bone conditions may be more likely to develop these tumors. There has been some research concerning previous injuries and the later development of chondrosarcomas. While early detection improves outlook, there are no established screening methods for chondrosarcomas.

Prognosis
The five-year survival rate of chondrosarcomas is 78%. However, if diagnosed while localized, this rate is 91%. If it has spread to surrounding tissues or organs as well the regional lymph nodes, the five-year survival rate is 75%. Unfortunately, if the cancer has spread to distant parts of the body, the survival rate is only 22%.

Significant Point

Chondrosarcoma is a common type of bone sarcoma, and is a slow-growing cancer of unknown origin. The slower the growth, the less likely this tumor is to metastasize to other areas of the body. A unique fact is that chondrosarcoma cells produce cartilage – this is unlike all other bone sarcomas.

Clinical Case

1. In which ages are chondrosarcomas most common?
2. What is the pathology of chondrosarcomas of the femur?
3. Why is surgery the primary treatment for chondrosarcomas?

A 53-year-old man with pain in his left femur was examined, and X-rays were taken. There was a radio-negative tumor of the distal third of the left femur. He had previously had a knee injury because of a minor car accident, but there were no abnormalities after he recovered from the injury. An MRI revealed an osteolytic lesion. An open biopsy was performed, identifying the tumor as a low-grade chondrosarcoma. The tumor was completely resected and a knee prosthesis placed, with an excellent clinical outcome. After three years of follow-up, the patient has had no recurrence.

Answers:

1. **Chondrosarcomas mostly occur in older adults and make up more than 40% of primary bone sarcomas in adults of all ages. The average age of diagnosis is 51 years, within a range of 20–70 years in the majority of cases. Males are slightly more affected than females, with peaks during the fifth and seventh decades.**
2. **Chondrosarcomas may form in the metaphysis or diaphysis of a long bone such as the femur. There are large lobules of hyaline cartilage, separated by fibrous tissue bands and anaplastic cells. Chondrosarcomas usually implant in surrounding tissues.**
3. **Surgical en bloc resection for low-grade chondrosarcomas can reduce risks of recurrence. Great care is required to avoid any spillage of tumor cells into the soft tissues, as part of biopsy or surgery. Low-grade tumors are usually curable. Since the tumors have a small amount of vascularity, chemotherapy and radiation are not extremely effective.**

Ewing Sarcoma

Ewing sarcoma is a round-cell bone tumor that is the second most common bone malignancy in patients under age 20. This tumor often occurs in periods during which the bones are quickly growing. Usually, the diaphysis of a long bone is affected, though Ewing sarcoma can also occur in flat bones. Most cases develop in the femur (most common), pelvis, and tibia (see Figure 11.7). The tumors start in the bone marrow, invade the bone cortex, and form soft-tissue masses.

Epidemiology
Approximately 1% of all childhood cancers are Ewing sarcomas. In the United States, only about 200 children and adolescents are diagnosed annually, with most occurring in adolescents. The peak incidence of Ewing sarcoma is between 10 and 25 years of age. It makes up 32% of bone malignancies in younger people. Ewing sarcomas also affect adults in their 20s and 30s. They are slightly more common in males than in females. Non-Hispanic or Hispanic Caucasians are mostly affected in comparison with all other racial or ethnic groups. These tumors seldom affect African Americans (less than 2% of this population).

Global statistics on Ewing sarcoma are lacking, but there are data for some countries. There are less than 100 cases diagnosed in the United Kingdom and Ireland annually. In Europe, incidence is just under two cases per million people (1.9 out of 1,000,000). Most cases occur between 10 and 20 years of age, with males slightly more affected than females. Caucasians from various countries are most often diagnosed.

Etiology and Risk Factors
The cause of Ewing sarcoma is uncertain. There are usually DNA changes that affect the gene known as *Ewing sarcoma RNA binding protein 1 (EWSR1)*. Risk factors include younger patient age, and ancestry, with people from European lineage being affected much more often than those from African or Eastern Asian lineage.

Clinical Manifestations
The most common symptoms of Ewing sarcoma are pain and swelling. Less often, there is anorexia, fever, and malaise. Soft-tissue masses are common. There may be tenderness near the

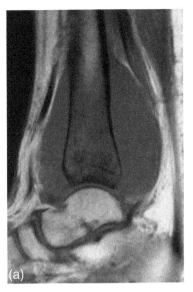
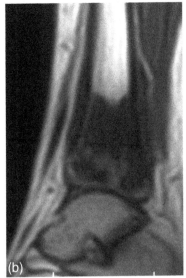
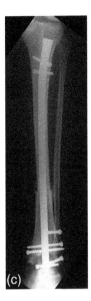

Figure 11.7 A 15-year-old girl with Ewing sarcoma of the left distal tibia. (a) Significant soft-tissue expansion is visible on MRI; (b) Dramatic response to preoperative chemotherapy is seen with extensive tumor shrinkage; (c) En bloc resection of the distal tibia and tibio-talar joint was performed, with reconstruction via bone allograft and multiple fixation. *Source*: Figure 42.6 from Page 624 of The American Cancer Society's Oncology in Practice – Clinical Management [9].

tumor site, bone pain, fatigue, and unintended weight loss.

Pathology

The majority of Ewing sarcomas develop in the extremities, though any bone can be affected. The disease is usually extensive, mostly involving the diaphyseal area, but sometimes affecting the entire bone. Between 15% and 20% occur around the metaphyseal area. Multiple layers of subperiosteal reactive new bone formation cause the onion skin-like appearance of the epidermis. It is classified by small, round blue cells. There is chromosomal translocation of the gene called *Ewing sarcoma (EWS, chromosome 11)* with fusion partner *Friend leukemia virus integration 1 (FLI1, chromosome 22)*. Additional fusion partners include *capicua transcriptional repressor (CIC)-double homeobox (DUX), envelope 1A (E1A), ETS transcription factor ERG*, and *ETS variant transcription factor 1 (ETV1)*.

Diagnosis

Diagnosis is based on imaging studies that reveal lytic destruction and especially a permeative infiltrating pattern that lacks clear borders. X-rays are usually not able to show all the bone areas that are affected. There is often a large soft-tissue mass surrounding the affected bone. An MRI provides better imaging and is helpful to guide treatment. CT scans are also helpful. Actual diagnosis of Ewing sarcoma is made by biopsy. The disease has been confused with some type of infection, because of similar appearance in imaging. It can also resemble Langerhans cell granulomatosis, a benign condition. Lesions that are aggressive in the ribs or diaphyses should be carefully evaluated. Accurate histology for diagnosis uses molecular markers. In laboratory tests, the **sedimentation rate** is elevated, and often, so is the lactic dehydrogenase (LDH) level – indicating a worsened outlook. A typical clonal chromosomal abnormality should be evaluated. Confirmation is made when an 11:22 chromosomal translocation is found in the tumor cells. At diagnosis or within one year, metastasis is often seen – usually to the lungs, various bones, bone marrow, lymph nodes, spleen, liver, and central nervous system. However, metastasis can occur to any organ.

Classic methods of diagnosis of Ewing sarcoma include electron microscopy, light microscopy, fluorescent in situ hybridization (FISH), and immunohistochemistry. Blood studies may reveal anemia, elevation of alkaline phosphatase, elevation of LDH, and leukocytosis. Today, reverse transcriptase polymerase chain reaction (RT-PCR) is being used for confirmation of diagnosis. Differential diagnoses include desmoplastic small round blue cell tumors, lymphoma, medulloblastoma, small cell osteosarcoma, and rhabdomyosarcoma.

Treatment

The treatment of Ewing sarcoma combines surgery, chemotherapy, and radiation therapy. Most patients are cured by this combination of treatments if the disease is primary and localized. Sometimes, even metastatic disease can be cured. Often, chemotherapy + surgical en bloc resection can provide better long-term results than chemotherapy + radiation therapy. For most patients, 3–4 cycles of chemotherapy are given for localized disease before surgery. Additional chemotherapy may require up to 17 cycles. Ewing sarcomas of all subtypes are highly sensitive to multi-agent chemotherapy. However, cure rates with only surgery + radiation are less than 15% for localized disease.

For localized Ewing sarcoma, chemotherapy consists of vincristine, doxorubicin (Adriamycin), and cyclophosphamide (VAC), which is alternated with ifosfamide and etoposide (I/E) for 10–17 cycles. When the maximum dose of doxorubicin is reached, dactinomycin is substituted. For adults, 10–14 cycles may be sufficient, and it is rare for an adult to tolerate 17 cycles, or regimens of 2 doses per 3 weeks. When there is no metastasis, there is no need to alternate I/E with VAC, or to use higher doses of alkylating agents, or to intensify the dosing regimen. For metastasizing Ewing sarcoma, other regimens include VAI (vincristine, Adriamycin, ifosfamide) and VIDE (vincristine, ifosfamide, doxorubicin, and etoposide). Choice of various agents is based on adverse effects. For example,

ifosfamide may cause renal tubular dysfunction, and cyclophosphamide can cause more blood toxicity. If there is only one site of recurrence, surgery, radiation, or both may be effective. If conventional chemotherapies fail, there can be combination therapies used. These include temozolomide + irinotecan, cyclophosphamide + topotecan, and gemcitabine + docetaxel. Patients should be enrolled in clinical trials as early as possible. Investigative treatments include immune checkpoint inhibitors, insulin-like growth factor receptor-1 (IGF1R) inhibitors, and poly adenosine diphosphate (ADP) ribose polymerase [PARP] inhibitors. For some patients, 12–18 months of chemotherapy is required after any surgery.

Prevention and Early Detection

There is no known prevention for Ewing sarcoma. Patients that may be at higher risk should discuss the factors that may make them more susceptible. There are no widely recommended screening tests available. Early detection can occur if the tumor causes symptoms early in its development (such as pain, swelling, or even warmth in the area).

Prognosis

In previous decades, Ewing sarcoma had five-year survival rates of only 5–10%. Today, a significant prognostic factor for Ewing sarcoma is the tumor's response to preoperative surgery and chemotherapy-induced necrosis. This factor is related to local as well as distant relapse. For localized disease, combined chemotherapy + surgery + radiation offers a 70% cure rate. However, truncal or pelvic disease only has a 40% survival rate over five years. Metastasis only to the lungs (stage IVA) has a 30–50% better prognosis than for involvement of other sites (stage IVB), in which it is less than 10% of patients. Poorer outcomes are associated with age over 15 years, larger tumor size, and tumor location within the axial or pelvic regions. The prognosis for metastasizing Ewing sarcoma is poor.

Significant Point

Ewing sarcomas form in the bones or soft tissues. Fortunately, about two-third of diagnosed patients survive the disease for many years. The most common subtype is Ewing sarcoma of the bone, with the less common varieties including *extraosseous Ewing tumor (EOE)* of the soft tissues, and *peripheral primitive neuroectodermal tumor (PPNET)*, which is much rarer.

Clinical Case – source: tumorsurgery. org/tumor-education/case-studies.aspx

1. Where do Ewing sarcomas usually develop?
2. What is the significance of the 11:22 chromosomal translocation?
3. What chemotherapy regimens are used for Ewing sarcoma?

A 16-year-old boy was taken to his pediatrician because of pain in his right hip and thigh. He had no other health complaints, and no history of fevers, night sweats, weight loss, or infections. All blood and urine laboratory tests were normal. An X-ray revealed a permeative lesion of his right proximal femur, with slight sclerosis. A CT scan showed that the lesion had extended through the proximal half of the femur, with slight thickening and expansion of the cortex. An MRI revealed significant edema, but no soft-tissue component. A biopsy was performed, showing a uniform collection of cells, and hypercellularity. The lesion had an 11:22 chromosome translocation. The diagnosis was Ewing sarcoma. Preoperative chemotherapy was given. During surgery, radial resection of the proximal half of the femur was done.

Reconstruction utilized a modular, segmental prosthetic device that also replaced the ball portion of the hip joint. Chemotherapy was given again after surgery. The patient recovered well, and after 18 months of follow-up, there has been no recurrence.

Answers:

1. **The majority of Ewing sarcomas develop in the extremities, though any bone can be affected. The disease is usually extensive, mostly involving the diaphyseal area, but sometimes affecting the entire bone. Between 15% and 20% occur around the metaphyseal area.**
2. **Confirmation of Ewing sarcoma is made when an 11:22 chromosomal translocation is found in the tumor cells.**
3. **Chemotherapy regimens for Ewing sarcoma include VAC, alternated with I/E (substitution of Adriamycin with dactinomycin); VAI; VIDE; temozolomide + irinotecan; cyclophosphamide + topotecan; and gemcitabine + docetaxel.**

Giant Cell Tumor of Bone

A malignant giant cell tumor is a rare primary tumor that usually develops at the very end of a long bone. Primary giant cell tumors of bone are much more common. Regardless, these tumors only make up 2–5% of the histologic types of bone tumors.

Epidemiology

Actual prevalence and incidence of malignant giant cell tumors is unknown. This is likely because of inaccurate diagnosis. In the few studies that have been undertaken, cumulate incidence of malignancy was only 4% of patients. This was subdivided into 1.6% having primary malignancies and 2.4% having malignant transformation from a primary benign form of the tumor. Giant cell tumor of bone occurs in many different age groups, but is rare below age 10 or above age 70. The majority of these tumors occur between ages 20 and 40. For some reason, this tumor affects females more than males, which is different from other bone tumors. There appears to be no significant racial or ethnic predilection for these tumors. Because of their rarity, there are no readily available global data.

Etiology and Risk Factors

The actual cause of malignant giant cell tumor of bone is unknown, but a few cases have been linked to *Paget disease of bone*. There are no other documented risk factors.

Clinical Manifestations

The most common symptoms of malignant giant cell tumor of bone include a visible mass, bone fracture, increased fluid in the joint closest to the affected bone, limited movement in the same joint, pain, and swelling. The symptoms can resemble other medical conditions, prompting extreme care during diagnosis.

Pathology

Giant cell tumor of bone has cells that release *RANKL*, which recruits cells. The giant cells are not neoplastic, while the neoplastic cells are primitive and mononuclear mesenchymal stromal cells. They look like **preosteoblasts**, expressing RANKL and preosteoblast markers such as alkaline phosphatase, **osteoclastin**, *runt-related family transcription factor 2 (RUNX2)*, and *transcription factor Sp7*. The giant cell tumors have well-defined borders, and may be expansive. There is cortical thinning or soft-tissue extension, with a "pushing" border that has a rim of reactive bone that is often not complete. Cut surfaces may have xanthomatous, fibrous, or hemorrhagic/cystic regions. In the largest of these tumors, necrosis may be visible. There is often a large and fleshy portion, with soft-tissue invasion.

Many osteoclast-like giant cells are distributed evenly, and many cells are larger than normal osteoclasts with more than 50 nuclei. Some areas have lower amounts of giant cells. Spindle and round or oval mononuclear cells also exist. They resemble macrophages and primitive mesenchymal cells, with poorly defined cytoplasm and mitotic activity (the neoplastic cells). The stroma is highly vascular, usually having reactive "woven" bone, and sometimes, fibrosis. Acute hemorrhage, hemosiderin, and xanthomatous histiocytes are common. In 10% of cases, secondary aneurysmal bone cyst (ABC)-like changes are present. There may be vascular invasion at the edges of the tumor, which is related to lung metastasis, but does not greatly alter the prognosis. The tumors resemble high-grade fibrosarcomas, osteosarcomas, and malignant fibrous histiocytomas.

Diagnosis

For diagnosis, X-rays can show malignant bone destruction, with mostly lytic destruction, as well as cortical destruction, soft-tissue extension, and pathologic bone fractures (see Figure 11.8). MRI and biopsy are needed for a confirmative diagnosis. To diagnose, there must be documentation of either a prior or coexisting benign giant cell tumor at the same location. Differential diagnoses include *Brown tumor of hyperparathyroidism, central giant cell granuloma, chondroblastoma, giant cell lesion of the small bones, nonossifying fibroma, primary aneurysmal bone cyst*, and *tenosynovial giant cell tumor.*

Treatment

Treatment of malignant giant cell tumor of bone is like that of osteosarcoma. However, the cure rate is lower. If a malignant giant cell tumor forms in a giant cell tumor that was previously benign, it is usually resistant to radiation therapy. Localized giant cell tumors can be managed well with repeated arterial **embolizations** using interferon or pegylated interferon. Because the tumor cells release RANKL, the chemotherapy agent called denosumab has

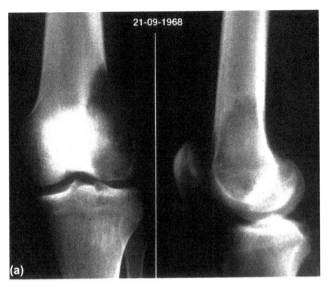

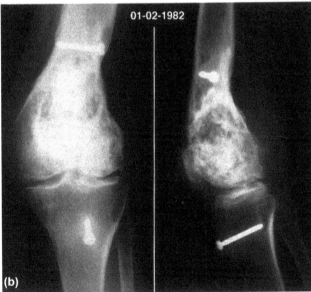

Figure 11.8 Primary malignancy in giant cell tumor of bone. (a) Anteroposterior; (b) lateral X-rays showing an expansile lytic lesion involving the medial condyle of the distal femur, with permeation of the cortex. *Source*: Figure 2 from American Cancer Society (ACS) Journals – Cancer [11].

been successful for treatment. This agent is a humanized monoclonal antibody. Up to 86% of patients have responded successfully to denosumab. In other studies, patients with resectable or unresectable disease, denosumab was effective in 96% of cases, and surgery was not needed. The agent has a long half-life. It is injected one per month, and there must be three weekly loading doses for it to reach optimal levels. Regarding surgery, if curettage is performed and no other therapy is given, 15–50% of these tumors recur, usually within two years. Aside from denosumab, antiosteoclast agents include the bisphosphonates.

Prevention and Early Detection

There is no known prevention for malignant giant cell tumor of bone, and no approved methods of early detection.

Prognosis

The prognosis of a malignant giant cell tumor of bone is poor. The average latent period for patients with secondary tumors is 7.9 years. Median recurrence-free survival is about five years. The five-year overall survival rate is 45.8%, and the 10-year overall survival rate is 36.1%. For primary malignant tumors, five-year survival is 56.2%, and for secondary malignant tumors, 40%. Pulmonary metastases occur in 69% of patients.

Significant Point

Though most primary or recurrent giant cell tumors of bone are benign, they can become malignant. However, malignant tumors of this type can also be primary. Identifying malignant giant cell tumors of bone is difficult because of a lack of clear diagnostic criteria. Extensive histologic sampling must be done to ensure an accurate diagnosis. There must also be close follow-up and timely treatment of any local recurrence.

Clinical Case

1. How do malignant giant cell tumors of the bone appear?
2. What is required for an accurate diagnosis?
3. What is the prognosis for malignant giant cell tumors of the bone?

A 32-year-old woman had developed very sharp pain in her right knee. An X-ray revealed fluid within the knee joint, but no other abnormalities. When the pain worsened, an MRI was ordered, and a lesion was seen. It was biopsied, and the pathology was consistent with a benign giant cell tumor of the bone. There was focal increased mitotic activity. Over time, the pain again worsened, and a focus of the tumor had eroded through the skin. The patient was given denosumab, but there was little improvement. A specialist ordered another MRI, which revealed a large, destructive mass at the right proximal tibia and soft tissues of the medial knee. There were also multiple lung nodules. The medical team was concerned that there had been a malignant transformation. An above-knee amputation was conducted, plus multiple lung wedge resections. The tumor was identified as a 19.0 cm solid necrotic, hemorrhagic, and fungating mass. It involved the epiphysis and metaphysis, extending proximally through the soft tissues, cortical bone, medullary bone, periosteum, and marrow cavity. A pathologic fracture had occurred. Histology revealed the tumor to be a high-grade malignant giant cell fibrosarcoma. The lung nodules were also consistent with this type of tumor. The patient recovered from the surgery and was fitted with a prosthetic leg, to which she slowly adjusted. However, tumors of this type are very likely to recur, so she remains under close observation.

Answers:

1. **These tumors have well-defined borders, and may be expansive. There is cortical thinning or soft-tissue expansion, with a "pushing" border that has a rim of reactive bone that is often not complete. Cut surfaces may have xanthomatous, fibrous, or hemorrhagic/cystic regions. In the largest of these tumors, necrosis may be visible. There is often a large and fleshy portion, with soft-tissue invasion.**

2. **MRI and biopsy are needed for a confirmative diagnosis. There must be**

documentation of either a prior or coexisting benign giant cell tumor at the same location.

3. The prognosis is poor. The average latent period with secondary tumors is 7.9 years. Median recurrence-free survival is about five years. The 5-year overall survival rate is 45.8%, and the 10-year overall survival rate is 36.1%. For primary malignant tumors, five-year survival is 56.2%, and for secondary malignant tumors, 40%. Pulmonary metastases occur in 69% of patients.

Metastatic Bone Tumors

Metastatic bone tumors are much more common than primary bone tumors, especially in adults. Any type of cancer can metastasize to the bones. However, metastases from carcinomas occur most frequently – especially when they first formed in the breasts, lungs, prostate, kidneys, thyroid, or colon. Breast cancer is the most common type of cancer to metastasize to the bones. Metastatic tumors usually do not spread to bones below the middle forearm or middle calf. However, if there is metastasis to these sites, it usually comes from primary tumors of the lungs or kidneys.

Epidemiology
Of all cancer patients, approximately 5.1% are diagnosed with metastatic bone tumors. This is equivalent to 18.8 cases out of every 100,000 people, annually, in the United States. According to the American Cancer Society, there are about 3,610 new cases diagnosed annually, and about 2,060 deaths occur from metastatic bone tumors. For patients below age 20, the most common primary cancers are endocrine cancers and soft-tissue sarcomas. Incidence is on the increase for prostate and stomach primary cancers. There appears to be no significant racial or ethnic predilection for metastatic bone tumors. Global data on metastatic bone tumors is lacking.

Etiology and Risk Factors
Bone metastasis occurs as cancer cells break away from an original tumor site. On reaching the bones, they begin to multiply. It is unknown why some cancers travel to the bones instead of more common metastatic sites such as the liver. Risk factors including having any of the types of cancer that more commonly spread to the bones. These include breast, kidney, lung, prostate, and thyroid cancers, as well as lymphoma and multiple myeloma.

Clinical Manifestations
The signs and symptoms of metastatic bone tumors may not develop for a long time, but usually involve various amounts of bone pain. Metastases can cause symptoms before a primary tumor has even been discovered, or can appear after a primary tumor has been diagnosed. Additional signs and symptoms of bone metastasis include bone fractures, bowel incontinence, hypercalcemia, nausea, vomiting, constipation, confusion, urinary incontinence, and weakness in the extremities.

Pathology
Metastatic bone disease is the most common cause of destructive bone lesions in adults. The most common sites of bony metastatic lesions include the spine, proximal femur, and humerus. Secondary to metastatic disease, pathologic fractures usually occur in the proximal femur, followed by the proximal humerus. The pathological mechanism of metastasis involves tumor cell intravasation, avoidance of immune surveillance, target tissue localization, extravasation into the target tissue, induction of angiogenesis, genomic instability, and decreased apoptosis. The *E cadherin cell adhesion molecule (CAM)* on tumor cells regulates release from the primary tumor focus into the blood stream, and *platelet-derived growth factor (PDGF)* promotes tumor migration. In target tissue localization, the *chemokine ligand 12 (CXCL12)* within stromal cell bone marrow functions as a "homing" chemokine to some tumor cells. It promotes bone targeting, as cells attach to the targeted

endothelial layer via the *integrin CAM* that is expressed on tumor cells. During extravasation, *matrix metalloproteinases (MMPs)* prompt invasion of the basement membrane and extracellular membrane. Angiogenesis is induced by expression of *VEGF*. In decreased apoptosis, *thrombospondin* inhibits tumor growth.

Osteolytic bone lesions have lytic actions. Tumor cells secrete *parathyroid hormone-related protein (PTHrP)*, stimulating release of RANKL from osteoblasts. The RANKL binds to the *RANK receptor* on osteoclast precursor cells. They differentiate to active osteoclasts, causing bony destruction. From resorbed bone, calcium, *insulin-like growth factor 1 (ILGF-1)*, and *transforming growth factor beta (TGF-B)* are released, stimulating tumor cells to release additional PTHrP. Osteoblastic lesions include prostate and breast cancer metastases. The lesions are due to tumor-secreted *endothelin-1 (ET-1)*, which binds to *endothelin A receptor (ETAR)* on the osteoblasts, stimulating them. The ET-1 decreases the *Wingless Int-1 (WNT)* suppressor *Dickkopf-related protein 1 (DKK-1)*, activating the WNT pathway and increasing osteoblast activity.

Diagnosis

Diagnosis of metastatic bone tumors involves a variety of different techniques. These include X-rays, whole-body radionuclide technecium-99 bone scanning, CT, MRI, PET-CT, clinical evaluation and testing, and biopsy. Metastatic bone tumors are considered whenever there is unexplained bone pain – but especially with known cancer, pain at multiple sites, radiographic abnormalities in multiple sites, and imaging results that suggest metastases. Breast cancer may be blastic or lytic, while prostate cancer is usually blastic and lung cancer is usually lytic. MRI and CT are very sensitive for certain metastatic bone tumors. Even so, when metastases are suspected, a less sensitive radionuclide whole-body scan is usually performed. Bone scans are better for early, asymptomatic bone metastases than plain X-rays, and the entire body can be scanned. Any lesions are presumed to be metastases if the patient has previously been diagnosed with a primary cancer. A needle biopsy of a single lesion is often done to confirm whether it is metastatic. For some tumors, whole-body PET-CT is often done, which is more specific for bone metastases than radionuclide bone scans. This procedure can identify metastases that are located outside of the skeleton.

If a patient has one or more bone lesions but has not previously been diagnosed with a primary cancer, diagnosis must include a comprehensive history, physical examination, CT of the chest/abdomen/pelvis, and based on the patient's gender, mammography, or a prostate-specific antigen (PSA) measurement. These procedures can identify the primary cancer in more than 85% of cases. Bone biopsy, especially using fine-needle or core biopsy, is required if a metastatic bone tumor is suspected and there has been no primary cancer diagnosed. Biopsy + immunohistologic staining may help identify a primary cancer type. Even so, identification is sometimes difficult after such testing, along with PET-CT and endoscopy, if indicated.

If a pathologic bone fracture has occurred, especially in the elderly, cancer must be considered. This is very true if the patient has had a diagnosed primary cancer. Sometimes the fracture is the first indication of an unknown primary cancer. In imaging, a destructive appearance may suggest cancer, though the abnormalities are sometimes very minimal. These include punctate calcifications, which can be easily missed. Unusually, there can be a fracture through a chondrosarcoma, osteosarcoma, or other primary bone tumor that results in a metastatic fracture. A musculoskeletal surgical oncologist or musculoskeletal radiologist is needed for the diagnosis of an atypical and destructive metastatic lesion. This is based on patient age and the appearance in imaging. Fracture may sometimes be present, most often along with punctate calcifications. These must be evaluated apart from a rare, primary bone tumor.

Treatment

Based on the type of organ tissue present, the treatment of metastatic bone tumors is varied.

Most commonly, radiation therapy is combined with chemotherapies or hormonal drugs. Symptomatic lesions, and lesions that are large and progressive to cause pain, fracture, or difficult stabilization are treated with radiation therapy. Bone destruction can be slowed by using radiation early. This ranges from one treatment of 8 Gy to multiple treatments, to 30 Gy treatment. Also, bisphosphonates such as denosumab, pamidronate, or zoledronate can be used. The tumors that usually heal with radiation therapy include the blastic breast cancer or prostate lesions. The lytic destructive lesions of lung cancer or renal cell carcinoma are less likely to heal. Denosumab blocks the RANKL. This slows progressive bone destruction, helping to prevent or relieve pain and fractures from metastases of various primary tumors. Denosumab can delay the first symptoms of skeletal metastatic disease and reduce metastatic events that affect the skeleton. These events include radiation therapy focused on the bone, repair of pathologic fractures before or after they occur, malignant hypercalcemia, and spinal cord compression.

For widespread bone destruction leading to fractures, surgical fixation or resection with reconstruction may be needed, stabilizing the bones and reducing complications. Once the primary tumor has been resected and there is only a small amount of bone metastasis, en block excision can be combined with chemotherapy, radiation therapy, or both. In rare cases, this is curative. These combined therapies are more effective if the metastatic lesion appears one or more years after the primary tumor. Via kyphoplasty or vertebroplasty, methyl methacrylate can be inserted into the spine. It reduces pain, while expanding and stabilizing compression fractures that lack epidural soft-tissue extension.

Prevention and Early Detection

The only prevention of metastatic bone tumors is to successfully treat the primary cancers from which they are derived. Some drugs such as the bisphosphonates can prevent or delay bone destruction from metastatic bone tumors. Today, early detection of metastatic bone tumors may be achieved via whole-body MRI and PET/CT. Radioactive tracers (isotopes or radiotracers) are used in PET/CT. Whole-body MRI can detect certain bone metastases before they have grown large enough that a radiotracer would be able to detect. Accuracy ranges from 95% to 100%, and there is no radiation exposure. With PET/CT, an isotope or radiotracer is injected, which bond with bone-seeking molecules. The isotope known as 18 F-fluoride has up to 100% accuracy for early detection of bone metastases.

Prognosis

Survival rates for metastatic bone tumors vary widely by cancer type and stage. The cancer with the lowest one-year survival rate after bone metastasis is lung cancer (10% of patients), while the highest one-year survival rate after bone metastasis is breast cancer (51% of patients). The survival rate is also decreased when there is metastasis to other sites as well as the bones. Common cancers with bone metastasis are further summarized as follows:

- Prostate cancer – 24.5% metastasize after five years, with a 6% survival rate
- Lung cancer – 12.4% metastasize after five years, with a 1% survival rate
- Kidney cancer – 8.4% metastasize after five years, with a 5% survival rate
- Breast cancer – 6% metastasize after five years, with a 13% survival rate
- Gastrointestinal cancers – 3.2% metastasize after five years, with a 3% survival rate

---

Significant Point

In lung cancer patients, about 30–40% will suffer from bone metastasis while they are being treated. Usually, the upper arms and legs, the pelvis, and the spine are affected by metastasis. The bones gradually weaken, and a fracture can occur with only slight trauma or injury.

Clinical Case

1. From which primary cancers do metastatic bone tumors most often develop?
2. What is the likelihood of death from metastatic bone tumors?
3. How can metastatic bone tumors be detected early?

A 51-year-old woman was assessed because of the development of malaise, fainting, epistaxis, and gingival bleeding. It was discovered that the patient had severe thrombocytopenia and anemia. Soon, ductal breast cancer was diagnosed, and it was found she also had extensive bone metastasis. The patient was started on hormonal therapy to treat the breast cancer. She did not improve over three months and developed severe mucosal bleeding. She was then started on steroids and IV immunoglobulin, resulting in a dramatic response and normalization of her thrombocytopenia and anemia. The bone metastasis was found to be treatable by surgery and radiation, along with adjuvant chemotherapy.

Answers:

1. **Metastatic bone tumors most often develop after cancers of the breasts, lungs, prostate, kidneys, thyroid, or colon. Breast cancer is the most common type of cancer to metastasize to the bones.**
2. **There are about 3,610 new cases of metastatic bone tumors diagnosed annually in the United States, and about 2,060 deaths occur.**
3. **Early detection of metastatic bone tumors may be achieved via whole-body MRI and PET/CT (which uses radioactive tracers). Whole-body MRI is 95–100% accurate. With PET/CT, using 18 F-fluoride, there is up to 100% accuracy.**

Key Terms

Blastic
Chondral
Codman triangle
Embolizations
Ewing sarcoma
Giant cell tumor
Lucent
Lytic
Maffucci syndrome
Multioculated
Nidus

Ollier disease
Osteoclastin
Osteosarcoma
Preosteoblasts
Punctate
Roentgenograms
Rotationplasty
Sclerotic rim
Sedimentation rate
Stromal cells
Sunburst sign

Bibliography

1   1MD. (2020). *Osteoid osteoma: Causes, complications, and long-term outlook*. Health Guides / 1MD. https://1md.org/health-guide/bone/disorders/osteoid-osteoma Accessed 2021.

2   American Cancer Society. (2021). *Key statistics for osteosarcoma*. American Cancer Society. https://www.cancer.org/cancer/osteosarcoma/about/key-statistics.html Accessed 2021.

3 American Cancer Society. (2021). *Key statistics about bone cancer*. American Cancer Society. https://www.cancer.org/cancer/bone-cancer/about/key-statistics.html Accessed 2021.

4 American Cancer Society. (2021). *Osteosarcoma risk factors*. American Cancer Society. https://www.cancer.org/cancer/osteosarcoma/causes-risks-prevention/risk-factors.html Accessed 2021.

5 American Cancer Society. (2021). *Can osteosarcoma be prevented?* American Cancer Society. https://www.cancer.org/cancer/osteosarcoma/causes-risks-prevention/prevention.html Accessed 2021.

6 American Cancer Society. (2021). *Can osteosarcoma be found early?* American Cancer Society. https://www.cancer.org/cancer/osteosarcoma/detection-diagnosis-staging/detection.html Accessed 2021.

7 American Cancer Society. (2021). *Key statistics for Ewing tumors*. American Cancer Society. https://www.cancer.org/cancer/ewing-tumor/about/key-statistics.html Accessed 2021.

8 American Cancer Society. (2021). *Ewing family of tumors – Early detection, diagnosis, and staging*. American Cancer Society. https://www.cancer.org/cancer/ewing-tumor/detection-diagnosis-staging.html Accessed 2021.

9 American Cancer Society. (2018). *The American Cancer Society's Oncology in Practice – Clinical Management*. Hoboken: Wiley-Blackwell. Figure 42.6 from Page 624.

10 American Cancer Society (ACS) Journals – Cancer. (2008). *High-grade surface osteosarcoma*. John Wiley & Sons, Inc. https://acsjournals.onlinelibrary.wiley.com/doi/full/10.1002/cncr.23340. Volume 112, Issue 7, p. 1592–1599. Figure 2. Accessed 2021.

11 American Cancer Society (ACS) Journals – Cancer. (2003). *Malignancy in giant cell tumor of bone*. John Wiley & Sons, Inc. https://acsjournals.onlinelibrary.wiley.com/doi/10.1002/cncr.11359. Volume 97, Issue 10, p. 2520–2529. Figure 2. Accessed 2021.

12 American Cancer Society (ACS) Journals – Cancer. (2000). *Small cell osteosarcoma of bone*. John Wiley & Sons, Inc. https://acsjournals.onlinelibrary.wiley.com/doi/full/10.1002/(SICI)1097-0142(19970601)79:11%3C2095::AID-CNCR6%3E3.0.CO;2-O. Volume 79, Issue 11, p. 2095–2106. Figure 8. Accessed 2021.

13 Association of Bone and Joint Surgeons, The. (2021). *Treatment and prognosis of chondroblastoma*. Clinical Orthopaedics and Related Research: September 2005 – Volume 438 – p. 103–109. The Association of Bone and Joint Surgeons. https://journals.lww.com/clinorthop/fulltext/2005/09000/treatment_and_prognosis_of_chondroblastoma.19.aspx Accessed 2021.

14 Beth Israel Lahey Health. (2021). *Osteochondroma (osteocartilaginous exostosis)*. Lahey Health System. https://www.lahey.org/health-library/osteochondroma Accessed 2021.

15 Bhushan, B. (2019). *Multiple Myeloma and Other Plasma Cell Disorders: Quintessential Disease Biology, Diagnostics and Therapeutics*. Jaipur: Bhushan.

16 BMC (Part of Springer Nature). (2016). *Non-ossifying fibroma: Natural history with an emphasis on a stage-related growth, fracture risk and the need for follow-up*. BioMed Central Ltd/Springer Nature. https://bmcmusculoskeletdisord.biomedcentral.com/articles/10.1186/s12891-016-1004-0 Accessed 2021.

17 Bone Cancer Research Trust – Until There's A Cure. (2021). *Ewing sarcoma is the second most commonly diagnosed form of primary bone cancer in children and young adults*. Bone Cancer Research Trust. https://www.bcrt.org.uk/information/information-by-type/ewing-sarcoma Accessed 2021.

18 Boston Children's Hospital. (2021). *Conditions – Osteoblastoma – Diagnosis & treatments*. Boston Children's Hospital / Harvard Medical School Teaching Hospital. https://www.childrenshospital.org/conditions-and-treatments/conditions/o/osteoblastoma/diagnosis-and-treatments Accessed 2021.

19 Cancer.Net / ACSO. (2021). *Bone cancer (sarcoma of bone): Statistics*. American Society of Clinical Oncology (ACSO) / Conquer Cancer – The ASCO Foundation. https://www.cancer.net/cancer-types/bone-cancer-sarcoma-bone/statistics Accessed 2021.

20 Cheng, X., Su, Y., and Huang, M. (2021). *Imaging of Bone Tumors in Shoulder and Elbow*. New York: Springer.

21 Children's Hospital of Philadelphia. (2021). *Osteoblastoma – What is osteoblastoma?* The Children's Hospital of Philadelphia. https://www.chop.edu/conditions-diseases/osteoblastoma Accessed 2021.

22 Children's Hospital of Philadelphia. (2021). *Nonossifying fibroma – What is nonossifying fibroma?* The Children's Hospital of Philadelphia. https://www.chop.edu/conditions-diseases/nonossifying-fibroma Accessed 2021.

23 Cidre-Aranaz, F. and Grunewald, T.G.P. (2020). *Ewing Sarcoma: Methods and Protocols (Methods in Molecular Biology, 2226)*. Totowa: Humana Press.

24 Czerniak, B. (2015). *Dorfman and Czerniak's Bone Tumors*, 2nd Edition. Amsterdam: Elsevier.

25 Denaro, V., Di Martino, A., and Piccioli, A. (2018). *Management of Bone Metastases: A Multidisciplinary Guide*. New York: Springer.

26 Drugs.com. (2021). *Chondrosarcoma – What is a chondrosarcoma?* Drugs.com https://www.drugs.com/health-guide/chondrosarcoma.html Accessed 2021.

27 Gasparetto, C. and Sivaraj, D. (2017). *Understanding Multiple Myeloma*. Burlington: Jones & Bartlett Learning.

28 Gidley, P.W. and DeMonte, F. (2018). *Temporal Bone Cancer*. New York: Springer.

29 Greenspan, A. and Borys, D. (2015). *Radiology and Pathology Correlation of Bone Tumors: A Quick Reference and Review*. Burlington: Lippincott, Williams, and Wilkins.

30 Harsh IV, G.R. and Vaz-Guimaraes, F. (2017). *Chordomas and Chondrosarcomas of the Skull Base and Spine*, 2nd Edition. Cambridge: Academic Press.

31 Healthline. (2018). *Outlook once cancer has spread to the bones*. Healthline Media – a Red Ventures Company. https://www.healthline.com/health/cancer-spread-to-bones-life-expectancy#outlook Accessed 2021.

32 Heymann, D. (2009). *Bone Cancer: Progression and Therapeutic Approaches*. Cambridge: Academic Press.

33 Jaffe, N., Bruland, O.S., and Bielack, S. (2010). *Pediatric and Adolescent Osteosarcoma (Cancer Treatment and Research, Book 152)*. New York: Springer.

34 Johns Hopkins Medicine. (2021). *Enchondroma – What is an enchondroma?* The Johns Hopkins University, The Johns Hopkins Hospital, and Johns Hopkins Health System. https://www.hopkinsmedicine.org/health/conditions-and-diseases/enchondroma Accessed 2021.

35 Johns Hopkins Medicine. (2021). *Giant cell tumor – What is a giant cell tumor?* The Johns Hopkins University, The Johns Hopkins Hospital, and Johns Hopkins Health System. https://www.hopkinsmedicine.org/health/conditions-and-diseases/giant-cell-tumor Accessed 2021.

36 Kleinerman, E.S. and Gorlick, R. (2020). *Current Advances in Osteosarcoma: Clinical Perspectives – Past, Present and Future (Advances in Experimental Medicine and Biology, 1257)*, 2nd Edition. New York: Springer.

37 Krishnan Unni, K. and Inwards, C.Y. (2009). *Dahlin's Bone Tumors: General Aspects and Data*, 6th Edition. Philadelphia: Lippincott, Williams, and Wilkins.

38 Mayo Clinic. (2021). *Patient care & health information – Diseases & conditions – Chondrosarcoma*. Mayo Foundation for Medical Education and Research (MFMER). https://www.mayoclinic.org/diseases-conditions/chondrosarcoma/symptoms-causes/syc-20354196 Accessed 2021.

39 Mayo Clinic. (2021). *Patient care & health information – Diseases & conditions – Ewing sarcoma*. Mayo Foundation for Medical Education and Research (MFMER). https://www.mayoclinic.org/diseases-conditions/ewing-sarcoma/symptoms-causes/syc-20351071 Accessed 2021.

40 Mayo Clinic. (2021). *Patient care & health information – Diseases & conditions – Bone metastasis.* Mayo Foundation for Medical Education and Research (MFMER). https://www.mayoclinic.org/diseases-conditions/bone-metastasis/symptoms-causes/syc-20370191 Accessed 2021.

41 Musculoskeletal Medicine for Medical Students. (2012). *Osteoid osteoma.* OrthopaedicsOne. https://www.orthopaedicsone.com/display/mskmed/osteoid+osteoma Accessed 2021.

42 National Cancer Institute – Center for Cancer Research. (2021). *Chondromyxoid fibroma.* U.S. Department of Health and Human Services/National Institutes of Health/National Cancer Institute/USA.gov. https://www.cancer.gov/pediatric-adult-rare-tumor/rare-tumors/rare-bone-tumors/chondromyxoid-fibroma Accessed 2021.

43 National Library of Medicine – National Center for Biotechnology Information. (2000). *Therapy and prognosis of enchondromas of the hand.* National Library of Medicine. https://pubmed.ncbi.nlm.nih.gov/11043135 Accessed 2021.

44 National Library of Medicine – National Center for Biotechnology Information. (2009). *The epidemiology of osteosarcoma.* National Library of Medicine. https://pubmed.ncbi.nlm.nih.gov/20213383 Accessed 2021.

45 National Library of Medicine – National Center for Biotechnology Information. (2015). *Bone cancer incidence by morphological subtype: A global assessment.* National Library of Medicine. https://pubmed.ncbi.nlm.nih.gov/26054913 Accessed 2021.

46 National Library of Medicine – National Center for Biotechnology Information. (1999). *Comparative frequency of bone sarcomas among different racial groups.* National Library of Medicine. https://pubmed.ncbi.nlm.nih.gov/11721448 Accessed 2021.

47 National Library of Medicine – National Center for Biotechnology Information. (2019). *Malignancy in giant cell tumor of bone: A Review of the Literature.* National Library of Medicine. https://pubmed.ncbi.nlm.nih.gov/30935298 Accessed 2021.

48 National Library of Medicine – National Center for Biotechnology Information. (2020). *Malignancy in giant cell tumor of bone in the extremities.* National Library of Medicine. https://pubmed.ncbi.nlm.nih.gov/33251099 Accessed 2021.

49 National Library of Medicine – National Center for Biotechnology Information. (2020). *Epidemiology of bone metastases.* National Library of Medicine. https://pubmed.ncbi.nlm.nih.gov/33276151 Accessed 2021.

50 Nebraska Hematology Oncology (NHO). (2021). *Treatment and prevention of bone metastases.* Nebraska Hematology Oncology. https://www.yourcancercare.com/types-of-cancer/bone-cancer/bone-metastases/treatment-and-prevention-of-bone-metastases Accessed 2021.

51 Ortho Bullets. (2021). *Metastatic disease of extremity.* Lineage Medical, Inc. https://www.orthobullets.com/pathology/8045/metastatic-disease-of-extremity Accessed 2021.

52 PathologyOutlines.com. (2021). *Bone & joints – Other tumors – Giant cell tumor of bone.* PathologyOutlines.com.https://www.pathologyoutlines.com/topic/bonegiantcelltumor.html Accessed 2021.

53 Peabody, T.D. and Attar, S. (2014). *Orthopaedic Oncology: Primary and Metastatic Tumors of the Skeletal System (Cancer Treatment and Research, Book 162).* New York: Springer.

54 Penn Medicine – Abramson Cancer Center. (2021). *Ewing sarcoma risks and prevention.* Penn Medicine / The Trustees of the University of Pennsylvania. https://www.pennmedicine.org/cancer/types-of-cancer/sarcoma/ewing-sarcoma/ewing-sarcoma-risks-and-prevention Accessed 2021.

55 Physiopedia. (2021). *Chondrosarcoma – definition/description.* Physiopedia / Physiospot / Physioplus. https://physio-pedia.com/Chondrosarcoma?utm_source=physiopedia&utm_medium=search&utm_campaign=ongoing_internal Accessed 2021.

56 PMC – US National Library of Medicine / National Institutes of Health. (2011). *Racial differences in the incidence of mesenchymal tumors associated with EWSR1 translocation.* National Center for Biotechnology Information, U.S. National Library of Medicine. https://www.ncbi.nlm.nih.gov/pmc/articles/PMC3051020 Accessed 2021.

57 Poitout, D.G. (2013). *Bone Metastases: Medical, Surgical and Radiological Treatment.* New York: Springer.

58 PrimeHealthChannel. (2013). *Bones, joints and muscles – Osteochondroma.* Prime Health Channel. https://www.primehealthchannel.com/osteochondroma.html Accessed 2021.

59 Randall, R.L. (2016). *Metastatic Bone Disease: An Integrated Approach to Patient Care.* New York: Springer.

60 Roessner, A., Althoff, J., Bassewitz, D.B.V., Bosse, A., Bouropoulou, V. et. al. (2012). *Biological Characterization of Bone Tumors (Current Topics in Pathology, Book 80).* New York: Springer-Verlag.

61 Schajowicz, F., Sundaram, M., Gitelis, S., and McDonald, D.J. (2012). *Tumors and Tumorlike Lesions of Bone: Pathology, Radiology, and Treatment*, 2nd Edition. New York: Springer.

62 ScienceDirect. (2021). *Case Report: Solitary enchondromas in a metatarsal bone, an incidental discovery.* International Journal of Surgery Case Reports, Volume 78, January 2021, p. 254–258. https://www.sciencedirect.com/science/article/pii/S2210261220312463 Accessed 2021.

63 Sik Kang, H., Mo Ahn, J., and Kang, Y. (2017). *Oncologic Imaging: Bone Tumors.* New York: Springer.

64 Sperling Medical Group. (2018). *Reading & research – 2 Proven ways to detect bone metastases early.* Sperling Radiology / Sperling Medical Group. http://sperlingmedicalgroup.com/2-proven-ways-to-detect-bone-metastases-early Accessed 2021.

65 Stanford Health Care. (2020). *Osteochondroma symptoms – What are the symptoms of osteochondroma?* Stanford Medicine / Stanford Health Care. https://stanfordhealthcare.org/medical-conditions/bones-joints-and-muscles/osteochondroma/symptoms.html Accessed 2021.

66 Wiley Online Library – Journal of the Sciences and Specialties of the Head and Neck. (2005). *Osteoblastoma of the mandible: Clinicopathologic study of four cases and literature review.* John Wiley & Sons, Inc. https://onlinelibrary.wiley.com/doi/abs/10.1002/hed.20192. Volume 27, Issue 7, p. 616–621. Accessed 2021.

67 Wiley Online Library – Orthopaedic Surgery. (2016). *Open surgery for osteoid osteoma with three dimension C-arm scan under the guidance of compute navigation.* John Wiley & Sons, Inc. https://onlinelibrary.wiley.com/doi/full/10.1111/os.12233. Volume 8, Issue 2, p. 205–211. Accessed 2021.

68 Wiley Online Library – Diagnostic Cytopathology. (2020). *Clear-cell chondrosarcomas: Fine-needle aspiration cytology, radiological findings, and patient demographics of a rare entity.* John Wiley & Sons, Inc. https://onlinelibrary.wiley.com/doi/full/10.1002/dc.24582. Volume 49, Issue 1, p. 46–53. Accessed 2021.

69 Wittig, J.C. (2014). *Osteoblastoma.* Tumorsurgery.org. http://tumorsurgery.org/tumor-education/bone-tumors/types-of-bone-tumors/osteoblastoma.aspx Accessed 2021.

70 Wu, J.S. and Hochman, M.G. (2012). *Bone Tumors: A Practical Guide to Imaging.* New York: Springer.

12

Kidney and Urinary Bladder Tumors

OUTLINE

Adenoma
Angiomyolipoma
Renal Cell Carcinoma
Renal Sarcoma
Wilms' Tumor
Metastatic Tumors
Urinary Bladder Cancer
      Transitional Cell Carcinoma
      Squamous Cell Carcinoma
      Adenocarcinoma
Key Terms
Bibliography

Adenoma

Adenomas of the kidneys are the most common neoplasms of the renal tubular epithelium. They are often found incidentally in adults during medical imaging for other reasons. Renal adenomas can be easily distinguished from simple cysts filled with fluids during ultrasonography. However, it may be difficult to differentiate large renal adenomas from renal cell carcinomas. Adenomas may be found because of the development of an abdominal mass, or when they cause symptoms. *Papillary adenomas* are the most common subtype. They are unencapsulated, with a diameter of 15 mm or smaller. *Tubular adenomas* and *alveolar adenomas* of the kidneys are less common than papillary adenomas. The tubular adenomas are hypervascularized and well-circumscribed, while the alveolar adenomas have structures that resemble the alveoli of the lungs. Other, even fewer common types of benign kidney tumors include oncocytomas, medullary fibromas, cystic nephromas, and metanephric adenomas.

Epidemiology

Papillary adenomas of the kidneys have been found in 7% of kidneys resected because of other tumors present. They are present in 25% or more of resected kidneys with renal cell carcinomas. This is a higher percentage than that of any other type of renal adenoma occurring along with a renal cell carcinoma. In autopsy studies, papillary adenomas of the kidneys are present in 7–40%, and incidence increases with age. There is a higher incidence in patients with chronic

Global Epidemiology of Cancer: Diagnosis and Treatment, First Edition. Jahangir Moini, Nicholas G. Avgeropoulos, and Craig Badolato.
© 2022 John Wiley & Sons Ltd. Published 2022 by John Wiley & Sons Ltd.

kidney disease, which is also true for papillary renal cell carcinomas. Papillary adenomas are very common in end-stage kidney disease, which is when the kidneys can no longer function on their own. Both males and females are equally affected, and there is no specific ethnic or racial predilection. There is little data available about papillary adenomas, likely due to their benign qualities.

Etiology and Risk Factors

The cause of papillary adenomas of the kidneys is unknown, but they may be secondary to renal injury. Chronic renal disease, chronic pyelonephritis, or a nearby mass tumor effect may be implicated. Risk factors include genetic disorders such as **von Hippel–Lindau syndrome**, chronic urinary dialysis, vascular kidney disease, and acquired cystic kidney disease.

Clinical Manifestations

Adenomas are often asymptomatic when they are found, but symptoms can include hematuria, abdominal or flank pain, or the development of a **paraneoplastic syndrome** that appears to be unrelated to the kidneys. The tumors grow slowly. Additional manifestations may include fatigue, low hemoglobin, constipation, nausea, hyperglycemia, urinary tract infections, and increased blood pressure.

Pathology

Renal adenomas develop in the cortex as pale yellow to gray discrete nodules. The microscopic appearance consists of complex, branched tubular and papillary structures that are lined by one layer of cells that have a bland appearance. There are small, regular nuclei and a tiny amount of cytoplasm. The cytologic appearance may be almost identical to that of low-grade papillary renal carcinomas. Lesions less than 3 cm in diameter seldom metastasize. However, metastatic lesions have been associated with primary tumors that were only about 1 cm in diameter. Papillary renal adenomas have cytogenetic

abnormalities that are like abnormalities in papillary renal cell carcinomas, but less extensive. These abnormalities include trisomy 7 and 17, and loss of the Y chromosome in males. There are sometimes gains of chromosomes 12, 16, and 20. Papillary adenomas are not known to metastasize, but are prevalent in damaged or injured kidneys. They may be related to a progenitor or stem cell-like tubular cell population that increases because of damage. Papillary adenomas may be precursor lesions to papillary renal cell carcinoma. Some adenomas have fine cytoplasmic granularity that is similar to that of papillary renal cell carcinomas. Foamy macrophages and calcifications may be seen. Most papillary adenomas are less than 0.5 cm in diameter and are well-circumscribed.

Diagnosis

Often, a CT scan with contrast is the first imaging method for renal adenomas, even though hemorrhagic cysts be similar in appearance. Abdominal X-rays may also be used. Doppler ultrasound is able to distinguish between adenomas and cysts. Papillary adenomas that are 15 mm or smaller are often not visible in CT scans. An MRI can also be done. In some cases, urinalysis, intravenous pyelogram, and vascular angiography may be required. Diagnosis can be done by biopsy or resection, but diagnosis via needle biopsy must be done very cautiously since the capsule and grade heterogeneity cannot be visualized. Core biopsy or open biopsy may be needed in some cases. Invasive diagnostic procedures include laparoscopy and laparotomy. Papillary adenomas are difficult to differentiate from other lesions only by using imaging. The nuclei are usually of a low grade (1 or 2), and the tumors are in direct contact with the renal parenchyma.

Treatment

Treatment of papillary adenomas of the kidneys is based on clinical manifestations. Usually, no treatment is required, but if required, total surgical excision is preferred. Surgery can be done endoscopically, via nephron-sparing surgery, or using tumor embolization.

Prevention and Early Detection

There is no currently known way to prevent papillary adenomas from developing. Regular medical screening, with tests and physical examinations, may allow for early detection.

Prognosis

Papillary adenomas are much more common than papillary renal cell carcinomas. Prognosis is good since they cannot metastasize, and prognosis may be excellent for smaller papillary adenomas if they are totally excised. For larger tumors, prognosis is based on the histological pattern and the patient's overall health status. The World Health Organization changed their size criterion from 5 mm to 15 mm in the 2016 classification update. This allowed for increased acceptance of donor kidneys for transplantation – kidneys with papillary lesions less than 15 mm in size would not be rejected.

Angiomyolipoma

Angiomyolipomas are perivascular epithelioid cell benign tumors. The classic form is a mesenchymal neoplasm that consists of thick dysmorphic blood vessels, smooth muscle, and adipose tissue in varying amounts. Some angiomyolipomas are extremely sclerotic. The epithelioid variant has sometimes been known to metastasize. Angiomyolipomas can also occur in sites outside of the kidneys, including the liver, lymph nodes, and rarely, the ovaries.

Epidemiology

Angiomyolipomas occur sporadically, or in patients with **tuberous sclerosis**. The sporadic cases are most common in middle-aged adults, and slightly more often in females. The tumors have also occurred in younger adults and the elderly. With tuberous sclerosis, angiomyolipomas occur in younger patients, with no female-to-male predilection. These tumors make up about 1% of all resected renal tumors.

Etiology and Risk Factors

The exact cause of angiomyolipomas is unknown. Solitary tumors may be caused by sporadic mutations of the *tuberous sclerosis complex subunit 1 and 2 (TSC1* and *TSC2)* genes, which indicates that affected patients do not have any preceding family history. Multiple angiomyolipomas occur along with tuberous sclerosis, and also when there is a positive family history of the tumors. Tuberous sclerosis complex is caused by genetic alterations of the TSC genes. When tuberous sclerosis is not present, there is a loss of **heterozygosity** of the genes. Tiny nodules with angiomyolipoma-like features may be precursor lesions. These lesions have been also seen in *TSC2/polycystic kidney disease contiguous gene syndrome*. Syndromic angiomyolipomas have been linked to **autosomal dominant** *polycystic kidney disease*, **Sturge–Weber syndrome**, *von Hippel–Lindau disease*, and **von Recklinghausen disease**. Hormones may be implicated in angiomyolipomas since they affect middle-aged females more than males, grow larger during pregnancy, can form after puberty, and there is high progesterone receptor activity visible in microscopic studies. Also, *lymphangioleiomyomatosis* is a related condition that occurs along with tuberous sclerosis – mostly in girls and young adult women. Risk factors for angiomyolipomas of the kidneys are unknown for the sporadic form, which makes up 80–90% of cases. The tuberous sclerosis-related form makes up only 10–20% of cases.

Clinical Manifestations

Angiomyolipomas are usually asymptomatic when they occur along with tuberous sclerosis, since they are often small when they are discovered. These tumors may be present along with renal cell carcinoma – especially clear cell carcinoma – in patients that do not have tuberous sclerosis. The classic variant can be complicated by hemorrhage if the tumor has become large.

Pathology

Angiomyolipomas arise from perivascular epithelioid cells, which have no known counterparts outside of the kidneys. They range from 0.5 to 25 cm in diameter. The tumors are circumscribed but not encapsulated, and have a "pushing" border. Cut surfaces have different colors. A red cut surface indicates the vascular component. A gray to white cut surface indicates the smooth muscle component, and a yellow cut surface indicates the adipose component. The tumor may involve the vena cava, renal vein, or intrarenal venous system. Rarely, the tumor is cystic. Usually, angiomyolipomas are unifocal and unilateral. Tuberous sclerosis is suggested by multiple or bilateral tumors.

In histology, the tumor has a classic triphasic appearance, with myoid spindle cells, mature adipose tissue, and blood vessels that are dysmorphic and thick-walled, without elastic lamina. The smooth muscle component is believed to originate from the vessel walls. It may be atypical, epithelioid, hypercellular, or **pleomorphic**. The vascular component has thick-walled hyalinized vessels. The fat component appears as mature adipose tissue and is preset in over 90% of angiomyolipomas. The epithelioid variant has only or mostly polygonal cells with clear or densely eosinophilic cytoplasm, and large, hyperchromatic bizarre nuclei. Multi-lobated nuclei and multinucleation are common. Also common is hemorrhage, mitotic figures, and necrosis. In cytology, there are oval to spindled cells plus cohesive stromal fragments, adipose tissue, and branching blood vessels within a hemorrhagic background, and no mitotic figures.

Diagnosis

Angiomyolipomas are often able to be correctly diagnosed only via imaging studies such as CT scan. The classic variant has a characteristic radiologic appearance because of its fat content. There is sometimes acute hemorrhage present as well. Radiologic findings are based on the amount of fat inside the tumor (see Figure 12.1). However, definitive diagnosis is by light microscopic examination of the kidney tissues. The *epithelioid* and *fat-poor* variants may require immunohistochemistry for diagnosis.

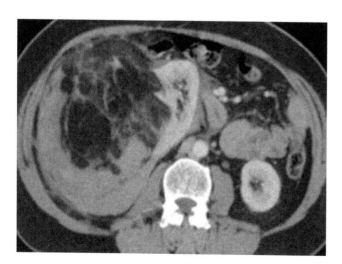

Figure 12.1 CT scan of a renal angiomyolipoma with large amounts of fat, accompanied by acute hemorrhage. *Source*: Figure 3 from BJU International - Diagnostics [17].

Treatment

Angiomyolipomas may be treated curatively with embolization or surgical excision. If the tumor is large or extends into the vena cava, **mTOR inhibitors** such as everolimus (Zortress) have been used successfully. Options for asymptomatic angiomyolipomas include endoscopic surgery, nephron-sparing surgery, and partial or complete nephrectomy. Dialysis may be required if kidney function is severely compromised because of renal failure. Retroperitoneal bleeding must be treated as an emergency situation. Post-operative care is needed until completely healed. Follow-up care with regular screening may be recommended.

Prevention and Early Detection

There is no established method of preventing angiomyolipomas. If the patient has a genetic disorder such as tuberous sclerosis, genetic testing and molecular testing of offspring during the fetal period may be indicated. With family history, genetic counseling helps to assess risks before having children. Regular medical screening with tests and physical examinations are recommended. It may be difficult to detect these tumors early in their development.

Prognosis

Prognosis is good for the classic variant of angiomyolipoma. Unfortunately, prognosis is not as good if the tumor has epithelioid or pleomorphic characteristics, since this means it is more aggressive. In extremely rare cases, there has been sarcomatous transformation with distant metastasis. The presence of retroperitoneal hemorrhage worsens prognosis. Patients with bilateral disease may have renal failure. Death has occurred because of contiguous organs – especially blood vessels.

Renal Cell Carcinoma

Renal cell carcinoma (RCC) is a malignant neoplasm of the kidney and the most common form. It is also classified as an *adenocarcinoma*. It may cause flank pain, hematuria, a fever of unknown origin, and a palpable mass. Many patients are asymptomatic however, and diagnosis is often suspected due to incidental findings. It is confirmed by CT or MRI, and sometimes by biopsy. Options for treatment include surgery, targeted therapies, experimental protocols, and if advanced, palliative therapy.

Epidemiology

RCC makes up 90–95% of primary malignant kidney tumors. In the United States, there are about 74,000 new cases per year, of which nearly 15,000 are fatal. Overall incidence is about 9.7 cases per 100,000 population, with males affected more than females (in a 3 : 2 ratio). People over age 65 have the most cases (in a common range of 50–70 years), and African Americans are affected more than any other racial group. Today, RCC is the ninth most common neoplasm in the United States. Globally, RCC makes up 2% of cancer diagnoses and deaths, and it has more than doubled in incidence in developed countries over the past 50 years. Countries with the highest rates of RCC include Belarus, Latvia, Lithuania, the Czech Republic, Estonia, Slovakia, metropolitan France, Hungary, Iceland, and Croatia (see Figure 12.2).

Etiology and Risk Factors

The exact cause of RCC is unknown. Risk factors include smoking (doubling the risk in 20–30% of cases), obesity, excessive use of **phenacetin**, familial syndromes such as von Hippel–Lindau disease, exposure to agents (asbestos, radiopaque contrast agents, cadmium, and products used in leather tanning and the petroleum industry), and in dialysis patients, acquired cystic kidney disease.

Clinical Manifestations

Signs and symptoms of RCC usually do not appear until late in its development, once the

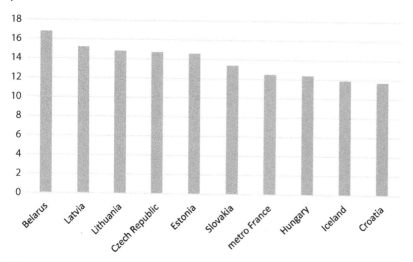

Figure 12.2 Countries with the highest rates of renal cell carcinoma, showing the number of cases per 100,000 population.

tumor is large and has metastasized. The most common sign is gross or microscopic hematuria. This is followed by flank pain, a fever of unknown origin, and a palpable mass. Hypertension may develop because of **pedicle** compression or segmental ischemia. About 20% of patients have paraneoplastic syndromes, including liver dysfunction described as **Stauffer syndrome**. Increased erythropoietin activity may cause **polycythemia**. Anemia may be present because of hematuria. Hypercalcemia often occurs, which may require treatment. Additional manifestations may include secondary **amyloidosis**, cachexia, and thrombocytosis.

Pathology

RCC usually appears as a relatively round mass made up of yellow tissue, with areas of fibrosis, hemorrhage, and necrosis. It may trigger the formation of thrombi in the renal vein, which sometimes invades the vena cava. Rarely, there is tumor invasion into the vein wall. It most often metastasizes to the lungs (60–75%), regional lymph nodes (60–65%, bones (39–40%), and brain (5–7%). Less often, metastases occur to the adrenal glands and liver. The clear cell subtype of RCC makes up 75% of cases, while the papillary subtype accounts for 13%, the chromophobe subtype makes up 5%, and the remainder 7% are miscellaneous RCCs (see Figure 12.3).

Figure 12.3 Renal cell carcinoma subtypes.

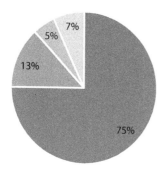

■ Clear cell ■ Papillary ▪ Chromophobe ▫ Miscellaneous

Diagnosis

A renal mass is often found incidentally during ultrasonography or a CT scan (see Figure 12.4). Diagnosis may be suggested by clinical manifestations and confirmed by an abdominal CT before and following the injection of a radiocontrast agent, or by MRI. An enhanced renal mass is strongly suggestive of RCC. Both CT and MRI can provide information about local extension as well as lymph node and venous involvement. An MRI also provides data about extension into the renal vein and vena cava, and has become the preferred technique over inferior vena **cavography**. The mass may be seen during ultrasound and intravenous urography, but these are less informative on the characteristics and extent of the disease compared with MRI and CT. The mass, regardless of malignancy, may be distinguished radiographically. Surgery is sometimes required for confirmation. If findings are not clear, needle biopsy is not sensitive enough for accurate diagnosis. It is only done if there is an infiltrative pattern and no discrete mass, if the mass may have metastasized from another known tumor, or to confirm diagnosis prior to chemotherapy for metastasis.

Prior to surgery, three-dimensional CT, MRI angiography, or CT angiography is done – especially before nephron-sparing surgery. These helps determine the number of renal arteries that are present and to determine the vascular pattern. These imaging methods have replaced aortography and selective renal artery angiography. Chest X-rays and liver tests are required. If an X-ray is abnormal, a chest CT is performed. Bone scanning is required if alkaline phosphatase is elevated. There will be measurement of blood urea nitrogen (BUN), calcium, creatinine, and serum electrolytes. Unless both kidneys are involved, the BUN and creatinine will not be affected. The tumor/node/metastasis (TNM) staging system is used for RCCs. At diagnosis, the disease is localized in about 45% of patients, is locally invasive in 30%, and has spread to distant sites in 25% (see Figure 12.5).

The staging for RCC is summarized in Table 12.1.

Treatment

The standard treatment method for localized RCC, which has a good chance to be curative, is radical nephrectomy. The kidney is removed along with the adrenal gland, perirenal fat, and the **Gerota fascia**. Open surgery and laparoscopic surgery offer similar results, but recovery is less intense with laparoscopy. Partial nephrectomy is done for many patients, even those with a normal contralateral kidney when the tumor is

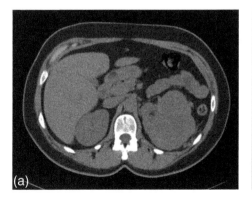
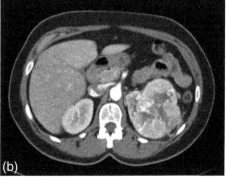

Figure 12.4 CT scan of a renal cell carcinoma (clear cell subtype). Left renal mass (a) before and (b) after intravenous contrast. *Source*: Figure 17.1 from Page 228 of The American Cancer Society's Oncology in Practice [8].

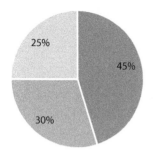

Figure 12.5   Renal cell carcinoma development at diagnosis.

■ Localized   ■ Locally invasive   ■ Distant

Table 12.1   TNM staging for renal cell carcinoma, according to the American Joint Commission on Cancer.

Stage	Tumor	Regional lymph node metastasis	Distant metastasis	Description
I	T1	N0	M0	The tumor is 7 cm across or less, and is only in the kidney.
II	T2	N0	M0	The tumor is larger than 7 cm across but is still only in the kidney.
III	T3 or T1 to T3	N0 or T1	M0	The tumor is growing into the renal vein or vena cava or into tissue around the kidney, OR the main tumor is of any size, and may be outside the kidney.
IV	T4 or Any T	Any N	M0 or M1	The main tumor has grown beyond Gerota's fascia and may be growing into the adrenal gland, and may or may not have spread to nearby lymph nodes, OR the main tumor is of any size and may have grown outside the kidney, and may or may not have spread to nearby lymph nodes, and has spread to distant lymph nodes and/or other organs.

between approximately 4 and 7 cm in size. Partial nephrectomy causes lower incidence of chronic kidney disease than radical nephrectomy. Though not primary treatments, other possibilities include nonsurgical tumor destruction by cryosurgery or radiofrequency ablation. These can often be done percutaneously. However, both procedures are still under review. Tumors of the renal vein and vena cava may be cured via surgery when there are no nodal or distant metastases. If it can be accomplished, bilateral disease can be treated with partial nephrectomy of one or both kidneys. Radiation therapy is no longer used along with nephrectomy, though **stereotactic** body radiation is being reviewed for small kidney tumors. Systemic therapies used adjuvantly have not yet prolonged survival in clinical trials, though improved disease-free survival has occurred with adjuvant sunitinib (Sutent) for high-risk patients.

Palliative treatments may include tumor embolization. For metastatic disease, resection can be palliative and prolong life if there are not many metastases – especially in a long time period between nephrectomy and metastases. Radiation therapy can be palliative if RCC metastasizes to the bones. Regarding chemotherapy, approximately 10–20% of patients respond well to interferon alfa-2b (Intron A) or interleukin-2, though response only lasts for a long time in under 5% of patients. For advanced tumors, effective targeted therapies include use of sunitinib, bevacizumab (Avastin), sorafenib (NexAVAR), cabozantinib (Cabometyx), pazopanib (Votrient), axitinib (Inlyta), and lenvatinib (Lenvima) – these are all tyrosine kinase inhibitors.

Newer chemotherapies for metastatic RCC include nivolumab (Opdivo) and pembrolizumab (Keytruda). Better overall survival has been achieved by combining nivolumab with ipilimumab (Yervoy), for untreated intermediate or poor risk metastatic disease. Combining pembrolizumab with axitinib also prolonged survival, progression-free survival, and response rate in all test patients. These combinations are now first-line treatments for metastatic RCC. Experimental treatments include stem cell transplantation, anti-angiogenesis therapy with thalidomide (Thalomid), various interleukins, and vaccine therapy. Progestins as well as traditional chemotherapy agents are ineffective – alone or in combinations. Cytoreductive nephrectomy prior to systemic therapy is controversial.

Prevention and Early Detection

It is uncertain whether RCC can be prevented, but reducing the likelihood of developing the disease can be achieved by avoiding or stopping smoking, maintaining a healthy weight by exercising, consuming a diet high in fruits and vegetables, and avoiding exposure to potentially harmful substances such as trichloroethylene. Many cases of RCC are discovered early, but since there are no recommended screening tests for people not at an increased risk, the tumors are often found after they have progressed and grown. Early detection has occurred via urinalysis and imaging tests for other medical reasons. For people with related inherited conditions, regular imaging tests are recommended. It is important to discuss any family history of kidney cancers.

Genetic testing may be able to determine an increased chance for developing RCC.

Prognosis

The prognosis for RCC varies widely based on staging. The five-year survival rate is about 81% for stage I disease, but only 8% for stage IV disease. Prognosis is worsened if the cancer is metastatic or recurrent, since treatments usually cannot cure the disease. However, they may be useful for palliation.

Significant Point

RCC is among the 10 most common cancers in men as well as women. It usually begins as just one kidney tumor, but can also start as multiple tumors, and can affect both kidneys at the same time. Today, targeted therapies are becoming more popular since they attack the specific components that the cancer cells need to have to survive and progress, such as the blood vessels and proteins of the tumors.

Clinical Case

1. How common is RCC in the United States, and what is changing about this cancer globally in developed countries?
2. What is the primary risk factor for RCC?
3. What occurs in a radical nephrectomy?

A 67-year-old man had a radical nephrectomy 8 years ago because of a RCC, with negative margins. After the surgery, he quit smoking, a habit he had for 23 years. Four years later, a CT scan revealed no evidence of recurrence. Today, the patient visits his physician because of dull right-sided flank plan and hematuria. A CT scan is done. There is a 7-cm mass in the renal fossa, up against the inferior vena cava and liver. A full metastatic evaluation is performed, which is negative. A percutaneous biopsy shows a recurrent clear cell RCC. The patient is treated with local sunitinib, which initially reduces the tumor size. Then it begins to enlarge again. The tumor is surgically resected, and the final surgical margins are negative for tumor cells.

Answers:

1. **RCC makes up 90–95% of primary malignant kidney tumors. In the United States, there are about 74,000 new cases per year, of which nearly 15,000 are fatal. Overall incidence is about 9.7 cases per 100,000 population. Globally this cancer makes up 2% of cancer diagnoses and deaths, and it has more than doubled in incidence in developed countries over the past 50 years.**
2. **Smoking is the primary risk factor for RCC, and it doubles the risk for the disease in 20–30% of cases.**
3. **In a radical nephrectomy, the kidney is removed along with the adrenal gland, perirenal fat, and the Gerota fascia.**

Renal Sarcoma

Renal sarcoma is a kidney tumor that is usually a secondary development from a retroperitoneal origin. Renal sarcomas that arise mostly within the kidneys are extremely rare. The morphological features are similar to soft tissue tumors. The most common subtype is *leiomyosarcoma*, which may form from the renal veins and their branches. There are also *synovial sarcomas, primitive neuroectodermal tumors, liposarcomas,* and the rarest, *angiosarcomas*. In total, there are 39 known subtypes but many of these are seldom seen in practice. Renal sarcomas only make up 0.3% of all renal malignancies.

Epidemiology

Renal sarcomas are rare adult malignancies that have been insufficiently studied regarding epidemiology and other factors. Overall, there are only about 0.5 renal sarcomas per 1 million people. There are only slight differences in incidence between males and females, with leiomyosarcomas more common in females, and angiosarcomas more common in males. Renal sarcomas mostly occur at a median age of 62 years.

Etiology and Risk Factors

There is no proven cause of renal sarcomas. However, risk factors include smoking, obesity, genetic predisposition, hypertension, kidney damage or injury, exposure to carcinogens, and chronic kidney illness.

Clinical Manifestations

Renal sarcomas may cause lower back pain, hematuria, a palpable mass, weakness, tiredness, lethargy, malaise, anorexia, nausea, insomnia, and in males, dilated testicular veins.

Pathology

The pathology of renal sarcomas depends upon the subtype. For example, leiomyosarcoma is a tan-colored tumor. Microscopic imaging reveals many spindle cells with an interlacing, fascicular pattern (see Figure 12.6). There are elongated, hyperchromatic nuclei and eosinophilic cytoplasm. Thin pink, curved fibers between the tumor cells are characteristic, and there is often fibroblastic differentiation. The tumor is often positive for smooth muscle actin, **caldesmon**, and **vimentin**.

Diagnosis

Renal sarcomas are often discovered when they are already in stage T3 (33% of cases). Stage T4 diagnoses make up only 14% of cases, and there is distant metastasis in 29% of cases. Diagnosis is

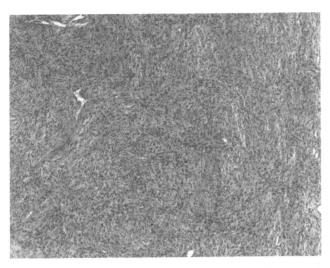

Figure 12.6 Histopathology of renal sarcoma, with spindle cells in an interlacing, fascicular pattern, plus elongated hyperchromatic nuclei and eosinophilic cytoplasm. *Source*: Figure 1 from Wiley Online Library – Clinical Case Reports [58].

prompted by an abdominal mass, and there must be an evaluation of the signs and symptoms since primary renal sarcomas mimic advanced RCCs.

Treatment

About 84% of T1 to T3 renal sarcomas are surgically resected, as are 71% of T4 renal sarcomas. Systemic chemotherapy is used in 32% of all cases. In 24% of cases, chemotherapy is combined with surgical resection.

Prevention and Early Detection

There is no proven method of preventing renal sarcomas except for avoiding the risk factors for the disease. Early detection of renal sarcomas may be difficult, since small kidney sarcomas cannot be seen or felt during a physical examination. There are no recommended screening tests for individuals not at an increased risk. No test has been shown to lower overall risks of death from this disease. The tumors have sometimes become quite large with no significant problems or pain.

Prognosis

Renal sarcomas have a one-year survival rate of 48%, while the three-year survival rate is at 24%, and the five-year survival rate is only at 13%. The best overall prognosis is for the primitive neuroectodermal tumor subtype (46–74% survival), and the worst prognosis is for the rare angiosarcomas (23–57% survival).

Significant Point

Renal sarcomas make up only 1–2% of primary renal cancers. Fibrosarcomas have a poor prognosis because of late diagnosis and presence of locally advanced involvement into the renal vein, or metastatic disease upon initial evaluation. The five-year survival rates are poor.

Clinical Case

1. How common are leiomyosarcomas, as part of the larger group of renal sarcomas?
2. How do these tumors appear during microscopic imaging?
3. How are these tumors correctly diagnosed?

A 58-year-old woman was evaluated because of left flank pain. Over time the pain worsened, so the patient was hospitalized. A left RCC was suspected, so a radical nephrectomy was performed, but complete resection could not occur since the tumor had directly invaded the abdominal wall and psoas muscle. This tumor was then diagnosed as a RCC with sarcomatoid changes. The patient was discharged, but five months later she developed left flank distention and severe back pain. A CT scan revealed another tumor, which was much larger than the first mass. The patient soon died. The autopsy revealed multiple tumors in the upper retroperitoneal space, left lobe of the liver, and invasion into the spleen, diaphragm, and gastric serosa. These lesions were diagnosed as leiomyosarcomas.

Answers:

1. **While leiomyosarcomas are the most common subtype of renal sarcomas, overall, these sarcomas are rare adult malignancies. There are only about 0.5 renal sarcomas per 1 million people.**
2. **These tumors appear in microscopic imaging with many spindle cells that have an interlacing, fascicular pattern.**
3. **Diagnosis is prompted by an abdominal mass, and there must be evaluation of the signs and symptoms since primary renal sarcomas mimic advanced RCCs.**

Wilms' Tumor

Wilms' tumor is an embryonal kidney cancer that is also called *nephroblastoma*. It consists of blastemal, epithelial, and stromal elements, and is the most common primary malignant kidney tumor in children. Growth of this tumor has implicated genetic abnormalities, though familial inheritance is only seen in 1–2% of all cases. Approximately 10% of cases occur along with genitourinary and other congenital abnormalities, as well as **hemihypertrophy**. *WAGR syndrome* combines Wilms' tumor, with **aniridia**, genitourinary malformations, and intellectual disability. The genitourinary malformations include cystic disease, renal hypoplasia, cryptorchidism, and **hypospadias**. Wilms' tumor is commonly diagnosed by imaging studies, and treated with surgical resection, chemotherapy, and radiation therapy.

Epidemiology

There are 500–650 new diagnoses of Wilms' tumor that occur annually in the United States. Wilms' tumor usually appears in children under the age of five years. Peak incidence is between two and three years of age. Less often, it occurs in older children, but is rare in adults. Wilms' tumor makes up approximately 6% of all cancers in children under 15 years of age. In patients under age 20, annual incidence in the United States is 6.3 cases per million females, and 5.3 cases per million males. The tumor is most common in African American children, with a slight female predominance. Of all racial or ethnic groups, Asian children are the least affected. Globally, Wilms' tumor affects about 1 child of every 10,000, but additional statistics are not well documented.

Etiology and Risk Factors

Most children with Wilms' tumor do not have any identified birth defects or inherited gene changes. However, there is a link between this tumor and birth defect syndromes as well as genetic changes. It appears that these changes occur during development in the womb, or early in the child's life. Risk factors for Wilms' tumor include younger patient age, the African American race, family history, **Denys–Drash syndrome**, trisomy 18, aniridia, **Frasier syndrome**, cryptorchidism, **Perlman syndrome**, **Bloom syndrome**, and hypospadias.

Clinical Manifestations

The most common sign and symptom of Wilms' tumor is a painless and palpable mass in the abdomen. Less often, there are abdominal pain, fever, hematuria, anorexia, nausea, and vomiting. Hematuria can be gross or microscopic. Hypertension may also be present. If the tumor metastasizes, it is usually to the regional lymph nodes and lungs. Less often, there is metastasis to the liver, brain, and bones.

Pathology

Wilms' tumor may arise from the renal medulla or cortex, and is usually well delineated from the parenchyma, which it often compresses. Unilateral cases usually occur at ages 3–4 years, while bilateral cases occur earlier, at 2.5–2.7 years. There is a chromosomal deletion of *Wilms' tumor 1 (WT1)*, a tumor suppressor gene, seen in some patients. Microscopically, Wilms' tumor consists of **blastemic**, epithelial, and stromal components. This is because primitive and undifferentiated blastemic cells may partially develop into epithelial or stromal tissue. Varying stages of differentiation may be present.

The sporadic form of Wilms' tumor occurs without any known genetic predisposition. The inherited cases only make up 1% of 2% of these tumors. They are transmitted in an autosomal dominant fashion. These tumors often have chromosomal gains, losses, or rearrangements. The most common findings are gains in chromosomes 6, 7, 8, 12, 13, and 18 as well as losses in chromosomes 11, 16, 22, and X. Approximately 10% of cases also show losses of other important genes, and are therefore accompanied by many congenital abnormalities.

Diagnosis

During physical examination, Wilms' tumor feels firm and smooth. It is usually a single mass on one side of the abdomen. Abdominal ultrasonography can determine whether a Wilms' tumor is cystic or solid, and if the renal vein or vena cava have been invaded. A complete blood count, liver and renal function tests, serum calcium level tests, and urinalysis are performed. Abdominal MRI or CT are commonly used to visualize the tumor (see Figure 12.7). They can determine tumor size and spreading to the regional lymph nodes, opposite kidney, or liver. A chest CT can detect metastatic pulmonary involvement upon initial diagnosis. Since imaging diagnosis is usually accurate, most patients then undergo nephrectomy instead of biopsy. A biopsy carries a risk of peritoneal contamination by the tumor cells, which could spread the cancer and result in a higher-stage cancer requiring more extreme therapy. During nephrectomy, the locoregional lymph nodes are sampled to determine pathological and surgical staging.

The most accepted staging system was created by the National Wilms Tumor Study Group (see Table 12.2). It is based on surgical findings and extent of disease at diagnosis. A high or low risk is assigned based on favorable or unfavorable histology (anaplasia).

Treatment

For unilateral Wilms' tumor, initial treatment is primary surgical resection, and then adjuvant chemotherapy. For stage III or IV tumors or metastases, chemotherapy is started 1–3 days after surgery. Surgical resection is curative for certain younger children with small tumors, and chemotherapy is not needed. Tumor histology and staging determine the choice of chemotherapy agent and the length of the treatment. Though depending upon individual risks, chemotherapy usually consists of dactinomycin

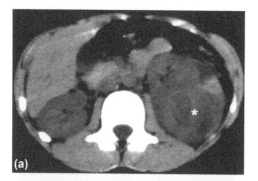

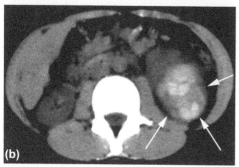

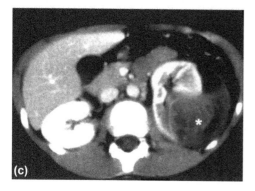

Figure 12.7 Wilms tumor in a nine-year-old boy: (a) and (b) show unenhanced axial images – the asterisk indicates the tumor at the lower pole of the left kidney, and the arrows indicate acute subcapsular hemorrhage; (c) is a contrast-enhanced axial image. Source: Figure 2 from American Cancer Society (ACS) Journals: Cancer [7].

(Cosmegen) and vincristine (Oncovin), with or without doxorubicin (Adriamycin). If the tumor is more aggressive, intensive chemotherapy with multiple agents is needed. If a child has very large tumors that cannot be resected, or bilateral tumors, chemotherapy is indicated. This is followed by a reevaluation, and possibly, surgical resection. For a child with higher-stage disease or tumors invading the regional lymph nodes, radiation therapy is indicated.

Prevention and Early Detection

There is no known method of preventing Wilms' tumor. However, in very rare cases, such as in children with Denys–Drash syndrome, physicians may recommend removal of the kidneys at a very young age, and then transplantation of donor kidneys. Early detection may be possible via ultrasound, but these tumors are usually found once they have become large enough to cause signs and symptoms. There are no blood tests or other tests that are useful for screening a healthy child for a Wilms' tumor. If a child has the related syndromes or birth defects, screening is very important. This involves physical examination and ultrasound every three or four months up until the age of seven years. If a parent is known to have a WT1 gene mutation, genetic testing can be performed to see if the mutation was passed on to the child.

Prognosis

The prognosis for Wilms' tumor is based on histology, staging, and the age of the patient. For children, prognosis is excellent. When the tumor is only within the kidney, cure rates range from 85% to 95%. Children with more advanced disease have cure rates that range from 60% with unfavorable histology to 90% with favorable histology. Wilms' tumor may recur, usually within two years of diagnosis. Children with recurrent cancer are often cured. The outcome following recurrence is better if the child first presents with lower-stage disease, the tumor recurs at a site that has not undergone radiation therapy, the relapse is more than one year after presentation, and in those that received less intensive treatment initially. A summary of the overall four-year survival rates for Wilms tumor is shown in Table 12.3.

Table 12.2 Staging of Wilms' tumor.

Stage	Characteristics
I 40–45% of cases upon diagnosis	The tumor is only in the kidney, and is completely resected during surgery
II 20–25%	The tumor ascends beyond the kidney or into the vessels of the renal sinus, and is usually totally resectable
III 20–25%	The tumor is non-hematogenous and only within the abdomen, with positive lymph nodes in the renal hila
IV 10%	There is hematogenous metastases, such as to the lungs, liver, bones, or brain
V 5%	There is bilateral disease at diagnosis or later, and each kidney must be staged

Table 12.3 Overall four-year survival rates for Wilms tumor.

Stage	With favorable histology	With unfavorable (anaplastic) histology
I	99%	83%
II	98%	81%
III	94%	72%
IV	86%	38%
V	87%	55%

Significant Point

There must be consideration of chemotherapy-induced cardiotoxicity for Wilms' tumor patients. This is especially true when doxorubicin is used. Congestive heart failure has occurred in 4.4% of patients treated with doxorubicin 20 years after the tumor was first diagnosed. There is a higher risk in females and patients that received lung or left abdominal radiation.

Clinical Case

1. What is the other term used for Wilms' tumor, and what does this tumor consist of?

2. What are the risk factors for Wilms' tumor?

3. What are the advantages of CT scans for this tumor?

A three-year-old African American boy was brought to his pediatrician because of right-sided abdominal swelling. Hematuria with clots occurred intermittently, causing the boy to cry during urination. After X-rays and a CT scan, the child was diagnosed with Wilms' tumor and hospitalized. He was given chemotherapy to shrink the tumor. The right side of his abdomen had a freely movable mass with smooth edges. It was easily palpated. The boy was hypertensive and anemic. A right nephrectomy was performed, and the tumor was fully resected. The patient recovered well and was discharged after 10 days. Histology confirmed the Wilms' tumor. Over one-year of follow-up there have been no serious complications or recurrence.

Answers:

1. **Wilms' tumor is also known as nephroblastoma, and consists of blastemal, epithelial, and stromal elements. It is the most common primary malignant kidney tumor in children.**

2. **Risk factors for Wilms' tumor include younger patient age, the African American race, family history, Denys–Drash syndrome, trisomy 18, aniridia, Frasier syndrome, cryptorchidism, Perlman syndrome, Bloom syndrome, and hypospadias.**
3. **Abdominal CT scans determine tumor size and spreading to the regional lymph nodes, opposite kidney, or liver. A chest CT can detect metastatic pulmonary involvement upon initial diagnosis. Since imaging diagnosis is usually accurate, most patients then undergo nephrectomy instead of biopsy.**

Metastatic Tumors

Metastatic tumors that affect the kidneys are also called *renal metastases*. The most common cancers that metastasize to the kidneys are various malignancy of other organs in the body. Renal metastases are sometimes mistaken for primary tumors.

Epidemiology

Renal metastases appear to occur in only 1% of all kidney tumors. The mean ages of patients are 56–61 years, with the male-to-female ratio being 1:1. However, there have been patients as young as 21 and as old as 75. Statistics on the prevalence and incidence of renal metastases are not well documented. There are no significant racial or ethnic differences in the occurrence of renal metastases. Global statistics are also lacking.

Etiology and Risk Factors

The causes of renal metastases are primary tumors of the skin (melanoma), lungs, colon, rectum, ears, nose, throat, breasts, soft tissues, thyroid, stomach, gynecological tract, intestines, pancreas, blood, and lymphatic system. Risk factors are the same as for the primary form of cancer from which the renal metastasis occurred.

Clinical Manifestations

Symptoms of renal metastases are often absent, even though there may be extensive interstitial invasion. About 30% of patients have flank pain, 16% have hematuria, and 12% have weight loss. Renal function may not be any different to that in normal patients. Proteinuria is insignificant or absent. Blood urea and creatinine levels are usually not increased unless there has been a complication such as a bacterial infection, hypercalcemia, or uric acid nephropathy.

Pathology

Most renal metastases (86%) are carcinomas, with adenocarcinomas being the most common subtype. There are also squamous cell carcinomas and small-cell carcinomas. Most carcinomas metastasize to the kidneys from the lungs. A small percentage (14%) of renal metastases are non-carcinomatous tumors such as sarcomas, germ cell tumors, and melanomas. New renal lesions in patients with advanced, non-curable cancer are more likely to be metastatic than primary. About 77% of renal metastases are solitary, but later, additional sites of metastasis develop. Approximately 69% of renal metastases develop in the cortex.

Diagnosis

Renal metastases are usually found when a primary tumor is being evaluated, or found incidentally in abdominal imaging studies. If there is not an identified primary tumor, the renal tumor is diagnosed in the same way as for renal cell carcinoma. In 88% of renal metastases, the primary tumor is diagnosed first. In 10% of cases, the primary and metastatic tumors are diagnosed at the same time, and only 2% of cases involve the metastatic tumor being diagnosed first. In 19% of cases, there is more than a 10-year interval between the time of initial primary tumor diagnosis and the diagnosis of renal metastases. About 37% of cases have no other known metastasis upon diagnosis. About 93% of patients have a renal mass. Less commonly, there are renal cysts or renal failure. Unfortunately, most renal metastases are diagnosed late in the course of malignancy. In radiographic imaging, metastases are usually multifocal, though those arising from the breasts, lungs, or colon may be large, solitary, and nearly identical to renal cell carcinomas. The preferred imaging method is CT scan, followed by ultrasound and IV urography. Compared with primary renal tumors, metastatic tumors are more often endophytic and solid with no difference in tumor size, CT enhancement patterns, or polar predominance.

Treatment

Treatment of renal metastases involves systemic chemotherapy. Surgery is only rarely performed, with ablation preferred over resection. Partial nephrectomy can be indicated, guiding the choice of systemic chemotherapy when a core needle biopsy cannot provide sufficient tissue for examination.

Prevention and Early Detection

There is no known method of preventing renal metastases except to effectively treat the primary form of cancer. Early detection sometimes occurs because of assessing the kidneys for other conditions, but often renal metastases are discovered late in their development.

Prognosis

The prognosis for renal metastases is usually poor. Median survival from time of renal metastatic diagnosis is 1.1 years, while median overall survival from primary tumor diagnosis is 3 years.

Significant Point

Renal metastases are often detected late in the course of malignancy, often without symptoms that seem to refer to the kidneys. Some patients have normal results from urinalysis or show either gross or microscopic hematuria, and sometimes, proteinuria. Metastases to the kidneys are often multifocal, but those arising from the lungs, colon, and breasts have been documented as large, solitary tumors.

Clinical Case

1. From where do most renal metastases originate?
2. What is the most common type of tumor appearing as a metastatic tumor in the kidneys?
3. What is the prognosis for renal metastases?

A 57-year-old woman had undergone a left mastectomy for breast cancer when she was 46 years of age. In a follow-up examination and endoscopy, it was found that she had a stomach tumor. A CT scan later revealed a large left renal tumor that had extended into the renal vein. The tumor closely resembled a renal cell carcinoma. Percutaneous biopsy confirmed metastasis from the breast cancer. The patient was treated with systemic chemotherapy and closely monitored.

Answers:

1. **The causes of renal metastases are primary tumors of the skin (melanoma), lungs, colon, rectum, ears, nose, throat, breasts, soft tissues, thyroid, stomach, gynecological tract, intestines, pancreas, blood, and lymphatic system.**

2. **Most renal metastases (86%) are carcinomas, with adenocarcinomas being the most common subtype. There are also squamous cell carcinomas and small-cell carcinomas.**
3. **The prognosis for renal metastases is usually poor. Median survival from time of metastatic diagnosis is 1.1 years, while median overall survival from primary tumor diagnosis is 3 years.**

Urinary Bladder Cancer

Urinary bladder cancer is the most common malignancy of the urinary tract. It is often known as **transitional cell carcinoma**. It is characterized by multiple growth that tend to recur in a more aggressive form.

Transitional Cell Carcinoma

Transitional cell carcinoma is the most common form of urinary bladder cancer (over 90% of cases), and begins in the urothelial cells lining the inside of the bladder. A small percentage are squamous cell carcinomas or adenocarcinomas. These cells also line other portions of the urinary tract, including the renal pelvis, ureters, and urethra. Sometimes, tumors also develop in these locations, so the entire urinary tract needs to be evaluated for tumors.

Epidemiology

In the United States, there are about 80,000 new cases of bladder cancer annually, with nearly 18,000 deaths. Urinary bladder cancer is the fourth most common cancer in men, but is three times less common in women. It is more prevalent in urban than in rural areas. Incidence increases with age, and the disease most often affects Caucasians. Worldwide, bladder cancer is diagnosed in about 275,000 people every year, and about 108,000 cases are fatal. In industrialized countries, the majority of cases are transitional cell carcinomas.

Etiology and Risk Factors

The exact cause of transitional cell carcinoma has not been identified, but the disease may have genetic factors.Risk factors for bladder cancer include smoking (causing more than 50% of new cases), excessive use of the analgesic called *phenacetin*, long-term use of cyclophosphamide (Cytoxan), chronic irritation due to chronic catheterization, and exposure to many different substances. These include benzidine, hydrocarbons, industrial chemicals (aniline dyes such as naphthylamine), tryptophan metabolites, and chemicals used in the electric, rubber, cable, pain, and textile industries. Other predisposing factors are chronic urinary tract infections and calculous disease.

Clinical Manifestations

Transitional cell carcinoma usually causes unexplained gross or microscopic hematuria. The patient may have anemia, and the hematuria is discovered during evaluation. Burning, dysuria, and urinary frequency, sometimes with pyuria, are often seen. Irritation from the tumor may mimic cystitis. With advanced carcinoma, pelvic pain develops after a pelvic mass becomes palpable.

Pathology

The majority of transitional cell carcinomas of the bladder are subclassified as *papillary carcinomas*. They are usually superficial and well-differentiated, growing outward. The less common *sessile* form is more insidious, often invading early in its development and then metastasizing. In more than 40% of cases, transitional cell carcinomas recur at the same site in the bladder, or in another site – especially if they are large, poorly differentiated, or multiple. Bladder cancer often metastasizes to the lymph nodes, bones, liver, and lungs. Tumor gene *p53* mutations may be linked to faster progression as well as resistance to chemotherapeutic agents. Within the bladder, *carcinoma in situ* is highly graded, yet non-invasive and often multifocal (see Figure 12.8). It often recurs.

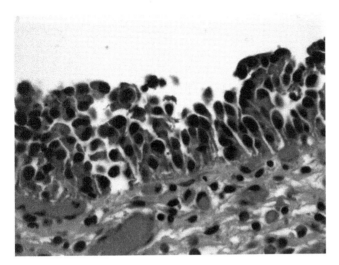

Figure 12.8 Transitional cell carcinoma of the bladder, in situ. *Source*: Figure 18.1 from Page 238 of the American Cancer Society's Oncology in Practice [9].

Diagnosis

When bladder cancer is suspected, urinalysis, excretory urography, cystoscopy, and urine cytology may be done to detect malignant cells. For diagnosis and clinical staging, biopsies of abnormal areas are required. Urinary antigen tests are not regularly used diagnostically, but may be used when cancer is suspected even though cytology is negative. After intravesical instillation of *hexyl-aminolevulinate*, cystoscopy with blue light aids in the detection of the cancer and improves recurrence-free survival, but not progression-free survival. Low-stage (T1 or more superficial) tumors make up 70–80% of bladder cancers, and for these, cystoscopy with biopsy is adequate for staging. If a biopsy reveals the tumor to be more invasive than a flat superficial tumor, another biopsy may be required that includes muscle tissue. A stage T2 or higher tumor that invades the muscle requires abdominal and pelvic CT as well as chest X-ray. This determines the tumor extent and evaluates for metastases. For invasive tumors, patients have bimanual examination. For men, this means rectal examination and for women, rectovaginal examination. These procedures are performed while the patient is under anesthesia for cystoscopy and biopsy.

Treatment

For superficial carcinoma, complete removal may be done via transurethral resection or **fulguration**. Risk of recurrence can be reduced by giving repeated instillations of chemotherapies such as gemcitabine [Gemzar] (with or without docetaxel [Taxotere]), and mitomycin C. Immunotherapies are used for carcinoma in situ and other high-grade superficial transitional cell carcinomas. These include post-transurethral resection instillation of *bacilli Calmette-Guérin (BCG)*. This is usually more effective than chemotherapy. The instillation can be performed in weekly or monthly intervals over a course of 1–3 years. For invasive transitional cell carcinomas, stage T2 or high tumors that penetrate the muscle usually are treated with radical cystectomy. This is removal of the bladder and nearby structures, with urinary diversion. A partial cystectomy may be done in less than 5% of patients. Before cystectomy, neoadjuvant chemotherapy with a regimen that includes cisplatin (Platinol) is preferred. Lymphadenectomy during surgery is used for staging, but its potential therapeutic benefits are controversial. Ongoing studies are examining limited versus extended lymphadenectomy in relation to survival.

After cystectomy, urinary diversion usually involves routing the urine stream through an ileal conduit, to an abdominal stroma, so that it can be collected in an external drainage bag. For many patients, alternatives include orthotopic neobladder or continent cutaneous diversion. In these procedures, an internal reservoir is created from the intestine. With orthotopic neobladder, this reservoir is connected to the urethra. The reservoir is emptied with the patient relaxes his or her pelvic floor muscles and increases abdominal pressure. The urine then passes through the urethra nearly the same as it did before the cystectomy and urinary diversion procedures. Urinary control is usually maintained during the day, but some amount of incontinence can occur at night. With continent cutaneous urinary diversion, the reservoir is attached to a continent abdominal stoma. The patient empties the reservoir via self-catheterization, regularly throughout the day. Bladder preservation methods, combining chemotherapy and radiation therapy, are sometimes preferred for older patients, or for those who do not want to undergo more aggressive surgery. These methods can provide five-year survival in 36–74% of cases, but 10–30% of patients will require salvage cystectomy. The patient must be monitored every 3–6 months for cancer progression or recurrence.

Prevention and Early Detection

There is no proven method of preventing transitional cell carcinoma, except to avoid the known risk factors. If discovered early, most cases of this cancer are curable. Early detection is aided by monitoring for fatigue, hematuria, unexplained weight loss, new or persistent back pain, and painful or frequent urination.

Prognosis

Prognosis of bladder cancer depends on the progressive and the staging of tumor. In the early stage of superficial bladder is rarely fatal. If the bladder musculature has been invaded, about 50% of patients survive for five years.

Significant Point

Transitional cells of the urinary bladder are able to change shape and stretch without breaking, allowing for the storage of urine. High-grade transitional cell carcinoma is the type of bladder cancer that is more likely to be life-threatening. However, this type of cancer is curable in most patients if it is superficial and confined to the renal pelvis or ureter.

Clinical Case

1. Where does transitional cell carcinoma of the bladder begin?
2. How common is bladder cancer in men as compared with women?
3. How recurrent is transitional cell carcinoma?

A 57-year-old man had been diagnosed with invasive transitional cell carcinoma of the bladder, and was scheduled for surgery. His symptoms had included burning upon urination and eventually, gross hematuria. Cystoscopy had revealed the tumor to be 3 cm in diameter. It involved the left ureteral orifice and extended to the left lateral bladder wall. The tumor was resected via the transurethral route and graded as a stage III tumor, with invasion of the muscularis propria. Chemotherapy included gemcitabine and cisplatin, which was successful. The patient remained disease-free after one year of follow-up.

Answers:

1. **Transitional cell carcinoma of the bladder begins in the urothelial cells lining the inside of the organ. These cells also line other portions of the urinary tract, including the renal**

pelvis, ureters, and urethra. Sometimes, tumors also develop in these locations, so the entire urinary tract needs to be evaluated for tumors.

2. Urinary bladder cancer is the fourth most common cancer in men, but is three times less common in women.

3. In more than 40% of cases, transitional cell carcinomas recur at the same site in the bladder, or in another site – especially if they are large, poorly differentiated, or multiple.

Squamous Cell Carcinoma

Squamous cell carcinoma of the bladder is less common than transitional cell carcinoma. These tumors usually occur in patients that have a parasitic bladder infestation, or chronic mucosal irritation. With chronic irritation, transitional cells of the bladder can change to squamous cells over time, which are flat and resemble scales. These cells can then become cancerous – especially with exposure to carcinogens or irritants.

Epidemiology

In the United States, only about 1–2% of all bladder cancers are squamous cell carcinomas. Most patients are in their 50s or 60s. Unlike transitional cell carcinoma, the male-to-female ratio for squamous cell carcinoma is nearly 1:1. African Americans are mostly affected, with 1.2 cases out of every 100,000 people, followed by Caucasians (0.6 cases per 100,000). For some reason, *global* cases of squamous cell carcinoma of the bladder are more prevalent than transitional cell carcinoma, unlike in the United States. Most cases occur in parts of the Middle East and Eastern Africa, where **schistosomiasis** is endemic. In these areas, squamous cell carcinoma of the bladder is the most common cancer in males. Patients in these areas tend to be younger than patients in the United States.

Etiology and Risk Factors

Chronic bladder infections and inflammation are likely causes of squamous **metaplasia** and **leukoplakia** of the urothelium. These are considered to be precancerous lesions. Risks for squamous cell carcinoma of the bladder include smoking, exposures to aromatic amines, *Schistosoma haematobium* (bilharzial) infections, and chronic cystitis. Schistosomiasis is also caused by *Schistosoma mansoni* and *Schistosoma japonicum*. Risks also include repeated use of urinary catheters and recurring infections – primarily in neuropathic bladder patients and even more so in patients with spinal cord injury. Risks may increase 0.38–10% after 10 years. There is a 1.8% risk for this carcinoma in patients being treated with cyclophosphamide for other cancers. This is linked to hemorrhagic cystitis developing about one year after treatment. Additional risk factors include pelvic irradiation and immunosuppression in transplant recipients. There may be an increased risk of squamous cell carcinoma in patients treated with intravesical BCG, if squamous dysplasia is present.

Clinical Manifestations

Signs and symptoms of squamous cell carcinoma of the bladder include hematuria, with or without lower urinary tract abnormalities. Other manifestations include frequent urination, pain or burning upon urination, urinary hesitancy, and lower back or pelvic pain.

Pathology

When viewed with a microscope, squamous cell carcinoma has cells that look very similar to the flat cells from the surface of the skin. The squamous cells have intracellular bridges, keratohyalin granules, and pearls. They must be distinguished from urothelial cancer that has squamous differentiation. Almost all of these carcinomas of the bladder are invasive. Metastasis is usually to the lymph nodes, bones, liver, adrenal glands, and lungs. Bilharzial squamous cell carcinoma is usually well-differentiated. There are nodular, exophytic, and fungating lesions. There is also a low prevalence of nodal or distant metastases. Patients with non-bilharzial squamous cell carcinomas usually have advanced stage disease when diagnosed. In more than 80% of cases, there is diffuse spread of the cancer, with muscle invasion. In 10% or more of all cases, metastasis already present upon diagnosis, indicated a worsened outlook. Common sites of metastasis include the regional lymph nodes, bones, intestines, and lungs.

Diagnosis

Diagnosis of squamous cell carcinoma is primarily with cystoscopy and biopsy. Patients are usually diagnosed when the carcinoma is at an advanced stage. Most tumors are moderate or high grade. During cystoscopy, the tumors are mostly ulcerative, often involving the trigone and lateral walls.

Treatment

Treatment is based upon staging. Superficial cancers are usually resected via endoscopy, similar to transitional cell carcinoma. If there is muscle invasion, radical cystectomy is preferred, offering a five-year survival rate of 23–46%. This relatively poor rate is usually because the cancer is quite advanced when discovered. Routine urethrectomy may also be done, since urethral recurrence is as high as 40%. Radiation therapy is a poor single therapy because the five-year survival rate is only 5–18%. Chemotherapy with epirubicin (Ellence) has provided a 50–60% response rate with locally advanced as well as metastatic disease. For advanced disease with nodal or distant metastases, palliative chemotherapy or radiation is used.

Prevention and Early Detection

There is no known prevention of squamous cell carcinoma of the bladder, though the form linked to bilharziasis is obviously preventable by avoiding water that has been contaminated with parasitic worms. Early detection of squamous

cell carcinoma involves cytology, cystoscopy, and biopsy.

Prognosis

The prognosis for squamous cell carcinoma of the bladder is poor due to the tumor's highly infiltrative characteristics, and the fact that it is often detected only after it has already become quite advanced.

Significant Point

Squamous cell carcinoma of the bladder is associated with chronic irritation from infections and long-term use of catheters. It is comparatively rare in the United States, and more common in countries in which bilharziasis (also referred to as schistosomiasis) is prevalent because of parasitic worms in contaminated water.

Clinical Case

1. What are the primary causes of squamous cell carcinoma of the bladder?
2. What are the risks for this type of cancer?
3. What are the treatment options?

A 43-year-old man was evaluated because of gross hematuria and pain during urination. Urinalysis revealed a filling defect in the bladder, and the patient underwent endoscopy, chest X-ray, and an abdominopelvic CT scan. Biopsy of the tumor revealed a grade 2 squamous cell carcinoma of the bladder. Total cystectomy and lymphadenectomy were performed. Unfortunately, the patient died six months later due to local recurrence of the tumor.

Answers:

1. **Squamous cell carcinoma of the bladder usually occurs in patients that have a parasitic bladder infestation, or chronic mucosal irritation. The causative bilharziasis (schistosomiasis) is most common in parts of the Middle East and Eastern Africa.**
2. **Risks include smoking, exposures to aromatic amines,** *Schistosoma haematobium* **(bilharzial) infections, and chronic cystitis. Risks also include repeated use of urinary catheters and recurring infections – primarily in neuropathic bladder patients and even more so in patients with spinal cord injury.**
3. **Treatment options include resection via endoscopy, radical cystectomy, routine urethrectomy, radiation therapy (though as a single therapy it gives poor results), and the chemotherapeutic agent called epirubicin.**

Adenocarcinoma

Adenocarcinoma of the urinary bladder may occur as a primary tumor, or in rare cases, as metastatic tumors from an intestinal carcinoma. Metastasis must be ruled out. The two general forms of bladder adenocarcinoma include those developing from the bladder itself (67% of cases) and those arising from the **urachus** (33%). Primary adenocarcinomas of the bladder are relatively rare. They may develop from intestinal metaplasia of the urothelium. These malignant glandular tumors are differentiated toward the colonic mucosa.

Epidemiology

Only about 1% of all bladder cancers are adenocarcinomas. The mean patient age at diagnosis is 67 years, within a range of 42–86 years. These tumors occur 66% of the time in males. There appears to be no distinct racial or ethnic predilection for these tumors. Globally, bladder adenocarcinomas appear to make up only 0.5–2% of all bladder cancers.

Etiology and Risk Factors

Adenocarcinomas may be caused by progression of extensive intestinal metaplasia known as **cystitis glandularis**, usually occurring at the trigone. They are primarily enteric. Etiology may be related to exstrophy with diffuse **intestinalization**. About 7% of cases develop into adenocarcinoma even after surgical repair. The diverticula sometimes develop adenocarcinomas, but less often than urothelial carcinomas. Other causes may include endometriosis, pelvic lipomatosis, and infection with *Schistosoma haematobium*. Risk factors for adenocarcinoma of the bladder include non-function of the organ itself, chronic irritation, **exstrophy**, and obstruction.

Clinical Manifestations

Signs and symptoms of adenocarcinomas of the bladder include hematuria and sometimes, mucusuria or dysuria. The mucusuria is more common with adenocarcinomas that developed from the bladder itself than with urachal adenocarcinomas.

Pathology

Adenocarcinoma cells are very similar to the gland-forming cells of colon cancer. Almost all adenocarcinomas of the bladder are invasive. In histology, the tumor is gland-forming and must be distinguished from urothelial carcinoma with glandular differentiation. The tumor usually forms in the lateral wall or the trigone of the bladder. The surface is covered with a gelatinous material. Microscopically, the glandular component predominates and usually resembles colonic carcinoma. Mucin is often produced, and the tumor often deeply invades the muscularis propria. The tumor is associated with an in-situ component. Intestinal metaplasia may be present. The urachal adeno-carcinomas usually have a mucinous or colloid appearance, with tumor cells floating in mucin. They may also have an enteric morphology. Additional morphologies include signet ring cell, adenocarcinoma not otherwise specified, and mixed.

Diagnosis

Prior to diagnosis, metastasis or extension from an intestinal adenocarcinoma must be considered. The staging is the same as for transitional cell carcinomas. Muscle invasion is present in 72% of cases upon diagnosis. The diagnosis of the urachal form of adenocarcinoma is based on the tumor being at the bladder dome, in most cases, or the anterior wall. The tumor is usually epicenter in the bladder wall. There is no florid cystitis glandularis in the bladder surface, and no known primary adenocarcinoma of the same morphology in another location. A *CT urogram* is a test that uses a CT scanner and a special contrast medium that helps to visualize the urinary system more clearly. The kidneys, bladder, and ureters can be examined in this type of test. It is usually performed on an outpatient basis.

Treatment

Treatment of bladder adenocarcinomas is with radical cystectomy. Adjuvant chemotherapy may be used. Treatment of urachal adenocarcinomas is with en bloc resection of the bladder, the urachal remnant, and the umbilicus.

Prevention and Early Detection -

There is no known method of prevention for bladder adenocarcinomas. Early detection followed by surgical resection can be curative and provide long-term survival.

Prognosis

The prognosis of adenocarcinoma of the bladder is poor due to the highly infiltrative nature of the tumor, and because it is often diagnosed after being extremely advanced. The five-year survival rate is only 18–47%. These tumors are often of a higher stage when discovered and as many as 40% of cases have already metastasized. Staging is the most important factor for prognosis. The prognosis of urachal adenocarcinomas is also poor, with five-year survival at 25–61%.

Significant Point

Adenocarcinomas of the urinary bladder are uncommon malignancies. They have various histologies and degrees of differentiation. The tumors are associated with chronic inflammation and irritation, and the majority of them are invasive.

Clinical Case

1. What are the two general forms of adenocarcinomas of the bladder?
2. What are the causes and risk factors of bladder adenocarcinomas?
3. What are the various morphologic patterns of these tumors?

A 59-year-old man went to see his physician because of painless gross hematuria. Physical examination, urinalysis, urine cytology, and a CT urogram were all performed. There were no palpable masses. Urine cytology showed that atypical cells were present. The CT urogram showed a midline bladder dome mass with perivesical extension. The patient was treated with transurethral resection of the bladder tumor and partial cystectomy.

Answers:

1. **The two general forms of bladder adenocarcinoma include those developing from the bladder itself (67%) of cases and those arising from the urachus (33%).**

2. Causes include cystitis glandularis, exstrophy with diffuse intestinalization, endometriosis, pelvic lipomatosis, and infection with *Schistosoma haematobium*. Risk factors include non-function of the bladder itself, chronic irritation, exstrophy, and obstruction.

3. Bladder adenocarcinomas may have enteric, not otherwise specified, mucinous, signet ring cell, hepatoid, and mixed morphologic patterns.

Key Terms

Amyloidosis
Angiomyolipomas
Aniridia
Autosomal dominant
Blastemic
Bloom syndrome
Caldesmon
Cavography
Cystitis glandularis
Denys–Drash syndrome
Exstrophy
Frasier syndrome
Fulguration
Gerota fascia
Hemihypertrophy
Heterozygosity
Hypospadias
Intestinalization
Leukoplakia
Metaplasia

mTOR inhibitors
Paraneoplastic syndrome
Pedicle
Perlman syndrome
Phenacetin
Pleomorphic
Polycythemia
Renal cell carcinoma
Renal sarcoma
Stauffer syndrome
Stereotactic
Sturge–Weber syndrome
Transitional cell carcinoma
Tuberous sclerosis
Urachus
Vimentin
von Hippel–Lindau syndrome
von Recklinghausen disease
Wilms' tumor

Bibliography

1 American Cancer Society. (2021). *Can Kidney Cancer Be Prevented?* American Cancer Society, Inc. https://www.cancer.org/cancer/kidney-cancer/causes-risks-prevention/prevention.html Accessed 2021.

2 American Cancer Society. (2021). *Kidney Cancer Stages – How is stage determined?* American Cancer Society, Inc. https://www.cancer.org/cancer/kidney-cancer/detection-diagnosis-staging/staging.html Accessed 2021.

3 American Cancer Society. (2021). *Kidney Cancer – Early Detection, Diagnosis, and Staging.* American Cancer Society, Inc. https://www.cancer.org/cancer/kidney-cancer/detection-diagnosis-staging.html Accessed 2021.

4 American Cancer Society. (2021). *Wilms Tumor – Causes, Risk Factors, and Prevention.* American Cancer Society, Inc. https://www.cancer.org/cancer/wilms-tumor/causes-risks-prevention.html Accessed 2021.

5 American Cancer Society. (2021). *Can Kidney Cancer Be Found Early?* American Cancer Society, Inc. https://www.cancer.org/cancer/kidney-cancer/detection-diagnosis-staging/detection.html Accessed 2021.

6 American Cancer Society. (2021). *What is Bladder Cancer?* American Cancer Society, Inc. https://www.cancer.org/cancer/bladder-cancer/about/what-is-bladder-cancer.html Accessed 2021.

7 American Cancer Society (ACS) Journals: Cancer. (2008). *Preoperative Wilms tumor rupture.* American Cancer Society, Inc. https://acsjournals.onlinelibrary.wiley.com/doi/full/10.1002/cncr.23535 113 (1): 202–213. Accessed 2021.

8 American Cancer Society The. (2018). *The American Cancer Society's Oncology in Practice – Clinical Management.* Hoboken: Wiley-Blackwell. Figure 17.1 from Page 228.

9 American Cancer Society The. (2018). *The American Cancer Society's Oncology in Practice – Clinical Management.* Hoboken: Wiley-Blackwell. Figure 18.1 from Page 238.

10 American Joint Commission on Cancer. (2018). *Kidney Cancer Stages.* American Cancer Society, Inc. https://www.cancer.org/cancer/kidney-cancer/detection-diagnosis-staging/staging.html Accessed 2021.

11 American Urological Association. (2021). *Renal Sarcomas.* American Urological Association. https://www.auanet.org/education/auauniversity/education-products-and-resources/pathology-for-urologists/kidney/mesenchymal-and-other-tumors/renal-sarcomas Accessed 2021.

12 American Urological Association. (2021). *Primary Bladder Adenocarcinoma.* American Urological Association. https://www.auanet.org/education/auauniversity/education-products-and-resources/pathology-for-urologists/urinary-bladder/non-urothelial-carcinomas/primary-bladder-adenocarcinoma Accessed 2021.

13 American Urological Association. (2021). *Urachal Adenocarcinoma.* American Urological Association. https://www.auanet.org/education/auauniversity/education-products-and-resources/pathology-for-urologists/urinary-bladder/non-urothelial-carcinomas/urachal-adenocarcinoma Accessed 2021.

14 Applied Radiology – The Journal of Practical Medical Imaging and Management. (2021). *Urachal adenocarcinoma.* Anderson Publishing. https://www.appliedradiology.com/articles/urachal-adenocarcinoma Accessed 2021.

15 Association of Community Cancer Centers. (2021). *Renal Cell Carcinoma.* Association of Community Cancer Centers. https://www.accc-cancer.org/home/learn/cancer-types/renal Accessed 2021.

16 Bhushan, B. (2020). *Urinary Bladder Cancers: Uro-oncology Series: Review and Self-assessment.* Jaipur: Bhushan.

17 BJU International – Diagnostics. (2012). *Renal angiomyolipoma.* Figure 3 from https://bjui-journals.onlinelibrary.wiley.com/doi/full/10.1111/j.1464-410X.2012.11618.x. 110 (S4): 25–27. Accessed 2021.

18 Bukowski, R.M., Figlin, R.A., and Motzer, R.J. (2009). *Renal Cell Carcinoma: Molecular Targets and Clinical Applications*, 2nd Edition. Totowa: Humana Press.

19 Campbell, S.C. and Rini, B.I. (2012). *Renal Cell Carcinoma: Clinical Management (Current Clinical Urology).* Totowa: Humana Press.

20 Coppes, M.J., Campbell, C.E., and Williams, B.R.G. (2013). *Wilms Tumor: Clinical and Molecular Characterization (Molecular Biology Intelligence Unit).* New York: Springer.

21 Dean, K. and Martin, B. (2014). *Renal Cell Carcinoma: An Essential Guide for Patients.* Scotts Valley: CreateSpace Independent Publishing Platform.

22 Detonic. (2020). *Renal sarcoma causes, symptoms, prognosis and treatment.* Detonic. https://detonic.shop/hypertension/renal-sarcoma-causes-symptoms-prognosis-and-treatment Accessed 2021.

23 Divatia, M.K., Ozcan, A., Guo, C.C., and Ro, J.Y. (2020). *Kidney Cancer: Recent Advances in Surgical and Molecular Pathology*. New York: Springer.

24 DoveMed. (2018). *Papillary Adenoma of Kidney*. DoveMed. https://www.dovemed.com/diseases-conditions/papillary-adenoma-kidney Accessed 2021.

25 DoveMed. (2018). *Angiomyolipoma of Kidney*. DoveMed. https://www.dovemed.com/diseases-conditions/angiomyolipoma-kidney Accessed 2021.

26 Finkel, K.W. and Howard, S.C. (2013). *Renal Disease in Cancer Patients*. Cambridge: Academic Press.

27 Hayat, M.A. (2010). *Methods of Cancer Diagnosis, Therapy, and Prognosis, Volume 6: Ovarian Cancer, Renal Cancer, Urogenitary Tract Cancer, Urinary Bladder Cancer, Cervical Uterine Cancer, Leukemia, Multiple Myeloma and Sarcoma*. New York: Springer.

28 Huang, W.C. and Becher, E. (2020). *Advanced and Metastatic Renal Cell Carcinoma (An Issue of Urologic Clinics: Surgery 47)*. Amsterdam: Elsevier.

29 Ishikawa, I. (2007). *Acquired Cystic Disease of the Kidney and Renal Cell Carcinoma – Complications of Long-Term Dialysis*. New York: Springer.

30 Journal of Clinical Oncology – An American Society of Clinical Oncology Journal. (2021). *Incidence and mortality of renal cell carcinoma in the U.S.: A SEER-based study investigating trends over the last four decades*. American Society of Clinical Oncology. https://ascopubs.org/doi/abs/10.1200/JCO.2018.36.6_suppl.604 Accessed 2021.

31 Journal of Clinical Oncology – An American Society of Clinical Oncology Journal. (2021). *Renal sarcomas: Epidemiology, treatment and outcomes*. American Society of Clinical Oncology. https://ascopubs.org/doi/abs/10.1200/JCO.2021.39.6_suppl.362 Accessed 2021.

32 Kwiatkowski, D.J., Whittemore, V.H., and Thiele, E.A. (2011). *Tuberous Sclerosis Complex: Genes, Clinical Features, and Therapeutics*. Hoboken: Wiley-Blackwell.

33 Lerner, S.P., Schoenberg, M.P., and Sternberg, C.N. (2008). *Treatment and Management of Bladder Cancer*. Boca Raton: CRC Press.

34 Lokeshwar, V.B., Merseburger, A.S., and Hautmann, S.H. (2010). *Bladder Tumors: Molecular Aspects and Clinical Management (Cancer Drug Discovery and Development)*. New York: Springer.

35 Mahdi, A.E. (2019). *The Role of HER2 Gene Mutation in Transitional Cell Carcinoma: Of Urinary Bladder, Using CISH Method*. Riga (Latvia): Noor Publishing.

36 Malouf, G.G. and Tannir, N.M. (2019). *Rare Kidney Tumors: Comprehensive Multidisciplinary Management and Emerging Therapies*. New York: Springer.

37 Medscape. (2021). *What is the global prevalence of bladder cancer?* WebMD LLC. https://www.medscape.com/answers/438262-38753/what-is-the-global-prevalence-of-bladder-cancer Accessed 2021.

38 Moffitt Cancer Center. (2021). *Squamous Cell Bladder Cancer*. Moffitt Cancer Center. https://moffitt.org/cancers/bladder-cancer/diagnosis/types/squamous-cell-bladder-cancer Accessed 2021.

39 Murphy, W.M., Grignon, D.J., and Perlman, E.J. (2004). *Tumors of the Kidney, Bladder and Related Urinary Structures (AFIP Atlas of Tumor Pathology Series 4)*. Arlington: American Registry of Pathology.

40 National Cancer Institute. (2021). *Transitional Cell Cancer of the Renal Pelvis and Ureter Treatment (PDQ®)-Health Professional Version*. U.S. Department of Health and Human Services/National Institutes of Health/National Cancer Institute/USA.gov. https://www.cancer.gov/types/kidney/hp/transitional-cell-treatment-pdq Accessed 2021.

41 National Comprehensive Cancer Network. (2019). *NCCN Guidelines for Patients – Kidney Cancer*. Plymouth Meeting: National Comprehensive Cancer Network.

42 National Library of Medicine – National Center for Biotechnology Information. (2020). *Epidemiology of Renal Cell Carcinoma.* National Library of Medicine. https://pubmed.ncbi.nlm.nih.gov/32494314 Accessed 2021.

43 National Library of Medicine – National Center for Biotechnology Information. (2011). *Diagnosis and treatment of primary adult renal sarcoma.* National Library of Medicine. https://pubmed.ncbi.nlm.nih.gov/22207927 Accessed 2021.

44 National Library of Medicine – National Center for Biotechnology Information. (2002). *Racial variation in the incidence of squamous cell carcinoma of the bladder in the United States.* National Library of Medicine. https://pubmed.ncbi.nlm.nih.gov/12394685 Accessed 2021.

45 National Library of Medicine – National Center for Biotechnology Information. (2010). *Clinical epidemiology of nonurothelial bladder cancer: Analysis of the Netherlands Cancer Registry.* National Library of Medicine. https://pubmed.ncbi.nlm.nih.gov/20083267 Accessed 2021.

46 Oak, S.N. and Parelkar, S.V. (2002). *Wilms' Tumor: Saga of a Century*, 2nd Edition. New Delhi: Jaypee.

47 PathologyOutlines.com. (2021). *Kidney tumor – Benign adult tumors – Papillary adenoma.* PathologyOutlines.com. https://www.pathologyoutlines.com/topic/kidneytumorrenalcortadenoma.html Accessed 2021.

48 PathologyOutlines.com. (2021). *Kidney tumor – Benign adult tumors – Angiomyolipoma.* PathologyOutlines.com. www.pathologyoutlines.com/topic/kidneytumorangiomyolipoma.html Accessed 2021.

49 PathologyOutlines.com. (2021). *Kidney tumor – Other tumors – Metastases.* PathologyOutlines.com. https://www.pathologyoutlines.com/topic/

kidneytumormalignantmetastases.html Accessed 2021.

50 PathologyOutlines.com. (2021). *Bladder, ureter & renal pelvis – Glandular neoplasms – Adenocarcinoma.* PathologyOutlines.com. https://www.pathologyoutlines.com/topic/bladderadeno.html Accessed 2021.

51 Pavone-Macaluso, M., Smith, P.H., and Edsmyr, F. (2012). *Bladder Tumors and Other Topics in Urological Oncology (Ettore Majorana International Science Series, 1).* New York: Springer.

52 Regional Cancer Care Associates. (2021). *Transitional Cell Carcinoma: An Aggressive Cancer.* Regional Cancer Care Associates. https://www.regionalcancercare.org/cancer-types/transitional-cell-carcinoma Accessed 2021.

53 Renal & Urology News. (2013). *Metastases to the Kidney May Be Mistaken for Primary Tumors.* Haymarket Media, Inc. https://www.renalandurologynews.com/home/news/urology/kidney-cancer/metastases-to-the-kidney-may-be-mistaken-for-primary-tumors Accessed 2021.

54 Riella, C., Czarnecki, P.G., and Steinman, T.I. (2017). *Polycystic Kidney Diseases – Colloquium Series on Integrated Systems Physiology, from Molecule to Function to Disease).* San Rafael: Morgan & Claypool Life Sciences.

55 RSNA Radiology. (1987). *Renal metastases: Clinicopathologic and radiologic correlation.* Radiological Society of North America. https://pubs.rsna.org/doi/10.1148/radiology.162.2.3797648 Accessed 2021.

56 ScienceDirect. (2021). *Kidney Adenoma.* Elsevier B.V. https://www.sciencedirect.com/topics/medicine-and-dentistry/kidney-adenoma Accessed 2021.

57 Wiley Online Library. (1993). *Medical and Pediatric Oncology – Epidemiology of Wilms tumor.* John Wiley & Sons, Inc. https://onlinelibrary.wiley.com/doi/abs/10.1002/mpo.2950210305 Accessed 2021.

58 Wiley Online Library – Clinical Case Reports. (2019). *Adult renal sarcoma*. Figure 1 from https://onlinelibrary.wiley.com/doi/full/10.1002/ccr3.1911. 7 (1): 47–50. Accessed 2021.

59 World Cancer Research Fund – American Institute for Cancer Research. (2018). *Kidney cancer statistics – Kidney cancer is the 14th most common cancer worldwide*. WCRF International. https://www.wcrf.org/dietandcancer/kidney-cancer-statistics Accessed 2021.

60 Zbar, B. (2013). *From Immunotherapy of Cancer to the Discovery of Kidney Cancer Genes – A Personal History. (Colloquium Series on the Genetic Basis of Human Disease.* San Rafael: Morgan & Claypool Life Sciences.

61 Zhou, M., Netto, G., and Epstein, J. (2012). *Uropathology: A Volume in the High Yield Pathology Series*. Philadelphia: Saunders.

13

Diagnostic Procedures

OUTLINE

Traditional X-rays
Computed Tomography
Positron Emission Tomography
Magnetic Resonance Imaging
Doppler and Duplex Doppler Ultrasonography
Transrectal Ultrasonography
Mammography
Nuclear Medicine
Endoscopy
Endoscopic Retrograde Cholangiopancreatography
Biopsy
Lumbar Puncture
Hematology Tests
Urinalysis
Genetic Testing
Key Terms
Bibliography

Traditional X-rays

X-rays are an electromagnetic radiation with wavelengths between about 0.005 and 10 nm. X-rays are produced when electrons traveling at high speeds strike certain materials, particularly heavy metals such as tungsten. They can penetrate most substances and are used to investigate the integrity of certain structures, to therapeutically destroy diseased tissue, and to make radiographic images for diagnostic purposes, as in radiography and fluoroscopy. Structures that are relatively radiopaque (allow few X-ray to pass through), such as bones and cavities filled with a radiopaque contrast medium, cast a shadow on the image receptor. In 1895, X-rays were discovered by physicist Wilhelm Conrad Röntgen in Germany. He was testing whether cathode rays could pass through glass or not, and saw that a nearby screen, coated with a chemical, began glowing. He named the rays "X-rays" since he did not know why they were causing this reaction. X-rays have wavelengths that are about 1,000 times shorter than those of light rays. Röntgen found that X-rays penetrate human skin but not substances that are of higher density, such as bones. The discovery became extremely important as a method of diagnosis in 1897. They were first used on a military battlefield to find bullets and fractured bones in soldiers. Traditional X-rays generate images of body tissues and structures. After passing through the body, they then pass through a detector, forming an image that

Global Epidemiology of Cancer: Diagnosis and Treatment, First Edition. Jahangir Moini, Nicholas G. Avgeropoulos, and Craig Badolato.
© 2022 John Wiley & Sons Ltd. Published 2022 by John Wiley & Sons Ltd.

represents shadow-like features, which are formed by internal body structures. X-ray detectors may put the images onto photographic film or into digital image collections, and the images are known as radiographs.

Patients are positioned so that the area of the body to be imaged is between the X-ray source and the detector. After turning on the X-ray machine, the radiation travels through the body and is absorbed in varying amounts by different tissues. This is based on the radiological density of the tissues, which is determined by the density and atomic number of the tissues. Bones, for example, contain calcium, which has a higher atomic number than most other tissues. This means that bones easily absorb X-rays, and are seen with the highest contrast by the X-ray detector compared with other

tissues. Bones appear brighter than other tissues, against the radiograph's black background. In the example of an osteosarcoma, Figure 13.1 shows the tumor involving the diaphysis of the femur. The dense mineralization has a "fluffy" appearance. X-rays travel less easily through fat, muscle, and air-filled structures, which are less radiologically dense. Therefore, these structures appear as a gray color in a radiograph.

Diagnostically, X-rays are used to image bone fractures, tumors, and other masses, certain types of injuries, pneumonia, calcifications, dental abnormalities, and foreign objects. Mammography uses X-rays to detect breast cancers and diagnose the type of tumor. The tumors are regular or irregular in shape, and slightly brighter on a black background, or slightly darker on a white

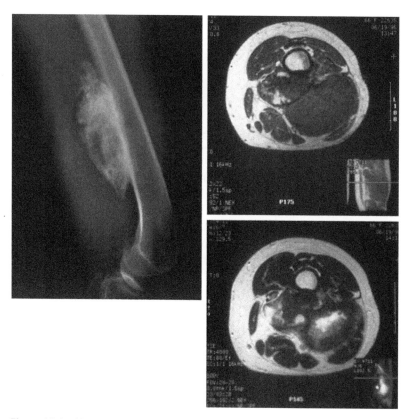

Figure 13.1 X-ray of a high-grade surface osteosarcoma of the femur. *Source*: Figure 2 (left image only) from American Cancer Society (ACS) Journals – Cancer [4].

background. Microcalcifications can also be seen, which appear as extremely bright "specks." Microcalcifications are benign, but sometimes indicate certain types of cancer. X-rays are also used as part of computed tomography, which utilizes computer imaging to create cross-sectional body images, and then combine them into three-dimensional images. **Fluoroscopy** utilizes X-rays with a fluorescent screen, generating real-time images of movements inside the body, or to view diagnostic procedures such as contrast agents that are swallowed or injected. Fluoroscopy can view the heart as it beats, and if contrast agents are used, radiologists can see the blood flow to the heart and through the blood vessels and organs. This technique is also used with a contrast agent to guide an internal catheter during the procedure called **cardiac angioplasty**.

The benefits of X-rays are much greater than the risks, which were discovered in 1904 after Clarence Dally, the assistant of Thomas Edison, died of skin cancer. He had worked extensively with X-rays, and other scientists reported cases of skin damage and burns due to exposure. X-ray scans can diagnose life-threatening conditions, including cancer. The risks concern repeated X-ray procedures over a patient's lifetime, in which there is an accumulation of the amount of radiation passing through the body. This increases cancer risks, but not significantly. For pregnant women, X-rays are avoided during the first trimester to prevent harm to the fetus. Instead, magnetic resonance imaging (MRI) or ultrasonography is preferred for these areas. In cancer treatment, radiation therapy uses X-rays as well as other forms of high-energy radiation to destroy cancer cells and tumors. This occurs by direct DNA damage. Radiation doses used in the treatment of cancer are much higher than those used for diagnostic imaging. Therapeutic radiation can be applied by an external machine or by placing radioactive materials into the body, either within or near cancer cells, or by injecting them into the bloodstream.

Significant Point

Traditional X-rays are best used for detecting bone fractures or bone and lung tumors. Most bone cancers appear irregular instead of solid, or may appear similar to holes in the bones. A chest X-ray is often done to see if bone cancer has spread to the lungs. Chest X-rays are best able to detect larger lung tumors. Abnormal lung growths appear in X-rays as relatively consolidated areas that are light gray. Confirmation of lung cancer is via computed tomography (CT), sputum cytology, and lung biopsy.

Clinical Case

1. **Why are bone cancers easily imaged by traditional X-rays?**
2. **How do the benefits of X-rays compare with the risks?**

A 16-year-old boy was taken to his pediatrician by his parents because of pain in his right hip and thigh. His overall health was very good, and he had no history of fever, night sweats, or weight loss. He also had no history of any serious infections. All blood and urine tests were in normal ranges. Several X-rays were taken of his hip and thigh, and a permeative lesion was found on the right proximal femur. The cortex of the femur was mildly thickened and expanded. A biopsy was performed, showing a small, round blue cell tumor with hypercellularity. The diagnosis was of Ewing sarcoma. The boy received preoperative chemotherapy, and there was a radical surgical resection of the proximal half of the femur. A reconstruction of that part of the bone was done with a prosthetic device, and the boy was given more chemotherapy after surgery. He recovered successfully, and there was no recurrence of the cancer.

Answers:

1. **Bones contain calcium, which has a higher atomic number than most other tissues. This means that bones easily absorb X-rays and are seen with the highest contrast by the X-ray detector compared with other tissues. Bones appear brighter than other tissues, against the radiograph's black background.**

2. **The benefits of X-rays are much greater than the risks. X-ray scans can diagnose life-threatening conditions, including cancer. The risks concern repeated X-ray procedures over a patient's lifetime, in which there is an accumulation of the amount of radiation passing through the body. This increases cancer risks, but not significantly.**

Computed Tomography

Computed tomography (CT) is also known as *computed axial tomography (CAT)*, and is a computerized X-ray imaging procedure. It allows for quick and noninvasive imaging, and is superior to MRI for visualizing fine bone details in many areas of the body. However, CT is not superior to MRI for visualizing the contents of body structures. A narrow beam of X-rays is aimed at a patient and quickly rotated around his or her body, which lies on a bed within a circular opening in a **gantry**. The bed moves slowly through the gantry as the X-ray tube rotates around. A CT machine is shown in Figure 13.2.

Film is not used to record CT images. Instead, specialized X-ray detectors pick up the X-rays leaving the patient's body and transmit them to the computer. The signals are processed after each full rotation, to generate cross-section images that look like "slices" of the body. These **tomographic images** contain highly detailed information in comparison with traditional X-rays. After many successive slices have been collected, the computer digitally combines them

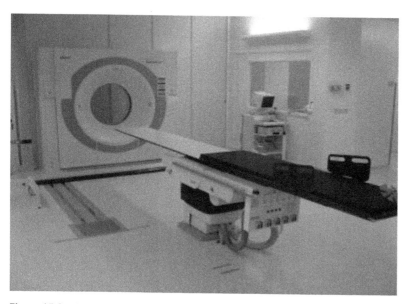

Figure 13.2 A computed tomography machine. *Source*: British Journal of Surgery (BJS) Society [9].

to form a three-dimensional image, which can aid in easily identifying and locating body structures, tumors, or other abnormalities. The thickness of the tissues in each image varies per each CT scanner, but is usually between 1 and 10 mm (see Figure 13.3). Image slices can also be viewed individually without being "stacked" together to form the 3D image. The multiple images allow physicians to find the exact location of any abnormality.

CT scans identify a variety of diseases or injuries as well as other abnormalities, and are useful to detect cancerous or benign tumors. A CT scan of the heart, for example, can detect numerous types of heart disease or abnormalities. For the skull, a CT can visualize injuries, clots that could lead to a stroke, tumors, and hemorrhage. It can reveal lung tumors, pulmonary embolism, emphysema, pneumonia, and excess fluid. For the bones, CT scans reveal fractures, erosion, and tumors in high detail.

Radiopaque contrast agents aid in detecting a variety of abnormalities. Non-contrast CT is used to quickly reveal conditions such as hemorrhage or gross structure alterations, with no danger of any adverse effects. The use of intrathecal agents with CT can show abnormalities of the central nervous system. When **CT angiography**

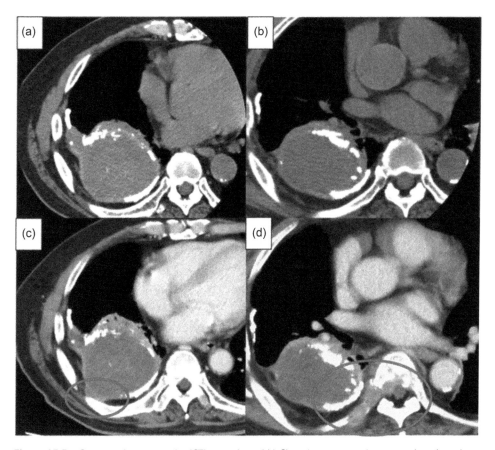

Figure 13.3 Computed tomography (CT) scan. (a and b) Chronic empyema is present but there is no evidence of cancer. (c and d) This scan, with contrast, was taken three months later, revealing irregular posterior pleural thickening and an abnormal right seventh costal mass. *Source*: Figure 1 from Wiley Online Library – Respiratory Case Reports [52].

is used, requiring a contrast agent, cerebral blood vessels can be visualized. This means that an MRI or another type of angiography will not be needed. However, adverse effects of contrast agents include contrast nephropathy and allergic reactions. Contrast-induced nephropathy with permanent irreversible kidney damage is rare, even in patients with mild to moderate kidney failure. Even so, intravenous contrast agents must be used very carefully for patients with abnormal kidney function. CT angiography is less common today, because of the development of MR angiography, but CT angiography is still the main imaging modality for acute stroke. CT has a high sensitivity, but limited specificity. The patient's medical history and a physical examination are also essential. Because soft body tissues have varying abilities to stop X-rays, CT scans may show them only faintly – requiring an intravenous contrast agent that will appear highly visible in the images produced. The contrast agents contain substances that stop the X-rays very well, increasing tissue visibility. For examination of the circulatory system, a contrast agent based on iodine is injected into the bloodstream, illuminating the blood vessels during imaging. For the digestive system, oral contrast agents such as barium sulfate may be used.

CT allows for the diagnoses of life-threatening conditions, aiding in earlier detection. However, since CT uses X-rays that produce ionizing radiation, it is important to be very careful in the amount of radiation that the patient is exposed to. The number of exposures to ionizing radiation during life increases the risks of developing cancer, though usually the risks are not significant. For a pregnant woman, CT can be used if the area being imaged is not the abdomen or pelvis – in that case MRI or ultrasonography would be used since they do not produce radiation. For children, the CT machine's settings are adjusted to appropriate levels.

The National Institute of Biomedical Imaging and Bioengineering is aiding in the development of a dedicated CT breast scanner that allows for 3D imaging and detection of tumors that would otherwise be hard to visualize. The amount of radiation produced is similar to a standard X-ray mammogram, and is advantageous because the breast does not need to be compressed. The patient lies face down on a special examination table with the breast being examined suspended in a special opening. The scanner is below, and rotates around the breast without X-rays passing through the chest. This reduces the amount of radiation needed. The actual X-rays in a CT machine are generated when a metal filament is heated until energized electrons escape from the **cathode** surface into a vacuum. An electric field accelerates the electrons, which acquire **kinetic energy**, as they are attracted to a positive **anode** target. Electrostatic or magnetic fields, or both, are used to focus the electron beam into a small area of the anode target, usually with a dimension of about 1 mm.

The use of CT for cancer patients is diverse. It can be used to screen for cancer, help diagnose tumors, provide information about staging, and guide a biopsy procedure. It is also used to guide cryotherapy, implantation of radioactive seeds, and radiofrequency ablation. CT helps in the planning of external-beam radiation therapy or surgery, to determine whether a tumor is responding to treatment, and to detect tumor recurrence. In cancer screening, CT is useful for colorectal cancer and lung cancer. In **CT colonography**, also called *virtual colonoscopy*, computed tomography can find large colorectal polyps as well as tumors. This process uses the same amount of radiation as in standard CT scans of the abdomen and pelvis. The CT colonography procedure has been found to be nearly identical in accuracy to standard colonoscopy, but is less invasive and has a lower risk of complications. When it discovers polyps or other abnormal growths, a standard colonoscopy is usually performed so that they can be removed. Unfortunately, most insurance companies do not yet cover CT colonography, even though it also produces images of organs and tissues outside of the colon – discovering other abnormalities.

Low-dose **helical CT** scans of the chest result in 20% less radiation exposure than standard X-rays. However, they are slightly less accurate. Even so, these CT scans are able to find other non-pulmonary abnormalities. Most insurance companies cover low-dose helical CT as a preventive care benefit for adults between 55 and 80 that have a 30-pack/year smoking history, if they still smoke or quit within the past 15 years. Total CT, also known as *whole-body CT*, creates images of almost the entire body – from the chin to below the hips. It is regularly used for diagnosed cancer patients, and sometimes in people without cancer symptoms that may be of higher risk for cancer. Follow-up tests are required, which can be expensive, uncomfortable, and even risky. Also, total CT exposes the patient to about four times higher volumes of ionizing radiation than standard CT.

There is also *combined positron emission tomography (PET)/CT*, in which *positron emission tomography* is also used. First, the CT scan creates images, and then PET creates images that include functional information about the chemical reactions active in cells and tissues. This is important because cancer cells often use different metabolic pathways than normal cells. The patient is given a radioactive substance (radiopharmaceutical) designed to target cancer cells. Since cancerous tumors metabolize glucose much more quickly than normal tissues, a radioactive form of glucose known as *fluorodeoxyglucose (FDG)* is used. The tumors take up more of the FDG and look different from normal tissues when the PET scan is completed. Other agents used in PET provide information on the level of oxygen in tissues, new blood vessel formation, bone growth, active division or growth of tumor cells, and the spreading of cancer. The PET/CT gives a more complete result about tumor location, growth, or spreading than either test can give alone. This may improve diagnoses, assess staging, plan treatment, and monitor patient responses. It also can reduce the amount of other imaging tests or procedures that will be required.

Significant Point

While X-rays were discovered in 1895 and became the first diagnostic imaging technology, CT was not created until the early 1970s. In the decades since, CT technology has continually improved, and is now faster and more highly detailed than ever before. In 1972, the scan time per CT "slice" took five minutes each. By 2005, the scan time took only 0.005 of a second.

Clinical Case

1. How are CT images recorded?
2. Why are contrast agents often required for CT scans?
3. How useful is CT for cancer patients?

A 70-year-old woman visited her physician complaining of increasing fatigue and muscle weakness. She also had low back pain, and recently developed pain in her arms and legs. The patient had a history of cirrhosis. Laboratory tests revealed a low platelet count and hypokalemia. The patient was given oral potassium and referred to a hematologist to be assessed for thrombocytopenia, but her platelet counts decreased even further, and she was hospitalized. A chest X-ray was taken, which was normal, and a CT scan of the patient's abdomen confirmed cirrhosis. The thrombocytopenia was attributed to the cirrhosis. Multiple platelet transfusions were given, and the hypokalemia did not respond to either oral or IV potassium supplementation. A bone marrow biopsy was performed, which showed metastatic small cell carcinoma. The patient had smoked throughout early adulthood but had quit at age 45. A contrast enhanced CT scan of her lungs revealed a mass in the left lung. Soon, the patient's hemoglobin and blood cell counts began to drop. She could not receive standard chemotherapy because of the severe thrombocytopenia and cirrhosis, and died within a few days from extensive metastatic spread.

Answers:

1. **Specialized X-ray detectors pick up the X-rays used in CT as they leave the patient's body and transmit them to a computer. The signals are processed after each full rotation, to generate cross-section images that look like "slices" of the body. After many successive slices have been collected, the computer digitally combines them to form a three-dimensional image, which can aid in easily identifying and locating body structures, tumors, or other abnormalities.**
2. **Because soft body tissues have varying abilities to stop X-rays, CT scans may show them only faintly – requiring an intravenous contrast agent that will appear highly visible in the images produced. The contrast agents contain substances that stop the X-rays very well, increasing tissue visibility.**
3. **The use of CT for cancer patients is diverse. It can be used to screen for cancer, help diagnose tumors, provide information about staging, and to guide a biopsy procedure. It is also used to guide cryotherapy, implantation of radioactive seeds, and radiofrequency ablation. CT helps in the planning of external-beam radiation therapy or surgery, to determine if a tumor is responding to treatment, and to detect tumor recurrence.**

Positron Emission Tomography

Positrons were first theorized in 1928, and are opposite to electrons since they carry a *positive charge*. Technology to use positrons in medical diagnostics was developed beginning in the 1950s. *Tomography* refers to images being constructed by combining image slices, and the term is based on the word *atom*. **Positron emission tomography** (PET) basically works as follows:

- The radioactive isotope called *fluorine-18* is produced in a particle accelerator, by colliding a proton beam into water that contains *oxygen-18*
- This is incorporated via chemistry in the glucose molecule called *fluorodeoxyglucose (FDG)*
- The FDG is administered to the patient
- As the FDG spreads and is metabolized, the fluorine decays and emits a positron
- The positron quickly finds an electron that is usually within 2 mm away
- It overcomes the electron and releases two gamma photons that quickly move away in opposite directions
- With the patient lying stationary inside a ring of gamma detectors, the two photons are detected in two separate locations, with the line connecting the locations revealing the axis upon which they moved
- The difference in the photon's arrival times reveals where on the axis they originated
- This information reveals the exact spot in the body where the electron annihilation occurred
- Multiple measurement of photons allows for triangulation, and eventually, an image is constructed
- A PET scan is basically a map of where glucose is being metabolized; since tumors are sites of high metabolism, they become very bright, and can be diagnosed and monitored – see Figure 13.4

done at a hospital or a center that has this type of technology. Before a PET-CT scan, patients may be required to drink only clear fluids, avoiding eating for a certain time period, avoid taking usual medications or supplements, discuss any medical conditions related to glucose such as diabetes mellitus, discuss any allergies, avoid heavy exercise, wearing loose clothing, removing anything with metal since the scan can be compromised, and to discuss insurance coverage.

The PET-CT scan begins with administration of a radioactive substance through intravenous injection. Body movements must be limited so that the substance does not move into body areas that are not being studied. The patient must wait for 30–90 minutes before the scan begins. In other situations, a contrast liquid may be swallowed or injected IV. The liquid is designed to make the images clearer. Immediately before the scan, the patient is asked to empty the bladder. The contrast liquid can make the injection site hot or itchy, and there is sometimes a metallic taste in the mouth, but these effects usually subside over several minutes. The patient must be told to alert the healthcare team to any serious reactions, such as difficulty breathing.

The technologist positions the patient on the scanning table – usually lying face up, but sometimes lying on the stomach or side – based on the area needing to be scanned. If a PET-CT scan is used to plan radiation therapy for treatment, the body position is even more important. To keep the body site very still, a mask or casting device is sometimes used. The PET-CT machine first slides the scanning table quickly through the hole in the center to determine whether the patient is in the correct position. It then slides slowly back and forth, and the patient can interact with the technician during the scan. Sometimes, the patient is required to hold his or her breath for a short time. The table can also be raised, lowered, or tilted as needed. The machine makes various clicking or **whirring** sounds of different volumes. The total

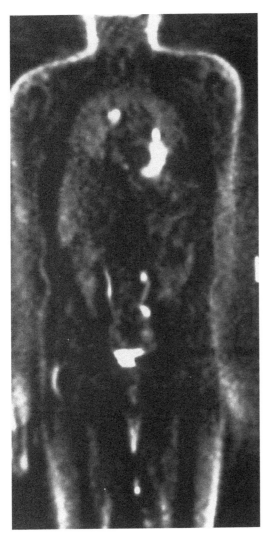

Figure 13.4 A positron emission tomography (PET) scan showing clinically undetected mediastinal melanoma metastases. *Source*: Figure 1 from American Cancer Society (ACS) Journals – Cancer [5].

Positron emission tomography is sometimes used along with CT, as a PET-CT scan. This combination technology helps to find the best biopsy site, learn if a cancer treatment is effective, checking for new cancer growth following treatment, and to plan radiation therapy. The benefits of PET-CT highly exceed the low risks of problems due to the radiation. The results of a PET-CT scan are evaluated by a radiologist or a nuclear medicine specialist. The scan can be appointment lasts for 1–3 hours. Once the radioactive substance reaches the area to be scanned, the actual PET-CT scan only takes about 30 minutes. This can vary if a larger body site needs to be scanned. The patient often remains on the scanning table until the technician makes sure that the images are clear. After the scan, the patient can usually resume normal activities immediately, including driving. Several glasses of water should be consumed to help remove the radioactive substance and contrast agent from the body.

Significant Point

Some types of cancer are unlikely to be visible on a PET scan, which is generally used for specific cancers affecting the lungs, breasts, brain, cervix, thyroid, and esophagus. PET scans are also usually used for melanoma and lymphoma. These scans show the tumors in a different color than the surrounding tissue activity.

Clinical Case

1. What components are used as part of PET?
2. Why is PET sometimes combined with CT?
3. How is a patient positioned on the scanning table?

A 40-year-old woman had developed numbness in her right arm and leg, and underwent an MRI that revealed a large mass lesion in the pons. The differential diagnosis was of a brainstem glioma, with hemorrhage. When a PET scan was performed, it showed the lesion to have centrally decreased activity, plus an outer rim with increased FDG uptake. This is most consistent with a brain lesion that has necrosis or central hemorrhage. Whole-body PET images showed increased FDG uptake in the right upper lung lobe. A biopsy of the brainstem lesion showed a poorly differentiated carcinoma, which had metastasized from the lung tumor. The patient underwent stereotactic radiosurgery and received fractionated whole-brain radiation therapy and responded well to these therapies. The lung cancer was treated with chemotherapy and immunotherapy, which were successful in stopping the growth of the tumor. Over six months of follow-up, she was doing fairly well, and her condition had not worsened.

Answers:

1. **In PET, the radioactive isotope called fluorine-18 is produced, which collides with a proton beam into water containing oxygen-18. This is incorporated via chemistry in the glucose molecule called fluorodeoxyglucose. A PET scan is basically a map of where glucose is being metabolized. Since tumors are sites of high metabolism, they become very bright.**

2. **The combination of PET with CT helps to find the best biopsy site, learn if a cancer treatment is effective, checking for new cancer growth following treatment, and to plan radiation therapy.**

3. **The technologist positions the patient on the scanning table – usually lying face up, but sometimes lying on the stomach or side – based on the area needing to be scanned. Body position is more important if the scan is used to plan radiation therapy for treatment. To keep the body site very still, a mask or casting device is sometimes used.**

Magnetic Resonance Imaging

Magnetic resonance imaging (MRI) produces three-dimensional and very detailed anatomical images. It is commonly used for detecting cancer and other diseases, for diagnosis, and for treatment monitoring. The technology is based on the excitation of protons and detection of changes in the direction of their rotational axes, within the water of body tissues. Powerful magnets produce a strong magnetic field. This forces protons within the body to align with the magnetic field. A radiofrequency current is pulsed through the patient's body, stimulating the protons. They spin out of equilibrium, against the pull of the magnetic field. Once the radiofrequency field is switched off, MRI sensors detect the energy that is released as the protons realign with the magnetic field. The amount of time this takes, along with the amount of energy released, is changed – based on the chemical nature of the molecules and their environment. Based on these magnetic properties, physicians are able to assess differences in various tissues. The procedure occurs with the patient lying inside an MRI machine, which is basically just a very large magnet. The patient is required to lie extremely still to avoid any blurring. Contrast agents – usually containing **gadolinium** – may be used via IV injection, either before or during the procedure. The agent increases the speed at which the protons realign with the magnetic field. The faster the realignment, the brighter the image. The use of IV contrast agents occurs for the following tumor-related conditions:

- Acoustic neuroma/Schwannoma
- Brain tumors
- History of cancer or metastasis
- Eye orbit cancer or mass tumors
- All soft tissue masses of the neck
- Spinal tumor or metastasis
- All abdominal protocols unless the biliary ducts are being evaluated
- Pelvic bone cancer or metastasis
- Pelvic fibroids
- Pelvic masses or tumors

- Ovarian cancer
- Uterine cancer
- Prostate cancer
- Bone tumors or metastasis
- Lymphoma of the extremities
- Soft tissue masses of the extremities

There are two basic imaging procedures that are part of MRI: T1-weighted and T2-weighted images, often called *T1 and T2 images*. The timing of the radiofrequency pulse sequences that create T1 images produces images that highlight fat tissues. The timing of the radiofrequency pulse sequences that create T2 images produces images that highlight fat tissues and water in the body. An easy way to remember this is that T1 highlights only one image (fat) and T2 highlights two images (fat and water). Both techniques highlight proton energy. In a T1-weighted image of the spinal cord, the cerebrospinal fluid (CSF) contains no fat, so it appears black – see Figure 13.5.

The MRI procedure does not use X-rays, so there is no damaging ionizing radiation. The scanners are especially good at imaging the soft tissues and non-bony areas of the body, including the brain, spinal cord, nerves, muscles, ligaments, and tendons. Therefore, MRI is preferred for such things as knee and shoulder imaging. Within the brain, MRI can visualize gray and white matter, and diagnose tumors and aneurysms. It is the method of choice if a patient needs frequent imaging – especially in the brain. Unfortunately, it is more expensive than X-ray or CT imaging. A special type of MRI is called *functional MRI (fMRI)*, which is used to visualize brain structures and their functions, for neurological conditions.

The extremely strong magnetic field of an MRI scanner attracts any object made of iron, certain types of steel, and other objects that respond to magnets. The patient is questioned about any type of metal implant. Any person with a pacemaker, implanted cardioverter-defibrillator, vagus nerve stimulator, insulin pump, loop recorder, cochlear implant, deep brain stimulator, or endoscopic capsule cannot have

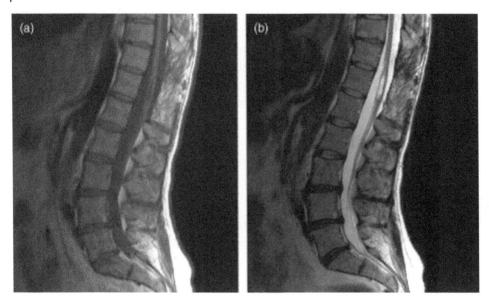

Figure 13.5 MRI of the spinal cord, using (A) T1-weighted imaging. Note that the CSF appears black because it contains no fat; and (B) T2-weighted imaging. Note that the CSF appears white because it contains water. *Source*: Figure 3 from Wiley Online Library – Journal of Medical Imaging and Radiation Oncology – Radiology – Pictorial Essay [53].

an MRI. The MRI scanner makes loud clicks and beeps that may require the patient to wear special ear protection. The scanner can also cause nerve stimulation, felt as twitching of various nerves. Also, a patient with severe renal failure who is on dialysis may not be able to tolerate gadodiamide or other gadolinium-containing contrast agents. Dialysis patients should only receive such agents when it is essential, and dialysis must be performed soon after the scan to remove the agent or agents quickly. The MRI procedure is generally avoided for a pregnant woman in her first trimester because the contrast agents could enter the fetal bloodstream and cause harm. Another consideration is that the long scan times inside the MRI machine may cause people with claustrophobia to panic. The patient should be familiarized with the MRI machine and process. Sedation or anesthesia can also relieve discomfort. Some patients do well when music is provided during the procedure, or if the eyes are closed or covered. A panic button may be offered if anxiety becomes overwhelming, so that the patient can alert the technician. The traditional MRI machine is closed at one end and fully surrounds the patient during the procedure. Because of claustrophobic patients, the *open MRI* was invented, which is open on the sides and does not fully surround the patient. This also reduces the noise level of the machine. Open MRI provides excellent images for many types of examinations, but cannot be used for every type, requiring use of traditional, closed MRI.

Some patients may not be able to eat for two or more hours before an MRI. Loose clothing should be worn, with no metal zippers, buttons, or any other components. Belts, earrings, clothes with snaps, and glasses should be removed. Often, the patient is asked to remove all clothing and wear only an examination gown. All jewelry must be removed. There will be discussion of all medications including herbs, supplements, and OTC drugs. Drug allergies and other medical conditions must be reviewed. Insurance coverage is also reviewed due to the cost of MRIs. The patient may be allowed to bring his or her own music, which can be played through headphones as the procedure occurs. The patient is informed that the contrast agent may feel cold as it spreads through the body, and that a metallic taste, slight headache, or nausea can occur. These are usually transitory.

The patient lies on the scanning table, face up with the arms at the side. His or her head is on a headrest. Small coils may be placed over and around the part of the body, which help send and receive radio waves, for a clearer image. The technologist then goes into a control room and can see the patient via a window or video cameras. An intercom system allows discussion between the technologist and patient. The scanning table slides through the hole of the MRI machine and the patient is asked to lie still. Each series of images takes up to 15 minutes, and 2–6 series may be required. Therefore, an MRI procedure can last up to 90 minutes, but this is discussed with the patient before the procedure. The part of the body being examined may feel warm during the MRI, which is normal. Once the procedure is finished, the patient may be required to remain on the table for a few minutes as the images are reviewed.

Significant Point

An MRI is excellent for the identification of brain and spinal cord tumors, prostate cancer, uterine cancer, certain liver cancers, and metastases to the bones or brain. Also, for women with dense breasts, "fast" MRI can detect breast cancers that 3D mammograms may miss. This technique is also known as *abbreviated MRI*. It is able to detect breast cancer at a very early stage, and provides high diagnostic accuracy with shorter image acquisition and interpretation time.

Clinical Case

1. Aside from the diagnosis of prostate cancer, for what other tumor-related conditions can MRI with contrast agents be used?
2. What are the two basic imaging procedures that are part of MRI?
3. How does the MRI procedure occur?

A 67-year-old man complained to his physician about urinary hesitation and nocturia. He was referred to a urologist, who performed a digital rectal examination, revealing enlargement of the prostate gland. The urologist ordered a prostate-specific antigen (PSA) test and found the level to be high. After biopsy, the patient was diagnosed with prostate cancer. An MRI with contrast was ordered to assess whether there was any metastasis. It showed bony metastasis to the L2 and L3 spine. The patient received radiation therapy to the spine.

Answers:

1. **MRI with contrast agents can also be used for acoustic neuroma/schwannoma, brain tumors, history of cancer or metastasis, eye orbit cancer or mass tumors, all soft tissue masses of the neck, spinal tumor or metastasis, all abdominal protocols unless the biliary ducts are being evaluated, pelvic bone cancer or metastasis, pelvic fibroids, pelvic masses or tumors, ovarian cancer, uterine cancer, bone tumors or metastasis, lymphoma of the extremities, and soft tissue masses of the extremities.**
2. **The two basic MRI imaging procedures are T1-weighted and T2-weighted imaging. T1 highlights only one image (fat), while T2 highlights two images**

(fat and water). Both techniques highlight proton energy.

3. **The patient lies on the scanning table, face up with the arms at the side. His or her head is on a headrest. Small coils may be placed over and around part of the body, which help send and receive radio waves, for a clearer image. The technologist then goes into a control room and can see the patient via a window or video cameras. An intercom system allows discussion between the technologist and patient. The scanning table slides through the hole of the MRI machine and the patient is asked to lie still. Each series of images takes up to 15 minutes, and 2–6 series may be required. The entire procedure can last up to 90 minutes.**

Doppler and Duplex Doppler Ultrasonography

Doppler ultrasonography is a noninvasive procedure that is often used to study the heart and blood vessels. It uses ultrasound with high-frequency waves and is based on the **Doppler effect**, for imaging the blood circulation. The Doppler effect is the dependence between the wave frequencies of transmitted sound. Used in medicine, Doppler ultrasonography studies the movements of erythrocytes in the blood vessels. It provides a color image of blood flow, along with information about blood flow direction, speed, and turbulence. This can be used for a wide variety of conditions, including cancer. Doppler ultrasonography is completely harmless and can be used as many times as necessary, since it is totally noninvasive and uses no radiation. All Doppler ultrasound machines have filters that cut out high amplitude, low-frequency Doppler signals that occur because of tissue movement, such as from blood vessel wall motion. Filter frequency can usually be adjusted

to exclude frequencies, such as those below 50, 100, and 200 Hertz (Hz). This limits the minimum flow velocities that can then be measured and discovered.

Duplex ultrasonography combines traditional ultrasound to create pictures from sound waves reflected in body tissues, with Doppler ultrasound to record the waves reflecting off of moving objects. As ultrasound passes through tissues and fluids but bounces back off certain body structures, the echoes allow the ultrasound machine to visualize deep body structures. A two-dimensional black and white image is produced. Ultrasound machines can show two different images simultaneously, and visualize the **grayscale image** of tissues with a color visualization of blood flow, based on the Doppler effect. The color is layered "over" the grayscale image (see Figure 13.6). This allows the technician to obtain data about blood flow in veins and arteries while observing surrounding tissues. A specific area of the image can be selected to detect localized blood flow by listening to the Doppler waveform. Duplex ultrasonography helps detect blockages in vessels, determine the width of vessels, and can diagnose aneurysms, arterial occlusion, blood clots, varicose veins, venous insufficiency, carotid occlusive disease, and renal vascular disease. It allows for real-time observations with no radiation and is completely noninvasive.

Ultrasound is an excellent way to discriminate between solid tumors and fluid-filled cysts, because they each have very different echo patterns. Most ultrasound waves pass through fluid-filled cysts, send back very few or only faint echoes, and result in the cysts appearing black on the display screen. Ultrasound waves bounce off solid tumors, creating echoes that result in a lighter-colored image. However, ultrasound cannot determine whether a tumor is cancerous. Ultrasound is often used as a needle biopsy of a tumor is being performed, to guide the needle into the tumor. Most ultrasound procedures take 20–30 minutes, but this depends on the type of evaluation being done and how difficult it may be to find any organ changes.

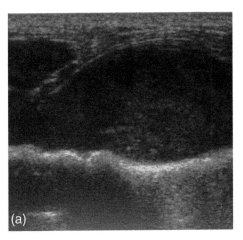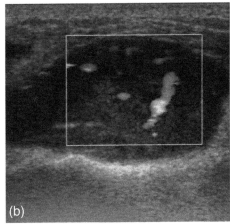

(a)

(b)

Figure 13.6 (a) Doppler ultrasonography of a desmoid tumor of the right foot, showing a homogeneous mass; (b) duplex Doppler ultrasonography showing substantial blood flow to the tumor. *Source*: Figure 3 from Wiley Online Library – Journal of Ultrasound in Medicine – Case Series [54].

Significant Point

Doppler ultrasonography studies the heart and blood vessels, providing color images detecting blood flow, and data about its direction, speed, and turbulence. Duplex Doppler ultrasonography combines traditional and Doppler ultrasonographic techniques, providing color images detecting blood flow, plus a two-dimensional grayscale image of tissues. It provides data on the presence of blood flow, direction, speed, and turbulence along with an image of surrounding tissues. Ultrasound is most successfully used to detect breast, abdominal, and testicular cancers.

Clinical Case

1. What is the basic difference between Doppler and duplex ultrasonography?
2. What images are produced by duplex Doppler ultrasonography?

3. How does ultrasound discriminate between solid tumors and fluid-filled cysts?

A 27-year-old champion bicyclist found a small mass and painless in his right testicle after winning a weekend bike race. When he was a baby, he had been diagnosed with an undescended right testicle. The man's physician performed a physical examination, followed by ultrasonography, which ruled out hydrocele or varicocele, and confirmed the presence of the testicular mass. Blood samples were drawn for tumor markers, and the man was staged with IIB testicular cancer, meaning it had spread to the nearby lymph nodes in his pelvis. An orchiectomy was performed, and the cancerous testicle was removed and replaced with a prosthesis. He also underwent two cycles of chemotherapy over six weeks, responding well to the treatment. The man returned to his normal lifestyle, enjoying his bike races, and even became a father within three years.

Answers:

1. **Doppler ultrasonography studies the movements of blood flow, in color.**

Duplex ultrasonography combines traditional ultrasound to create pictures from sound waves reflected in body tissues, with Doppler ultrasound to record the waves reflecting off of moving objects.

2. **Duplex Doppler ultrasonography** allows two different images to be shown simultaneously, and to visualize the grayscale image of tissues with a color visualization of blood flow, based on the Doppler effect. The color is layered over the grayscale image. This allows the technician to obtain data about blood flow in veins and arteries while observing surrounding tissues.

3. **Ultrasound is an excellent way to discriminate between solid tumors and fluid-filled cysts, because they each have very different echo patterns. Most ultrasound waves pass through fluid-filled cysts, send very few or only faint echoes, and result in the cysts appearing black on the display screen. Ultrasound waves bounce off of solid tumors, creating echoes that result in a lighter-colored image.**

Transrectal Ultrasonography

Transrectal ultrasonography (TRUS) is used for the diagnostic assessment of the prostate gland. An ultrasound transducer is placed into the patient's rectum and sound waves are used to scan the prostate gland in two planes. The resulting images help to guide biopsies of the prostate gland. This procedure may be recommended after an abnormal digital rectal examination or if the PSA level is elevated. The procedure is expensive, and rarely detects prostate cancers on its own. Therefore, it is commonly used only to guide a biopsy. During the procedure, the patient lies on his side. After it is completed, the images produced may indicate cancer by irregular, dark patches that appear on the prostate.

Mammography

Mammography is the process of using machinery to assess breast tissue, to produce a *mammogram*. The machine uses X-rays that are of lower, safer doses than those used in traditional X-rays. Since these X-rays do not penetrate breast tissue easily, the machine has two plates, which are used to flatten or compress the breast. This spreads the tissues apart and provides a better image. Digital mammograms are more common today than the traditional film-printed mammograms. Mammography is currently the only examination approved by the US Food and Drug Administration (FDA) to help screen for breast cancer in asymptomatic patients. A **screening mammogram** uses X-rays of each breast, usually from two different angles, to find any signs of breast cancer when there are no symptoms or problems. The two views of each breast are as follows: one from above (cranial–caudal view), and one from an oblique or angled view (mediolateral–oblique view). Table 13.1 summarizes guidelines for screening mammograms according to the American Cancer Society and the International Agency for Research on Cancer.

A **diagnostic mammogram** is done when there are breast symptoms or changes in breast tissue have been found in a screening mammogram. Extra images of the breast in question may be needed, including from latero-medial view toward the center of the chest and then from the center of the chest outward. Sometimes, diagnostic mammograms are used to screen women previously treated for breast cancer. The newer three-dimensional (3D) mammogram is also known as **digital breast tomosynthesis**. Each breast is compressed one time, and the machine takes many X-rays while it moves in an arc over the breast. A connected computer puts the images together, creating a series of thin slices, allowing viewing of the breast tissue in three dimensions. A standard 2D mammogram can also be taken at the same time, or reconstructed from the 3D images. In many studies, 3D mammography appears to reduce the need for follow-ups, finds more breast cancers, and may be of

Table 13.1 Guidelines for screening mammograms.

Age group	American Cancer Society guideline	International Agency for Research on Cancer guideline
40–49 yr with average risk	Women 40–44 yr of age *should have the choice* to start having screening mammograms every year if they wish. Risks and benefits must be considered. Women 45–49 yr of age *must* have a screening mammogram every year.	There is limited evidence that screening mammograms reduce mortality from breast cancer in women 40–49 yr of age.
50–74 yr with average risk	Women 50–54 yr of age *must* have a screening mammogram every year. For those age 55 or older, screening mammograms are *recommended* either once per year or every 2 yr. Women aged 55 and older should start having screening mammograms every 2 yr, but can continue to have them once per year if they desire. Clinical breast examination to screen for breast cancer is not recommended.	There is insufficient evidence that screening mammograms reduce breast cancer mortality to an extent that the benefits greatly outweigh risks of radiation-induced cancer from the procedures. However, there is solid evidence that clinical breast examination results in tumors being detected in greater numbers while they are in a lower stage.
75 yr or older with average risk	Screening mammograms should continue as long as overall health is good, and life expectancy is 10 yr or more.	This is not addressed.

help for women with higher breast density. Continuing studies of 3D mammography in comparison with 2D mammography are ongoing.

The *Breast Imaging Reporting and Data System (BI-RADS)* is used to describe mammography results. There are seven categories, as follows:

- 0 – Incomplete – additional imaging evaluation, comparison, or both are required – the radiologist may have seen something that appeared abnormal, but more tests are required. Options include another mammogram with spot compression, in which compression is applied to a smaller area during the procedure, magnification, special mammogram viewing, or ultrasound. Also, the radiologist may want to compare a new mammogram with previous ones to assess any changes.
- 1 – Negative – no significant abnormalities. The breasts are symmetrical with no masses, structural distortions, or suspicious calcifications. Nothing bad has been found.
- 2 – Benign finding – also a negative result, but there may be benign calcifications, benign lymph nodes, or calcified fibroadenomas. This

category ensures no other technician will misinterpret the benign finding as suspicious.
- 3 – Probably benign finding – a shorter follow-up time is suggested – there is a higher than 98% chance of findings being benign, and they are not expected to change. The area in question should be followed-up within six months, and regularly after that until the finding is proven to be stable – usually at least over two years. This helps avoid unneeded biopsies. If the area does change, it allows for early diagnosis.
- 4 – Suspicious abnormality – biopsy should be considered – the findings do not definitely look like cancer, but the radiologist feels that a biopsy is needed. Subdivisions of this category include:
  - 4A – 2–10% likelihood of cancer
  - 4B – 10–50% likelihood of cancer
  - 4C – 50–95% likelihood of cancer
- 5 – Highly suggestive of malignancy – findings look like cancer of 95% chance or higher, and a biopsy is strongly recommended.
- 6 – Known biopsy-proven malignancy – only used for findings already proven to be cancer

via previous biopsy. Mammograms used this way help determine cancer responses to treatment.

The BI-RADS reporting system also assesses breast density – the amount of fibrous and glandular breast tissue in comparison with fatty tissue. Breast density is classified into four groups, as follows:

- 1 – almost all fatty tissue
- 2 – scattered areas of dense fibrous and glandular tissue
- 3 – more of the breast consists of dense fibrous and glandular tissue, known as being *heterogeneously dense* – this makes it hard to see small tumors in or around the dense tissue
- 4 – *extremely dense*, making it very hard to see tumors in the tissue

Though the benefits of mammography are extensive, there are a few outcomes that may not be desired. These include the following:

- *False-positive results* – an abnormality is seen that is potentially positive for cancer, leading to anxiety and psychological distress. Additional testing that is needed can be expensive, time-consuming, and painful. False-positive results are more common in younger women, those with dense breasts, those that had earlier breast biopsies, those with family history of breast cancer, and women taking estrogen. The chance for a false-positive result increases with the number of mammograms a woman has undergone. Over 50% of women screened yearly, over 10 years, experience a false-positive result, and many then undergo a biopsy.
- *Overdiagnosis and overtreatment* – ductal carcinoma-in-situ and small cancers that are symptomatic or non-life-threatening can be excessively diagnosed. Treatment results in "overtreatment."
- *False-negative results* – occur when mammograms appear normal, but breast cancer is actually present. Screening mammograms miss about 20% of breast cancers. False-negative

results can delay treatment and provide a false sense of security to the patient. These results may be due to high breast density, and occur more in younger women due to more breast density than older women.

Significant Point

Diagnostic mammography takes a longer time than screening mammography, and the total dose of radiation is higher since more X-ray images are required, from several angles. Technologists can magnify suspicious areas, producing a detailed picture that greatly aids in accurate diagnoses.

Clinical Case

1. How is a screening mammogram performed?
2. According to the American Cancer Society, what are the guidelines for screening mammograms for a 40-year-old woman?
3. What are the four classifications of breast density?

A 40-year-old woman underwent a screening mammogram, which showed an abnormality in her right breast, which was not palpable. Surgical biopsy revealed a 0.9-cm grade 4B infiltrating ductal carcinoma, with associated ductal carcinoma-in-situ. There were cancer cells found at the posterior margin. Because the cancer was multicentric, breast conservation surgery could not be done, and a mastectomy had to be performed, followed by reconstructive surgery. Since the woman was in good overall health, she was able to recover very well with no serious adverse events. She continues to live a normal life, and has had no recurrence of cancer over three years of follow-up.

Answers:

1. **The mammogram machine uses X-rays that are of lower, safer doses than those used in traditional X-rays. Since these X-rays do not penetrate breast tissue easily, the machine has two plates, which are used to flatten or compress the breast. This spreads the tissues apart and provides a better image. A screening mammogram uses X-rays of each breast, usually from two different angles, to find any signs of breast cancer when there are no symptoms or problems. The two views of each breast are as follows: one from above (cranial–caudal view), and one from an oblique or angled view (mediolateral–oblique view).**

2. **Actually, for a woman who is 40–49 years of age with average risk for breast cancer, she should be given the choice to start having screening mammograms every year if desired. Risks and benefits must be considered.**

3. **According to the BI-RADS reporting system, breast density is classified as group 1 (almost all fatty tissue), group 2 (scattered areas of dense fibrous and glandular tissue), group 3 (more of the breast consists of dense fibrous and glandular tissue, known as being heterogeneously dense – this makes it hard to see small tumors in or around the dense tissue), and group 4 (extremely dense, making it very hard to see tumors in the tissue).**

Nuclear Medicine

Nuclear medicine is an area of medical specialty, in which artificial radionuclides are applied for the diagnosis, therapy, and biomedical research of cancer. These radioactive drugs bind to cancer cells and destroy them. Nuclear medicine helps with cancer staging and treatment effectiveness determinations. It can usually be done on an outpatient basis and is painless. Some of the most common nuclear medicine scans for cancer include the following:

- Bone scans – for cancers that may have metastasized from other sites; they discover bone changes much earlier than X-rays can; they are performed a few hours after a tracer is administered; the radionuclide takes 2–3 hours to be absorbed and the patient is asked to drink a lot of water to flush out excessive tracer that does not accumulate in the bones; the actual scan takes about 60 minutes
- Gallium scans – use Gallium-67 as a tracer, to find cancer in certain organs or the entire body; there may be several days between the injection of Gallium and the actual scan, and some patients must be scanned more than once; each individual scan takes 30–60 minutes
- Multigated acquisition (MUGA) scans – monitors heart function before, during, and after certain chemotherapies; adverse heart affects may require a change in chemotherapy; patients should not smoke or drink caffeinated beverages for 24 hours before these scans; for these scans, the patient lies on a flat table and the scanning camera is positioned above the chest; MUGA scans can take up to three hours based on the number of images that are required
- PET scans – usually use a form of radioactive glucose, with cancer cells taking up larger amounts than normal cells; the patient cannot consume any sweetened liquids for several hours before the test; after the patient waits for one hour to allow the tracer to collect, the actual scan takes about 20–30 minutes
- Thyroid scans – radioactive iodine is swallowed by the patient, which eventually collects in the thyroid gland, for diagnosis as well as treatment of thyroid cancer; the patient must avoid iodine-containing substances, and be evaluated for any allergies to iodine or

seafood; the patient takes the radioactive tracer as a pill or liquid about 24 hours before the procedure. For a thyroid scan, the patient sits in a chair and faces the scanner, which is placed in front of the neck; the patient's chin rests on top of the scanner, and the scan takes less than 30 minutes

The results of nuclear scans are usually available in a few days. Another type of tracer, a *synthetic monoclonal antibody*, may be used in a scan since it adheres to substances on cancer cell surfaces. A radioactive substance is attached to the **monoclonal antibody**, which is injected IV. Once reaching tumor cells, they "light up" when viewed through a specialized scanner.

Images are based on metabolism and body chemistry instead of physical structures. Liquid radionuclides, which release low levels of radiation are used as *tracers*, and are also called **radiopharmaceuticals**. Tissues affected by cancer may absorb more or less of the tracers. Specialized cameras use the pattern of radioactivity to create images showing where the tracers travel and collect. Tumors can be revealed as *hot spots* – areas of increased cellular activity and tracer uptake. Sometimes, tumors appear as *cold spots* – areas of less cellular activity and decreased uptake. Nuclear scans do not always reveal extremely small tumors, and are not always able to identify malignancy from a benign tumor. The images are not extremely detailed, but nuclear scans can reveal certain tissue and organ abnormalities. Nuclear scans are often used with other types of imaging. For example, if a bone scan reveals skeletal hot spots, X-rays of the affected bones are then performed since they show structural details more clearly.

Tracers may be administered orally or intravenously. They collect over a few seconds in many circumstances but may take several days for this to occur. Gamma rays are sent out and then picked up by a *gamma camera, rectilinear scanner*, or **scintiscan**. A computer processes the signals into 2D or 3D images, sometimes with color to increase the clarity.

Significant Point

Nuclear medicine is a therapy option for patients with meningiomas, neuroendocrine tumors, lymphoma, prostate cancer, and thyroid cancer. Options include radioimmunotherapy (for non-Hodgkin lymphoma, prostate cancer, melanoma, leukemia, colorectal cancer, and high-grade brain glioma), radioactive iodine therapy (for thyroid cancer), brachytherapy (for bile duct, brain, breast, cervical, and many other cancers), and Y90 radioembolization (for liver cancer).

Clinical Case

1. What are the indications for nuclear medicine?
2. What are the various types of nuclear medicine?
3. How do tumors appear in thyroid scans?

A 73-year-old woman told her physician about a lump in her neck and difficulty to swallow. Physical examination revealed a palpable, non-tender neck mass. Laboratory testing revealed normal thyroid-stimulating hormone levels. An ultrasound revealed a 3-cm mass in the right lobe of the thyroid gland, and there were three lymph nodes ranging from 0.2 to 0.8 cm in diameter. An ultrasound-guided fine-needle aspiration biopsy of the thyroid mass was performed, and papillary thyroid carcinoma was diagnosed. A thyroid scan allowed visualization of the entire mass to determine resectability. A total thyroidectomy was performed, and the diseased lymph nodes were also removed. The patient underwent treatment with an ablative dose of radioactive iodine, and levothyroxine was started. Within six months, her hormone levels had normalized, and she had no other medical problems.

Answers:

1. **In nuclear medicine, artificial radionuclides are applied for the diagnosis, therapy, and biomedical research of cancer. These radioactive drugs bind to cancer cells and destroy them.**
2. **The various types of nuclear medicine include bone scans, gallium scans, multigated acquisition (MUGA) scans, PET scans, and thyroid scans.**
3. **Tumors can be revealed as hot spots – areas of increased cellular activity and tracer uptake, or as cold spots – areas of less cellular activity and decreased uptake.**

Endoscopy

Endoscopy is a diagnostic procedure that allows for the visualization of internal organs and cavities of the body with an endoscope. The GI structures that can be examined through the procedure include the esophagus, stomach, duodenum, colon, pancreas, and the biliary tract with the aid of X-ray film and fluoroscopy. Endoscopy can also be used to obtain samples for cytological and histological examination and to follow the course of a disease. An *upper endoscopy* allows the examination of the esophagus, stomach, and duodenum. An endoscope is used in the procedure. It is a thin, flexible tube with a light and a small camera on its end. The endoscope is inserted into the mouth, down the throat, and into the esophagus. Images are viewed on a screen to search for tumors or other abnormalities. There is also a channel through the endoscope that allows tools to be passed to remove tissue samples, for later examination under a microscope. Some endoscopes use colored light to find precancerous conditions in the lining of the esophagus. This is called *narrow band imaging*. Most often, endoscopic procedures are performed by gastroenterologists. Before the procedure, the patient may be required to avoid eating foods or drinking anything, including water, for up to eight hours prior. The stomach and duodenum must be totally empty. Also, the patient may be required to avoid taking aspirin or other OTC pain medications for seven days prior, since they can increase the risk of bleeding during the procedure.

During the upper endoscopy, the patient is given anesthesia and a sedative through an intravenous needle. The anesthesia blocks the awareness of pain while the sedative relaxes the patient. The throat of the patient may be sprayed with a local anesthetic to numb it, or the patient may receive a liquid anesthetic to gargle with, to help prevent gagging. A mouthpiece may be inserted to hold the mouth open during the procedure. The patient lies either on the left side or on the back. As the endoscope is inserted there is a slight pressure throughout the esophagus. The endoscope inflates the stomach by blowing air inside it, allowing for better imaging of the stomach lining. The patient can breathe without assistance during the procedure, and often falls asleep. An upper endoscopy usually takes 20–30 minutes. The endoscope is gently removed after the procedure and the patient is taken to a recovery room. After the procedure, the patient remains awake for up to two hours as the medications' effects wear off. He or she is not allowed to drive a vehicle, so someone else must take the patient home. Usually, patients can return to normal activities the following day. Adverse effects of the procedure may include a sore throat, bloating or cramping due to the air blown into the stomach, and some discomfort from lying still for a long time. Rare but serious adverse effects include severe pain in the throat or chest, fever, shortness of breath, and difficulty swallowing.

A *lower endoscopy* allows for the visualization of the lower GI tract, which includes the rectum, sigmoid colon, and other parts of the colon. If the colon and rectum are examined, this is known as a **colonoscopy**, which can reveal polyps or tumors such as adenomas or malignant tumors (see Figure 13.7). Prior to a colonoscopy, the patient may not be allowed to eat, and can only drink clear liquids for 1–3 days. Usually, there are only clear liquids for one day, and sometimes other dietary changes, on an individualized basis. Laxatives or an enema may also be prescribed. The procedure takes 30 minutes or longer. For both a colonoscopy and sigmoidoscopy, the patient lies on the left side. A sedative is given for a colonoscopy via an IV line. The endoscope is inserted into the rectum, sometimes causing pressure and cramping. The endoscope transmits images to a video screen, which can be printed out. Biopsies, polyp removal, or other treatments may be done. After the procedure, the patient is allowed to rest. There may be some discomfort due to trapped air, which is relieved by changing position and passing the air. **Sigmoidoscopy** is the inspection of the rectum and sigmoid colon by the aid of a sigmoidoscope. This procedure usually takes about 20 minutes. Sigmoidoscopy usually does not require a sedative.

The most common types of endoscopies are listed in Table 13.2.

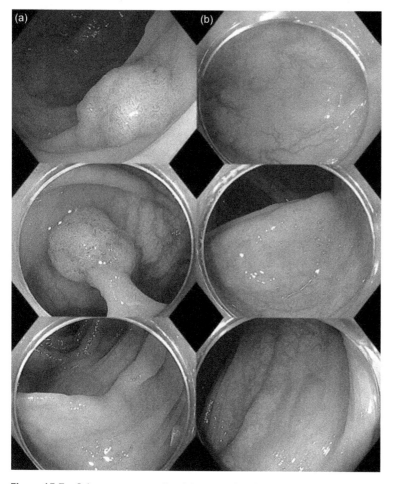

Figure 13.7 Colonoscopy, revealing (a) conventional tubular/tubulovillous adenomas; (b) sessile serrated adenomas. *Source*: Figure 1 from Wiley Online Library – Internal Medicine Journal – Clinical Perspectives [55].

Table 13.2 Common types of endoscopy.

Procedure	Area or organ viewed
Anoscopy	Anus and/or rectum
Arthroscopy	Joints
Bronchoscopy	Trachea and lungs
Colonoscopy	Colon and large intestine
Colposcopy	Vagina and cervix
Cystoscopy	Bladder
Esophagoscopy	Esophagus
Gastroscopy	Stomach and duodenum
Laparoscopy	Stomach, liver, female reproductive organs
Laryngoscopy	Larynx
Neuroendoscopy	Areas of the brain
Proctoscopy, sigmoidoscopy	Rectum and sigmoid colon
Thoracoscopy	Pleura and structures covering the heart

Clinical Case

1. What is narrow band imaging as used in endoscopy?
2. What are indications of upper endoscopy?
3. What are the potential adverse effects of this procedure?

A 59-year-old woman underwent an upper endoscopy to assess symptoms that included difficulty swallowing, chest pain, chronic coughing, stomach pain, and nausea. She was diagnosed with a 7-cm esophageal squamous cell carcinoma that involved over two-third of the circumference of the esophageal lumen. The patient had concurrent chronic obstructive pulmonary disease making her of high risk for surgical resection. Therefore, an endoscopic en-bloc resection was performed, and the entire tumor was able to be removed. Even though the tumor was large in size, it was still a superficial T1a cancer, and the endoscopic resection was curative. The patient remains cancer free to date.

Answers:

1. **Some endoscopes use colored light to find precancerous conditions in the lining of the esophagus. This is called** *narrow band imaging.*
2. **Upper endoscopy is indicated for the examination of the esophagus, stomach, and duodenum for a variety of conditions that include cancer, gastritis, and ulcers; as well as to obtain samples for cytological and histological examination.**
3. **Adverse effects of an upper endoscopy may include a sore throat, bloating or cramping due to the air blown into the stomach, and some discomfort from lying still for a long time. Rare but serious adverse effects include severe pain in the throat or chest, fever, shortness of breath, and difficulty swallowing.**

Endoscopic Retrograde Cholangiopancreatography

Endoscopic retrograde cholangiopancreatography (ERCP) is a procedure combining upper endoscopy with X-rays to treat abnormalities of the bile ducts and pancreatic ducts. This procedure is performed when the bile or pancreatic ducts have been narrowed or blocked due to gallstones, infections, pancreatitis, trauma, surgical complications, pancreatic pseudocysts, and tumors or cancers. Before the procedure, the patient may be asked to stop taking medications that affect blood clotting or that may interact with sedatives. During the ERCP procedure, sedatives are usually used for the patient's comfort. The patient receives a liquid anesthetic gargle or spray to prevent gagging. General anesthesia is used. This procedure can be performed on a pregnant patient as long as precautions are taken to protect the fetus from radiation. The patient lies on the examination table and the endoscope is passed all the way down the esophagus and stomach to reach the duodenum. Images send video to a monitor, and air is pumped into the stomach and duodenum for better visualization.

The specialist locates the opening where the bile and pancreatic ducts empty into the duodenum. A catheter is slid through the endoscope and into the ducts. A contrast medium is injected to make the duct more easily visible. Fluoroscopy is used to examine the ducts and search for blockages or narrowed areas. Other tools may be passed through the endoscope to open blocked or narrowed ducts, break up or remove stones, perform a biopsy, remove ductal tumors, or to insert stents to hold the ducts open. Also, temporary stents can be inserted to stop bile leaks occurring after gallbladder surgery. The ERCP procedure usually takes 1–2 hours. The patient remains in recovery for 1–2 hours, requires a person to drive him or her home, and may require overnight hospitalization. Adverse effects may include bloating, nausea, and sore throat. The day after the procedure, the patient can return to a normal diet, but should remain at home and rest. Potential complications of ERCP include pancreatitis, infection, hemorrhage, respiratory or cardiac problems, perforations, tissue damage from X-ray exposure, and only rarely, death. Patients with complications are usually treated in a hospital. Patients must call their physician if they have blood or black stools, chest pain, fever, worsening abdominal pain, breathing problems, swallowing problems, intensifying throat pain, and vomiting – especially if it is bloody or very dark in color. The ERCP procedure is most useful in the diagnosis of esophageal, stomach, intestinal, gallbladder, pancreatic, bile duct, or liver cancers.

Biopsy

A biopsy is the removal of a small piece of living tissue from an organ or other parts of the body for microscopic examination to confirm or establish a diagnosis, estimate prognosis, or follow the course of a disease. This procedure is the primary method of diagnosing most types of cancer. A biopsy may be recommended when something suspicious is found during a physical examination or other tests. The type of biopsy that is needed is based on the location of a possible tumor. There are a variety of different types of biopsies, which include the following:

- Image-guided biopsy – used when a tumor cannot be palpated, or when the area is deep inside the body; a needle is guided to the tumor location via one of the imaging techniques listed below; the actual biopsy of choice can use a fine needle, core, or vacuum-assisted technique, based on the amount of tissue needed and possible diagnosis.
  - Ultrasound-guided biopsy
  - Fluoroscopy-guided biopsy
  - CT-guided biopsy
  - X-ray-guided biopsy
  - MRI-guided biopsy
- Vacuum-assisted biopsy – a suction device collects a tissue sample through a special needle; multiple or large samples can be collected; it may or may not require imaging guidance

- Shave biopsy – a sharp tool is used to remove tissue from the surface of the skin
- Punch biopsy – a sharp, circular tool is inserted into the skin, and a sample is taken from below the skin surface
- Laparoscopic biopsy – a thin tube with a video camera (a laparoscope) is inserted into the abdomen through a small incision, to view abnormal areas; a small needle can also be inserted to take tissue samples
- Bone marrow aspiration and biopsy – bone marrow aspiration removes a sample of bone marrow fluid with a needle, while bone marrow biopsy removes a small amount of solid tissue, also with a needle; these procedures assess for blood disorders or cancers, which include leukemia, lymphoma, and multiple myeloma; the pelvic bone is a common site that is used
- Liquid biopsy – a minimally invasive procedure that tests blood samples for cancer; it is less risky than a tissue biopsy and can be performed multiple times; it can also allow assessment of tumor progress and success of treatment; currently, this procedure is not commonly done for most cancer patients

Biopsies are performed by a variety of health care practitioners, based on the area of the body being examined. These individuals include surgeons, radiologists, oncologists, gastroenterologists, dermatologists, gynecologists, family practice physicians, and other specialists. For many biopsy procedures, the patient lies on his or her stomach or back, or may even be allowed to sit up. The patient may be required to hold the breath as the needle is inserted, and remain still. Usually, some type of anesthesia is used. Local anesthesia is injected into the specific area. Conscious sedation or monitored anesthesia is injected intravenously and may be combined with a local or regional anesthesia. Minimally invasive biopsies require no recovery time. More invasive procedures may require some amount of recovery time. If sedation is used along with anesthesia, the patient will usually need someone to drive him or her home. The patient should contact the biopsy facility if he or she develops an infection, severe pain, fever, or

bleeding. Results of a biopsy are often given within 2–3 days, but a result requiring a more complicated analysis may take 7–10 days. Chapter 14 discusses biopsy techniques such as *fine-needle aspiration, core-needle biopsy, open biopsy*, and *endoscopic biopsies* in greater detail.

Lumbar Puncture

A **lumbar puncture**, or *spinal tap*, evaluates intracranial pressure as well as CSF composition. It can assess diseases, infections, CNS cancer, leukemia, and multiple sclerosis. Lumbar puncture allows for the therapeutic reduction of intracranial pressure, and also the administration of radiopaque agents for **myelography**, and intrathecal drugs. The entire procedure usually takes about 30 minutes to perform. For lumbar puncture, the patient is usually placed in the lateral decubitus position (see Figure 13.8). For a patient who cannot maintain this position, assistants may be needed to help hold the patient's body. Sometimes, the spine is better flexed if the patient (especially if obese) sits on the side of the bed and leans over a tray table. A puncture site of about 20 cm in diameter is cleaned with iodine, and then wiped with sterile gauze. This prevents the iodine from entering the subarachnoid space.

A lumbar puncture needle, with a *stylet*, is inserted into the L3–L4 interspace. The needle is pointed rostrally, toward the patient's umbilicus, and kept perfectly parallel to the floor. As the needle enters into the subarachnoid space, there is usually an audible popping sound. The stylet is removed, allowing CSF to flow outward. The opening pressure is measured with a *manometer*. Four tubes are filled with approximately 2–10 ml of CSF. The puncture site is covered with a sterile adhesive strip. Up to 10% of patients experience a post-lumbar puncture headache. Hydration is the mainstay of its treatment and prevention. When the CSF is normal, it is clear and lacks color. It will be cloudy or turbid if there are 300 or more cells per microliter, which may suggest bacterial meningitis. Bloody fluid may indicate a traumatic puncture or subarachnoid hemorrhage.

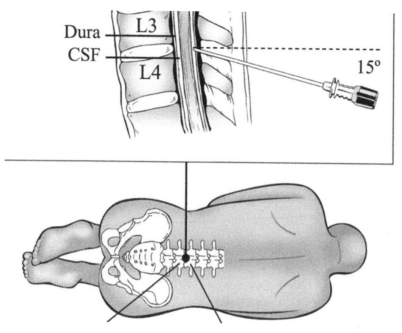

Figure 13.8 Lumbar puncture location between L3 and L4, and a patient in the lateral decubitus position. *Source:* Alzheimer's Association – Alzheimer's & Dementia: Diagnosis, Assessment & Disease Monitoring – CSF Biomarker [1].

Significant Point

Lumbar punctures are not usually done to diagnose brain tumors. However, they may be performed to determine the extent of a tumor by looking for cancer cells in the CSF. They are often done when a tumor has previously been diagnosed as an ependymoma or another type that commonly spreads through the CSF. These tumors include medulloblastomas, germ cell tumors, pineal parenchymal tumors, and gliomas.

Clinical Case

1. What can a lumbar puncture assess?
2. What position is used for lumbar puncture?

3. Where is the lumbar puncture needle inserted, and how much CSF is collected?

A 76-year-old woman complained of increasing leg numbness and weakness. An MRI revealed a pia mater intramedullary lesion of the high thoracic spine. To assess the extent of any cancer cells, a lumbar puncture was performed. The cancer cells found in the CSF indicated that the spinal cancer was metastatic from the lungs. Surgery was performed for the spinal tumor, and the patient's symptoms subsided. There was no spinal recurrence over three months of follow-up, and the patient began radiation therapy for the lung tumor. She responded well, with only slight nausea and tiredness.

Answers:

1. **A lumbar puncture can assess CNS infections, and other conditions. These include brain cancer, spinal**

cancer, leukemia, and non-cancerous conditions such as meningitis, inflammation, and multiple sclerosis.

2. The patient is usually placed in the lateral decubitus position. For a patient who cannot maintain this position, an assistant may be needed to help hold the patient's body. Sometimes, the spine is better flexed if the patient (especially if obese) sits on the side of the bed and leans over a tray table.

3. A lumbar puncture needle, with a stylet, is inserted into the L3–L4 interspace. The needle is pointed rostrally, toward the patient's umbilicus, and kept perfectly parallel to the floor. When the stylet is removed, the cerebrospinal fluid flows outward, and four tubes are filled with approximately 2–10 milliliters of CSF.

Hematology Tests

There are a variety of hematology tests used to diagnose cancer. They include the *complete blood count (CBC)*, *blood protein tests*, *tumor marker tests*, and *circulating tumor cell tests*. The CBC measures various types of blood cells in a sample of the patient's blood. Blood cancers can be detected if there are too many or too few cells of certain leukocytes, or if abnormal cells are found. Confirmation of this test and other blood tests may be done by bone marrow biopsy. For blood protein testing, **electrophoresis** is used to examine proteins in the blood. Figure 13.9 shows different serum protein electrophoresis (SPEP) for a normal patient and a patient with multiple myeloma. Abnormal immunoglobulins are elevated in the multiple myeloma patient known as a distinctive "M-spike."

In tumor marker tests, the focus is on finding tumor markers in the blood, which are manufactured by tumor cells. However, tumor markers are also produced by some normal cells, and levels can be highly elevated even without the presence of cancer, limiting the potential for tumor marker tests being accurate. Only rarely are these tests sufficient to confirm cancer being present. Examples of tumor markers include PSA, cancer antigen 125 (for ovarian cancer), calcitonin (for medullary thyroid cancer), alpha-fetoprotein (for liver cancer), and human chorionic gonadotropin (HCG) for ovarian and testicular cancers.

Circulating tumor cell tests are relatively new, and detect cancer cells that have broken away from the original site of cancer and are circulating through the bloodstream. These are also known as **liquid biopsies**, approved by the FDA

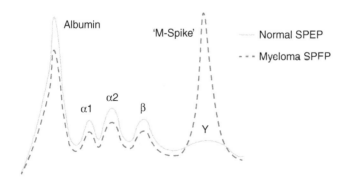

Figure 13.9 Multiple myeloma serum protein electrophoresis. Note the differences in peaks between a normal patient (solid line) and a multiple myeloma patient (dotted line), with the distinctive "M-spike," which indicates excessive immunoglobulin. *Source*: Wiley Online Library – European Journal of Haematology – Review Article [56].

to guide treatment decisions for cancer patients including *Guardant360 CDx* and *FoundationOne Liquid CDx*. They utilize genetic changes in tumors as a treatment-guiding feature. Targeted therapies and immunotherapies work the best against tumors with specific **genetic chambers** that identify genetic changes such as mutations. They accomplish this by scanning DNA shed into the blood by the tumors, which is called **cell-free DNA**. Both of these tests were approved in 2020 for patients with any solid cancer, including lung and prostate cancer, but not for actual blood cancers. Liquid biopsies are sometimes an alternative to traditional biopsies, and are less invasive and faster to perform. Specifically, Guardant360 CDx was approved for non-small cell lung cancer and can assess changes in over 60 different genes. FoundationOne Liquid CDx was approved for non-small cell lung cancer as well as prostate cancer, assesses **microsatellite instability**, and can identify changes in over 300 genes.

Significant Point

The new liquid biopsies have been shown to be accurate in 93% of blood samples, and can accurately predict where in the patient's body that the cancer first developed – in 96% of the samples. The false-positive rate is only 0.7%. This means that less than 1% of patients have an inaccurate diagnosis of cancer from using these tests. Earlier detection of over 50% of cancers could save millions of lives every year, on a global scale.

Clinical Case

1. What are the common hematology tests used to diagnose cancer?
2. What is the relationship between electrophoresis and multiple myeloma?
3. What do circulating tumor cell tests (liquid biopsies) detect?

A 55-year-old man visits his physician, complaining of fatigue after any type of physical exertion. Blood tests reveal low hemoglobin levels. A SPEP was then performed, showing a monoclonal immunoglobulin A protein of 1.5 grams per deciliter. A bone scan revealed occult lytic lesions in the patient's skull and in both humeri bones. A bone marrow biopsy showed 30% involvement by abnormal plasma cells. The diagnosis was multiple myeloma.

Answers:

1. **The common hematology tests used to diagnose cancer include the CBC, blood protein tests, tumor marker tests, and circulating tumor cell tests.**
2. **For blood protein testing, electrophoresis is used to examine proteins in the blood. In cases of multiple myeloma, abnormal immunoglobulins may be elevated.**
3. **Liquid biopsies detect cancer cells that have broken away from the original site of cancer and are circulating through the bloodstream. They utilize genetic changes in tumors as a treatment-guiding feature. Liquid biopsies are sometimes and alternative to traditional biopsies, and are less invasive and faster to perform. The two newly approved tests can assess and identify changes in over 60–300 different genes.**

Urinalysis

Urinalysis provides information on body function, and is often used in the diagnosis of cancer. Potential signs of cancer include hematuria. The presence of bilirubin in the urine may indicate liver cancer, or that a bile duct is blocked by a tumor. An increased number of epithelial cells in the urine can also be an indication of cancer, though this condition can also indicate infection or inflammation. When abnormal urinalysis results occur, a follow-up urinalysis may be ordered for confirmation of the abnormality, or other tests may be performed.

While bladder cancer is the most obvious type of cancer to find in urine, there can also be remnants of cervical, kidney, and prostate cancer present. The two primary ways for cancer cells to move into the urine is through the kidneys, or from the bladder and ureters. Molecules that are able to pass through the filtering system of the kidneys and enter the bladder must be very small. Therefore, they are usually molecular building blocks such as proteins, which are part of cancer cells. Another clue does not come directly from a tumor. New studies show that the human papillomavirus, responsible for most cases of cervical cancer, can be detected in the urine. More significant clues include actual cancer cells or their DNA. If these are present in the urine, they have traveled directly from the bladder or ureters.

According to the Translational Genomics Research Institute in February of 2021, a study was conducted that determined that cell-free DNA in urine is a possible method of detecting cancer. The study focused on the analysis of short strands of cell-free DNA in urine. It is now known that these **DNA fragments** are not randomly degraded, and indicate a difference between a healthy patient and one that has developed cancer. Tissue samples were evaluated, which came from children with various types of cancer, and from adults with pancreatic cancer. Certain regions of the genome are protected from fragmentation in the urine of healthy individuals. However, the same regions of the genome are more fragmented if cancer is present. The differences in the fragmentation between various test subjects were very small. The lengths of the DNA fragments were similar, and the regions of the genome where the fragmentation occurred were consistent. The new discovery will likely help people with all types of cancers, but is extremely encouraging for pancreatic cancer patients. The next step is to test much larger populations of cancer patients, identifying differences in the findings between genders, ages, and when other conditions are present concurrently.

Significant Point

The most significant sign of cancer when a urinalysis is performed is the presence of blood. Fortunately, only about 20% of people with blood in the urine actually have cancer. A relatively new discovery is that three key proteins linked to *pancreatic cancer* can be present in the urine. This has great promise for being a way to find this cancer earlier, which until this time has not often occurred, resulting in the death of most patients with the disease.

Clinical Case

1. What types of cancer may be discovered via urinalysis?
2. What does it mean if actual cancer cells or their DNA are present in the urine?
3. What is the significance of the recent discovery of cell-free DNA in the urine?

A 27-year-old man went to his local emergency department after seeing blood in his urine. He stated that he has had no problems urinating, but has experienced slight abdominal pain for the past four months. His family history includes colon cancer (his father). The patient had no history of smoking, and only drinks alcohol at social events occasionally. Urinalysis revealed tumor cells to be present, which resemble those of adenocarcinoma. A CT scan identified a partially calcified mass at the dome of the urinary bladder, plus infiltration of the adjacent lower abdominal mesentery. A cystoscopy with transurethral resection of the bladder tumor was performed. A right ureteral stent was placed, and the bladder tissue was biopsied. Unfortunately, it was too extensive to be completely resected. The diagnosis was of a primary mucinous adenocarcinoma of the bladder.

Answers:

1. **Aside from bladder cancer, urinalysis is able to detect liver, bile duct, cervical, kidney, and prostate cancers.**

2. **The presence of actual cancer cells or their DNA in the urine means that they have traveled directly from the bladder or ureters.**

3. **Cell-free DNA in urine is a possible method of detecting cancer. Short strands of cell-free DNA are not randomly degraded, and indicate a difference between a healthy patient and one that has developed cancer. Certain regions of the genome are protected from fragmentation in the urine of healthy individuals. However, the same regions of the genome are more fragmented if cancer is present.**

Genetic Testing

Genetic testing is a procedure that searches for specifically inherited variants in an individual's genes. Genetic variants may result in beneficial or neutral effects, but also harmful, uncertain, and unknown effects upon disease development. Harmful genetic variants are linked to an increased risk of cancer. Inherited genetic variants contribute to 5–10% of all cancers. In some families, cancers occur in several members, yet may not be due to an inherited genetic variant. Shared environments or lifestyles such as tobacco use may cause similar cancers to develop among family members. However, the types of cancer that develop, non-cancerous conditions that occur, and ages when the cancer usually develop may be suggestive of an inherited susceptibility to cancer. Genetic testing can also be performed to determine whether family members that have not yet developed a cancer have the same inherited genetic variant as another family member known to carry a cancer susceptibility predisposing

variant. **Tumor DNA sequencing** is another type of genetic testing that can be done to assess if cancer cells of diagnosed individuals have genetic changes that may be used to guide treatment. Most of these cancer cell changes occur randomly. The factors that determine whether an individual with a genetic variant will actually develop cancer include the **penetrance** of the variant, and the varied **expressivity** of a hereditary cancer syndrome. Lifestyle and environment also influence disease expression. There are over 50 hereditary cancer syndromes. Most are due to harmful variants inherited in an autosomal dominant fashion. For most of these syndromes, genetic testing is available. Tests are also available for some inherited genetic variants not associated with identified syndromes, but which also increase cancer risk. These include inherited variants in the following genes:

- *BRIP1* – increased risk of ovarian cancer
- *CHEK2* – increased risks of breast and colorectal cancers
- *PALB2* – increased risks of breast and pancreatic cancers
- *RAD51C* and *RAD51D* – increased risk of ovarian cancer

People that should consider genetic testing for risks of cancer are those in which the personal or family histories include the following:

- Cancer diagnosed at an unusually young age
- Several different types of cancer in the same individual
- Cancer in both of a set of paired organs, such as the breasts or kidneys
- Several first-degree relatives with the same type of cancer, family members with breast or ovarian cancer, and family members with colon and endometrial cancer
- Unusual cases of a specific cancer type, such as male breast cancer
- Presence of birth defects that are associated with inherited cancer syndromes, such as benign skin growths and skeletal abnormalities linked to neurofibromatosis type 1 (NF1)

- Having a racial or ethnic background with increased risks to an inherited cancer susceptibility syndrome, and one or more of the above features
- Having several family members with cancer

Any family member that actually has or had cancer should receive genetic testing first, since it is more informative, followed by other family members to see if they share the same genetic traits. Genetic counseling is recommended before any genetic testing for a hereditary cancer syndrome. It may also be performed after genetic testing, especially when a positive result occurs. Genetic counseling covers may aspects of genetic testing, including:

- Hereditary cancer risk assessments
- Appropriateness, benefits, and harms of testing
- Implications of positive, negative, and uncertain results
- Possibilities that a test may find a variant whose effect upon cancer risk is unknown
- Psychological risks and benefits of genetic test results
- Risk of passing genetic variants to children

- Family impact of genetic testing
- The most appropriate tests to perform
- Explanation of the actual tests, their accuracy, and their interpretation

Genetic testing is performed on a small sample of body fluids or tissues – usually blood cells, and sometimes saliva cells from the inside of the cheek. Also, skin cells are sometimes tested. Results usually take several weeks or more to be returned.

A *positive result* means that a genetic variant associated with an inherited cancer susceptibility syndrome was found. There is an increased risk of developing cancer in the future, which may be lowered by more frequent follow-ups, medications, surgeries, changing lifestyle choices, and making decisions about having offspring. A *negative result* means that no specific variant was found. A *true negative* result does not mean there is no cancer risk, but that the risk is probably nearly the same as for the general population. In a *variant of uncertain significance*, the result does not clarify risks and is usually not considered in making health-care decisions. In a *benign variant* result, there is no association with any increased risk of cancer.

Key Terms

Anode
Atomic number
Biopsy
Cardiac angioplasty
Cathode
Cell-free DNA
Colonoscopy
Computed tomography
CT angiography
CT colonography
Diagnostic mammogram
Digital breast tomosynthesis
DNA fragments
Doppler effect

Doppler ultrasonography
Duplex ultrasonography
Electrophoresis
Endoscopy
Expressivity
Fluoroscopy
Gadolinium
Gantry
Genetic chambers
Grayscale image
Helical CT
Kinetic energy
Liquid biopsies
Lumbar puncture

Magnetic resonance imaging
Mammography
Microsatellite instability
Monoclonal antibody
Myelography
Nuclear medicine
Penetrance
Positron emission tomography
Positrons

Radiopharmaceuticals
Scintiscan
Screening mammogram
Sigmoidoscopy
Tomographic images
Transrectal ultrasonography
Tumor DNA sequencing
Whirring

Bibliography

1 Alzheimer's Association – Alzheimer's & Dementia: Diagnosis, Assessment & Disease Monitoring – CSF Biomarker. (2017). *Consensus guidelines for lumbar puncture in patients with neurological diseases.* John Wiley & Sons, Inc. https://alz-journals.onlinelibrary.wiley.com/doi/full/10.1016/j.dadm 8 (1): 111–126, Figure 3. Accessed 2021.

2 American Cancer Society and International Agency for Research on Cancer. (2016). *Breast Cancer Screening Guidelines for Women.* Columbus Regional Health. https://www.crh.org/docs/default-source/default-document-library/breast-cancer-screening-guidelines.pdf?sfvrsn=65d326a1_0 Accessed 2021.

3 American Cancer Society. (2021). *Understanding Your Mammogram Report.* American Cancer Society, Inc. https://www.cancer.org/cancer/breast-cancer/screening-tests-and-early-detection/mammograms/understanding-your-mammogram-report.html Accessed 2021.

4 American Cancer Society (ACS) Journals - Cancer. (2000). *High grade surface osteosarcoma – A clinicopathologic study of 46 cases.* John Wiley & Sons, Inc. https://acsjournals.onlinelibrary.wiley.com/doi/full/10.1002/(SICI)1097-0142(19990301)85:5%3C1044::AID-CNCR6%3E3.0.CO;2-A. Figure 2 (left image only). Accessed 2021.

5 American Cancer Society (ACS) Journals – Cancer. (2000). *Positron emission tomography scanning in malignant melanoma – Clinical utility in patients with Stage III disease.* John Wiley & Sons, Inc. https://acsjournals.online library.wiley.com/doi/full/10.1002/1097-0142%2820000901%2989%3A5%3C1019%3A%3AAID-CNCR11%3E3.0.CO%3B2-0. 89 (5): 1019–1025, Figure 1. Accessed 2021.

6 Atlas, S.W. (2016). *Magnetic Resonance Imaging of the Brain and Spine*, 5th Edition. Philadelphia: Lippincott, Williams, and Wilkins.

7 Baron, T.H., Kozarek, R.A., and Carr-Locke, D.L. (2018). *ERCP*, 3rd Edition. Amsterdam: Elsevier.

8 Bennett, P.A. (2020). *Diagnostic Imaging: Nuclear Medicine E-Book*, 3rd Edition. Amsterdam: Elsevier.

9 British Journal of Surgery (BJS) Society. (2011). *Randomized clinical trial comparing the effect of computed tomography in the trauma room versus the radiology department on injury outcomes.* John Wiley & Sons, Inc. https://bjssjournals.onlinelibrary.wiley.com/doi/abs/10.1002/bjs.7705. 99 (S1): 105–113. Accessed 2021.

10 Brun del Re, R. (2010). *Minimally Invasive Breast Biopsies (Recent Results in Cancer Research)*. New York: Springer.

11 Bushong, S.C. and Clarke, G. (2014). *Magnetic Resonance Imaging: Physical and Biological Principles*, 4th Edition. Maryland Heights: Mosby.

12 Chalazonitis, A., Feida, E., and Gkali, C. (2018). *Contrast Enhanced Digital Mammography: Basic Principles and Interpretation of Clinical Cases.* Riga (Latvia): Scholars' Press.

13 Chandrasekhara, V., Elmunzer, B.J., Khashab, M.A., and Muthusamy, V.R. (2018). *Clinical Gastrointestinal Endoscopy: Expert Consult*, 3rd Edition. Amsterdam: Elsevier.

14 Chun, H.J., Yang, S.K., and Choi, M.G. (2019). *Therapeutic Gastrointestinal Endoscopy: A Comprehensive Atlas*, 2nd Edition. New York: Springer.

15 Cohen, J. (2017). *Comprehensive Atlas of High-Resolution Endoscopy and Narrowband Imaging*, 2nd Edition. Hoboken: Wiley-Blackwell.

16 Cotton, P.B. and Leung, J.W. (2020). *ERCP: The Fundamentals*, 3rd Edition. Hoboken: Wiley-Blackwell.

17 Dattoli, M.J. (2019). *Advanced Imaging for Prostate Cancer: A Primer on 3D Color-Flow Power Doppler Ultrasound, Multiparametric MRI and CT Fusion Techniques*. Sarasota: Dattoli Cancer Foundation.

18 Deeg, K.H., Rupprecht, T., and Hofbeck, M. (2014). *Doppler Sonography in Infancy and Childhood*. New York: Springer.

19 DeMaio, D.N. (2017). *Mosby's Exam Review for Computed Tomography*, 3rd Edition. Maryland Heights: Mosby.

20 Dixon, A.M. (2007). *Breast Ultrasound: How, Why and When*. London: Churchill Livingstone.

21 Downey, R. (2020). *Lung Cancer: Advances in Diagnosis and Treatment*. Forest Hills: Foster Academics.

22 Epstein, J., Reuter, V., and Amin, M.B. (2016). *Biopsy Interpretation of the Bladder (Biopsy Interpretation Series)*, 3rd Edition. Philadelphia: Lippincott, Williams, and Wilkins.

23 Ganjel-Azar, P., Jorda, M., and Krishan, A. (2011). *Effusion Cytology: A Practical Guide to Cancer Diagnosis*. New York: Demos Medical Publishing.

24 Henson, J.W. and Resta, R.G. (2021). *Diagnosis and Management of Hereditary Cancer: Tabular-Based Clinical and Genetic Aspects*. Cambridge: Academic Press.

25 Hoda, S.A., Rosen, P.P., Brogi, E., and Koerner, F.C. (2017). *Rosen's Diagnosis of Breast Pathology by Needle Core Biopsy*, 4th Edition. Philadelphia: Lippincott, Williams, and Wilkins.

26 Juweid, M.E. and Hoekstra, O.S. (2011). *Positron Emission Tomography (Methods in Molecular Biology #727)*. Totowa: Humana Press.

27 Lee, L.S. (2015). *ERCP and EUS: A Case-Based Approach*. New York: Springer.

28 Lerner, S.P., Schoenberg, M.P., and Sternberg, C.N. (2015). *Bladder Cancer: Diagnosis and Clinical Management*. Hoboken: Wiley-Blackwell.

29 Lille, S. and Marshall, W. (2018). *Mammographic Imaging: A Practical Guide*, 4th Edition. Philadelphia: Lippincott, Williams, and Wilkins.

30 Metcalfe, P., Kron, T., and Hoban, P. (2007). *Physics of Radiotherapy X-Rays and Electrons*. Madison: Medical Physics Publishing.

31 Mettler, F.A. and Guiberteau, M.J. (2018). *Essentials of Nuclear Medicine and Molecular Imaging*, 7th Edition. Amsterdam: Elsevier.

32 Miller, L.C. and Lehmann, T.L. (2020). *Improving Mammography Image Quality: Two-Part Collection*. San Diego: Mammography Educators.

33 Mostbeck, G.H. (2012). *Duplex and Color Doppler Imaging of the Venous System (Medical Radiology Diagnostic Imaging)*. New York: Springer.

34 Muggia, F., Santin, A.D., and Oliva, E. (2018). *Uterine Cancer: Screening, Diagnosis, and Treatment*, 2nd Edition. *(Current Clinical Oncology Series)*. New York: Springer.

35 Mulhall, J.P. and Jenkins, L.C. (2016). *Atlas of Office Based Andrology Procedures*. New York: Springer.

36 O'Malley, J.P., Ziessman, H.A., and Thrall, J.H. (2020). *Nuclear Medicine and Molecular Imaging: The Requisites in Radiology*, 5th Edition. Amsterdam: Elsevier.

37 Patel, U. and Rickards, D. (2002). *Handbook of Transrectal Ultrasound and Biopsy of the Prostate*. Boca Raton: CRC Press.

38 Romans, L.E. (2018). *Computed Tomography for Technologists: A Comprehensive Text*, 2nd Edition. Philadelphia: Lippincott, Williams, and Wilkins.

39 Ruggieri, P. and Lakhani, A. (2018). *Colon & Rectal Cancer: From Diagnosis to Treatment*, 3rd Edition. Omaha: Addicus Books.

40 Russo, A., Giordano, A., and Rolfo, C. (2017). *Liquid Biopsy in Cancer Patients: The Hand Lens for Tumor Evolution (Current Clinical Pathology)*. Totowa: Humana Press.

41 Schaffner, F., Merlin, J.L., and von Bubnoff, N. (2020). *Tumor Liquid Biopsies (Recent Results in Cancer Research)*. New York: Springer.

42 Schiff, D., Arrillaga, I., and Wen, P.Y. (2018). *Cancer Neurology in Clinical Practice: Neurological Complications of Cancer and Its Treatment*, 3rd Edition. New York: Springer.

43 Science Daily. (2021). *Cell-free DNA in urine as potential method for cancer detection*. The Translational Genomics Research Institute. https://www.sciencedaily.com/releases/2021/02/210218094524.htm Accessed 2021.

44 Seeram, E. (2015). *Computed Tomography: Physical Principles, Clinical Applications, and Quality Control*, 4th Edition. Philadelphia: Saunders.

45 Seiberlich, N. and Gulani, V. (2020). *Quantitative Magnetic Resonance Imaging (Advances in Magnetic Resonance Technology and Applications Volume 1)*. Cambridge: Academic Press.

46 Shah, R.B. and Zhou, M. (2019). *Prostate Biopsy Interpretation: An Illustrated Guide*, 2nd Edition. New York: Springer.

47 Shaikh, K., Kirshnan, S., and Thanki, R. (2021). *Artificial Intelligence in Breast Cancer Early Detection and Diagnosis*. New York: Springer.

48 Shimada, H. (2019). *Biomarkers in Cancer Therapy: Liquid Biopsy Comes of Age*. New York: Springer.

49 Treglia, G. and Giovanella, L. (2020). *Evidence-based Positron Emission Tomography: Summary of Recent Meta-analyses on PET*. New York: Springer.

50 Van Meir, E.G. (2009). *CNS Cancer: Models, Markers, Prognostic Factors, Targets, and Therapeutic Approaches (Cancer Drug Discovery and Development)*. Totowa: Humana Press.

51 WHO Classification of Tumours Editorial Board. (2016). *WHO Classification of Tumours of the Central Nervous System*, 4th Edition. Geneva: World Health Organization.

52 Wiley Online Library – Respiratory Case Reports. (2019). *Computed tomography imaging-based observation of the aggressive growth of angiosarcoma: A case study*. John Wiley & Sons, Inc. https://onlinelibrary.wiley.com/doi/10.1002/rcr2.479. 7 (8): Figure 1. Accessed 2021.

53 Wiley Online Library – Journal of Medical Imaging and Radiation Oncology – Radiology – Pictorial Essay. (2014). *Magnetic resonance imaging of intramedullary spinal cord lesions: A pictorial review*. John Wiley & Sons, Inc. https://onlinelibrary.wiley.com/doi/full/10.1111/1754-9485.12202. 58 (5): 569–581, Figure 3. Accessed 2021.

54 Wiley Online Library – Journal of Ultrasound in Medicine – Case Series. (2014). *Sonographic Appearances of Desmoid Tumors*. John Wiley & Sons, Inc. https://onlinelibrary.wiley.com/doi/full/10.7863/ultra.33.8.1519. 33 (8): 1519–1525, Figure 3. Accessed 2021.

55 Wiley Online Library – Internal Medicine Journal – Clinical Perspectives. (2015). *Colorectal cancer screening*. John Wiley & Sons, Inc. https://onlinelibrary.wiley.com/doi/full/10.1111/imj.12636. 45 (1): 1–15, Figure 1. Accessed 2021.

56 Wiley Online Library – European Journal of Haematology – Review Article. (2017). John Wiley & Sons, Inc. https://onlinelibrary.wiley.com/doi/full/10.1111/ejh.13003. 100 (3): 221–228, Figure 3. Accessed 2021.

57 Yeh, C.H. (2020). *Liquid Biopsy – A New Frontier in Cancer Dx: Enabling Circulating Cell-free Nucleic Acid Diagnostic to Empower Cancer Management*. Chisinau: Eliva Press.

58 Zhang, J. and Knopp, M.V. (2020). *Advanced in PET: The Latest in Instrumentation, Technology, and Clinical Practice*. New York: Springer.

Part III

Treatment of Cancers

14

Surgical Oncology

OUTLINE

Biopsy Techniques

To diagnose cancer, there are many different types of biopsy options. The chosen method is decided upon so that the needed information can be obtained for diagnosis, whether it is benign or malignant. Options are based on the type of abnormal lesion, whether or not it is palpable, and the procedures that are performed by the individual facility. A medical oncology team usually refers patients to a surgical oncology team or an interventional radiology team. Especially with palpable lesions, surgical oncology teams usually perform biopsies. An interventional radiology team performs biopsies to obtain enough

tissue for imaging studies. Biopsy techniques include fine-needle aspiration, core-needle biopsy, open biopsy, and endoscopic biopsies.

Fine-Needle Aspiration

When there is a solid, palpable lesion, surgical oncologists may utilize **fine-needle aspiration** to obtain tissue. This is commonly done for lesions in the breast, thyroid, and lymph nodes. Mediastinal lymph node staging can be determined via this method. Fine-needle aspiration is often sufficient to diagnose lung cancer, and is performed via bronchoscopy or a transthoracic approach, though the amount of tissue collected

Global Epidemiology of Cancer: Diagnosis and Treatment, First Edition. Jahangir Moini,
Nicholas G. Avgeropoulos, and Craig Badolato.
© 2022 John Wiley & Sons Ltd. Published 2022 by John Wiley & Sons Ltd.

is often not enough for molecular study. For pancreatic cancer, to determine lymph node status, endoscopic ultrasonography-guided fine-needle aspiration biopsy is done. For liver cancer, fine-needle aspiration via endoscopic ultrasound can be diagnostic in 45–86% of cases. Gastrointestinal cancers can be correctly diagnosed 80% of the time via endoscopic ultrasound-guided fine-needle aspiration. The pretreatment diagnosis of salivary gland cancer is often done via fine-needle aspiration. For cervical cancer, fine-needle aspiration or biopsy can reveal evidence of enlarged or fixed lymph nodes. The procedure is also performed in cases of vaginal cancer if there are palpable inguinal or femoral lymph nodes.

For most fine-needle aspiration procedures, a 20-gauge needle and 10-mL syringe are usually chosen. First, the skin is prepared using alcohol, povidone-iodine (Betadine), or chlorhexidine, plus a local anesthetic that is usually 1% lidocaine with no epinephrine. The needle in inserted into the lesion. It is moved backward and forward using negative syringe pressure so that cellular material can be collected in the hub of the needle. The material is then placed onto several slides, usually without a fixative agent, to be reviewed by a cytopathologist.

The results of fine-needle aspiration can be positive, uncertain, or negative. Fine-needle aspiration does not provide any histologic differences required for definitive treatment. An additional biopsy is sometimes required to confirm malignancy, and to provide enough needed information about the lesion. Confirmative accuracy is often less than desired. False-negative results sometimes occur. With an extremely suspicious lesion, but when fine-needle aspiration does not indicate malignancy, a second biopsy is needed. This is usually of larger scope, removing a greater amount of tissue for pathological study. To make sure that aspiration of the lesion occurs, ultrasound- or MRI-guided imaging may be used.

When a lesion is cystic, fine-needle aspiration provides fluid that can be clear, cloudy, **purulent**, or bloody. When the fluid is clear and of any color except red, this often confirms a benign, cystic lesion. Such cysts are common in the thyroid and breast tissues. If the fluid is cloudy or bloody, several slides are prepared for examination. When the fluid is purulent, it is placed into a culture tube for evaluation. Sebaceous cysts provide thick white or yellow material that resembles cottage cheese.

Significant Point

In fine-needle aspiration, biopsy is generally safe and complications are not common. It is most often performed because of a lump that is just under the skin. Fine-needle aspiration is often recommended for cysts, solid nodules or masses, and enlarged lymph nodes. To assess possible cancers, fine-needle aspirations are often performed on the breasts, thyroid gland, and lymph nodes.

Clinical Case

1. For which types of cancer is fine-needle aspiration commonly performed?
2. What must occur if a fine-needle aspiration procedure gives uncertain results?
3. What different features of fluid extracted from the body via fine-needle aspiration may exist, and what procedures may follow?

An 88-year-old woman was examined because of voice hoarseness, and was found to have left-sided vocal cord paresis. A CT scan revealed bilateral thyroid nodules, with the largest being 2.5 cm in diameter. A fine-needle aspiration of this nodule revealed it to be suspicious of papillary thyroid cancer. It was located behind the carotid artery. An ultrasound revealed a suspicious lymph node in the left side of the patient's neck. A total thyroidectomy was performed, with central and lateral neck dissection. The voice hoarseness was totally resolved after surgery. The final diagnosis was of multi-focal medullary thyroid cancer, with no lymphovascular invasion. Over one year of follow-up, the patient remained disease-free.

Answers:

1. **Fine-needle aspiration is commonly performed when there is a solid, palpable lesion, such as those of the breast, thyroid, and lymph nodes. It is also used for lung, pancreatic, liver, GI tract, salivary gland, and cervical cancers.**
2. **If fine-needle aspiration gives uncertain results, an additional biopsy may be done to confirm malignancy and provide enough needed information about the lesion.**
3. **When a lesion is cystic, fine-needle aspiration provides fluid that can be clear, cloudy, purulent, or bloody. When the fluid is clear and of any color except red, this often confirms a benign cystic lesion. If the fluid is cloudy or bloody, several slides are prepared for examination. When the fluid is purulent, it is placed into a culture tube for evaluation.**

Clinical Case

1. When is a biopsy usually recommended?
2. What occurs during a fine-needle aspiration biopsy?
3. Aside from fine-needle aspiration biopsy, what are the other types of available biopsy options?

A 45-year-old woman noticed a lump in her left breast during a monthly self-examination. Her physician documented a fixed round lump with irregular borders, in the upper outer quadrant of her left breast. There was also left axillary edema. The patient's older sister had died of breast cancer a few years previously. A diagnostic mammogram and fine-needle aspiration biopsy are performed, and it is determined that the patient has stage II breast cancer. A lumpectomy with lymph node dissection was performed successfully, followed by administration of tamoxifen, and the patient has had no problems or recurrence over one year of follow-up.

Answers:

1. **A biopsy may be recommended when something suspicious is found during a physical examination or other tests. Though other tests may be suggestive of cancer, only a biopsy can confirm the diagnosis. A small amount of tissue is removed for examination under a microscope. The type of biopsy that is needed is based on the location of a possible tumor.**
2. **A fine-needle aspiration biopsy is a minimally invasive procedure. A thin, hollow needle attached to a syringe collects a small amount of tissue. This may be done for a palpable mass, and may or may not require imaging guidance.**
3. **Aside from fine-needle aspiration biopsy, other biopsy options include image-guided biopsy (via ultrasound, fluoroscopy, CT, X-rays, and MRI), core-needle biopsy, vacuum-assisted biopsy, excisional biopsy, shave biopsy, punch biopsy, endoscopic biopsy, laparoscopic biopsy, bone marrow aspiration and biopsy, and liquid biopsy.**

Core-Needle Biopsy

Because fine-needle aspiration is often insufficient in quantity and quality to give a complete cancer diagnosis, a solid tissue biopsy is often needed. It can provide tissue samples allowing for closer and more extensive examination of biologic, genetic, molecular, and pathologic markers. A **core-needle biopsy** is often performed for this reason. It uses an 11–14 gauge-cannulated needle, within a spring-loaded device such as a **biopsy gun**, which is manually operated. Enlarged lymph nodes and other nearby structures may require biopsy guidance with ultrasound. Before a core-needle biopsy, the skin above the lesion is sterilized with a 1% lidocaine without epinephrine. A small cut of about 2–3 mm is made in the exposed skin so that the core needle can be inserted once. The needle then rests against the solid, palpable lesion. In some cases, mammography, MRI, or ultrasound may be needed to guide the procedure. Based on tissue integrity, 4–6 pieces of tissue may need to be removed in total. The final step in the biopsy procedure is application of a steri-strip to the site, and then a sterile dressing to aid in healing.

Needle biopsies always require a correlation between anticipated results and the actual pathologic findings. A lesion is not guaranteed to be benign just because there was a negative biopsy reading. If the lesion is highly suspicious yet the biopsy is negative or inconclusive, an open biopsy may be required, so that more tissue can be obtained and the diagnosis correctly confirmed. If **atypia** is found, which may be a precursor to actual neoplasia, an open biopsy must be done for complete diagnosis and accurate treatment. Open surgical excisions remove enough tissue for the pathology laboratory, while determining that no adjacent cells are malignant.

Significant Point

Core-needle biopsy is a standard method used to diagnose or rule out breast cancer. It can be used for palpable masses or nonpalpable abnormal findings seen in mammography or other types of imaging. Core-needle biopsy is accurate, does not involve actual surgery, and has only a small chance of infection or bruising. The tissue removed during the procedure provides important information on tumor type and grade.

Clinical Case

1. Why are solid tissue biopsies often needed?
2. Why is core-needle biopsy often performed?
3. What must occur if a core-needle biopsy is negative or inconclusive, but the lesion is highly suspicious?

A 63-year-old woman with no family history of breast cancer was told during a recent mammogram that she had dense breast tissue. A small area of distortion was seen in her left breast. An ultrasound found a mass in the same area, and a core-needle biopsy was performed. The diagnosis was invasive ductal carcinoma. An MRI was done to evaluate the extent of the cancer. There were also abnormal lymph nodes, and further biopsy revealed that they contained metastatic cancer cells. A left mastectomy was performed, along with radiation therapy to the axillary lymph nodes, and chemotherapy. The patient is cancer-free over two years of follow-up.

Answers:

1. **Because fine-needle aspiration is often insufficient in quantity and quality to give a complete cancer diagnosis, a solid tissue biopsy is often needed.**
2. **Solid tissue biopsy can provide tissue samples allowing for closer and more extensive examination of biologic, genetic, molecular, and pathologic markers. A core-needle biopsy is often performed for this reason.**
3. **If a lesion is highly suspicious but a core-needle biopsy is negative or inconclusive, an open biopsy may be required, so that more tissue can be obtained and the diagnosis correctly confirmed.**

Open Biopsy

Using a skin incision, an **open biopsy** removes part or all of a lesion. Open biopsies may be *incisional* or *excisional*. Incisional biopsies remove part of a lesion, while excisional biopsies remove all of a lesion. When a lesion is not palpable but must be removed, needle localization helps isolate it, using guide wires. This aids in the complete removal of all structures that can be seen in imaging. Needle localization uses radiographic images to identify lesions that must be removed. These images may be obtained via computed tomography, mammography, MRI, or ultrasound.

For open biopsy with needle localization, a radiologist places one or two thin guide wires through the skin above the lesion. Each wire has a hook at the end, which secures it in the correct place. As the open biopsy proceeds, the surgeon creates an excision where the wire leaves the skin, then follows the wire down to the lesion so that it can be removed. Needle localization is often required for excisional biopsies of lesions that cannot be palpated, based on location, accessibility, and the probable accuracy. For the cancer known as *melanoma*, use of excisional biopsy instead of incisional, punch, or shave biopsy can affect the outcome of the disease. Various studies have found that excisional biopsies provided the highest accuracy of **Breslow thickness** compared with various incisional biopsies that can fail to determine the actual pathologic depth of a lesion.

Significant Point

An excisional open biopsy allows for an entire tumor to be checked for cancerous cells, instead of just a part of it. The procedure is also referred to as a wide local incision, or if performed on a breast, a lumpectomy. For suspected melanoma, excisional biopsy is the preferred method, and the procedure may be followed by skin grafting or the use of rotation flaps of skin from other sites. However, most cutaneous melanoma excisions can be closed without placing a skin graft.

Clinical Case

1. What are the two types of open biopsies?
2. With open biopsy, what is done when a lesion is not palpable?
3. How are guide wires used in open biopsy?

A 45-year-old man was evaluated because of a dark brown mole on his right leg that had recently changed in appearance. The mole had become slightly raised, with irregular borders. The man had regularly used tanning booths for the last seven years, and never wore sunscreen during his work on construction sites. He had no personal or family history of skin cancer. Examination revealed the mole to be 10 mm in diameter. There was no sign of lymphadenopathy. The mole was asymmetrical, had a lighter color near its center, and did not appear similar to any other mole on the patient's skin. The physician was highly suspicious of melanoma, so an excisional open biopsy was performed, including the subcutaneous fat, with a 10-mm margin. The mole was only 0.28 mm in thickness. Histopathology revealed obvious proliferation of atypical melanocytes at all levels of the epidermis, extending into the papillary dermis. Diagnosis was confirmed as a superficial spreading malignant melanoma. The patient did not develop any additional melanoma over one year of follow-up.

Answers:

1. **Open biopsies may be incisional or excisional. Incisional biopsies remove part of a lesion, while excisional biopsies remove all of a lesion.**
2. **When a lesion is not palpable but must be removed, needle localization helps isolate it, using guide wires. This aids in the complete removal of all structures that can be seen in imaging. Needle localization uses radiographic images to identify lesions that must be removed.**
3. **For open biopsy with needle localization, a radiologist places one or two**

thin guide wires through the skin above the lesion. Each wire has a hook at the end, which secures it in the correct place. As the open biopsy proceeds, the surgeon creates an excision where the wire leaves the skin, then follows the wire down to the lesion so that it can be removed.

Significant Point

An endoscopic biopsy is performed through a fiber-optic endoscope through a natural body orifice or a small incision. The endoscope can view areas for abnormal or suspicious features, obtain tissue samples, or even remove an entire lesion.

Endoscopic Biopsies

Another option for biopsy is accessing internal areas by using an endoscope within the alimentary canal. For example, endoscopic biopsy of an early stomach tumor is shown in Figure 14.1. For example, gastrointestinal cancers can be viewed, biopsied, or even totally removed. Also, there are procedures that can penetrate the colonic or gastric walls to access the upper and lower abdominal and peritoneal areas. These procedures allow for biopsies without requiring an open incision into the abdomen. Also, the respiratory tract can be accessed endoscopically to biopsy lesions in nearby organs. These are called *luminal openings*. Surgeons use flexible or rigid tubes that are very thin and have lights near the tip. Another method involves using laparoscopic techniques to access lesions nearly everywhere in the body. Laparoscopy is often used in place of less appropriate or more difficult biopsy options.

An endoscope is a long, thin tube with a close-focusing telescope on the end. It is used to view areas of the body for abnormal or suspicious tissues, and to obtain samples of them. Endoscopic procedures are named for the area or organ that will be visualized, removed, or both, as follows:

- Alimentary tract endoscopy – GI tract
- Arthroscopy – joint cavities
- Bronchoscopy – bronchial system
- Cystoscopy – bladder
- Laparoscopy – abdominal cavity
- Laryngoscopy – trachea
- Mediastinoscopy – middle part of the chest

Cardiopulmonary Factors

The cardiopulmonary system must be clear for all surgical procedures, and especially when general anesthesia or conscious sedation is used. The patient must be evaluated about personal or family histories of angina, stroke, congestive heart failure, myocardial infarction, diabetes mellitus, and renal insufficiency. This information helps to fully understand the likelihood of any possible complications. The heart can be weakened by previous use of anthracyclines, biologic agents, or taxanes. A two-dimensional **echogram** can provide accurate assessment of the function of the heart before any general anesthesia is used for surgery. Also, pulmonary disease must be ruled out or evaluated as to its seriousness before surgery. For example, a patient with cancer has a higher chance of having pleural effusions, pneumonia, and toxicity caused by previous chemotherapy agents. For most types of cancer, it is important to perform anterior and posterior chest X-rays to assess pulmonary function or disease, and any additional imaging that may be needed before surgery. Head and neck cancers may result in a patient developing aspiration pneumonia. Pulmonary cancers can cause obstructive pneumonia or **pneumothorax**. If a patient has previously been treated with radiation therapy, there may be **interstitial pneumonitis**, which can become chronic fibrotic disease. If a patient has physical or imaging limitations, pulmonary function studies may be required before surgery or any advanced type of imaging.

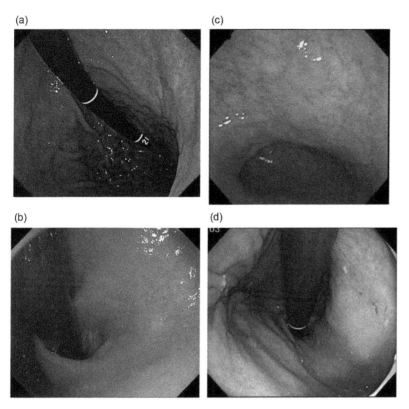

Figure 14.1 (a) Early stomach cancer seen during an endoscopic biopsy; (b) there is concavity of faded color at the atrophic border of the lesser curvature of the cardia; (c) reddish lesion in severely atrophic mucosa in the posterior wall of the upper corpus; (d) the cancer in severely atrophic mucosa, with intestinal metaplasia in the greater curvature of the middle corpus. *Source*: Figure 9 from Wiley Online Library [27].

Hematologic Factors

A complete blood count should be performed and carefully evaluated before surgery. For a patient with severe anemia – less than 7 g/ dL, blood transfusions may be needed before or during surgery. This is especially true if a large amount of blood is likely to be lost during surgery. Epoetin alfa is human erythropoietin produced in cell cultures by using recombinant DNA. It can greatly increase hemoglobin by causing hematopoiesis. Before hip or knee replacement, or other major surgeries, preoperative epoetin alfa results in significant increases in hemoglobin before, during, and after surgery. For immunocompromised patients, an absolute neutrophil count (ANC) of 1500 mm^3 per microliter or more can be protective, preventing infections from developing.

To maintain a circulating level of platelets and stop excessive bleeding during and following surgery, there must be a stable platelet count of 50,000 mm^3 per microliter or more. The platelet count may be elevated by administering 5–10 units of platelets before surgery. Platelets are administered just before surgery begins, and platelet counts are performed as needed during surgery if the entire procedure is longer than 2–3 hours. Administering preoperative prednisone and IV immunoglobulins can prevent autoimmune thrombocytopenia during surgery.

An evaluation for possible bleeding is done before surgery for any patient with a current history of cancers of the bone marrow or liver with malignant infiltration, chemotherapy, malnutrition, or anticoagulant therapy. Prothrombin time (PT) or partial thromboplastin time (PTT) can be done to determine the patient's anticoagulant status. If a patient is taking anticoagulants for current or past clotting abnormalities, there must be a discussion about possible surgical risks and how to address them. The patient may have to taper off the anticoagulants before surgery or be hospitalized before surgery, during which oral anticoagulants are stopped. An option is to use heparin therapy instead. When heparin is used, it is discontinued 1–2 hours before surgery and restarted immediately afterward. Heparin quickly anticoagulates blood, so this method is better than stopping oral anticoagulants for several days before surgery and then restarting them afterward. In emergent situations, tapering may not be done due to lack of time. Therefore, vitamin K can be injected before surgery to quickly support blood clotting.

Gastrointestinal Factors

Malnutrition is another important factor since it impairs healing, strength of tissues, and overall survival following surgery. It varies based on different primary or metastatic cancer sites. Food consumption can be impaired because a patient may have nausea, pain, stomatitis, or tumors of the GI tract or oropharynx. Therefore, cancer patients can become extremely malnourished and dehydrated. Anemia can develop from bleeding, coagulopathy, or malabsorption with vitamin D deficiencies. Correcting or improving such nutritional deficiencies before surgery may improve healing and disease progression, or prevent infections. Prior to extensive abdominal surgery, nutritional supplements can improve outcomes, and postsurgical enteral nutrition may also be needed for a short period of time. Severe deficiencies due to a tumor obstructing the alimentary tract can be improved by use of IV fluids with balanced nutrients or hyperalimentation. Sometimes, deficiencies must be corrected with medications or with oral or IV supplements before surgery can begin.

Geriatric Factors

With the growing elderly population in most countries, there is a larger problem with adverse effects and complications related to cancer. A person's actual age may not be reflective of their body functioning, or the likelihood of treatment complications. One example is with older females with breast cancer. There may be wide variations concerning their functional status, coexisting conditions, physical health, and general concerns due to age. To correctly predict a patient's ability to handle treatment, chances of the treatment being successful, and to assess any other coexisting conditions besides cancer, there needs to be assessment of cognitive issues, dizziness or fainting, weakened health status, incontinence, and all other possible risks. There needs to be more studies of geriatric patients in relation to cancer and all of these factors. This age group is often excluded from clinical studies simply because of the higher risks for negative outcomes.

For primary or metastatic cancers, a *comprehensive geriatric assessment* (CGA) should be performed in a geriatric-focused facility. This examines the patient's functional status, cognitive and mental health, physical health, environmental conditions, and social factors. The CGA usually involves health-care professionals from multiple areas so that risks concerning health conditions, life expectancy, and death can be considered properly. There is measurement of comorbidities, fatigue, nutrition, socioeconomics, polypharmacy, delirium, dementia, falling, abuse or neglect, spontaneous fractures, constipation, failure to thrive, **sarcopenia**, pressure ulcers, and skin changes. Polypharmacy in the elderly is very important in relation to surgery, since multiple medications have the potential to interact and cause negative surgical outcomes. Changes in how the liver metabolizes drugs, and how the kidneys eliminate them, can also negatively impact surgical outcomes. There are methods of predicting any postoperative complications that may occur within one month after surgery. Full geriatric assessments require multiple visits with the health-care team. Before or after any sentinel events, there may be a need for reassessment of the patient. Personalized care allows for the comparison of the patient's worries about cancer and its treatment.

Common problems that must be considered when surgery is required for an elderly patient include hypertension, artery blockages, and disease of the brain, heart, lungs, liver, or kidneys. An older person's brain is more vulnerable to anesthesia, and two major anesthesia-related surgery risks are *postoperative delirium* and *postoperative cognitive dysfunction*. Postoperative delirium is temporary and causes confusion, disorientation, lack of awareness of surrounding, memory problems, and inattention. Postoperative delirium may not begin until a few days after surgery, may improve slightly and then worsen again, and usually subsides after about seven days. Postoperative cognitive dysfunction is more serious, and can result in long-term memory loss as well as difficulty learning, thinking, and concentrating. The only way to determine if this condition is present is by conducting a mental test on the elderly patient prior to surgery, since some of these problems may already be present. The risks for postoperative cognitive dysfunction are increased if a patient has previously had congestive heart failure or other heart disease, lung disease, a stroke, Alzheimer's disease, or Parkinson's disease.

A major issue when surgery is needed for an elderly individual is whether or not he or she is considered "frail." The term *frailty*, in this regard, is defined by meeting three of the following:

- Losing 10 or more pounds within one year
- Self-reported physical exhaustion
- Muscle weakness, measured by having a weak strength when gripping an object with the hands
- Slowing down of normal walking speed
- Having low physical activity

People that are considered frail by medical criteria have higher risks for surgical complications. Interventions may involve a physical therapy and/or exercise program to improve muscle strength, reduce exhaustion, and increase physical activity. Nutrition should also be addressed to improve health status.

Aging causes changes in the heart and blood vessels. The heart becomes unable to beat as fast during physical activity or in times of stress, compared with earlier life. The number of heartbeats per minute – the heart rate – does not, however, change significantly as we age. **Arteriosclerosis** is increased stiffness of larger arteries, and results in hypertension, which then increases the risks of developing **atherosclerosis**. Since there are modifiable risk factors for atherosclerosis, it is not considered a part of normal aging. As plaque builds up inside the walls of the arteries, they harden and narrow, limiting flow of oxygen-rich blood to the tissues. Heart disease reduces blood flow to the heart muscle. If the heart becomes weakened or damaged, heart failure may result. Heart damage is caused by heart attacks, chronic diabetes mellitus and hypertension, and chronic heavy alcohol use. Age-related changes in the heart's electrical system can lead to arrhythmias. When heart valves become stiffer than normal, they can cause pulmonary edema, ascites, or edema on legs, and feet. The heart chambers may also increase in size, due to chronic hypertension. With aging, people become more sensitive to salt, which can also cause hypertension and edema of the ankles and feet. Thyroid disease and chemotherapy may also weaken the heart.

Lung disease affects approximately one of every seven elderly people. Moderate to severe respiratory problems affect about 33% of the elderly, and 17% of people between ages 60 and 79 have asthma or chronic obstructive pulmonary disease (COPD). Other common geriatric pulmonary conditions include pneumonia, pulmonary embolism, and lung cancer. Chronic lung disease is a risk factor for postoperative pulmonary complications, and predicts death within one year in relation to cardiovascular events. Anesthesia used during surgery decreases respiration. If lung disease is present, its effects are more significant. Postsurgical pain medications (narcotics) can also decrease respiration, which in the elderly has the potential to trigger sudden cardiac arrest. Surgery alone has the potential to have lung complications – especially when the surgery involves the lungs, heart, and abdomen. Risks and concerns of lung disease include the following:

- Previous hospitalization related to lung disease that included assisted breathing with a ventilator
- Worsening of COPD that resulted in hospitalization
- Current lung infections
- Coughing and presence of sputum
- Past and current smoking history

With liver disease, surgery can also be complicated. There must be a careful evaluation of an elderly individual's liver function and overall health before any surgical procedure, since compromised liver function can be severely affected and worsened by surgery. Evaluations include the severity of existing liver disease, the type of surgery to be performed and the need for it to be done urgently, and the type of anesthesia that will be used. The surgical team evaluates whether the patient has any nausea, vomiting, jaundice, night sweats, itching, weight loss or gain, ascites, recent GI bleeding, and memory or sleep changes. During the surgical procedure, hypotension must be closely monitored. The most serious event is if the patient experiences decreased hepatic blood flow, which leads to hepatic ischemia and necrosis, liver decompensation or failure, and the release of inflammatory mediators that may trigger multiple organ failure. When liver disease is serious, surgery is often avoided if possible.

Individuals with chronic kidney disease that need surgery must also be carefully evaluated, since perioperative morbidity and death occur more often. With kidney disease, cardiovascular events are the most common cause of death. Patients with end-stage renal disease that undergo heart surgery have a 10–20% chance of dying during or after the procedure. Age over 60 or coexisting diabetes mellitus increases these percentages. Since more than 50% of elderly people above age 75 have some degree of kidney disease, planned surgeries must always take into account the level of kidney function that exists.

Significant Point

Elderly patients have higher risks of complications during and after many types of surgery. Surgical risks are increased if a person has smoked for many years, has not exercised sufficiently, eats a lot of red meat or fried foods, is on medication for hypertension, has high cholesterol, has had a heart attack, or is diabetic or pre-diabetic. Elderly adults are much more likely to require rehabilitation after surgery, develop sleep disturbances, develop delirium, or take a much longer time to recover than younger patients.

Clinical Case

1. With elderly patients, what types of risks must be assessed?
2. What is a CGA?
3. What is measured as part of the CGA?

An 81-year-old woman underwent colon surgery, for sigmoid diverticulitis, under general anesthesia. Four days later, she remained in a state of delirium. She had a history of smoking two packs of cigarettes per day for 45 years, and continued to smoke up until the day of surgery. The patient also had hypertension and peripheral vascular disease for which she had stents previously placed into her iliac arteries and left femoral artery three years previously. Her medications, before surgery, included clopidogrel, simvastatin, bromazepam, valsartan, and bisoprolol. Prior to her surgery, her cardiopulmonary status was satisfactory. After surgery, the patient was disoriented, used bad language when talking to hospital staff members, threw some of her food at them, stated that she could hear people whispering negative things about her, and also moved slower than normal. Soon, the patient was evaluated as to the cause behind her delirium, and it was discovered she had developed postoperative peritonitis, for which she was treated with broad-spectrum antibiotics. Once the peritonitis resolved, the patient's behavior returned to normal, and she became oriented as to her surroundings. She was eventually discharged and taken home by her family, with no further problems.

Answers:

1. **To correctly predicts a geriatric patient's ability to handle surgery and to be successful in treatment. It must be to assess any other coexisting conditions besides cancer, there needs to be assessment of cognitive issues, dizziness or fainting, weakened health status, incontinence, and all other possible risks.**
2. **The CGA is a tool used to examine an elderly patient's functional status, cognitive and mental health, physical health, environmental conditions, and social factors.**
3. **The CGA measures comorbidities, fatigue, nutrition, socioeconomics, polypharmacy, delirium, dementia, falling, abuse or neglect, spontaneous fractures, constipation, failure to thrive, sarcopenia, pressure ulcers, and skin changes.**

Medications Affecting Surgery

To avoid anesthesia-related complications or excessive bleeding, there may be a need to discontinue some medications, or to administer preoperative drugs to the patient. The anesthesia team needs to assess in detail any personal or family history concerning complications from previous anesthesia – especially hyperthermia that results from its use. Though rare, anesthesia-related hyperthermia is often hereditary, causing a high fever and hypoxia that can result in circulatory collapse and death. All medications the patient is taking must be reviewed carefully. To avoid any withdrawal or rebound effect, there should be no abrupt changes to the use of alpha agonists, beta-blockers, barbiturates, or opioids. Additional medications that may need to be taken differently before surgery include insulin, oral hypoglycemics, angiotensin-converting enzyme (ACE) inhibitors, corticosteroids, and calcium-channel blockers.

There should be careful assessment and possible dosing changes for drugs affecting platelet aggregation or prolonging bleeding. Any OTC drugs or herbal remedies, and all antithrombolytic or antiplatelet agents must be discussed. These drugs must be stopped or reduced immediately before surgery – especially if the patient has a hypercoagulable state, artificial heart valves, valvular disease, atrial fibrillation, or has had any thromboembolic events. A few days before surgery, there may be a need to switch from oral to IV anticoagulants.

Significant Point

Medications that are continued on the day of surgery include most heart and blood pressure medications. However, anticoagulants are stopped three days prior to surgery, and aspirin or NSAIDs are stopped 5 – 10 days prior to surgery. Doses of insulin are usually adjusted, but some oral diabetic medications are stopped. Steroid medications should be continued during and after surgery, though the doses may be changed. Some dietary supplements can interfere with medications that may be required after surgery, so they must be discussed.

Anesthesia

Before a surgical procedure, the health-care team and patient discuss anesthesia, control of pain, and what will be done to manage any surgical adverse effects related to the patient's type of cancer. The surgical plan and the patient's overall health are also discussed. Based on preexisting comorbidities, anesthesia can cause heart abnormalities, pneumonia, throat soreness, or vomiting. For cancer patients, anesthesia may be local, epidural, or spinal, regional with peripheral nerve blocks, or general. Often, combinations of these are needed, based on the patient's anxiety and comorbidities. When orthopedic surgery is performed, a peripheral nerve block is often performed, to totally numb a body part or an entire limb. Nerve blocks can persist for 6–36 hour, depending on the surgical site. Opioid and nonsteroidal analgesics will be required after this period to treat pain. Regional epidural anesthesia causes numbness below the nerve roots that are injected. In epidural anesthesia, a catheter can be placed so that medications can continuously or intermittently injected, even postoperatively (see Figure 14.2). Epidural and general anesthesia are often combined for thoracic procedures and other extremely painful surgeries. The drugs numb the injured nerves to increase pain control and reduce systemic adverse effects. Spinal anesthesia is given by puncturing the dural sac between the L3 and L4 vertebrae, with local anesthetics injected into the cerebrospinal fluid (CSF). The anesthetics reach the lower abdomen and extremities along with causing the adverse effects of general anesthesia. The patient can remain awake or semiconscious and breathe without assistance. Spinal anesthesia is therefore relatively safe, based on which area of the body requires surgery.

Anesthesia helps patients relax, stops pain from being perceived, causes amnesia or sleepiness, and brings about altered consciousness or unconsciousness. It also controls blood pressure, breathing, and heart rhythm. General anesthesia causes a reversible loss of consciousness. Therefore, surgeons can operate while the patient has a secure airway and remains motionless. Preoperative, operative, and postoperative vital signs, including body temperature, are closely monitored. Pain management combines anesthesia, analgesics, and anti-nausea medications. After surgery is completed, the patient's symptoms, including pain are managed carefully. Once a patient awakens from surgery, can

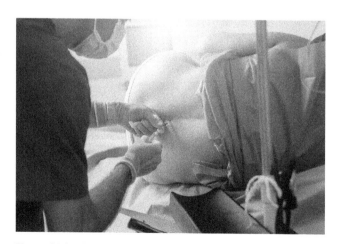

Figure 14.2 Epidural anesthesia procedure. *Source:* Unnumbered figure. Wiley Spinal [29]. Roman Zaiets/ Shutterstock.

swallow, and is not experiencing nausea or vomiting, ice chips and cold water can be given frequently. This helps relieve sore throat that is related to dryness caused by oxygen supplementation, breathing through the mouth, or from use of an endotracheal tube during surgery. Prolonged fatigue throughout the body can occur because of general anesthesia. Spinal anesthesia can cause a severe headache and nausea because it disrupts the spinal tract by introducing medications or losing CSF. Anesthesia-induced headache can be prevented or relieved by having the patient lie flat upon the bed.

Significant Fact

The most common complications after general anesthesia are nausea and vomiting. Additional complications include sore throat, hoarseness, dry mouth, shivering or chills, fever, sleepiness, muscle aches, and itching. Serious complications that may require immediate medical attention include confusion, delirium, difficulty urinating, infections, ileus, respiratory problems, aspiration, aspiration pneumonia, blood clots, and malignant hyperthermia.

Resection

For malignant tumors, surgical resection is often the first step of treatment. However, it is used along with systemic treatments and/or radiation therapy. The goals of surgical resection are to achieve a cure, as much as this may be possible. Traditionally, open en bloc resection of primary tumors is done, with achievement of negative margins around them. Removal of regional or draining lymph nodes also occurs, but this can cause distal **lymphedema**. For certain cancers, open en bloc resection can be replaced by less

invasive techniques. These include endoscopic microsurgery, robotic-assisted, and laparoscopy. Esophageal tumors may consist of premalignant cells with high-grade dysplasia, or malignant cells that came from squamous tissue (squamous cell carcinoma) or glandular tissue (adenocarcinoma). Tumors may only be within the superficial mucosa, or extend into the muscularis mucosa or submucosal layer. The medical oncology team may decide to begin neoadjuvant chemotherapy and radiation therapy prior to surgery. These techniques can greatly reduce tumor depth and width, or even shrink it completely, simplifying surgery. Adjuvant therapy is focused on increasing disease-free survival or overall survival.

Some extensive surgical resections take a long period of time and result in extended hospitalizations, intensive home care, and nutritional problems that can be life-threatening. Sometimes, radiation therapy harms normal tissues to a significant degree, resulting in complications. Based on a tumor's location and size, there may be a need to combine surgery with chemotherapy, radiation therapy, hormones, or biologic therapies. Though surgery is often a primary form of treatment, it may not occur first, since neoadjuvant chemotherapy, radiation therapy, hormone therapy, which all of these may reduce tumor size. Surgical resection must be evaluated as to its potential outcomes, margin status, survival of the patient, and possible recurrence of the cancer.

Tumor Margins

Tumor margins are microscopic three-dimension (3-D) edges of a tumor near to noncancerous tissues. For all cancer surgeries, clear margins must be achieved to prevent local recurrence or systemic disease. The definitions of the tumor margins are consistent with the primary tumor site, to prevent buried cancer cells from remaining. Some tumors require larger margins, of several centimeters, and others require much smaller margins. Tumor margins are calculated based on tumor size and location, pathologic subtype, and the depth of invasion. Pathologic examination of tumor margins is important to ensure that all malignant cells have been removed. Radiation therapy can eradicate remaining microscopic cells for many cancers. It may be difficult for pathological examination of tumor margins to be completed, as surgery is ongoing.

Significant Point

For a pathology sample, an extra area of normal tissue surrounding a tumor – the tumor margin – is also removed for study. It is examined for cancer cells. If positive, there are cancer cells at the edge of the margin, and more surgery is needed. If described as "close," there are cancer cells in the tumor margin, but they do not extend all the way to the edge. Additional surgery may still be required.

Sentinel Lymph Node Biopsy

Sentinel lymph node biopsy (SLNB) was developed in the late 1990s. When performed by an experienced surgical team, it can provide excellent and accurate results. Cancer sites that are assessed via SLNB include cervical, thyroid, penile, head/neck, and breast cancers, as well as melanoma. The procedure is an option to examine the axilla for tumors that may drain to the lymph node basins. Nodes that can be examined include the *ipsilateral axillary* or inguinal lymph nodes. The procedure involves injections of radioactive sulfur colloid and blue dye, to identify areas of radioisotope uptake. For most solid tumors, the regional lymph nodes are the most common site of metastasis. Surgical resection of the proximal lymph node basin occurs to determine staging of the cancer – even if no tumor cells are evident in the lymph nodes. If there is a visible or palpable tumor in the axilla, for example, or if cancer has been verified in the sentinel lymph node, dissection of the lymph node will be done. Systemic biologic therapy, chemotherapy, or hormonal therapy may be able to eradicate cancer cells in clinically benign lymph nodes, avoiding extensive resection. An adverse effect of SLNB is that the patient's urine and stool can be blue-colored for up to 24 hours after the procedure.

Significant Point

Sentinel lymph node biopsy (SLNB) is a procedure to remove and check the first lymph node where a cancer would be expected to spread. Since it removes less lymph node to assess cancer spread than in other procedures, SLNB lowers the risk of developing lymphedema. Before this procedure became available, all women with early-stage breast cancer had to have most of the lymph nodes removed from under their arms, resulting in arm swelling, lymphedema, infection, and pain.

Minimally Invasive Procedures

Minimally invasive surgical procedures use incisions of less than 1–2 cm to provide laparoscopic access with special instruments and techniques. This is based on certain body structures, including cavities, organs, joints, and bones. Body cavities require carbon dioxide insufflation to make room for the instruments to move and so that structures can be visualized, using tiny cameras,

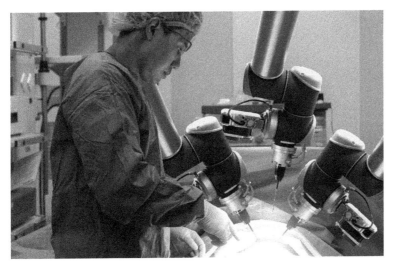

Figure 14.3 Robotic surgery. *Source*: Figure 1 from Wiley Online Library – The AJT Report [28].

fiber-optic lights, high-definition monitors, and microscopes. Other laparoscopes allow surgical instruments to be passed into body structures (see Figure 14.3). Robotic surgery offers advantages including performing surgery with more precise instruments, through very small incisions. Results of surgery are usually better compared with traditional or scope-assisted procedures. The surgeon has a 3-D, multi-level area to work within, plus a better field of vision than with scope-assisted techniques. One centimeter in diameter surgical "arms" plus highly sensitive electronics allow for precise movements.

In robotic surgery, the surgeon sits at a machine, apart from the patient, as the robotic arms perform the desired work. The surgeon manipulates joysticks on a console as a computer coordinates the robotics. Everything is visualized through a fiber-optic camera. Instruments can be introduced through laparoscopic techniques, with the robot holding the ports. Better range of motion is possible than with traditional laparoscopy, which also lacks 3-D imaging. Robotic surgery allows for better

visualization and access, and more precise dissection – especially near to nerves, arteries, and veins. A malignant tumor can be removed with more precision, including all cancerous tissue. Robotic surgery takes slightly longer than traditional surgery, but many patients are still able to return home the same day, or on the next day. However, robotic surgery may not be available in many locations, and it requires extensive training.

Significant Point

An experienced surgeon always performs robotic surgery. It results in smaller and fewer scars, less pain, lower risk of infection, and a much faster recovery period. The Food and Drug Administration cleared the first surgical robot for general minimally invasive surgeries in 2000, and in 2005, for gynecologic cancer surgeries.

Clinical Case

1. What is used in body cavities to make room for surgical instruments?
2. What are the differences in the surgeon's views between robotic surgery and traditional laparoscopy?
3. Why is robotic surgery generally preferred over more traditional forms of surgery?

A 62-year-old man had been diagnosed with transitional cell carcinoma of the bladder. He had previously undergone a left nephrectomy for renal carcinoma, using traditional open surgery. The patient is on dialysis due to his remaining kidney functioning poorly. It was determined that a bladder resection was needed. Due to the risk of future cancer of the prostate and remaining kidney, it was decided to remove them during the same procedure. The entire procedure was performed with a minimally invasive robotic-assisted technique, using five 1-cm incisions, plus a single larger incision through which the organs were removed. The organs were removed in one piece, along with the ureter. The patient was able to return home within two days and returned to normal activities quickly. Over one year of follow-up, he is still cancer-free.

Answers:

1. **Body cavities require carbon dioxide insufflation to make room for surgical instruments to move and so that structures can be visualized, using tiny cameras, fiber-optic lights, high-definition monitors, and microscopes.**

2. **In robotic surgery, the surgeon has a 3-D, multi-level area to work within, plus a better field of vision than with scope-assisted techniques. Traditional laparoscopy does not provide 3-D imaging.**

3. **Robotic surgery offers advances including performing surgery with more precise instruments, through very small incisions. Results are usually better compared with traditional or scope-assisted procedures. Tiny surgical "arms" plus highly sensitive electronics allow for precise movements. Better range of motion is possible than with traditional laparoscopy. More precise dissection can be done – especially near to nerves, arteries, and veins. A malignant tumor can be removed with more precision, including all cancerous tissue.**

Emergent Surgery

Emergent surgery is another term for emergency surgery, often occurring after another surgery that results in bleeding. Emergent surgery may be needed as part of reconstructive surgery, to reestablish a flap of skin, or to remove a bowel obstruction. Another use of emergent surgery is to remove spinal bony metastasis that impinges on the spinal cord. This must be done quickly to decompress spinal cord pressure, to avoid possibly permanent paralysis of the lower limbs, or less often, the upper limbs.

Key Terms

Arteriosclerosis
Atherosclerosis
Atypia
Biopsy gun

Breslow thickness
Core-needle biopsy
Echogram
Emergent surgery

Fine-needle aspiration
Interstitial pneumonitis
Lymphedema
Open biopsy
Pneumothorax

Purulent
Sarcopenia
Sentinel lymph node biopsy
Tumor margins

Bibliography

1 Amin, M.B., Edge, S.B., Greene, F.L., Byrd, D.R., Brookland, R.K., et. al. (2017). *AJCC Cancer Staging Manual*, 8th Edition. New York: Springer.

2 Brun del Re, R. (2010). *Minimally Invasive Breast Biopsies (Recent Results in Cancer Research)*. New York: Springer.

3 Chu, Q.D., Gibbs, J.F., and Zibari, G.B. (2014). *Surgical Oncology: A Practical and Comprehensive Approach*. New York: Springer.

4 Cohen, T.N., Ley, E.J., and Gewertz, B.L. (2020). *Human Factors in Surgery: Enhancing Safety and Flow in Patient Care*. New York: Springer.

5 D'angelica, M.D. and Pawlik, T.M. (2020). *Management of Metastatic Liver Tumors (Surgical Oncology Clinics)*. Amsterdam: Elsevier.

6 Delman, K.A., Lowe, M.C., and Pawlik, T.M. (2020). *Melanoma (Surgical Oncology Clinics)*. Amsterdam: Elsevier.

7 Feig, B.W. and Ching, C.D. (2018). *The MD Anderson Surgical Oncology Handbook*, 6th Edition. Philadelphia: Lippincott, Williams, and Wilkins.

8 Gervais, D.A. and Sabharwal, T. (2011). *Interventional Radiology Procedures in Biopsy and Drainage (Techniques in IR Series)*. New York: Springer.

9 Govindan, R. and Morgensztern, D. (2021). *The Washington Manual of Oncology*, 4th Edition. Philadelphia: Lippincott, Williams, and Wilkins.

10 Hunter, J.G., Spight, D.H., Sandone, C., and Fairman, J.E. (2018). *Atlas of Minimally Invasive Surgical Operations*. New York: McGraw-Hill Education/Medical.

11 Jaffe, R.A., Schmiesing, C.A., and Golianu, B. (2019). *Anesthesiologist's Manual of Surgical Procedures*, 6th Edition. Philadelphia: Lippincott, Williams, and Wilkins.

12 Junaid, M., Kazi, M., and Qadeer, S. (2013). *Toluidine Blue: A Head and Neck Perspective– Intraoperative Assessment of Tumor Margins*. New Delhi: Lap Lambert Academic Publishing.

13 Karakousis, C.P. (2015). *Atlas of Operative Procedures in Surgical Oncology*. New York: Springer.

14. Khatri, V.P., Petrelli, N.J., and Pawlik, T.M. (2019). *Precision Medicine in Surgical Oncology (Surgical Oncology Clinics, Volume 29–1)*. Amsterdam: Elsevier.

15 Latifi, R. (2020). *Surgical Decision Making in Geriatrics: A Comprehensive Multidisciplinary Approach*. New York: Springer.

16 Lonser, R.R. and Elder, J.B. (2018). *Surgical Neuro-Oncology (Neurosurgery by Example)*. Oxford: Oxford University Press.

17 Luchette, F.A. and Barraco, R.D. (2018). *Surgery and the Geriatric Patient (Clinics in Geriatric Medicine, 35)*. Amsterdam: Elsevier.

18 Malawer, M.M., Wittig, J.C., Bikels, J., and Wiesel, S.W. (2015). *Operative Techniques in Orthopaedic Surgical Oncology*, 2nd Edition. Philadelphia: Lippincott, Williams, and Wilkins.

19 Mariani, G., Vidal-Sicart, S., and Valdes Olmos, R.A. (2020). *Atlas of Lymphoscintigraphy and Sentinel Node Mapping: A Pictorial Case-Based Approach*, 2nd Edition. New York: Springer.

20 Moore, F.D., Rhee, P.M., and Fulda, G.J. (2018). *Surgical Critical Care and Emergency Surgery: Clinical Questions and Answers*, 2nd Edition. Hoboken: Wiley-Blackwell.

21 Moran, C.A., Kalhor, N., and Weissferdt, A. (2020). *Oncological Surgical Pathology Volume 1*. New York: Springer.

22 Morita, S.Y., Balch, C.M., Kumberg, V.S., Pawlik, T.M., Posner, M.C., and Tanabe, K.K. (2017). *Textbook of Complex General Surgical Oncology*. New York: McGraw-Hill Education/ Medical.

23 Poston, G.J., Wyld, L., and Audisio, R.A. (2016). *Surgical Oncology: Theory and Multidisciplinary Practice*, 2nd Edition. Boca Raton: CRC Press.

24 Rosenthal, R.A., Zenilman, M.E., and Katlic, M.R. (2000). *Principles and Practice of Geriatric Surgery Volume 1*. New York: Springer.

25 Soreide, K. and Stattner, S. (2021). *Textbook of Pancreatic Cancer: Principles and Practice of Surgical Oncology*. New York: Springer.

26 Stanford Health Care. (2020). *Endoscopic Biopsy*. Stanford Health Care. https:// stanfordhealthcare.org/medical-tests/b/ biopsy/types/endoscopic-biopsy.html Accessed 2021.

27 Wiley Online Library. (2016). *Basic principles and practice of gastric cancer screening using high-definition white-light gastroscopy*. John Wiley & Sons, Inc. https://onlinelibrary.wiley. com/doi/full/10.1111/den.12623 from Digestive Endoscopy, 28(S1): 2–15. Figure 9. Accessed 2021.

28 Wiley Online Library – The AJT Report. (2020). *Robotic Surgery for Obese Patients*. John Wiley & Sons, Inc. http://onlinelibrary.wiley. com/doi/full/10.1111/ajt.15780. 20 (2): 325–326. Accessed 2021.

29 Wiley Spinal. (2018). *Anesthesia Given Right*. Epimed International. https://www. wileyspinal.com/. Unnumbered figure near the top. Accessed 2021.

30 Wright, F.C., Escallon, J.M., Cukier, M., Tsang, M.E., and Hameed, U. (2020). *Surgical Oncology Manual*, 3rd Edition. New York: Springer.

31 Zimmermann, A. (2017). *Tumors and Tumor-Like Lesions of the Hepatobiliary Tract: General and Surgical Pathology*. New York: Springer.

15

Radiation Therapy

OUTLINE

The Purpose of Radiation Therapy
Radiobiology
    Cellular Response to Radiation
    The Cell Cycle and Radiosensitivity
Cell Death
Factors Affecting the Biology of Cancers
    Oxygen Effect
    Dose Rate
    Relative Biologic Effectiveness
    Radiosensitivity
    Apoptosis
    Linear Energy Transfer
    Fractionation
Types of Radiation Therapy
    External Beam Radiation Therapy
    Stereotactic Radiosurgery
    Adaptive Planning
    Charged Particle External Beam Radiation Therapy
    Heavy Charged Particle External Beam Radiation Therapy
    Brachytherapy
    Radionuclide Therapy
    Intraoperative Radiotherapy
Combined-Modality Therapy
Hyperthermia
Accidental Radiation Exposure
    Acute Radiation Syndrome
    Cutaneous Syndrome
    Gastrointestinal Syndrome
    Hematopoietic Syndrome
    Cerebrovascular Syndrome
    Radiation on the Embryo and Fetus
    Radiation and Malignancies
Special Populations
    Pregnant Women
    Children
    Elderly
Key Terms
Bibliography

Global Epidemiology of Cancer: Diagnosis and Treatment, First Edition. Jahangir Moini, Nicholas G. Avgeropoulos, and Craig Badolato.
© 2022 John Wiley & Sons Ltd. Published 2022 by John Wiley & Sons Ltd.

The Purpose of Radiation Therapy

Radiation therapy is highly important in cancer treatment. Approximately 60% of cancer patients receive radiation therapy to achieve a cure, to control the disease, or for palliation. Radiation can cure a tumor in its early stages, though many patients require long-term and intensive treatment. If total radiation doses are very high, toxicities are more severed. Chemotherapy is often used along with radiation therapy, increasing the **therapeutic index**. For cancers such as early Hodgkin disease or skin cancer, radiation is often used alone. A cure or destruction of the tumor may not be possible for some cancers and tumors that are in later stages. If this is the case, months to years of radiation therapy may be able to control the disease. Cancers that can be controlled by radiation therapy with chemotherapy or surgery include recurring breast cancer, lung cancer, and certain sarcomas.

If palliation is the goal, radiation therapy can prevent pathologic fractures, relieve pain, and help the patient to regain mobility. Radiation is often applied to metastatic bone lesions from primary sites. These include the lungs, breasts, and prostate gland. The pain relief is often excellent, and a patient often may receive multiple palliative radiation to different bones over several years. For bone metastases, radiation therapy vastly improves the quality of life. Palliative radiation also relieves symptoms from brain metastasis or spinal cord compression. Palliative radiation can reduce or even eliminate hemorrhage, obstruction, superior vena cava syndrome, fungating lesions, and ulceration. *Anticipatory radiation* treats asymptomatic lesions that could become symptomatic. Examples include treating a vertebral lesion to prevent likely spinal cord compression, or treating a mediastinal mass to avoid development of superior vena cava syndrome. For patients with small cell lung cancer, radiation may also be used prophylactically to prevent brain metastases from occurring. For non-malignant tumors, radiation can prevent heterotopic ossification in the joints. Post-operatively, radiation can stop keloids from recurring after surgeries.

Radiobiology

Ionizing radiation has radiobiologic effects because of the events that occur in sequence after absorbing the energy. The body sequentially reacts to these events. Radiation affects the cells, followed by the tissues, organs, or the whole body – based on the site of treatment. The biologic influences of radiation upon cells take into account biochemical, genetic, and kinetic factors. The dose, rate, and type at which radiation is administered also results in different effects. These can be classified as acute, subacute, or late – based on severity and incidence.

Cellular Response to Radiation

At the cellular level, radiation can have direct or indirect effects, based on **target theory**. When any key cellular molecules are damaged, a **direct hit** has occurred, due to energy being directly aimed into the DNA or RNA. There are four types of damage after high-dose radiation of DNA molecules *in vitro*, as follows:

- Change or loss of a base – adenine, cytosine, guanine, or thymine
- Breaking the hydrogen bond between the two chains of the DNA molecule
- Breaking one or both chains of the DNA molecule
- Cross-linkage of the chains after they are broken

Unrepaired breaks or changes in a base result in mutations, and then impaired function of the cell or cellular death. An indirect hit occurs when ionization happens, mostly in the intracellular water that surrounds the cells' molecular structures. If this happens, radiation absorbed by the water molecules results in a **free radical** being formed, as an electron is "pushed out" of its orbit around the ion. These free radicals can trigger many chemical reactions and produce new cell-toxic compounds. The ionizing effects of radiation upon intracellular water are explained in Table 15.1.

Therefore, the free radicals resulting from radiation interacting with water can trigger many chemical reactions inside cells. They are believed to be a primary factor in the production of cellular damage. Most experts agree that direct hits that damage the DNA and cause chromosomal abnormalities make up the most effective and deadly injuries of those produced by ionizing radiation. Even so, the relative ratio of water to DNA in a single cell means that the likelihood of indirect damage from ionization of intracellular water is much greater than the likelihood of damage from a direct hit. Radiation damage significantly causes cancer cells to become unable to reproduce. Radiation can also damage cellular carbohydrates, enzymes, and proteins while altering cell membrane

permeability. This may add to the total effects of radiation at the cellular level. Table 15.2 summarizes the biologic effects of radiation upon cells.

The Cell Cycle and Radiosensitivity

In the mitosis (M) and growth 2 (G2) phase of the cell cycle, radiosensitivity is at its maximum (see Figure 15.1). In early research, the sensitivity of cells to radiation was suggested to be directly proportional to their reproductive activities, and *inversely* proportional to their amount of differentiation. A differentiated cell does not undergo mitosis, and is functionally or morphologically specialized, such as red blood cells. An undifferentiated cell only has a few specialized characteristics, such as erythroblasts, lymphoblasts, and stem cells. Their main purpose is to divide, creating new cells so that their numbers

Table 15.1 Ionizing effects of radiation upon intracellular water.

Effect	Equation
The final products of water molecule (HOH) ionization are a pair of ions (H^+ and OH^-), plus free radicals (H° and OH°), which can damage the cell.	$HOH + e^- \rightarrow HOH^-$
The free electron (e^-) is captured by another water molecule to form the second ion.	$HOH + e^- \rightarrow HOH^-$
Since HOH^+ and HOH^- from these reactions are not stable, quick breakdown occurs in the presence of other, normal water molecules. This forms another ion and a free radical.	$HOH^+ \rightarrow$ $H^\circ + OH^\circ$ and $HOH^- \rightarrow OH^- + H^\circ$
The resulting ions (H^+ and OH^-) have slight potential for cell damage via chemical reactions. So, they are more likely to recombine and form HOH. The free radicals (H° and OH°) are highly reactive, and also may recombine to form water. However, free radicals are more likely to experience chemical interactions with other free radicals, to form cytotoxic agents.	$OH^\circ + OH^\circ \rightarrow H_2O_2$ (hydrogen peroxide)

Table 15.2 Biologic effects of radiation upon cells.

Factor	Effect
Mitosis	Delayed, to allow for DNA to be repaired
If one strand of a DNA double helix is damaged	Repair can occur accurately
If both strands of a DNA double helix are damaged	Repair can usually not occur
Incorrect repair of damaged DNA	A mutation will occur
Severe DNA damage cannot be repaired	The cell will die (apoptosis)

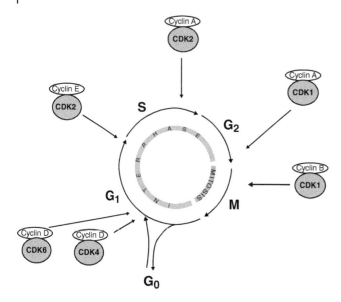

Figure 15.1 Stages of the cell cycle. *Source*: Wiley Online Library – Cell Proliferation [34].

can be maintained. With radiation effects highest during mitosis, the undifferentiated cells are generally the most sensitive. In contrast, well-differentiated cells are mainly resistant to radiation. When radiation is used, there are changes in mitotic activity. These are described as *delayed onset or complete inhibition*. With delayed onset of mitosis, damage occurs during prophase, but repair can occur, and cell division happens. Differently, in complete inhibition of mitosis – also called **cell sterilization** – the cell can no longer divide, but it still may live with being able to reproduce.

Cell Death

The two major forms of cell death are *mitotic* and *apoptotic*. Other types include *autophagic, necrotic*, and *senescence* cell death. The forms of cell death are further summarized as follows:

- *Mitotic cell death* – occurs after one or several cell divisions; often with much smaller doses of radiation needed to cause interphase death

- *Apoptotic cell death* – there must be active metabolic processes; nearby cells must phagocytize cell remnants; the entire process occurs in a few hours
- *Autophagic cell death* – occurs at the intracellular level, via removal of damaged proteins
- *Necrotic cell death* – membrane integrity is lost and the cell increases in size; there is a release of lyposomal enzymes, and an inflammatory response is generated; this type of cell death may be a pathologic response to vascular damage, and a pathway for cells that do not have an effective apoptotic pathway
- *Senescence death* – is believed to be a gradual decline in physiology of cell; with cancer cells, they become unable to divide over time

---

Significant Point

In mitotic cell death, there is a *mitotic catastrophe*, which kills cancer cells after radiation or drug-induced DNA damage. Within the cell nucleus, the genetic damage cannot be repaired. Cell division no longer can occur, the cell dies. Mitotic catastrophe is not related to apoptosis, and is seen in cells that lack functional apoptotic pathways. It can also be triggered by agents that affect the stability of microtubule spindles, or by defective cell cycle checkpoints.

Clinical Case

1. Is radiation a good option for Hodgkin lymphoma?
2. What are the four types of DNA damage caused by radiation therapy?
3. What is mitotic cell death?

A 61-year-old man went to his physician because of low back pain that recently began to affect his left hip. The pain sometimes woke him up at night, and he constantly would feel fatigued during the day. He had lost weight recently without any changes to his diet or physical activity. The physician questioned the patient about family history of any cancer, and discovered that the patient's mother died of breast cancer. The patient had no other significant medical problems, did not smoke, and rarely drank alcohol because it seemed to make his pain worse. After many tests were performed, the patient was diagnosed with Hodgkin lymphoma, with metastasis to the lumbar spine. The patient underwent surgery to remove malignant lymph nodes in his pelvis, and was started on radiation therapy, which had excellent results. The patient experienced minimal adverse effects, and the disease went into remission.

Answers:

1. **For cancers such as early Hodgkin disease, radiation is often used alone. Cancers of the lymphoid organs have high radiosensitivity.**

2. **The four types of damage after high-dose radiation of DNA molecules include: change or loss of a base (adenine, cytosine, guanine, or thymine), breaking the hydrogen bond between the two chains of the DNA molecule, breaking one or both chains of the DNA molecule, and cross-linkage of the chains after they are broken.**
3. **Along with apoptotic cell death, mitotic cell death is the other major form, and occurs after one or several cell divisions, often with much smaller doses of radiation needed to cause interphase death.**

Factors Affecting the Biology of Cancers

The factors that affect cancer biology come directly from application of radiation. These factors also help in determining treatment outcomes. The factors include the oxygen effect, dose rate, relative biologic effectiveness, radiosensitivity, apoptosis, linear energy transfer, and fractionation.

Oxygen Effect

Tumors that are well-oxygenated have a much more intense response to radiation than those that are poorly oxygenated. The existence of **oxygen tension** from 20 to 40 mm Hg during radiation therapy significantly increases the target cells' radiosensitivity. The oxygen effect may be related to oxygen being able to combine with free radicals formed during ionization. This produces new, toxic combinations. Another theory is that the presence of oxygen during radiation therapy stops the reversal and repair of chemical changes that occur from ionization. Therefore, the oxygen effect involves modification of the radiation dose required to produce the needed amount of biologic damage. The oxygen enhancement ratio (OER) expresses the amount of the oxygen effect. The OER is a ratio of a radiation dose when hypoxia is present – to the radiation dose when oxygen is present and the amount needed to cause the same biologic effect. Hypoxic cells are highly radioresistant. If they are present, radiation therapy is of less effectiveness. For example, head, neck, and cervical cancers have worsened survival rates if the tumors are hypoxic. There is a relationship between hypoxia and anemia, as lower levels of hemoglobin are linked to increased rates of hypoxia.

Dose Rate

The dose rate describes how quickly machinery or other equipment delivers a given dose during cancer treatment. This is very important if therapy is fractionated over many days or weeks, such as in *standard external beam therapy*. Low dose rates are much less effective in causing fatal cell damage than higher dose rates. This is generally true since low dose rates allow cell repair to occur before the fatal dose has been reached, as part of fractionated treatments.

Relative Biologic Effectiveness

Since different types of radiation have various energy loss rates, biologic responses from radiation therapy will also be different. Relative biologic effectiveness (RBE) compares a dose of test radiation with a dose of standard radiation that results in the same biologic response. RBE is expressed in the following formula:

$$RBE = \frac{\text{Dose of reference radiation to produce a specific biologic effect}}{\text{Dose of test radiation to produce the same biologic effect}}$$

Radiosensitivity

Remember that ionizing radiation is of most effectiveness on cells that are undifferentiated and experiencing active mitosis. According to various clinical and laboratory studies, this is usually true in all types of body tissues.

Apoptosis

Apoptosis is programmed cell death. It occurs in normal as well as malignant cells, different from how cells die of hypoxia. Failure of normal apoptosis means that malignant cells can survive and proliferate without control. Ionization and direct DNA damage result in cell death during mitosis of most cells that receive radiation. The process of apoptosis is accelerated by radiation therapy. This is especially true in the germ cells, lymphocytes, salivary gland cells, and small-bowel crypt cells.

During a radiation procedure, biochemical, genetic, and molecular substances; basic fibroblast growth factors (bFGF); and protein kinase C (PKC) inhibitors all play an important role in radiation-induced apoptosis. Examples of substances that play roles in this include *tumor protein 53 (p53), B-cell lymphoma 2 (BCL-2)*, and the *retinoblastoma protein (pRb)*. The presence or absence of these and many other substances may enhance responsiveness in different cell lines. Continuing research is focused on the identification of the pathways that result in apoptosis. If these pathways can be manipulated, radiation oncology can be increased in its therapeutic beneficial ratio.

Significant Point

Apoptosis is an orderly process in which the genome of cells is broken down. The cell fragments into smaller pieces, to be consumed by phagocytes. Apoptosis consists of an initiation phase and an execution phase. The initiation phase is started by extracellular or intracellular signals, such as loss of growth factors, hypoxia, and radiation. Intracellular signals include DNA damage, effects of chemotherapy, malfunction of telomeres, and viral infections.

Linear Energy Transfer

Linear energy transfer (LET) is the rate at which energy is lost from various forms of radiation, as it travels through any type of matter. X-rays and gamma rays are classified as *low-LET radiation*, which is only slightly ionizing. It follows a random pathway resulting in a few direct hits in the nucleus of the cell. However, alpha particles, negative pions, and neutrons are classified as *high-LET radiation*. This has a higher chance of interacting with matter, resulting in more direct hits inside cells.

Fractionation

Fractionation divides the total required radiation dose into equal fractions, with an understanding that each dose may need to be higher because of the need to deliver doses in multiple fractions. One dose of radiation has a greater biologic effect than the same dose delivered in a divided or fractionated procedure. The single dose will not spare normal tissues, however, while killing the tumor. *Hyperfractionation* uses smaller doses per fraction. Treatment is done two times per day, with at least six hours in between. There are four R's of radiobiology that must be understood regarding the biologic and chemical effects of fractionation upon tumors as well as normal body tissues. These are *repair, redistribution, repopulation,* and *reoxygenation,* which are further explained as follows:

- *Repair* – fractionation allows for repair of intracellular sublethal damage by normal cells, in between the daily-dose fractions. A dose is delivered that is enough to stop tumor cells from being repaired, but allows normal cells to recover before the next dose is administered. Some tumor cells can also undergo repair between the daily doses, but they may also become reoxygenated, which makes them more radiosensitive to the next dose of radiation. While some tumor cells can be somewhat repaired between doses, the continuing daily doses usually result in tumor control.

- *Redistribution* – within the cell cycle, redistribution of cell age because of daily radiation therapy is important, since more tumor cells become radiosensitive. With additional daily doses, more and more tumor cells experience delays in the cell cycle, and reach mitosis as the next dose is given. This increases the amount of cancer cells that die.

- *Repopulation (new growth)* – this occurs in normal tissues through cell division during fractionated treatments. Dose fractionation permits this repopulation to occur, sparing normal tissues from some late adverse effects that could occur if the process were inhibited. Tumor cells that can divide during fractionated radiation therapy usually cannot survive due to the effects of radiation. Therefore, fractionation kills tumor cells while sparing normal tissues.

- *Reoxygenation* – while normal tissues are usually highly oxygenated, tumors usually are normal to hypoxic to anoxic in relation to oxygen levels. Radiosensitivity is closely related to oxygen tension in tumor cells, with hypoxic or anoxic cells usually being radioresistant, while oxygenated cells are radiosensitive. Dose fractionation permits the cells to become oxygenated while the tumor is shrinking.

Sensitivity of affected cells define the responses of tissues and organs to radiation therapy. There are more than one cell type present. Each cell category has varying degrees of radiosensitivity. Tissue response is also based on the balance of parenchymal versus stromal substances present in the tissue. The parenchyma is made up of cells with features of the tissue or organ. In the testis for example, the cells are radiosensitive, so ionizing radiation has strong effects upon the parenchyma. Oppositely, the parenchyma of the spinal cord is comparatively radioresistant. Therefore, responses to radiation in the spinal cord are based on indirect effects upon the stroma – primarily, the vasculature that supplies the parenchyma. In Table 15.3, there is a list of body organs categorized by their degrees of radiosensitivity, determined by parenchymal hypoplasia.

Table 15.3 Radiosensitivity of body organs based on parenchymal hypoplasia.

Radiosensitivity level	Body organs
High	Blood, bone marrow, intestines, lymphoid organs, ovaries, testes
Somewhat high	Bladder, cervix, corneas, esophagus, oral cavity, rectum, skin
Medium	Fine vasculature, growing bone and cartilage, optic lenses, stomach
Somewhat low	Adrenal glands, kidneys, liver, mature bone or cartilage, pancreas, pituitary gland, respiratory organs, salivary glands, thyroid gland
Low	Brain, muscles, spinal cord

Significant Point

Fractionation of radiation therapy usually occurs over multiple weeks. Radiation doses are divided into multiple fractions, to maximize destruction of malignant cells while minimizing damage to healthy tissues. Dividing the total dose of radiation into multiple fractions maximizes the likelihood of irradiating cells when they are in the most radiosensitive period of the cell cycle. It also allows cells that are closer to sources of oxygen to be killed first.

Clinical Case

1. What is fractionation, as used in radiation therapy?
2. How does radiation therapy accelerate tumor cell death?
3. What are the four R's of radiobiology that must be understood concerning the use of fractionation in radiation therapy?

A 66-year-old woman was taken to the emergency department because of vaginal bleeding, passing of large clots, and severe abdominal pain. She was hospitalized and found to have a large cervical mass that was later diagnosed as invasive, well-differentiated carcinoma. The patient was severely anemic and received three blood transfusions. A CT scan revealed the mass to be 8.6 cm in diameter. A cystoscopy was performed, and the final diagnosis was stage IIB cervical cancer. Daily pelvic radiation therapy was started, plus weekly chemotherapy (intravenous cisplatin). The bleeding almost totally stopped very soon, and the abdominal pain lessened considerably. The patient still remained fatigued but was able to be discharged within 10 days.

Answers:

1. **Fractionation divides the total required radiation dose into equal fractions, with an understanding that each dose may need to be higher because of the need to deliver doses in multiple fractions.**
2. **Ionization and direct DNA damage result in tumor cell death during mitosis of most cells that receive radiation – especially in germ cells, lymphocytes, salivary gland cells, and small-bowel crypt cells. During a radiation procedure, biochemical, genetic, and molecular substances; basic fibroblast growth factors; and protein kinase C inhibitors all play an important role in radiation-induced apoptosis.**
3. **The four R's of radiology include repair, redistribution, repopulation, and reoxygenation. Fractionation**

allows for repair of intracellular sublethal damage by normal cells, in between the daily-dose fractions. In the cell cycle, redistribution of cell age because of daily radiation therapy is important, since more tumor cells become radiosensitive. Repopulation occurs in normal tissues through cell division during fractionated treatments. While normal tissues are usually highly oxygenated, tumors usually are normal to hypoxic to anoxic in relation to oxygen levels. Dose fractionation permits the cells to become oxygenated while the tumor is shrinking.

Types of Radiation Therapy

Radiation therapies are cancer treatments that use beams of intense energy to kill cancer cells. X-rays are most commonly used, but protons and other types of energy can also be used. In most cases, the term *radiation therapy* refers to *external beam radiation therapy*. In all forms of radiation therapy, tumor cells are killed by destroying the genetic material that controls their growth and division. Radiation therapy damages healthy as well as cancerous cells, and the goal of radiation therapy is to kill as many cancer cells as possible while minimizing damage to normal cells. Other types of radiation therapy include stereotactic radiosurgery, charged particle external beam radiation therapy, heavy charged particle external beam radiation therapy, brachytherapy, radionuclide therapy, and intraoperative radiotherapy.

External Beam Radiation Therapy

External beam radiation therapy (EBRT) is used for nearly every type of malignant cancer. It may be curative, adjuvant, or palliative. A linear accelerator is usually used to deliver EBRT. The expensive and very large machine is also known as a *linac*. A **linear accelerator** converts electricity to high-energy X-rays. It does this by accelerating electrons to a very high speed and then allowing them to pass through *tungsten*, or another high-density material. As the electrons interact with the material, they are bent or slowed, resulting in a beam of high-energy X-rays. This is known as the *Bremsstrahlung effect*. Also, the electrons can be allowed to not interact with the high-density material, and be "shot" out of the accelerator as a beam. Additionally, EBRT can be delivered from a machine containing Cobalt-60 or another radioactive material, generating continuous high-energy gamma rays, which are physically the same as X-rays.

Regardless of the beam that is created, it is shaped to match the shape of the tumor or other clinical factors. Beam shaping is attained by multiple "leaves" (beam shapers), controlled by computer software and individual motors. The leaves are 2–10 mm in width. Each leaf can be stationary or movable, to achieve dynamic beam shaping. Accurate positioning of the patient and the machinery optimizes treatment. The patient lies on a table made of carbon fiber. This allows X-ray beams to traverse it easily. The table can be moved to any needed angle. Immobilization devices keep the patient still. They are locked into the table to improve accuracy and reproducibility of positioning.

Electrons are used for superficial treatments. There is minimal exposure to deeper tissues, so electrons are perfect to treat skin and breast tumors. X-rays may be used for deeper tumors, and their use is much more common. Penetration depth is determined by the energy of the electron or X-ray beam. Linacs can usually generate beams of several electron and X-ray energies, allowing optimal treatment flexibilities. The Cobalt-60 machine only provides fixed, natural energies, emanating as Cobalt-60 decays. The first step in treatment planning is a simulation. During a simulation, the best positioning for the patient is determined. The required immobilization devices are created. A CT or MRI scan is then performed. The images are loaded into software allowing the radiation oncology team to develop a virtual treatment, to assess all possible treatment delivery options. There are several types of EBRT, as follows:

- *Three-dimensional conformal radiotherapy (3DCRT)* – via the planning CT scan, the 3D representation of the tumor and normal tissues are used, along with all possible beam angles, patient angles, and non-movable beam shapes; this form of EBRT is used frequently today – often for breast or lung cancer
- *Intensity-modulated radiation therapy (IMRT)* – the beam shape is dynamically changed during treatment, with dynamic movements of the leaves; it adds an almost limitless amount of treatment options, with every shape being possible for as long as needed; this form of EBRT utilizes *inverse planning* that uses a series of goals for treatment, with software creating the best dynamic beam shaping for the patient; the series of goals include dose–volume relationships for the tumor or tumors plus surrounding normal tissues, and a prioritization score for each organ – for example, the amount of Gray (Gy) that each organ can receive, or how much of the tumor must receive a full dose; IMRT is successfully used for thymic cancer (see Figure 15.2) as well as for sinonasal and nasopharyngeal cancers, malignant pleural mesothelioma, soft tissue sarcomas, and anal cancer
- *Image guidance (basic)* – after reproducing patient positioning from the simulation, a series of X-ray images are obtained using the linac; these verify that patient positioning, beam shaping, and beam angles match the treatment plan; after the images are approved by the radiation oncologist, treatment begins; if adjustments are required, they are made before the actual treatment starts; the images are repeated regularly – often weekly – to assure there are no changes; image-guided radiotherapy is successfully used for thymic cancer
- *Image guidance (advanced)* – sometimes, more detailed and frequent forms of image guidance are done, with more visualization than on plain X-rays; radio-opaque markers called **fiducials** can be placed into the organ of interest; when the X-ray is taken, the markers are visualized; the location of the soft tissue organ can be precisely assessed and its position adjusted so that it is with 1 mm of the correct location; this form of EBRT is often used for liver, lung, pancreas, and prostate cancers – especially along with stereotactic body radiotherapy (SBRT); fiducial-based image guidance is usually performed before each treatment; another type of advanced image guidance is done with a CT scan by using the linac, before treatment; this is called a *cone beam CT (CBCT)* and can be done daily; position of the tumor can be noted, as well as variations in internal anatomy that could affect proper dosing; the tumor position can be adjusted to within 2 mm accuracy for soft tissues; other adjustments can be made for normal tissue changes
- *Image-guided IMRT and image-guided 3DCRT* – daily image guidance can be combined with IMRT or 3DCRT, but this is not a common practice in radiation oncology; if it is done, image-guided IMRT is used for head, neck, and prostate cancers, and image-guided 3DCRT is used for lung cancers

---

Significant Point

EBRT is the most common type of radiation therapy used for cancer treatment. It allows for very careful delivery of radiation to a target site, is often done as an outpatient procedure, and may last for many weeks. All of the various types of EBRT are used to deliver the highest prescribed dose of radiation to a tumor while sparing normal tissue surrounding it. Each type uses a computer to analyze tumor images to calculate the most precise dose and the best treatment path.

(a)

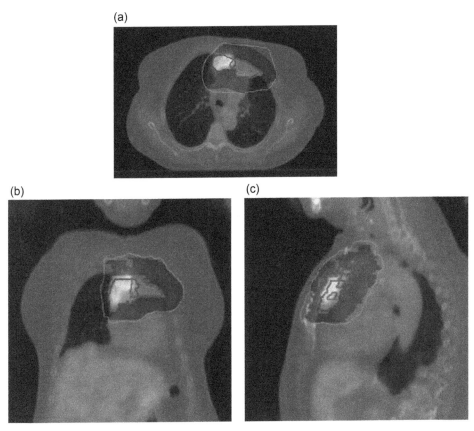

(b)   (c)

Figure 15.2 Three-dimensional intensity-modulated radiation therapy (IMRT) for stage IIB thymic carcinoma after thymectomy with a positive margin in (a) axial, (b) coronal, and (c) sagittal planes. The preoperative PET scan has been fused to the CT simulation scan for target delineation purposes. The red line shows the preoperative gross tumor volume. The pink line shows the postoperative tumor bed. The clinical target volume is green, and the planning target volume is blue. The orange line indicates the total irradiated area. *Source*: Figure 2.1 from Page 24 of The American Cancer Society's Oncology in Practice [1].

Adverse effects of the various forms of EBRT (based on the area of the body being treated) include skin fibrosis, altered taste, mucositis, osteoradionecrosis, and chronic dry mouth.

Stereotactic Radiosurgery

Stereotactic radiosurgery (SRS) is a procedure that uses many extremely focused radiation beams to target tumors and other abnormalities in the brain, neck, lungs, liver, spine, and other areas. A similar procedure, **stereotactic body radiotherapy** (SBRT) is also known as *stereotactic ablative body radiosurgery (SABR)*. It offers the same features of EBRT

along with precise tumor localization throughout an entire treatment. It accounts for movements of the patient plus internal organ movements, via rigid immobilization and tracking of the target organ. Both procedures are so precise that a margin of tissue around a tumor does not also need to be treated. A much higher dose of radiation can be used in a single treatment. This means there is a need for fewer treatments. Biologically significant higher doses yield better tumor control. The SRS procedure often focuses on brain irradiation, and it is often used for brain metastases as well as benign and malignant brain tumors. The SRS procedure is delivered using a linac or the dedicated unit called the **Gamma**

Knife. The SBRT procedure is applied in the body, often for liver, lung, and prostate cancers, as well as for certain metastases. The high radiation doses per treatment yield greatly improved tumor control than expected for the doses used. This is especially true for renal cell carcinoma, but also for melanoma and prostate cancer.

For T1, and T2 lymph node negative lung tumors, in patients that cannot have surgery because of other comorbidities, SBRT is effective. Delivery over 3–5 fractions can achieve almost 90% disease control. The SBRT procedure is good for peripheral tumors and is being studied for centrally located tumors. It is also being studied for use along with systemic therapy for early-stage non-small cell lung carcinoma. For lung cancer, other surgical options include three-dimensional conformal radiotherapy (3DCRT), advanced image guidance radiation therapy, image-guided 3DCRT, and stereotactic body radiotherapy.

For stage IV disease, stereotactic radiosurgery can be used for patients with low volume brain metastasis, when there are less than four lesions. This therapy can also be used for brain lesions that progress after whole brain radiotherapy has been administered. Availability of stereotactic radiosurgery has greatly improved survival for patients with lung cancer that has metastasized to the brain. Stereotactic radiosurgery is also commonly used to treat pituitary tumors.

Clinical Case

1. Which types of radiation therapy are options for lung cancer?
2. How does stereotactic radiosurgery work?
3. Can stereotactic radiosurgery be used for stage IV lung cancer?

A 71-year-old woman began experiencing a constant, nonproductive cough whenever she exercised. A CT scan and biopsy confirmed an isolated early-stage lung tumor. The patient did not want to have surgery if at all possible, so the medical team decided that stereotactic radiosurgery was a good option. The procedure was undertaken, and was curative, using minimized radiation doses and adverse effect risks to the patient's lungs, heart, and esophagus. She recovered well and was able to resume her exercise regimen soon after returning home.

Answers:

1. **Radiation therapies that are options for lung cancer include three-dimensional conformal radiotherapy (3DCRT), advanced image guidance radiation therapy, image-guided 3DCRT, stereotactic radiosurgery, and stereotactic body radiotherapy.**
2. **Stereotactic radiosurgery is a procedure that uses many extremely focused radiation beams to target tumors and other abnormalities. It is so precise that a margin of tissue around a tumor does not also need to be treated, and a much higher dose of radiation can be used in a single treatment. This means there is a need for fewer treatments. Biologically significant higher doses yield better tumor control. The procedure is delivered using a linac or the dedicated unit called the Gamma Knife.**
3. **For stage IV lung cancer, stereotactic radiosurgery can be used for patients, even with low volume brain metastasis – when there are less than four lesions.**

Adaptive Planning

Another benefit of cone beam CT-based image guidance is identifying significant decreases in tumor volume because of treatment – as they occur. With these decreases, normal tissues occupy the space where the tumor had been, and therefore, they can be exposed to larger-than-intended doses of radiation. The radiation oncologist can use adaptive planning by repeating the planning CT simulation and then re-planning a smaller volume radiation procedure. This decreases risks of toxicity from radiotherapy.

Charged Particle External Beam Radiation Therapy

Charged particle EBRT uses protons because a proton beam will not deliver radiation to body tissues beyond a specific intended depth. The proton beam also delivers a lower entry dose before reaching the target depth – compared with X-rays. Therefore, much lower doses of radiation are delivered to tissues not extremely close to the tumor. However, tissues that are very close to the tumor still receive radiation. It is currently unknown about the benefits of delivering lower doses of radiation to these tissues via protein EBRT. It is theorized that proton therapy should have a lower risk of radiation-linked secondary malignancies. One of the leading uses of proton therapy is for pediatric radiation oncology. Other common uses are treatment of eye tumors, skull-based tumors, and recurring head and neck cancers. All techniques used for X-rays are either part of proton therapy or are being developed. Proton treatment centers have grown in popularity throughout the world.

Heavy Charged Particle External Beam Radiation Therapy

A new development in radiation therapy is the use of beams of heavy charged particles, such as carbon ions. The particles are more damaging over short distances. They provide more tumor cell death with only single "hits." This may overcome resistance of hypoxic tumors to X-rays and protons. However, there are not many particle beam facilities in existence as of today.

Brachytherapy

Brachytherapy involves the implantation of radioactive materials, within seeds, pellets, or wires, into or close to tumors. This treatment method can be curative in head, neck, cervical, vaginal, rectal, penile, and prostate cancers. It is also used as an adjunct to surgery for recurring tumors, soft tissue sarcomas, and uterine cancers. Brachytherapy allows for very high doses of radiation to be delivered into a tumor. The level of radiation exposure decreases quickly as the distance away from the radioactive source increases. This creates a good ratio of *dose:tumor* versus *dose:normal* tissues. There are three important elements regarding the use of brachytherapy, as follows:

- There must be a localized tumor or tumor bed that can be encompassed by the radiation emitted from the implanted radioactive materials
- There must be a method for safely and effectively placing the radioactive materials into the tumor or tumor bed
- The normal tissues in or very near the implant, within the volume of the tumor, can tolerate the provided doses

Brachytherapy is not applicable when treatment to a body region is required, such as an entire breast, or the pelvis. Brachytherapy may involve *permanent* and *temporary* implants. Permanent implants have radioactive materials of low energy. This means that radiation is delivered within 5–10 mm of the source. There is a half-life providing complete delivery of the therapeutic dose over weeks to months. This allows the patient to return home immediately after the radioactive materials have been placed. The radioactivity decays into a non-radioactive element, and can remain in the patient's body throughout life with no problems. Permanent brachytherapy is most often used for prostate cancer.

Temporary implants use radioactive materials that deliver radiation for a shorter period of time. There is high energy, and the patient should not go out into public places while the implants are in place. There are two forms of temporary implants: *low-dose-rate (LDR)* and *high-dose-rate (HDR)* implants. The LDR implants usually deliver therapeutic doses over a 24–48-hour implant session. The patient usually needs 1–2 sessions, which require an inpatient stay. The HDR implants deliver therapeutic doses over only 5–45 minutes, resulting in a higher biologic effect per dose to the normal tissues. The treatment is divided into 2–6 treatments, over 1–6 weeks. The treatments can be performed on an outpatient basis. In recent years, there has been increased use of outpatient multi-faction HDR implants compared with temporary LDR inpatient treatments.

Significant Point

Traditional brachytherapy delivers low doses of radiation; the newest variations use high doses. The radiation used for brachytherapy is generated electronically and designed with a high level of precision. Brachytherapy requires a much shorter treatment time than other traditional radiation procedures. Prostate brachytherapy usually involves an outpatient procedure, and has comparable results to radical prostatectomy.

Clinical Case

1. What is the procedure of brachytherapy and its indication?
2. How much radiation can be used during brachytherapy?
3. What are the permanent and temporary implants used in brachytherapy?

A 56-year-old African American man was referred by his physician to a urologist because of rising PSA levels. The patient also had decreased force of his urine stream, and hesitancy. Transrectal ultrasound and biopsy revealed a differentiated adenocarcinoma of the prostate gland, with no local invasion. It was considered very low risk, and it was determined that LDR brachytherapy would be an excellent treatment option. Brachytherapy seeds were implanted, and they remained within the prostate with no misplacement elsewhere in the patient's body. The procedure was successful, and the prostate cancer was cured.

Answers:

1. **Brachytherapy involves the implantation of radioactive materials, within seeds, pellets, or wires, into or close to tumors. It can be curative in head, neck, cervical, vaginal, rectal, penile, and prostate cancers. Brachytherapy can also be used as an adjunct to surgery for recurring tumors, soft tissue sarcomas, and uterine cancers.**
2. **Brachytherapy allows for very high doses of radiation to be delivered into a tumor. The level of radiation exposure decreases quickly as the distance away from the radioactive source increases. This creates a good ratio of dose:tumor versus dose:normal tissues.**
3. **Permanent implants have radioactive materials of low energy, and radiation is delivered within 5–10 mm of the source, over weeks to months. Permanent brachytherapy is most often used for prostate cancer. Temporary implants use radioactive materials that deliver radiation for a shorter period of time. There is high energy, and the patient should not go out into public places while the implants are in place. There are LDR and HDR implants. The HDR implants are used more often today, delivering therapeutic doses over only 5–45 minutes, with 2–6 treatments occurring over 1–6 weeks, on an outpatient basis.**

Radionuclide Therapy

Radionuclide therapy, also called *unsealed source radiotherapy*, delivers radioactive materials directly into the patient. This can occur intravenously, intraarterially, or orally. The materials are not sealed within a seed, pellet, or wire. This type of radiation therapy is important for treating thyroid and liver cancers, lymphomas, and bone metastases – especially from prostate cancer. Nuclear medicine physicians or radiation oncologists usually provide unsealed source radiotherapy. The radioactivity is delivered to tumors in one of three ways, as follows:

- Tumor or normal tissue biochemistry – radium-223 for bone metastases, iodine-131 for thyroid cancer
- Attachment to a monoclonal antibody, targeted to a tumor-expressed antigen – such as yttrium 90-ibritumomab for CD20-positive lymphoma
- Direct, selective delivery into an artery that feeds the tumor – yttrium-90-microspheres into a hepatic artery branch, for liver tumors

The therapeutic radiation must travel only a short distance, from the radioactive materials. It is delivered via **beta particles** (equivalent to electrons) such as I-131 or Y-90, or via alpha particles such as Radium-223. From I-131, gamma rays are also delivered, which allows it to be imaged.

Intraoperative Radiotherapy

Intraoperative radiotherapy can be delivered via an external radiation source. This includes mobile electron beam machines, mobile low-energy X-ray machines (electronic brachytherapy machines), linacs, and via brachytherapy using intraoperative HDR or intraoperative catheter placement. After the operation, the catheters are loaded with LDR sources. Intraoperative radiotherapy is often used to treat tumors along with surgical resections. This is especially done in areas that are difficult to treat with conventional radiation therapies. These include previously irradiated sites and retroperitoneal sarcomas. Intraoperative radiotherapy is being studied to treat breast cancer along with lumpectomy.

Combined-Modality Therapy

Combined-modality therapy (CMT) uses biotherapy, chemotherapy, radiation, and surgery concurrently, or at alternating intervals. This therapy can be extremely successful and improve disease-free survival, local-regional disease control, and overall survival rates. Organ function can also be preserved. Quality of life is improved regardless of whether the therapy is to control or cure cancer, or to provide palliation. As far back as 1999, studies proved that platinum-based chemotherapy given along with daily radiation for cervical cancer provided a 30–50% increased survival rate. This changed the standard of care for cervical cancer. Chemotherapeutic agents used because of their radiosensitizing effects include: carboplatin, cisplatin, docetaxel, 5-fluorouracil (5-FU), mitomycin-C, navelbine, and paclitaxel. Agents that may also be useful include: actinomycin D, bleomycin, doxorubicin, etoposide, methotrexate, and vinblastine. Cisplatin and 5-FU are commonly used radiosensitizing agents. For brain tumors, the drug called temozolomide is often used.

In CMT, a greater kill rate of tumor cells can be obtained by either radiation or chemotherapy alone. However, there is a potential for acute and late toxicities to be more common, which must be evaluated, documented, and managed quickly. The chemotherapy agent may cause toxicities that are similar or different from those of radiation therapy alone. Acute toxicities are most likely in the GI tract, integumentary, and myeloproliferative systems. Late toxicities are most common at the actual site of radiation therapy. In lung cancer patients, for example, there may be fibrosis, pneumonitis, or both. In rectal cancer patients, there may be proctitis.

In combination regimens, targeted therapies are beginning to have promising results. The monoclonal antibody called cetuximab is approved for locally or regionally advanced squamous cell carcinoma of the head and neck, concurrently with radiation therapy. Adverse effects of cetuximab include acneiform rash, pruritus, and an infusion reaction during administration. It is important to distinguish between radiation skin reactions and acneiform rash since their treatments are different. Ongoing study focuses on targeted agents for head and neck, colorectal, and lung cancers. The newer agents are different from traditional chemotherapies because of different adverse effect profiles.

A difficult aspect is determining the best timing, sequencing, and dose of each chemotherapy agent with radiation therapy. Some agents must be administered immediately before or after another type of treatment. Often, surgery can be done before or after administration of chemotherapy and radiation. Before radiation, surgery, or both, chemotherapy can be given (induction or neoadjuvant), to reduce tumor size. This can result in a smaller radiation treatment field or less tissues that need to be surgically removed. This method can also reduce risks for metastasis. Concurrent chemotherapy is given during radiation therapy. This may be daily, weekly, or continuous infusion based on the agent, its dose, and its toxicities. Chemotherapy helps increase tumor cell death and maximize tumor responses to radiation. *Sequential therapy (the sandwich technique)* is another form of concurrent therapy. It has been done in clinical trials for lung, head, and neck cancers. A split course of radiation is given, and during planned pauses in radiation therapy, chemotherapy is given. Also, adjuvant chemotherapy can be given after a course of radiation is done, to control subclinical disease and micrometastases.

Based on the site of the cancer, radiation therapy can also be given before or after surgery. Preoperative radiation can help shrink tumors, meaning that there can be less extensive surgical resection, increasing the likelihood for the target organ to be preserved. However, surgical staging is often affected since the tumor has reduced in size. The patient can experience healing problems at the site of irradiation. After surgery, radiation is delivered to reduce risks of local recurrences. CMT is used to treat cancers such as squamous cell tumors of the anus, cervix, head, neck, lungs, and rectum. Chemotherapy with radiation in varying schedules can be done for cancers of the bladder, esophagus, pancreas, and stomach. It is crucial to correctly manage symptoms since each treatment has unique adverse effects, which can be synergistic, or can worsen adverse effects of other treatments.

> **Significant Point**
>
> CMT for cancer usually involves some combination of radiation therapy, chemotherapy, and surgery. These combinations are utilized when it is possible to improve the likelihood of a cure, or to decrease risks of significant complications. One example of CMT is to administer radiation therapy for cancers of the mouth or throat, followed by neck dissection to remove lymph nodes from the neck.

Hyperthermia

In clinical trials, the use of hyperthermia is being studied. Heat may be applied along with radiation and chemotherapy. Body tissues are exposed to temperatures up to 113°F, to damage and kill cancer cells while only causing minimal injury to normal tissues. Hyperthermia can shrink tumor cells by killing cancer cells and damaging the proteins and structures inside the cells. Heat can be applied locally to a small area, or regionally to larger areas of the body. There is also whole-body hyperthermia for metastatic cancer that has spread widely. The U.S. Food and Drug Administration (FDA) approved the first hyperthermia system in 2011, called the *BSD-2000 Hyperthermia System*, created by *BSD Medical*. It uses focused electromagnetic energy to apply therapeutic heating to deep tumors, more than 3 cm under the skin surface.

Hyperthermia has additive and synergistic effects after radiation therapy has already been done. It appears that hyperthermia complements the effects of radiation in relation to inhibited DNA repair, sensitivity of the cell cycle, plus effects of hypoxia and deprivation of nutrients. Tumor tissues are sensitized more than normal tissues. Supportive biologic effects include increased sensitivity to radiation during the S phase of the cell cycle, reoxygenation, and inhibited DNA repair. Hyperthermia has been used to treat cancers of the brain, head, neck, breasts, cervix, and rectum as well as various sarcomas and melanoma. Regional hyperthermia is applied in a machine that uses multiple antennas and widely spread applicators to distribute power density and temperature (see Figure 15.3).

The smaller devices are used for superficial areas, such as for melanoma, while the regional or deep applicators are used for deeper-located tumors, such as cancers of the cervix and rectum. Treatments last from 60 to 90 minutes. Tumors are heated for 30 minutes or longer, usually to temperatures between 104°F and 109.4°F. Thermometry catheters are placed either into the actual tumor, onto the skin, or within a body orifice. Heating is achieved via low- or high-frequency microwaves, radiofrequencies, or ultrasound. With increased temperature, blood flow increases in the tissues. *Thermotolerance* is a temporary reaction to thermal stress. It causes surviving, heated cells to be more resistant to further heat stress. It may develop during or after heat stress, lasting for several days. Heat treatments are given two times per week, once per week, or monthly. This is based on the combinations between hyperthermia, radiation, and chemotherapy. Common adverse effects include first- or second-degree superficial or subcutaneous burns. With regional deep hyperthermia, there is cardiovascular stress because of changes in blood pressure and pulse.

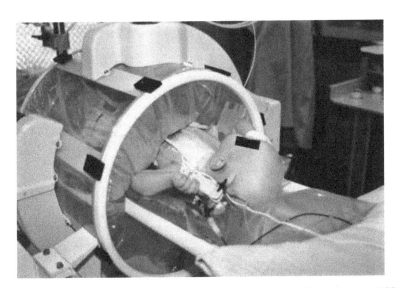

Figure 15.3 Regional hyperthermia device. *Source:* American Cancer Society (ACS) Journals – Cancer [2].

Hyperthermia has additive and synergistic effects with chemotherapy as well as radiation. Drug delivery and reoxygenation are increased by higher perfusion rates. This increases the effectiveness of radiation therapy. Except for 5-FU and possibly other antimetabolites, most chemotherapy agents are best used with concurrent administration with the heat therapy, or if the chemotherapy is administered immediately before the heat therapy.

Significant Point

Hyperthermia is usually used along with other forms of cancer therapy. It makes some cancer cells more sensitive to radiation, and can also harm other cancer cells that are not damaged by radiation. Hyperthermia and radiation therapy are often administered within one hour of each other. Most studies have revealed that these combination treatments provide a significant reduction in tumor size. Effectiveness of hyperthermia is related to the temperature that is reached, the length of treatment, and the characteristics of the target cells and tissues.

Clinical Case

1. How does hyperthermia work in cancer treatment?
2. In what way does hyperthermia complement radiation therapy?
3. How long do hyperthermia treatments last?

A 69-year-old woman with recurrent breast cancer was evaluated by a radiation oncologist, who recommended that hyperthermia with radiation therapy be used. His reasoning was based on the fact that hyperthermia makes tumor cells more sensitive to radiation, which improves tumor control while minimizing damage to healthy tissues. The procedure was performed, and the patient remained taking hormonal therapy afterward. There was no recurrence of the cancer this time.

Answers:

1. **In hyperthermia, body tissues are exposed to temperatures up to 113°F, to damage and kill cancer cells while only causing minimal injury to normal tissues. Hyperthermia can shrink tumor cells by killing cancer cells and damaging the proteins and structures inside the cells. Heat can be applied locally, regionally, or to the whole body.**
2. **Hyperthermia has additive and synergistic effects after radiation therapy has already been done. It appears that hyperthermia complements the effects of radiation in relation to inhibited DNA repair, sensitivity of the cell cycle, plus effects of hypoxia and deprivation of nutrients.**
3. **Hyperthermia treatments last from 60 to 90 minutes. Tumors are heated for 30 minutes or longer. Treatments are given two times per week, once per week, or monthly, based on combinations between hyperthermia, radiation, and chemotherapy.**

Accidental Radiation Exposure

Because of background radiation from environmental radioactive substances and cosmic rays, chronic low-dose exposure to radiation affects us all. The amount we receive is varied based on location on the planet and the surrounding environmental factors. On average, each human being receives about 3 millisieverts (mSv) of background radiation per year. This is a safe level of radiation exposure and basically is unavoidable. People that work in the radiation industry are exposed to higher levels, but they are still considered within safe limits. They use **dosimeters** to monitor levels of exposure. These devices are also used by personnel that work with brachytherapy and radiopharmaceuticals. Accidental radiation exposure or low-dose exposure occurs in nuclear power plants or in those that handle **isotopes**. Common injuries from these exposures include chromosomal translocations and bone marrow and skin changes.

Radiation levels must be monitored, using *as low as reasonable achievable* guidelines. Aside from dosimeters, **ring badges** may be worn that monitor exposure, as well as **pocket ion chambers**. Most data on radiation exposure have come from nuclear reactor accidents or the atomic bombs used in World War II. Data is also available from radiation treatment procedure documentation. It is basically known that it takes less time for leukemia to develop after accidental radiation exposure than it takes for solid tumors to develop.

Acute Radiation Syndrome

In *acute radiation syndrome*, prodromal signs and symptoms occur immediately after exposure. The prodromal phase lasts only two days, signified by various fever, GI symptoms, and tachycardia. Symptoms are more severe when the radiation dose is larger. Next, there is a latent phase, from day 2 to 20, with illness manifesting in days 21–60. Symptoms are linked to the actual syndrome being experienced. In low-dose exposure, the latent phase can last for weeks. With higher doses, the prodromal and latent phases may be short, with the patient immediately developing a syndrome that can be fatal. The four types of syndromes caused by acute radiation syndrome are: cutaneous, gastrointestinal, hematopoietic, and cerebrovascular.

Cutaneous Syndrome

Acute radiation exposure causes cutaneous syndrome. Symptoms include edema, erythema, and desquamation. If cutaneous syndrome is advanced, there may be ulceration of the epidermis or dermis.

Gastrointestinal Syndrome

After total body exposure to 10 gray or more, death occurs within a few days to weeks. This length of time is based on the amount of GI damage. The intestinal villi are highly sensitive to radiation. The villi disappear and there is a complete loss of normal cell-renewal processes. Symptoms include anorexia, nausea, vomiting, severe diarrhea, and lethargy before death. Sepsis is another critical feature. Treatment is generally supportive, using antiemetics, antimotility agents, antibiotics, intravenous fluids, narcotics, and total parenteral nutrition.

Hematopoietic Syndrome

Hematopoietic failure occurs after total body radiation exposure, in one dose between 300 and 800 **centigray** (cGy). Stem cells are highly susceptible and are sterilized almost immediately. As blood circulating cells die off over a few weeks, bone marrow replacement becomes insufficient, and crisis symptoms appear. Usually, within three weeks of exposure, the patient has fatigue, petechiae, mouth ulcerations, chills, and fever. These are all related to distraction of blood cells. Treatment usually includes isolation, antibiotics, blood transfusions, and growth factors. Unless the bone marrow recovers or there is a successful bone marrow transplantation, the patient will die.

Cerebrovascular Syndrome

Following total body exposure of more than 10 Gy, cerebrovascular symptoms appear. These symptoms may present as visual impairment, seizures, lack of coordination, disorientation, hypotension, kidney failure, respiratory distress, and coma. There are short prodromal and latent phases. If exposure is from high doses, GI symptoms develop almost immediately. Death from neurovascular failure occurs within hours to a few days. Treatment is generally supportive, consisting of oxygen, anticonvulsants, intravenous fluids, narcotics, and sedatives.

Radiation on the Embryo and Fetus

Most data on radiation exposure to embryos and fetuses have come from animal studies, for obvious ethical reasons. Information on human fetal exposure has been documented because of children that were in utero during the atomic bombs dropped on Japan in 1945. Additional data have been provided from medical radiation exposure during the twentieth century – before its impact on embryos and fetuses was understood. Radiation is a teratogen. A developing embryo or fetus is sensitive to its damaging effects, because of quickly dividing cells during development. Organogenesis and the fetal period have high sensitivities to radiation. There are three primary effects of radiation upon a developing embryo, as follows:

- Intrauterine growth retardation
- Death during the embryonic, fetal, or neonatal periods
- Congenital malformations

Frequency and severity of radiation exposure-related effects are based on the stage of gestation at exposure; organ systems that are exposed, the LET of the radiation, the total dose or absorbed-dose equivalent, the dose rate, and fractionation. Radiation is usually lethal to an embryo during preimplantation or soon afterward. A surprising fact is that a surviving embryo experiences normal growth since, at this time of gestation, cells are only dividing and not differentiating.

During organogenesis, the embryo has the highest risk of developing malformations due to radiation exposure. Neonatal death often follows radiation exposure, since many abnormalities that result from such exposure are not compatible with life. If radiation exposure occurs after six weeks of development, there is usually growth retardation, microcephaly, and

mental retardation. Other abnormalities include blindness, clubfoot, hydrocephalus, alopecia of the scalp, and spina bifida.

Radiation and Malignancies

Chronic and low-dose exposure to radiation is known to have carcinogenic effects. While acute exposures are rare, chronic low-dose exposure occurs from the environment or in relation to certain types of work. Therapeutic doses of radiation that are usually given (2500–6500 cGy) are still considered less carcinogenic than lower doses given over significantly longer periods of time. It is theorized that a cell that survived low-dose radiation exposure, but was damaged or altered, can undergo carcinogenic mutation if other conditions are present. Also, a cell that has been destroyed or sterilized by therapeutic radiation doses is likely to be not capable of any malignant changes. Malignancies associated with radiation exposure include hematologic and solid tumors. Individual factors contributing to carcinogenesis include geographic location, genetics, health history, and lifestyle. Child and adult cancer survivors have a higher risk for secondary malignancies based on previous treatments and their genetics. After receiving radiation therapy, patients must be encouraged to continue to have regular screenings and physical examinations. They must be taught the correct self-examination techniques. Lifestyle

---

Significant Point

It is very important to understand that radiation exposure that occurs in an embryo or fetus can increase the risk of development of cancer later in life. Unborn babies are highly sensitive to the cancer-causing effects of radiation. Large radiation doses to a fetus early in development are more likely to cause birth defects – especially to the brain.

choices may need to be changed to decrease the chances of a secondary malignancy.

Special Populations

There are special populations that must be considered in regard to radiation therapy. These include pregnant women (including effects upon the developing fetus), children, and the elderly.

Pregnant Women

Pregnant women requiring radiation therapy must be carefully treated since a developing fetus is highly sensitive to radiation. It is preferable to avoid radiation therapy during the first trimester, which is when the fetus is most highly sensitive. Each individual patient must be evaluated concerning whether treatment is needed, how it should be done, what needs to be treated, and when treatment must occur.

Children

Children are highly sensitive to radiation because it can affect their growth and intellectual development. Also, radiation therapy in children increases risks for treatment-related cancers. However, benefits outweigh the risks, so radiation therapy is often used for a variety of childhood malignancies. There is a large amount of study on pediatric cancers and the links between them and radiation therapy.

Elderly

Radiation therapy in the elderly is generally well-tolerated. However, the patient's overall health status, functionality, and specific organ functions must be evaluated. Many oncological studies have not included elderly patients. This complicates oncological knowledge of radiation use for these patients. Even in the extreme elderly, radiation therapy appears to be better tolerated than chemotherapy.

Key Terms

Apoptosis
Beta particles
Brachytherapy
Cell sterilization
Centigray
Charged particle EBRT
Combined-modality therapy
Direct hit
Dosimeters
External beam radiation therapy
Fiducials
Fractionation
Gamma Knife

Free radical
Gray
Isotopes
Linear accelerator
Osteoradionecrosis
Oxygen tension
Pocket ion chambers
Ring badges
Stereotactic body radiotherapy
Stereotactic radiosurgery
Target theory
Therapeutic index

Bibliography

1 American Cancer Society. The. (2018). *The American Cancer Society's Oncology in Practice*. Hoboken: John Wiley & Sons, Inc. Figure 2.1 from Page 24.

2 American Cancer Society (ACS) Journals – Cancer. (2000). *Hyperthermia for the treatment of patients with malignant germ cell tumors*. John Wiley & Sons, Inc. https://acsjournals.

onlinelibrary.wiley.com/doi/full/10.1002/(SICI)1097-0142(19980215)82:4%3C793::AID-CNCR24%3E3.0.CO;2-S. Volume 82, Issue 4, p. 793–800, Figure 2. Accessed 2021.

3 Baronzio, G.F. and Hager, E.D. (2006). *Hyperthermia in Cancer Treatment: A Primer (Medical Intelligence Unit)*. New York: Springer.

4 Bellon, J.R., Wong, J.S., MacDonald, S.M., and Ho, A.Y. (2016). *Radiation Therapy Techniques and Treatment Planning for Breast Cancer: A Practical Guide on Treatment Techniques (Practical Guides in Radiation Oncology)*. New York: Springer.

5 Cefaro, G.A., Genovesi, D., Perez, C.A., and Vinciguerra, A. (2008). *A Guide for Delineation of Lymph Nodal Clinical Target Volume in Radiation Therapy*. New York: Springer.

6 Chinol, M. and Paganelli, G. (2016). *Radionuclide Peptide Cancer Therapy*. Boca Raton: CRC Press.

7 Cognetta, A.B., Jr and Mendenhall, W.M. (2013). *Radiation Therapy for Skin Cancer*. New York: Springer.

8 Darafsheh, A. (2021). *Radiation Therapy Dosimetry: A Practical Handbook*. Boca Raton: CRC Press.

9 Fanti, S. and Lopci, E. (2016). *Diagnostic Nuclear Medicine and Radionuclide Therapy*. Bologna: Societa Editrice Esculapio.

10 Gibbons, J.P. (2019). *Khan's The Physics of Radiation Therapy*, 6th Edition. Philadelphia: Lippincott, Williams, and Wilkins.

11 Hahn, G.M. (2012). *Hyperthermia and Cancer*. New York: Springer.

12 Hall, E.J. and Giaccia, A.J. (2018). *Radiobiology for the Radiologist*, 8th Edition. Philadelphia: Lippincott, Williams, and Wilkins.

13 Heron, D.E., Soifull Hug, M., and Herman, J.M. (2018). *Stereotactic Radiosurgery and Stereotactic Body Radiation Therapy (SBRT)*. New York: DemosMedical.

14 Hoffman, G. (2019). *Radiotherapy: Theory and Practice*. Forest Hills: Foster Academics.

15 Hoisak, J.D.P., Paxton, A.B., Waghorn, B., and Pawlicki, T. (2020). *Surface Guided Radiation Therapy*. Boca Raton: CRC Press.

16 Issels, R.D. and Wilmanns, W. (2012). *Application of Hyperthermia in the Treatment of Cancer (Recent Results in Cancer Research, Book 107)*. New York: Springer-Verlag.

17 Joiner, M.C. and van der Kogel, A.J. (2018). *Basic Clinical Radiobiology*, 5th Edition. Boca Raton: CRC Press.

18 Kaider-Person, O. and Chen, R. (2018). *Hypofractionated and Stereotactic Radiation Therapy*. New York: Springer.

19 Knapp, F.F., (Russ) and Dash, A. (2016). *Radiopharmaceuticals for Therapy*. New York: Springer.

20 Koontz, B.F. (2017). *Radiation Therapy Treatment Effects: An Evidence-Based Guide to Managing Toxicity*. New York: DemosMedical.

21 Li, X.A. (2020). *Adaptive Radiation Therapy*. Boca Raton: CRC Press.

22 McDermott, P.N. and Orton, C.G. (2018). *The Physics & Technology of Radiation Therapy*, 2nd Edition. Madison: Medical Physics Publishing.

23 Medgadget. (2011). *BSD-2000 hyperthermia system receives FDA HDE marketing approval*. Medgadget, Inc. https://www.medgadget.com/2011/11/bsd-2000-hyperthermia-system-receives-fda-hde-marketing-approval.html. Accessed 2021.

24 Meola, A. and Chang, S.T. (2020). *Stereotactic Radiosurgery (SRS) – Procedure, Results and Risks*. Hauppauge: Nova Science Publishin Inc.

25 Minev, B. (2011). *Cancer Management in Man: Chemotherapy, Biological Therapy, Hyperthermia and Supporting Measures*. New York: Springer.

26 National Cancer Institute. (2021). *Hyperthermia in cancer treatment*. U.S. Department of Health and Human Services/National Institutes of Health/National Cancer Institute/USA.gov. https://www.cancer.gov/about-cancer/treatment/types/surgery/hyperthermia-fact-sheet Accessed 2021.

27 Pang, C.L.K. (2015). *Hyperthermia in Oncology*. Boca Raton: CRC Press.

28 Petrovich, Z., Brady, L.W., Apuzzo, M.L., and Bamberg, M. (2003). *Combined Modality Therapy of Central Nervous System Tumors*

(Medical Radiology/Radiation Oncology). New York: Springer.

29 Saha, G.B. (2013). *Physics and Radiobiology of Nuclear Medicine*, 4th Edition. New York: Springer.

30 Stigbrand, T., Carlsson, J., and Adams, G.P. (2008). *Targeted Radionuclide Tumor Therapy: Biological Aspects*. New York: Springer.

31 Trifiletti, D.M., Chao, S.T., Sahgal, A., and Sheehan, J.P. (2019). *Stereotactic Radiosurgery and Stereotactic Body Radiation Therapy: A Comprehensive Guide*. New York: Springer.

32 Valkovic, V. (2019). *Radioactivity in the Environment*, 2nd Edition. Amsterdam: Elsevier.

33 Washington, C.M., Leaver, D.T., and Trad, M. (2020). *Washington & Leaver's Principles and Practice of Radiation Therapy*, 5th Edition. Maryland Heights: Mosby.

34 Wiley Online Library – Cell Proliferation. (2003). *The cell cycle: A review of regulation, deregulation, and therapeutic targets in cancer*. https://onlinelibrary.wiley.com/doi/epdf/10.1046/j.1365-2184.2003.00266.x. John Wiley & Sons, Inc. Volume 36, Issue 3, p. 131–149, Figure 1. Accessed 2021.

35 Xia, P., Godley, A., Shah, C., Videtic, G.M.M., and Suh, J.H. (2018). *Strategies for Radiation Therapy Treatment Planning*. New York: DemosMedical.

16

Chemotherapy

Global Epidemiology of Cancer: Diagnosis and Treatment, First Edition. Jahangir Moini,
Nicholas G. Avgeropoulos, and Craig Badolato.
© 2022 John Wiley & Sons Ltd. Published 2022 by John Wiley & Sons Ltd.

Pharmacology of Chemotherapeutic Drugs

Many chemotherapeutic drugs are unique in comparison with other types of drugs, since the main goal is to cause the death of tumor cells. Since normal cells and tumor cells may be similar, chemotherapy often causes healthy tissues to be destroyed along with tumors. Having the most effectiveness and lowest toxicities are the pharmacological focuses of chemotherapeutic drugs.

Principles of Pharmacokinetics

Pharmacokinetics, the study of how drugs move throughout the body, differs significantly between individual people. It is very closely related to each drug's physical and chemical properties. Outcomes of pharmacokinetics are also based on the patient's physiology and the type of cancer that is present. The serum **half-life** is the period of time needed for a drug's serum concentration to decrease by one-half. Understanding a chemotherapeutic agent's half-life is important to determine the time needed for a dose to be eliminated from the body. This is equivalent to 3–4 half-lives of the drug. **Clearance** is based on an organ's blood flow – usually the kidneys or liver – and how effective they are in removing the drug from the bloodstream. When a drug is cleared by more than one body organ, *total clearance* is the sum of the individual clearances of each involved organ. Total clearance determines the drug's steady-state concentration. It is an independent factor from half-life. Clearance is affected by protein binding, enzyme function, and changes in blood flow to an organ. The drug *cyclophosphamide* is extremely dependent upon metabolizing enzymes to be activated and inactivated. Induction or inhibition of metabolizing enzymes can cause faster or slower drug clearance.

A drug's **volume of distribution** (V_D) compares the amount of drug present to the serum concentration. This is different between individual patients. It is related to the drug's ability to bind to proteins, and to be distributed in the extravascular compartments – known as *tissue binding*. Changes in protein binding from hypoalbuminemia or drug interactions can alter the removal of drugs that are highly protein-bound, such as *etoposide* and *teniposide(Vumon)*. Pharmacokinetic variabilities help explain response and toxicity differences in patients given similar doses and schedules of the same drug. The four major principles of pharmacokinetics include *absorption, distribution, metabolism,* and *elimination*, which are further explained as follows:

- *Absorption* – a drug's absorption from the gastrointestinal tract (GI) should be enough so that there is sufficient bioavailability. Most anticancer drugs have poor, unpredictable bioavailability. Therefore, most are given by injection, ensuring accurate doses and the best possible systemic exposure. Oral anticancer drugs include the following:
  - Alkylating agents – *cyclophosphamide (Cytoxan), chlorambucil (Leukeran), melphalan (Alkeran)*
  - *etoposide (Toposar)*
  - *lomustine (Gleostine)*
  - *methotrexate (Trexall)*
  - *procarbazine (Matulane)*

Oral distribution is not ideal for some of these drugs. However, the amount reaching the systemic circulation (and even more important, the tumor) is enough to cause a response. Some drugs are given as *prodrugs*, which are easily absorbed from the GI tract, then converted to an active cytotoxic agent. *Capecitabine (Xeloda)* and *temozolomide (Temodar)* are such oral prodrugs. In vivo, they are transformed into biochemically equivalent agents – respectively, *fluorouracil* and *dacarbazine*. Newer oral anticancer drugs offer better predictability of their bioavailability.

- *Distribution* – mostly based on a drug's ability to penetrate various tissues, and the amount of **affinity** for binding to plasma proteins. Highly lipophilic drugs usually are more easily taken up by lipophilic tissues – including bone marrow, fat, and tissues of the central nervous system. *Nitrosoureas* include *carmustine (Gliadel)* and *lomustine*. They are used for brain malignancies since they easily penetrate the blood-brain barrier, and for blood malignancies since they easily penetrate the bone marrow. In many cancer patients, there are often decreased plasma protein levels – primarily, albumin. This may be due to nutritional deficiencies or decreased albumin synthesis in the liver. Cytotoxic activities of highly protein-bound agents such as etoposide and teniposide may be increased in this situation, due to a higher percentage of the drug remaining unbound in the bloodstream. Increased unbound fraction of a drug can occur when two highly bound drugs are given concurrently – such as etoposide given with *warfarin (Coumadin)* or *phenytoin (Dilantin)*. Methotrexate is abnormally distributed if a patient has ascites and pleural effusions. This delays its clearance while enhancing hematologic and mucosal toxicities.

- *Metabolism* – the liver is the main site of activation, inactivation, or catabolism of drugs. Some of these enzymatic processes also occur in tumor cells and normal cells. Drugs that must be systemically or intracellularly activated before becoming cytotoxic include anthracycline antibiotics, *capecitabine, carmustine, cyclophosphamide, dacarbazine (DTIC-Dome), hexamethylmelamine (Hexalen), ifosfamide (Ifex), ixabepilone (Ixempra), lomustine*, nitrosoureas, *procarbazine*, and *temozolomide*. The antimetabolites *fluorouracil (Adrucil)* and *cytarabine (Cytosar-U)* are phosphorylated into active nucleotides within tumor cells. *Cisplatin* undergoes intracellular **chemical aquation**, generating a positively charged species that will form **adducts** with DNA molecules. Cyclophosphamide and ifosfamide are transformed into active alkylating species by microsomal enzymes in the liver. Some agents are metabolized into inactive compounds, which are excreted. Metabolic conversion rates can be changed by drug-induced or tumor-induced liver dysfunction, genetic variances in drug

metabolism, or drug-induced changes of enzyme function. If liver function or metabolic enzymes change, this may cause less cytotoxic activity, higher treatment-related toxicity, or both. Activation and/or degradation of many agents utilizes the cytochrome P450 (CYP) family of microsomal enzymes. The CYP subfamily is identified as CYP 3A4. It helps metabolize several drugs used to treat cancer or support cancer care. Cyclophosphamide is activated by the CYP 2B6 subfamily, and has high **inducibility** by antiepileptic drugs such as *phenobarbital (Luminal)* and phenytoin. There is genetic polymorphism in several CYP enzyme subfamilies, including CYP 2D6 and CYP 1A2. In the CYP 2D6 subfamily, there are *extensive, poor*, and *ultra-rapid metabolizers*. Most people are extensive metabolizers. Poor metabolizers make up 5–10% of the Caucasian population, and just 1–2% of the African American and Asian populations. The CYP 2D6 group does not metabolize any anticancer drugs currently known, but does metabolize opiate narcotics, antidepressants, and beta blockers. *Doxorubicin* and *vinblastine* competitively inhibit CYP 2D6, which can lead to a narcotic overdose. Another metabolic factor is the **P-gp efflux pump**. Interactions with this are important in the disposition of drugs used to treat cancer and support care. There is overlap in substrate, inhibitor, and inducer specificity for P-gp and CYP 3A4. This can limit bioavailability and toxicity. Herbs and nutrients can also affect CYP enzymes and alter pharmacokinetics. These include St. John's wort, green tea, fish oil, ginger, and probiotics.

- *Elimination* – for most drugs and their metabolites, the kidneys are the primary organs of elimination. Many anticancer drugs depend on adequate kidney function for elimination. Extreme decreases in kidney function can result in excessive toxicity of drugs such as *bleomycin (Blenoxane), carboplatin (Paraplatin),* cisplatin, cyclophosphamide, *eribulin (Halaven),* etoposide, methotrexate, *oxaliplatin (Eloxatin), pemetrexed (Alimta), pralatrexate (Folotyn)*, and *streptozocin (Zanosar)*. Cisplatin and methotrexate are mostly eliminated by the kidneys, and are actually nephrotoxic. So, reduced kidney function can cause enhanced toxicity if they are given along with additional declines in kidney function. The vinca alkaloids are mostly eliminated by the biliary tract.

Pharmacogenomics

Genetic polymorphism partly explains variability in pharmacokinetics and pharmcodynamics. **Pharmacogenomics** are the inherited differences in drug disposition and effects. In the CYP family of microsomal enzymes, extreme polymorphism has been found in relation to the isoenzymes CYP 3A4, 2C9, and 2D6. Examples of drug-metabolizing enzyme polymorphisms that have clinical oncologic applications include the following:

- Thiopurine-S-methyltransferase deficiency – an inherited condition that results in severe intolerance to *mercaptopurine (Purinethol)*
- Dihydropyrimidine dehydrogenase (DPD) deficiency – this is a rate-limiting enzyme that catabolizes fluorouracil; there can be severe and sometimes fatal toxicity; a blood test is available that detects DPD deficiency, identifying the polymorphism; however, the test is expensive and not widely used.

Genetic polymorphism also describes pharmacodynamic differences. *Tamoxifen (Nolvadex)* is an anti-estrogen used to reduce recurrences of breast cancer – whether adjuvant or metastatic. The CYP 2D6 enzyme aids in biotransformation of tamoxifen to the activate metabolite called *endoxifen.* An extreme genetic polymorphism results in patients being poor, intermediate, or extensive metabolizers. There may be a three-times-higher risk, in poor metabolizers, for breast cancer recurrence, compared with extensive metabolizers. Patients concurrently receiving CYP 2D6 inhibitors, which include antidepressants, may be at risk for cancer recurrence due to reduced metabolic activation of tamoxifen.

Targets of anticancer drugs may be intracellular molecules or structures, including DNA, enzymes, and microtubules. Tumor cells must have an adequate blood supply for optimal chemotherapy. Drugs are transported intracellular though passive, facilitated, or active transport. These can speed up the drug entering the cell or speed up its removal. Systemic drug exposure is also important. A measure of systemic drug exposure is the area under the *serum concentration–time curve (AUC).* The AUC depends upon drug administration and elimination, so changes in these can greatly affect results of treatment. A more rapid clearance rate may mean that larger doses are needed. For a drug such as *carboplatin,* a target AUC is used along with the patient's renal function to predict the best dose.

Chemotherapeutic drugs have traditionally been dosed based on the patient's weight and height (body surface area or BSA), or just on the patient's weight. Individualized dosing is now preferred. Drugs must have certain pharmacokinetic and pharmacodynamic characteristics, calculated via a formula so that the best and most accurate dosing can be accomplished. For example, with *carboplatin,* which is significantly eliminated by the kidneys, clearance is very closely related to the glomerular filtration rate (GFR). Therapeutic efficacy and toxicity can be assessed by an area under the concentration–time curve. Doses can be adjusted based mostly on kidney function and not on the patient's BSA. Carboplatin's primary blood toxicity is thrombocytopenia. Impaired renal function is related to more severe thrombocytopenia. Therefore, for carboplatin, the *Calvert formula* is used, avoiding overdosing when there is impaired kidney function. The formula also maximizes carboplatin's effects when kidney function is above average. The target AUC = 5–7 for single-agent carboplatin; 4–5 for carboplatin with other myelosuppressive drugs (estimated creatinine clearance used for GFR may underestimate dose). The formula is as follows:

Carboplatin dose = AUC × (GFR + 25)

The AUC is calculated as milligrams per milliliter, multiplied by minutes. The GFR is calculated as milliliters per minute. The Calvert formula is often used in adult patients with solid tumors such as ovarian or lung cancer.

Creatinine clearance is measured using the 24-hour urinary collection procedure, or often is calculated using the *Cockcroft–Gault* or *Jelliffe methods*, as follows:

Cockcroft–Gault method

For adults with stable kidney function, and no obesity, the estimated creatinine clearance = [(140 minus age) × actual weight in kg] divided by (72 × serum creatinine in milligram/ deciliter). For females, the result is multiplied by 0.85. For patients from 1 to 20 years, (0.55 × length) divided by serum creatinine. For children under one year of age, (0.45 × length) divided by serum creatinine.

Jelliffe method

For adults with stable kidney function, and no obesity, 98 minus [0.8 × (age minus 20)] divided by serum creatinine in milligram/deciliter. For females, multiply the result by 0.9. To adjust for BSA in any patient, multiply by BSA/1.73.

Drug Interactions with Chemotherapy

When one drug's effects (therapeutic or toxic) are modified by another drug, a drug interaction has occurred. Most interactions are due to changes in pharmacokinetics of the **object drug**, caused by a **precipitating** drug. Changes in metabolism of the object drug, and its distribution and elimination, are usually the cause for pharmacokinetic changes. Less often, interactions are due to overlapping toxicities, including GI intolerance or myelosuppression. Some interactions are beneficial, improving therapy or avoiding toxicity. Most interactions have undesired outcomes, such as worsened adverse effects or less-than-optimal therapeutic response. Clinically significant drug interactions in cancer chemotherapy are summarized in Table 16.1.

Most drug interactions do not cause clinically significant problems or toxicities. They are evaluated based on their overall effect upon therapy and care of the patient. The mechanisms of drug interactions should be assessed. For example,

the cyclosporine and calcium-channel blockers such as *verapamil* are strong inhibitors of the CYP 3A4 enzymes used for the elimination of doxorubicin and etoposide. Cyclosporine and verapamil are also inhibitors of the P-gp-mediate drug resistance for these chemotherapy drugs and natural products. This means that the overall therapeutic response or toxicity reflects both mechanisms of action. When more drugs are needed for therapy, the chance of serious interactions increases. For a patient taking only a few drugs, incidence of all types of interactions is estimated at 3–5%, but in hospitalized patients taking 10–20 medications, interactions are as high as 20%. The risk of drug interactions for cancer patients is relatively high. Toxic outcomes are more likely because of concurrent use of drugs with steep dose–response curves and narrow therapeutic indices. Patients receiving chemotherapies must be continuously monitored for significant drug interactions.

Significant Point

Many members of the public are unaware that common herbal medications can reduce the effectiveness of chemotherapy drugs, or even lead to toxic conditions in the body. Usually, dangerous interactions occur with oral dosage forms of chemotherapies, which are often taken by patients at home. Major interactions have occurred with antidepressants, anticoagulants, antiemetics, antacids, antibiotics, NSAIDs, antifungals, and antivirals.

Antineoplastic Drugs

Chemotherapeutic drugs have long been classified by biological source, chemical structure, and mechanism of action. Cytotoxic drugs are generally grouped by where in the cell cycle they are most toxic. *Cell-cycle-specific agents* are those

Table 16.1 Clinically significant drug interactions in cancer chemotherapy.

Chemotherapy drug	Interacting drug	Effects
Arsenic trioxide	Beta blockers, cisapride, dolansetron, terfenadine	Additive toxicity
Asparaginase	Methotrexate	Reduced toxicity
Bleomycin	Cisplatin	Reduced renal elimination, increased pulmonary toxicity
Busulfan	Phenytoin	Increased metabolic clearance, reduced bone marrow cytotoxicity
Capecitabine	Warfarin	Increased AUC and elimination half-life, doubling international normalized ratio, prolonged prothrombin time
Carmustine	Phenytoin	Reduced phenytoin blood level and antiseizure effects
Cisplatin	Carbamazepine, mesna, phenytoin, sodium thiosulfate, valproic acid	Reduced oral absorption of anticonvulsants, reduced blood levels, chemical incompatibility, reduced cytotoxic and toxic effects; sodium thiosulfate may be used as an antidote for cisplatin toxicity
Corticosteroids (dexamethasone, hydrocortisone, methylprednisolone)	Aminoglutethimide, mitotane	Increased metabolic clearance, reduced therapeutic effect
Cyclophosphamide	Allopurinol	Reduced renal elimination of alkylating metabolite, increased toxicity
CYP 3A4 metabolized drugs (cabazitaxel, dexamethasone, docetaxel, irinotecan, paclitaxel, vinca alkaloids)	Aprepitant	Reduced metabolism, increased cytotoxic effects
Doxorubicin	Verapamil, cyclosporin	Increased AUC, reduced metabolic clearance
Etoposide	Highly protein-bound drugs, phenobarbital, phenytoin	Reduced protein binding, increased myelotoxicity, increased metabolic clearance
Epirubicin (and possibly, other anthracycline compounds)	Paclitaxel (if administered before epirubicin)	Increased neutropenia, thrombocytopenia, and AUC
Fluorouracil	Alfa-interferon	Reduced metabolic clearance, increased cytotoxicity
FOLFOX regimen (fluorouracil, leucovorin, oxaliplatin)	Warfarin	Increased international normalized ratio
Ifosfamide	Antifungals (itraconazole, ketoconazole), phenobarbital	Increased metabolic activation and toxicity
Interleukin-2 (IL-2)	Corticosteroids	Blocked antitumor effects, reduced tumor response rate

(Continued)

Table 16.1 (Continued)

Chemotherapy drug	Interacting drug	Effects
Mercaptopurine	Allopurinol; Warfarin	Reduced metabolic clearance, increased serum levels, prolonged bone marrow suppression; Antagonized anticoagulant effects
Methotrexate	Cotrimoxazole; Nonsteroidal anti-inflammatory drugs (NSAIDs), salicylates	Reduced renal clearance, additive antifolate activity, increased bone marrow toxicity; Reduced renal clearance and protein binding, increased bone marrow and GI toxicity
Mitotane	Warfarin	Increased metabolic clearance
Paclitaxel	Cisplatin	Reduced total-body clearance, increased myelotoxicity
Procarbazine	Ethanol	Blocks metabolism of alcohol, with a disulfiram-like reaction
Tamoxifen	Warfarin	Unknown; enzyme inhibition and/or protein-binding displacement
Vinblastine	Phenytoin	Reduced phenytoin blood levels
Vincristine	Asparaginase	Increased risk of peripheral neurotoxicity

that affect one portion of the cell cycle. Most drugs have effects on no specific phase of the cell cycle, however. They are called *cell-cycle-non-specific agents*. Though antineoplastic drugs in the same class have similar characteristics, there can still be major differences in their indications, pharmaceutical properties, and toxicities. Patients with a form of cancer that is less responsive to a standardized treatment may receive combinations of biological, cytotoxic, and targeted therapies.

Classic Alkylating Agents

Alkylating agents were some of the first drugs used to treat cancer, and are still important in today's chemotherapy. They include drugs with single-agent tumoricidal activity and others that are important as part of combination chemotherapy. Alkylating agents contribute electrophilic alkyl groups, attacking nucleophilic sites on DNA and other biological macromolecules that are rich in electrons. Most often, the site of DNA alkylation is the N-7 position of guanine.

Such DNA adducts may produce many different types of lesions. These include nucleotide-base deletions, ring openings, and strand breaks. With alkylating agents, cytotoxicity and mutagenicity usually occur from these DNA adducts, plus interfering replication and transcription. Many DNA lesions can be restored by repair enzymes. If repairs are only partial, additional DNA damage may occur. Alkylators are non-cell-cycle-phase-specific. Most of them are active in G0, the resting phase, and are usually considered to be mutagens with potential carcinogenicity. This means that health-care workers must avoid exposure to these agents while working with them.

Nitrogen mustard, or *mechlorethamine*, was the first alkylating agent used for cancer therapy. It spontaneously experiences molecular rearrangement in aqueous solution, forming a reactive species, with two chloroethyl groups that can form cross-links with DNA strands. Nitrogen mustard has an extremely short half-life. Within a few minutes of administration, it is usually undetectable in the bloodstream. It must be handled with caution to prevent exposure to health-care staff and to prevent extravasation as it is administered. Dose-limiting toxicities can be severe, including myelosuppression, and fast-onset nausea and vomiting. Primarily, mechlorethamine is used as part of **MOPP chemotherapy** (with vincristine (Oncovin), procarbazine, and prednisone) to treat Hodgkin's lymphoma. It is also used topically, to treat mycosis fungoides and skin cancer, and via intracavitary instillation, to treat malignant pericardial or pleural effusions. Usually given orally, the following drugs are additional examples of alkylating agents:

- *Busulfan (Myleran)* – also available for injection for certain indications; a bifunctional alkylating, with two reactive groups on opposing ends of the molecule, forming DNA adducts – resulting in strands that are cross-linked; used for chronic myelogenous leukemia (CML), and also as part of a high-dose conditioning regimen for allogeneic or autologous stem-cell transplantation
- *Chlorambucil (Leukeran)* – absorbed completely from the GI tract, with a predictable myelotoxicity profile; it is commonly used for chronic lymphocytic leukemia (CLL)
- *Melphalan (Alkeran)* – also available for injection for certain indications; developed as a targeted drug for selective uptake in tumors that use phenylalanine and tyrosine (such as malignant cells that produce melanin); absorption from the GI tract is varied, but slowed if taken with food, so it should be taken on an empty stomach; may be injected if the oral route is not appropriate for the patient; the parenteral form is also used as a conditioning regimen for autologous stem-cell transplantation in multiple myeloma patients; a 50% dose reduction is considered if there is greatly decreased kidney function

There are other examples of the "classic" alkylating agents, with varying types of activation and mechanisms of action. *Cyclophosphamide* and *ifosfamide* have multi-step activation in vivo,

with liver microsomal and cellular enzymes systems, generating reactive chemical species. For cyclophosphamide, the two active metabolites that cause most of the drug's cytotoxicity are *phosphoramide mustard* and *acrolein*. This latter metabolite mostly induces hemorrhagic cystitis, occurring in about 10% of patients. This complication is avoided by adequately hydrating the patient and encouraging frequent urination over the first 24 hours after cyclophosphamide is administered. Ifosfamide causes a much higher incidence of urotoxicity than cyclophosphamide. This may be due to an altered pharmacokinetic profile, resulting in more urotoxic metabolite precursors than with cyclophosphamide. Cystitis is prevented by concurrent use of *mesna*, which inactivates urotoxic metabolites in the bladder. Cyclophosphamide and ifosfamide use the kidneys and liver for elimination, so their toxicity may be extended if the patient has reduced function of these organs.

Thiotepa (Tepadina) has numerous functions, inducing many types of DNA damage that includes **interstrand cross-links**. The drug can be given in various ways. It is used intravenously for breast cancer, intraperitoneally for refractory ovarian cancer, intrapleurally for malignant pleural effusions, and intravesically for superficial bladder cancer. The agents known as *nitrosoureas* decompose in aqueous solutions, forming two reactive intermediates. These are a chloroethyldiazohydroxide and an isocyanate group. The first intermediate forms adducts with DNA, inducing interstrand cross-links. The isocyanate groups deplete glutathione while inhibiting the repair of DNA. The nitrosoureas are unique in that they are extremely lipid soluble, easily crossing the blood-brain barrier. Therefore, they are very active for CNS tumors, and are also indicated for Hodgkin's lymphoma, non-Hodgkin's lymphoma (NHL), and malignant melanoma. These agents may result in severe, chronic myelosuppression due to high lipophilicity.

Bendamustine (Treanda) was developed in the 1960s, and it was not completely assessed to be an antineoplastic drug until the 1990s. It has a nitrogen mustard group and a unique benzimi-dazole ring, with purine-analog effects. There is partial in vitro cross-resistance with the other alkylating agents. The dose-limiting toxicity of bendamustine is myelosuppression. Up to 40% of patients have grade 3 or 4 myelosuppression. Blood system troughs (nadirs) usually occur in the third week of a 28-day treatment regimen. Additional adverse effects include anaphylaxis, infusion reactions, and severe skin or allergic reactions. The GI events are mild to moderate, including diarrhea, nausea, and vomiting. If the tumor burden is high, the patient must be monitored for tumor lysis syndrome. Bendamustine is approved for CLL, and for NHL that is refractory to single-agent therapy with *rituximab (Rituxan)*.

Clinical Case

1. Why was the alkylating agent *melphalan* initially developed?
2. In which phase of the cell cycle are most alkylating agents active?
3. What are other examples of the classic alkylating agents?

A 53-year-old woman's malignant pleural effusion was diagnosed as a metastasis from an occult cancer of the ovary via a pathological study even though there was a lack of evidence upon imaging. The patient refused IV chemotherapy. After tamoxifen was ineffective, oral melphalan was able to cause remission of the tumor. The patient's only adverse effect was the development of mucositis, which was not severe.

Answers:

1. **Melphalan was developed as a targeted drug for selective uptake in tumors that use phenylalanine and tyrosine, such as malignant cells that produce melanin.**
2. **Most alkylating agents are active in G0, the resting phase of the cell cycle, and are usually considered to be mutagens with potential carcinogenicity.**
3. **Other examples of the classic alkylating agents include busulfan, chlorambucil, cyclophosphamide, ifosfamide, thiotepa, and bendamustine.**

Platinum Analogs

The *platinum analogs* are compounds that contain platinum, such as *cisplatin, carboplatin*, and *oxaliplatin*. They are highly activated agents used for many different types of cancer. Inside the cells, these platinum compounds experience a substitution reaction. One water molecule is switched with a chloride ion, in the process of aquation. This allows them to react with macromolecules that have strong binding sites – such as DNA. Cytotoxicity and antitumor activity are well-linked with the cisplatin-induced DNA adducts and formation of intrastrand DNA cross-links. Cisplatin and the other platinum analogs are somewhat similar to the alkylating agents, but their cytotoxicity is likely due to combined mechanisms of action such as DNA inhibition and protein synthesis, altered cell membrane transport, and suppressed mitochondrial function.

The current platinum analogs are mostly eliminated by the kidneys. Cisplatin is removed from the bloodstream in free as well as protein-bound forms, using a triphasic elimination method. In the first two phases, the free, unbound form is eliminated. Since 90% is excreted by the kidneys, the patient must have normal kidney function to prevent drug accumulation and excessive toxicity. If a patient previously was given cisplatin, he or she may have a higher risk of carboplatin toxicity, and must be assessed for kidney function. Intraperitoneal cisplatin causes peak levels up to 21 times higher than peak plasma levels with similar doses. Concurrent IV sodium thiosulfate can prevent severe systemic toxicities. Carboplatin and oxaliplatin elimination have a similar triphasic elimination pattern. Cisplatin and carboplatin are effective for similar tumors, but oxaliplatin + fluorouracil and leucovorin is the only platinum analog with high effectiveness against colorectal cancer.

There are differences between the platinum analogs regarding dosing, administration, and adverse effects. The dose-limiting toxicity of cisplatin is nephrotoxicity. Acute kidney failure can occur in 24 hours. Patients at greatest risk are those that do not receive sufficient hydration. Nephrotoxicity can usually be avoided by adequate hydration and giving furosemide, mannitol, or both diuretics. Carboplatin and oxaliplatin are not actually nephrotoxic, and hydration or diuresis are rarely needed. With the platinum compounds, nausea and vomiting are common. Vomiting is often worse and lengthier with cisplatin. Combination antiemetics are usually needed. Dose-limiting myelosuppression is seen much more often with carboplatin than with cisplatin. Neurotoxicity and ototoxicity are common adverse events of cisplatin.

More than 74% of patients taking oxaliplatin experience peripheral sensory neuropathy. Acute neuropathies mostly include peripheral sensory neuropathy and neuropathy that is caused by exposure to cold temperatures. More continued sensory neuropathies have occurred over two weeks or longer, including dysesthesia, paresthesia, and numbness in various body sites. The IV administration of calcium and magnesium immediately before and after oxaliplatin infusion was first believed to reduce incidence of grade 2 sensory neuropathies, but this was not proven, and is no longer done.

Miscellaneous Alkylating Agents

Miscellaneous drugs with alkylating-like effects include *dacarbazine (DTIC-Dome)*, *temozolomide (Temodar)*, and *procarbazine (Matulane)*. Dacarbazine can act as an antimetabolite, by

inhibiting the incorporation of purine nucleoside into DNA. It does not show activity that is specific to any cell-cycle phase, killing cells in all phases. Dacarbazine is very sensitive to light, and decomposes into active and inactive compounds with light exposure. Significant adverse effects include nausea and vomiting, which can decrease with repeated use. Other toxicities include a flu-like syndrome, photosensitivity, and myelosuppression. Dacarbazine may cause veno-occlusive disease of the liver, with fever and acute liver necrosis.

Temozolomide is a newer agent that must be dealkylated to produce an unstable intermediate, decomposing quickly and releasing methyldiazonium. Temozolomide is usually given orally, having extreme activity against malignant brain tumors such as anaplastic astrocytoma or glioblastoma multiforme. It is usually very effective also for advanced metastatic malignant melanoma. An injectable form is also available if the patient cannot take oral medications. Altretamine is an oral agent approved for recurrent ovarian cancer. It is also used for endometrial cancer. Its mechanism of action is unknown. Common adverse effects include myelosuppression, nausea, vomiting, and peripheral neuropathy.

Procarbazine is given orally along with other cytotoxic agents, for brain tumors and Hodgkin's lymphoma. In relation to an ability to inhibit the enzyme called *monoamine oxidase*, procarbazine can cause a hypertensive crisis, severe headache, sweating, and coma. The patient must not eat foods high in tyramine, such as aged cheese, chocolate, liver, and wine. Another interaction is with alcohol, which can cause a disulfiram-like reaction, with nausea, vomiting, sweating, and palpitations.

Anthracycline Antibiotics

Anthracyclines are highly colored compounds called *rhodomycins*, with antineoplastic and antimicrobial functions. The anthracyclines include *daunorubicin*, *doxorubicin*, *epirubicin (Ellence)*, and *idarubicin (Idamycin)* as well as the similar agent *anthracenedione (mitoxantrone)*. These agents have many mechanisms of cytotoxicity, which include covalent DNA binding, intercalation, formation of free radicals, and inhibition of the topoisomerase II enzyme. Most of their cytotoxic actions are believed to be from free radical formation and inhibition of topoisomerase II. Anthracyclines interfere with DNA unwinding catalyzed by topoisomerase II. By inhibiting this enzyme's ability to reconnect DNA strands, a *cleavable complex* is produced, creating double-strand DNA breaks.

Anthracyclines generate oxygen radical via donation of one electron to an oxygen molecule, which generates a superoxide. This is converted to hydrogen peroxide by superoxide dismutase, and then to a hydroxyl radical. Hydroxyl radicals are the most reactive compounds in existence. They quickly attack cell membrane lipids and DNA. An iron-anthracycline complex can produce hydroxyl radicals from hydrogen peroxide. Most normal body tissues as well as tumor cells have enzymes that can detoxify hydrogen peroxide – except for heart muscle cells. Therefore, cardiac tissue cannot detoxify hydrogen peroxide, and a reactive hydroxyl radical may be generated. The drug–iron complex is believed to be important in the cytotoxicity of the anthracyclines. In cardiac tissue, formation of hydroxyl radicals may be greatly decreased by using *dexrazoxane*, an edetate analog that effectively chelates iron.

Anthracyclines are metabolized into active and inactive compounds in the liver. The primary metabolites of most anthracyclines are alcohols such as *doxorubinicinol*. These have antitumor activities, but not as strongly as those of the originating compound. Anthracycline doses must be reduced if there is liver dysfunction – especially with elevated bilirubin levels. Doses do not need to be adjusted with kidney failure since clearance of anthracyclines is only slight. Cardiac toxicity from anthracyclines can cause acute electrocardiogram (ECG) changes and arrhythmias. These are worsened in patients that have heart disease. A common and often treatment-limiting cardiotoxicity is the development of cardiomyopathy, resulting in congestive heart failure. Up to 10% of patients receiving a cumulative dose of doxorubicin over 550 mg/m^2 develop this toxicity. In most cases, cardiac function is monitored via serial measurements of left ventricular function and ECG. Prolonged doxorubicin infusions and cardioprotective drugs such as dexrazoxane (Zinecard) may be helpful.

Mitoxantrone (Novantrone) may cause less alopecia, nausea, and vomiting. Cardiac toxicity appears to be less than with doxorubicin. There may be no difference in incidence of cardiomyopathy with doses similar to those used for doxorubicin. Since daunorubicin, doxorubicin, epirubicin, and idarubicin are vesicants, they all may induce severe extravasation, with pain, reddening, and tissue necrosis. Mitoxantrone is an irritant, so extravasation is less common. Additional toxicities include mucositis, alopecia, nausea, and vomiting.

Newer anticancer agents include versions of doxorubicin and daunorubicin processed with liposomal encapsulation. They offer different therapeutic and toxicity profiles. The mechanism of action is not believed to be different. The liposomal formulation changes the pharmacokinetics. There is a longer half-life and greater uptake by tumor cells. These two newer therapies are used for Kaposi's sarcoma as part of acquired immunodeficiency syndrome (AIDS). Liposomal doxorubicin is also indicated for advanced breast cancer. It is combined with vincristine to treat multiple myeloma. Liposomal doxorubicin is used for recurrent ovarian cancer. These newer agents cause less alopecia, nausea, vomiting, or neurotoxicity than the older agents. Cardiac toxicity is less dose limiting as well. Cumulative doses over 1,000 mg/m^2 have been administered with no significant alterations of left ventricular function. About 7% of patients with a first dose of liposomal doxorubicin develop an infusion reaction, with back pain, chest tightness, and flushing. Treatment usually does not have to be discontinued. It may be addressed with the administration of diphenhydramine, then restarting the infusion using at a slower rate. Fairly often, liposomal doxorubicin causes palmar or plantar skin eruptions, involving pain, swelling, redness, and skin desquamation. *Valrubicin (Valstar)* is a semisynthetic doxorubicin analog, with similar effects for stopping the synthesis of DNA and RNA. It is given intravesically into the bladder. Systemic exposure it reduced by the bladder wall's integrity. Valrubicin is used for therapy of Bacillus Calmette-Guerin (BCG)-resistant carcinoma in situ of the bladder. It has shown high response rates but contains an agent called *Cremophor EL*, able to cause hypersensitivity reactions.

Miscellaneous Antitumor Antibiotics

Bleomycin is a polypeptide, made up of low-molecular-weight-proteins isolated from a fungus called *Streptomyces verticullus*. Via **intercalation**, a drug–iron–oxygen complex binds to DNA, generating oxygen radicals that result in single- and double-stranded DNA breaks. The G_2 (premitotic) and mitotic phases of the cell cycle are when tumor cells are most sensitive to the effects of bleomycin. The drug has been utilized to synchronize cells into the G_2 and S phases of the cycle. This allows other antineoplastic drugs that act in the same phases to be more effective. Bleomycin is also effective when combined with other chemotherapy agents since it lacks extreme myelosuppressive effects. The drug is extremely dependent upon renal clearance to be eliminated. Doses must be reduced by 50–75% in patients that have a creatinine clearance of less than 50 mL per minute. Also, kidney function of patients that have previously received kidney-toxic drugs or those currently receiving cisplatin must be closely monitored. The pulmonary toxicity of bleomycin may cause coughing, dyspnea, and pleuritic chest pain. Those at higher risk for pulmonary fibrosis from the drug include people aged 70 or older, those who have had mediastinal radiation therapy, and those with preexisting pulmonary disease. Cumulative doses greater than 450 units is linked to increased chances for bleomycin-induced fibrosis, but significant pulmonary toxicity has also occurred with lower doses. To reduce possible pulmonary toxicity, bleomycin can be given via the intracavitary route, controlling ascites and/or pleural effusions.

Dactinomycin, also called *actinomycin D* and sold under the trade name *Cosmegen*, binds via intercalation to DNA, causing single-strand breaks similar to the breaks caused by doxorubicin. The drug is only used for pediatric tumors and gestational trophoblastic neoplasms. It is not greatly metabolized, and mostly excreted unchanged in the bile and urine. *Mitomycin-C*, also called simply *mitomycin*, is sold under the trade name *Mutamycin*. The drug is activated to an alkylating agent, with cytotoxicity caused by the formation of cross-links with DNA. This results in the inhibition of DNA synthesis and tumor cell death. Mitomycin-C is more highly activated in hypoxic tissues, such as those of solid tumors. There is poor metabolism in the liver of this drug. Renal clearance is only minor regarding the drug's elimination from the body. It degrades at a pH below 6, so when it is used intravesicularly to treat bladder cancer, a pH above 6 must be maintained so that it remains effective. Mitomycin causes a delayed, cumulative myelosuppression, but more serious is the development of a hemolytic-uremic syndrome that cannot usually be reversed, and can cause kidney failure. Mitomycin is a vesicant, and often causes bluish streaks above veins that are distal to the site of administration.

Folate Antagonists

Folate antagonists, or *antifolates*, are structural analogs of nucleotide bases – the building blocks of DNA and RNA. The folate antagonists inhibit nuclei acid synthesis, or they can be incorrectly incorporated into the DNA double helix. Examples such as *methotrexate (Trexall)* and *trimetrexate (generic only)* inhibit the enzyme called *dihydrofolate reductase (DHFR)*. This enzyme catalyzes the reduction of folic acid (dihydrofolate) into tetrahydrofolic acid (tetrohydrofolate). Reduced folates are one-carbon donors required for purine and pyrimidine bases to be synthesized. When methotrexate inhibits DHFR, there is depletion of the intracellular reduced folates, which blocks de novo synthesis of nucleotide bases. Other folate-dependent enzymes are also inhibited, including *thymidylate synthase*, which catalyzes uracil into thymidine. As folate-dependent enzymatic reactions are arrested, cytotoxicity occurs. The arrested reactions affect DNA, RNA, and protein synthesis.

In the S phase, quickly proliferating cells are most damaged by methotrexate-induced reduction of folate depletion. Longer exposure of tumor cells to methotrexate allows more cells to enter the DNA synthesis cell phase, and more tumor cells die. Most cells are able to function with very small amounts of DHFR, maintain enough reduction of folates. So, a high intracellular level of antifolate drugs must be maintained so that complete enzyme inhibition occurs. Large amounts of methotrexate may achieve thus – the same amounts used to treat sarcomas and malignant lymphomas. These high doses are only possible with timely administration of folinic acid (leucovorin), which avoids the methotrexate-induced enzyme blockage, saving normal cells by giving them the reduced folates required for protein and nucleic acid synthesis.

Methotrexate has been widely studied regarding its pharmacokinetics. A simple blood assay is used to monitor the drug's possible toxicity when moderate to high doses are given. Methotrexate, at low to moderate doses, is well-absorbed orally. It is mostly eliminated via renal excretion, through glomerular filtration and active secretion within the proximal tubules. Doses must be reduced in patients with impaired renal function. Blood levels are monitored after each dose. High blood levels of methotrexate can cause myelosuppression and mucositis. Leucovorin therapy is continued until the methotrexate levels become normalized. Patients with a creatinine clearance of 10–50 mL/min must receive 30–50% of the original dose. If the creatinine clearance is less than 10 mL/min, only 15% of the original dose is given.

Methotrexate interacts significantly with drugs that decrease the GFR. Pharmacokinetics of the drug are altered by distribution into third-space fluid collections, such as ascitic accumulation within the peritoneal cavity. Elimination is lengthened. Toxicity is increased in these conditions due to slow redistribution of methotrexate from the peritoneum to the blood.

Toxicities of methotrexate also include hepatotoxicity, nephrotoxicity, and pulmonary fibrosis. Hepatotoxicity may be due to high doses, signified by acute and reversible peaks in liver function enzymes. Methotrexate is a prophylactic as well as a treatment for meningeal leukemia, but is not well-distributed into the CSF. Therefore, a preservative-free formulation must be injected into the CSF via lumbar puncture or an intraventricular device. With intrathecal administration, toxicities include nuchal rigidity, severe headache, fever, and vomiting. If severe, there may be demyelinating encephalopathy.

Pemetrexed (Alimta) is a different type of folate antagonist, since it inhibits many enzymes involved in the synthesis of nucleotides. These include DHFR, glycinamide ribonucleotide formyltransferase, and thymidylate synthase. Pemetrexed is combined with cisplatin to treat non-resectable malignant pleural mesothelioma. It is also used along for recurring non-small cell lung cancer. Severe hematologic toxicity has been linked to patients with poor nutritional status. With folic acid supplementation, plus vitamin B12, much less toxicity was seen. All patients taking pemetrexed must receive these supplements. Additional adverse effects include nausea, vomiting, diarrhea, fatigue, and skin rash. The day before, the day of, and the day after pemetrexed administration should include the administration of dexamethasone, which can prevent skin rashes. Pemetrexed is mostly excreted in the urine. Between 70% and 90% of each dose is eliminated unchanged in the first 24 hours after being taken. If there is a creatinine clearance above 45 mL/min, doses do not require adjustment. A delayed clearance of the drug can occur with co-administration of nephrotoxic drugs or drugs eliminated by the kidneys. So, caution is needed in these situations.

Raltitrexed (Tomudex) is a quinazoline folate analog. It selectively inhibits thymidylate synthase. The drug is available in Canada and Europe, to treat colorectal cancer. In the United States, trials have not been consistent regarding improvement in outcomes, compared with fluorouracil-based agents. However, the drug is also under study in the United States to treat head and neck cancers, mesothelioma, and pancreatic cancer. *Pralatrexate (Folotyn)* is a newer drug with higher affinity for the reduced-folate carrier type I (RFC-I) transporter system. This mechanism is mostly used for the uptake of the drug into selected cells. It may also be a pathway of resistance in cells that have decreased expression of RFC-I. Pralatrexate is used to treat patients with refractory or relapsed peripheral T-cell lymphomas. The most common adverse reactions include mucositis, neutropenia, thrombocytopenia, and temporary elevations in serum transaminases. The patient must receive supplementation with folic acid and vitamin B12. Kidney function is monitored before each cycle of treatment. Doses are adjusted to allow for creatinine clearance reductions from baseline. Liver function is monitored to assess any impairment. Dose adjustments may be needed if liver function is altered. Pralatrexate + gemcitabine has been studied clinically to treat NHL, but is not yet approved.

Purine Analogs

Purine analogs form as thiopurines, such as 6-mercaptopurine (6-MP) and 6-thioguanine (6-TG), are converted into their monophosphates. These inhibit pure synthesis, causing an accumulation of nucleic acid precursors. These allow the conversion of 6-MP and 6-TG into active nucleotides. The triphosphate nucleotides are incorporated into DNA, causing strand breaks related to cytotoxicity. Methotrexate acts synergistically with these 6-thiopurines, blocking urine synthesis and

enhancing thiopurine activation. *Fludarabine (Fludara)* highly resists deactivation and has increased solubility compared with other adenine arabinoside analogs. After IV administration, it is quickly dephosphorylated into F-ara-A (9-beta-D-arabinofuranosyl-2-fluoroadenine). This form enters cells through nucleotide-specific membrane transport. The main mechanism of action is inhibition of DNA polymerases that are part of DNA synthesis and repair. Fludarabine is preferred to treat CLL and indolent NHL. In the first trials, 4-times daily doses over 5–7 days caused extreme neurotoxicity, including cortical blindness, seizures, coma, and death. Follow-up trials showed that lower doses could be safe over five days. Common toxicities were immunosuppression and myelosuppression. Prophylactic therapy for *Pneumocystis jiroveci* pneumonia is required concurrently. Rarely, a life-threatening and possibly fatal autoimmune hemolytic anemia has occurred. When fludarabine had to be used again in patients, with or without previous steroid administration, death has occurred. Fludarabine is toxic to stem cells and must be avoided in patients that may be candidates for autologous stem-cell transplantation.

Cladribine (2-CdA or Leustatin) is a deoxyadenosine purine nucleotide analog. Similar to fludarabine, it resists deactivation. The drug enters lymphocytes by a nucleotide transporter system, accumulating until becoming lymphotoxic. After phosphorylation, the drug is converted into cladribine triphosphate, falsely incorporated into DNA, and eventually affects DNA synthesis and repair. Cladribine can cause complete remission in up to 91% of hairy cell leukemia patients. The drug can also be effective for CLL and NHL, but remissions are short term. A dose-limiting effect is myelotoxicity. Recovery can take 3–5 weeks after one course of therapy. In patients with CLL receiving multiple cycles of cladribine, a severe autoimmune hemolytic anemia plus fatal bone marrow aplasia has occurred. However, cladribine causes less immunosuppression and opportunistic infections than fludarabine.

Clofarabine (Clolar) is a similar agent, incorporated into DNA to cause chain termination and inhibited DNA synthesis. For cytotoxicity to occur, intracellular activation into clofarabine triphosphate is required. Clofarabine is approved as single-agent treatment of refractory or relapsed acute lymphoblastic leukemia (ALL) in children and adults under age 21. One study revealed that a five-day regimen of clofarabine + cyclophosphamide + etoposide caused a response rate of 44% in children that were refractory to standard induction therapy. However, 6 of the 25 tested patients died of treatment-related hepatotoxicity, infection, and multi-organ failure. With or without cytarabine, clofarabine has been successful for patients under age 60 with post-induction or induction failures for acute myeloid leukemia. The patient should be monitored closely for tumor lysis syndrome, inflammatory responses, or capillary leak syndrome.

Nelarabine (Arranon) is a prodrug for ara-G, also called deoxyguanosine analog 9-bega-D arabinofuranosylguanine. This is a cytotoxic agent that inhibits DNA synthesis. The drug is quickly demethylated by adenosine deaminase (ADA) into ara-G. It has benefited patients with T-cell ALL, with response rates between 33% and 60%, complete remissions being induced, and a one-year survival rate of 28% for adult patients. Nelarabine is also approved for T-cell lymphoblastic lymphoma that is refractory to other chemotherapies, or has relapsed. Neurotoxicity is dose-limited, and may include altered mental status, headache, and seizures. *Pentostatin (Nipent)* is also called 2-deoxycoformyciin. It was developed to potently inhibit adenosine deaminase, and blockage of this enzyme results in deoxyadenosine accumulation – leading to cytotoxicity. Pentostatin is used to treat many lymphocytic diseases, including CLL, prolymphocytic leukemia, and T-cell lymphoma. Significant immunosuppression can continue for over one year after the drug has been discontinued. Additional adverse events include dermatologic and GI toxicity, and ocular abnormalities.

Pyrimidine Analogs

Pyrimidine analogs include 5-fluorouracil, also called *fluorouracil*. This fluoropyrimidine experiences significant metabolism intracellular. It becomes an active metabolite known as *fluoro-deoxyuridine monophosphate (FdUMP)*, which binds covalently with thymidylate synthase (TS). It inhibits the enzyme from synthesizing *deoxythymidine triphosphate (dTTP)*, which is a precursor of DNA synthesis. Additional metabolic pathways assist the conversion of fluorouracil into *fluorouridine triphosphate (FUTP)*, which can be incorporated into RNA, plus conversion of FdUMP into the triphosphate form, which can be incorporated into DNA. Cytotoxicity of fluorouracil in these pathways depletes dTTP and results in false incorporation of various metabolites into DNA and RNA. Fluorouracil + leucovorin enhances the reaction, increasing the cytotoxic effects of fluorouracil.

Fluorouracil is quickly cleared by the liver, having a plasma half-life of only 6–20 minutes. Clearance rates can vary widely, however. The drug is metabolized by dihydropyrimidine dehydrogenase into *dihydrofluorouracil* in the liver and elsewhere. If a patient is deficient in this enzyme, there are much higher levels of fluorouracil, and toxicity. If fluorouracil or floxuridine are given directly into the hepatic artery or portal vein, liver metastases experience direct exposure to the drug. Yet, only slight systemic exposure occurs due to the drug's high first-pass clearance. Based on the schedule of administration, the major dose-limiting toxicity can be different. If the drug is given by rapid bolus injection, myelosuppression is more significant. With prolonged infusions over 2–5 days, mucositis and GI toxicity are more common. Intrahepatic administration of fluoropyrimidines may cause biliary sclerosis and cholestatic jaundice. Fluorouracil has caused chest pain, electrocardiogram changes that resemble those of myocardial ischemia, and elevated cardiac enzymes. This syndrome may be linked to fluorouracil-induced coronary vasospasm.

Oral fluoropyrimidines have been avoided due to irregular bioavailability. Therefore, the following three approaches have become popular:

- *Capecitabine* – approved for metastatic breast or colorectal cancer; it is a prodrug that experiences many metabolic steps in the liver and body tissues, to become fluorouracil; it is a cytotoxic metabolite more highly concentrated in tumor cells than normal cells, due to larger concentrations of thymidine phosphorylase, which converts the drug into fluorouracil; major dose-limiting adverse effects include diarrhea, hand-and-foot syndrome, and stomatitis
- *Ftorafur* – a fluorouracil prodrug studied for colorectal cancer, but ultimately discontinued
- *Uracil* – also studied for colorectal cancer; note that ftorafur and uracil were administered together as "UFT," which did not have better effects than infused fluorouracil + leucovorin; uracil was also discontinued

Cytarabine (Cytosar-U) was first isolated from a sponge known as *Cryptothethy acrypta*. The parent drug is phosphorylated into arabinofuranosylcytosine triphosphate (ara-CTP). This competes with the substrate deoxycytidine triphosphate (dCTP), inhibiting DNA polymerase-alpha. The DNA polymerases are important enzymes for the synthesis and repair of DNA. The metabolite ara-CTP can also be incorporated into DNA, interfering with chain polymerization as well as DNA strand repair. Like other antimetabolites, the S phase of the cell cycle is when normal tissues and tumor cells are most sensitive to cytarabine. The drug is quickly converted to an inactive metabolite, uracil arabinoside (ara-U) by an enzyme called cytidine deaminase. This is present in many tissues, such as the GI epithelium and liver. Cytarabine is usually given via continuous infusion. This maintains cytotoxic levels even though the drug is quickly inactivated, and so that all cycling cells can be exposed to the maximum cytotoxic effects during the S phase.

Cytarabine can be used alone or with methotrexate to treat meningeal leukemia. To obtain high enough concentrations in the CSF, direct intrathecal administration is required. Small amounts of the drug are needed intrathecally since deamination in the CSF is minimal. Toxicities include GI epithelial injury and myelosuppression. High doses are used for refractory acute myelogenous leukemia (AML), and 20% of patients have cerebral and cerebellar dysfunction. This is more common in patients above age 50, signified by ataxia, confusion, slurring of the speech, and coma. High doses of cytarabine also cause conjunctivitis, which may be prevented using ophthalmic steroid drops.

Gemcitabine (Gemzar) is a pyrimidine analog of deoxycytidine. It is intracellularly converted to its diphosphate and triphosphate metabolites. Gemcitabine diphosphate inhibits ribonucleotide reductase, inhibiting de novo nucleotide synthesis. Gemcitabine triphosphate inhibits DNA synthesis via competition with the deoxycytidine triphosphate substrate for DNA polymerase, and being incorporated into DNA. Reduced intracellular deoxycytidine triphosphate due to gemcitabine diphosphate increases the incorporation of gemcitabine triphosphate into DNA, via *self-potentiation*. Due to this, the half-life of gemcitabine is lengthened, and infusions cannot exceed 30 minutes in duration. Longer infusions cause higher degrees of myelotoxicity. Other serious adverse effects include elevated liver transaminases, nausea, vomiting, and skin rash that may or may not include pruritus.

Vinca Alkaloids

Vinca alkaloids were first isolated from plant materials. They are present in small amounts in the *periwinkle* plant. Vinca alkaloids are very similar in chemical structure, but have widely differing antitumor effects and toxicities, and are summarized as follows:

- *Vinblastine (Velban)* – used mostly for germ cell tumors and advanced Hodgkin's lymphoma; it is myelotoxic and neurotoxic

- *Vincristine (Oncovin)* – has a broad spectrum of activity; used for leukemia, lymphoma, breast cancer, lung cancer, and multiple myeloma; it is neurotoxic but has very low myelotoxicity; cells are sensitive to low concentrations of this drug; duration of exposure determines the amount of cytotoxic effect; vincristine is mostly metabolized by the liver and concentrated in the bile; 70% is excreted in the feces, and 10% in the urine; dose modified is assessed with hepatic dysfunction – especially with biliary obstruction
- *Vinorelbine (Navelbine)* – the newest of these drugs, used for breast cancer and non-small cell lung cancer; it is myelotoxic and neurotoxic
- *Vindesine (Eldisine)* – is available throughout Europe, but is only used in clinical trials in the United States

The vinca alkaloids are *tubulin-interactive agents*, and the cytotoxic effects mostly interfere with microtubule formation and function. These processes are needed for the mitosis cell-cycle phase, and for cell division. The microtubules also maintain cell shape and intracellular transport. Vinca alkaloids bind to certain sites on tubule to prevent the formation of tubulin dimers, and inhibiting the formation of microtubule structures. Mitotic arrest is the main mechanism of cell death, but the vinca alkaloids may have cytolytic effects upon resting cells during the G0 phase, and other cells during the G1 or S phase. Though vinca alkaloids are widely used, there is little information about their pharmacology and pharmacokinetics. Vinblastine and vinorelbine share similar pharmacokinetics. Excretion mostly occurs via the biliary tract. All vinca alkaloids have a long terminal elimination phase half-life of 1–4 days.

These agents' peripheral neurotoxicity is often a cumulative dose-limiting effect. Toxicity first appears as sensory impairment, such as stocking-and-glove distribution, and paresthesias. Later, patients may develop motor dysfunction and neuritic pain. Continued therapy causes foot and wrist drop, ataxia, loss of deep tendon reflexes, and paralysis. Discontinuation of vinca alkaloids is the only effective way to manage these symptoms. If vincristine is accidentally administered intrathecally, there will be ascending paralysis that causes death. Older patients often complain of abdominal pain and constipation. For vinblastine and vinorelbine, myelosuppression is also a dose-limiting toxicity. Since the vinca alkaloids are vesicants, extravasation must be avoided.

Taxanes

Taxanes are important antitumor agents effective against many cancers. They are chemically complex and difficult to synthesize. The only source for *paclitaxel (Taxol)* until the 1990s was extraction and isolation from the bark of the Pacific yew tree called **Taxus brevifolia**. Later, a semisynthetic process that used a taxane precursor was created. Paclitaxel is poorly soluble in water, so its injectable formulation must contain 50% polyoxyethylated castor oil (Cremophor EL) to have aqueous solubility. This causes problems with administration, since the drug can strip hepatotoxic plasticizer from infusion devices made of PVC plastic. The drug is the cause of most severe hypersensitivity reactions. Paclitaxel and *docetaxel (Taxotere)* bind mostly to microtubules instead of tubulin dimers. They inhibit disassembly of microtubules, which is needed for normal functioning of their structures. Cells have many disorganized microtubules in all cell-cycle phases because of paclitaxel. Though the taxanes have unique antimicrotubule effects upon cells, cell death is still of unclear cause. The mechanism of action and cytotoxicity of docetaxel are similar to those of paclitaxel.

Paclitaxel and docetaxel are believed to be primarily eliminated via liver metabolism and biliary excretion. They are excreted at less than 5% via the urine. The clearance of paclitaxel is lowered by up to 30% if the drug is given after cisplatin was previously administered. The interaction causes increased peak plasma concentrations of paclitaxel. There is more extreme myelotoxicity than when paclitaxel is given after cisplatin, in comparison with reversing the administration of the drugs. Therefore, paclitaxel is advised to be given before cisplatin, and also given before carboplatin if that drug is indicated. Taxanes have high protein binding of 90–95%. Extreme toxicities include myalgias, total body alopecia, myelosuppression, hypersensitivity, and neurotoxicity. The nails may separate, especially if paclitaxel is administered as a one-hour infusion every week. Hypersensitivity has occurred in about 10% of patients receiving paclitaxel in the early clinical trials. All of these reactions are most common within 10 minutes of initial infusion. Manifestations include extreme facial flushing, dyspnea, bronchospasm, and hypotension. To prevent a major hypersensitivity, a corticosteroid such as dexamethasone, an antihistamine such as diphenhydramine, and an H2-blocker such as cimetidine can be given before a taxane is administered. Paclitaxel can be given parenterally with safety. Infusions last for 1 hour, 3 hours, or 24 hours. The shorter infusion rates have been shown to cause less neutropenia than the 24-hour infusion.

Toxicity is different between docetaxel and paclitaxel. Hypersensitivity reactions are less common with docetaxel. Severe reactions only occur in under 1% of patients. Skin reactions include macular or papular lesions, desquamation, erythema, and pruritus. These occur in 50–70% of patients. The patient's nails may become orange in color and also may thicken. More significantly, fluid retention and weight gain occur in 6% of patients. To prevent and reduce fluid retention as well as hypersensitivity reactions, corticosteroids are given in a three-day regimen.

Nanoparticle albumin-bund paclitaxel, also called *nab-paclitaxel* and *Abraxane*, is synthesized via homogenization of paclitaxel with human serum albumin. Total doses of nab-paclitaxel can be much higher than the maximum doses of conventional paclitaxel. No hypersensitivity reactions occurred with nab-paclitaxel. The drug is approved for treating metastatic breast cancer that does not respond to other chemotherapy or relapses within six months – unless it is contraindicated. Nab-paclitaxel is further approved along with gemcitabine to treat metastatic pancreatic adenocarcinoma, and along with carboplatin to treat metastatic non-small cell lung cancer.

Cabazitaxel (Jevtana) is a semisynthetic taxane. It is created using a precursor that is extracted from **yew tree needles**. Cabazitaxel binds to tubulin, promoting its formation of microtubules, while at the same time, inhibiting breakdown of the microtubules. Unlike the other taxanes, cabazitaxel is not a good substrate for the P-gp efflux pump. It may be successful in treating multidrug-resistant tumors. Overall survival is longer in the group receiving cabazitaxel. Progression-free survival and tumor- and prostate-specific antigen response rates is also better. The patient must be given premedication with H_1 and H_2 antihistamines and corticosteroids, to prevent hypersensitivity reactions. Dose-limiting toxicities of cabazitaxel include myelosuppression and neurotoxicity.

Another newer taxane is called *paclitaxel poliglumex (PPX)*. The paclitaxel component is conjugated to L-glutamic acid, making it water soluble. This reduces hypersensitivity reactions and allows the drug to preferentially target tumors. This drug overcomes conventional paclitaxel's poor aqueous solubility, and avoids hypersensitivity reactions. The polymer conjugates are absorbed by tumor cells as well as the reticuloendothelial system. Free paclitaxel is released intracellularly by **esterolysis**. The tumor is exposed to five times more of the drug when this form is used. In one trail, PPX was compared with docetaxel for patients with non-small cell lung cancer. There was no large difference in median survival or progress of the cancer. However, there were less adverse effects with PPX. These included allergic reactions and alopecia, and the drug did not have to be administered as often as docetaxel. While PPX is effective for advanced malignant tumors, it is uncertain if it is more beneficial regarding adverse effects and outcomes compared with conventional taxanes – as first-line treatments or for refractory cancer.

Omacetaxine mepesuccinate (Synribo) is a taxane derived from the evergreen tree known as *Cephalotaxus harringtonia*. The drug inhibits *breakpoint cluster region-tyrosine-protein kinase (Bcr-Abl)*. Bcr-Abl kinase is required for CML's initiation, maintenance, and progression. Omacetaxine is used to treat the chronic or accelerated phase of CML that resists or is intolerant to two or more tyrosine kinase inhibitors. The drug has provided major cytogenetic responses in 18.4% of chronic-phase CML patients, and a total hematologic response of 14.3% in those with accelerated-phase CML. However, induction therapy is made more complicated because of the twice per day subcutaneous administration that lasts for two weeks. Treatments can be self-administered at home as long as a home care specialty pharmacy is involved.

Clinical Case

1. What type of drug classification contains docetaxel and paclitaxel?
2. To what do docetaxel and paclitaxel mostly bind?
3. What are the extreme toxicities of these agents?

A 72-year-old man went to his dermatologist because of skin ulcers and purpura located on his head. Skin biopsy confirmed the presence of angiosarcoma. The tumor was circumscribed, so extended resection was performed and weekly docetaxel chemotherapy was started. Two months later, the tumor recurred. Radiation therapy and biweekly paclitaxel were initiated. Complete remission occurred within another two months. However, seven months later, the tumor recurred again and there was frequent bleeding. Combination therapy with low-dose radiation and the anti-vascular endothelial growth factor receptor agent called *pazopanib* was started, and the lesion disappeared within three weeks. After four months, however, the patient developed thrombocytopenia. Frequent platelet transfusions were not effective, and the pazopanib was stopped. The bleeding resolved. Unfortunately, lung and spinal metastases were found, and the patient died within six weeks, of respiratory failure.

Answers:

1. **Docetaxel and paclitaxel are classified as taxanes, important antitumor agents that are effective against many cancers. They are chemically complex and difficult to synthesize.**
2. **Docetaxel and paclitaxel mostly bind to microtubules instead of tubulin dimers. They inhibit disassembly of microtubules, which is needed for normal functioning of their structures. Though these taxanes have unique antimicrotubule effects upon cells, cell death is still of unclear cause.**
3. **Extreme toxicities of these agents include myalgias, total body alopecia, myelosuppression, hypersensitivity, and neurotoxicity.**

Hormonal Therapies

Hormonal therapies are some of the oldest methods of treating cancer. At first, tumors sensitive to these therapies did not respond significantly, but today these therapies are very successful for a large variety of tumors. The most commonly used hormonal agents and their main indications are summarized in Table 16.2.

The most common hormonal therapies include steroids, steroid analogs, and enzyme inhibitors. They are believed to work by inhibiting the stimulation of steroid-specific receptors

Table 16.2 Common hormonal agents and indications.

Agents	Indications
Corticosteroids	
Prednisone (Deltasone)	Breast cancer, multiple myeloma
Hydrocortisone (Cortef)	Hodgkin's disease
Dexamethasone (Dex)	Leukemias
Methylprednisolone (Solu-medrol)	Malignant lymphomas
Androgens	
Fluoxymesterone (Halotestin), Testosterone (generic only)	Breast cancer
Estrogens	
Conjugated estrogens (Premarin), diethylstilbestrol (DES), estradiol (Estrace)	Prostate cancer Breast cancer
Antiestrogens, progestins	
Medroxyprogesterone (Provera)	Endometrial cancer
megesterol (generic only)	Breast cancer
Estrogen-receptor antagonists	
Fulvestrant (Faslodex), tamoxifen (Nolvadex), toremifene (Farestron)	Breast cancer
Aromatase inhibitors	
Aminoglutethimide (AG)	Breast cancer
Anastrozole (Arimidex), exemestane (Aromasin), letrozole (Femara), mitotane (Lysodren)	
Luteinizing hormone-releasing hormone analogs	
Goserelin (Zoladex)	Prostate cancer
Histrelin (Vantas), leuprolide (Lupron), triptorelin (Trelstar)	Breast cancer
Gonadotropin-releasing hormone antagonist	
Abarelix (Plenaxis)	Prostate cancer
Antiandrogens	
Bicalutamide (Casodex), flutamide (Eulexin), nilutamide (Nilandron),	Prostate cancer

on cell surfaces. By blocking these receptors, tumor cells cannot receive normal hormonal growth stimulation. This decreases tumor growth.

Antiestrogens

Tamoxifen (Soltamox) is often used for adjuvant treatment of breast cancer and for metastatic breast disease that involves estrogen-receptor-positive tumors. The main mechanism of action is the blocking of estrogen stimulation of tumor cells. This occurs via inhibition of the translocation and nuclear binding of the estrogen receptor. Tamoxifen is an estrogen antagonist in breast tissues, but is an estrogen agonist in bone, lipids, and endometrium. The primary toxicity involves hot flashes, which affect 50% of women taking tamoxifen. Additional adverse effects include slight increases in the occurrence of thromboembolism and endometrial cancer. In one large study, tamoxifen was compared with a placebo. The tested women that had a risk for developing a breast malignancy were 50% less likely to develop cancer if tamoxifen was taken daily. Megestrol has also been used for metastatic breast cancer, but today is mostly used for the anorexia and cachexia that are related to cancer.

Fulvestrant (Faslodex) is an injectable anti-hormonal agent given once monthly. It is used to treat estrogen-receptor-positive metastatic breast cancer after previous treatment with tamoxifen has failed. Fulvestrant binds to estrogen receptors, to block hormone-dependent and hormone-independent activities, and to prevent estrogen-induced growth of tumor cells. Fulvestrant has equivalent treatment success with *anastrozole (Arimidex)* regarding survival length, tumor progression, and responses of patients that have locally advanced metastatic cancer after the disease has progressed while taking tamoxifen or other endocrine treatments. Like anastrozole, fulvestrant is generally well-tolerated, with few adverse effects. It was first approved for once monthly IM dosing in a low dose, which has since been doubled because it offers better control of metastatic disease.

Aromatase Inhibitors

Aromatase inhibitors work by suppressing post-menopausal estrogen synthesis. They inhibit peripheral conversion of androgens into estrogens. Aromatase is an enzyme in the CYP group, which catalyzes the final step of estrogen synthesis. Aromatase inhibitors primarily are used to treat hormonally sensitive breast cancer. Ovarian manufacture of estrogen is not affected, so these agents are only used in postmenopsual women or in those that have had an **oophorectomy**. *Aminoglutethimide* was the first aromatase inhibitor. It is used rarely today because it is poorly tolerated and affects the synthesis of corticosteroids. Newer aromatase inhibitors are classified as *steroidal* or *nonsteroidal*. Steroidal inhibitors irreversibly bond with the aromatase enzyme. Nonsteroidal inhibitors reversible bond with the heme iron site, allowing return of enzymatic activity once the inhibitor is removed. *Exemestane (Aromasin)* is a steroidal inhibitor, while *anastrozole* and *letrozole (Femara)* are nonsteroidal inhibitors. They all are potent and just as effective as aminoglutethimide, but they affect synthesis of aldosterone, corticosteroids, and thyroid hormone only slightly – making them less toxic. The nonsteroidal inhibitors cause toxicities such as arthralgia, differential lipid profile effects, and loss of bone mineral density. Anastrozole does not greatly affect lipids, but letrozole increases total cholesterol and low-density lipoproteins significantly. Exemestane has a better effect upon bone density. It can prevent bone loss, but also has weak androgenic features that can cause acne and weight gain. Compared with tamoxifen, anastrozole and letrozole are better for adjuvant therapy and to treat metastatic breast cancer. Tamoxifen followed by anastrozole is more effective than tamoxifen alone – this was tested over five years of treatment.

Gonadotropin-Releasing Hormone Analogs

Gonadotropin-releasing hormone analogs – specifically the *luteinizing hormone-releasing hormone (LH-RH) agonists* – are synthetic versions of naturally occurring hormones. At first, they cause an increase in testosterone levels that is secondary to stimulating LH release. Over time, the pituitary gland is desensitized, and there is a large decrease in production of androgens and estrogens. *Leuprolide (Lupron)* and *goserelin (Zoladex)* are commonly used to treat breast and prostate cancers. All LH-RH agonists can be administered as slow-release depot injections or pellets. They are intended for monthly use, or every three or four months, or once per year. Castration levels of testosterone occur in 3–4 weeks with leuprolide, and in 1 month with goserelin. For ovarian suppression that will allow treatment with tamoxifen in a postmenopausal woman who has hormone-receptor-positive breast cancer, goserelin is used.

Antiandrogens

Antiandrogens are indicated for men with hormone-responsive metastatic prostate cancer. They can be the first therapy, or used along with a gonadotropin-releasing hormone analog.

Antiandrogens prevent flare reactions that occur when LH-RH agonist therapies are started to treat active prostate disease. Antiandrogens work by binding to androgen receptors, blocking effects of dihydrotestosterone upon prostate cancer cells. *Flutamide (Eulexin)* was the first-ever antiandrogen. Its common adverse effects included diarrhea, **gynecomastia**, and sometimes, hepatotoxicity. Additional antiandrogens include *bicalutamide (Casodex)* and *nilutamide (Nilandron)*, which are of equivalent strength as flutamide. These two drugs are tolerated better by most patients, since they cause less diarrhea and have a dosing schedule that is simpler.

Significant Point

Antiandrogens work by blocking the effects of androgens such as testosterone, by binding to androgen receptors. They are effective against ovarian, adrenal gland, and prostate tumors. These agents include drugs such as apalutamide, bicalutamide, darolutamide, enzalutamide, flutamide, and nilutamide. New research has shown that these agents may also be effective against certain types of breast cancer.

Chemotherapy-Induced Adverse Effects

According to the National Cancer Society, chemotherapy-induced adverse effects are addressed via the *Common Terminology Criteria for Adverse Events (CTCAE)*. Criteria of adverse events are graded as 1 through 5, with 1 being the mildest classification, and 5 indicated death from an adverse effect of chemotherapy. Adverse effects of chemotherapy include bone marrow suppression, anemia, insomnia, cognitive dysfunction, fatigue, thrombocytopenia, neutropenia, tumor lysis syndrome, GI tract toxicity, integumentary toxicity, cardiotoxicity, neurotoxicity, pulmonary toxicity, nephrotoxicity, and hepatotoxicity.

Bone Marrow Suppression

Bone marrow suppression is also referred to as *myelosuppression*, in which there are low blood cell counts. It is the most common dose-limiting adverse effect of traditional chemotherapeutic agents, but does not occur with all of them. Normally, the bone marrow makes erythrocytes, leukocytes, and platelets. Leukocytes are also called white blood cells (WBCs). Erythrocytes are known as red blood cells (RBCs), and platelets are called thrombocytes. The WBCs include the following subtypes:

- *Neutrophils* – which fight infection
- *Basophils* – which are part of the inflammatory response
- *Eosinophils* – which increase with allergic reactions
- *Lymphocytes* – which include immune cells (B and T cells)
- *Monocytes* – which ingest bacteria and other foreign bodies

Platelets are cell fragments that help stop bleeding and they are essential for the clotting process that occurs in plasma when blood vessels are ruptured.

When some or all of these cells are decreased in number, myelosuppression is present. Often, the neutrophils are the most affected cells, since they only survive for 6–12 hours, and experience rapid turnover into new cells. After chemotherapy is administered, the neutrophil count is usually at its lowest in 10–14 days. This low point is called a **nadir**. The neutrophil count usually returns to normal within 3–4 weeks.

Anemia

Anemia is a condition in which the blood's oxygen-carrying capacity is too low to support normal metabolism. It is a sign of some disorder rather than a disease in itself. Its hallmark is blood oxygen levels that are inadequate to support normal metabolism. In anemic patient, there is also a decrease in the total number of RBCs and a decrease in the amount of hemoglobin. This leads to hypotension, pallor, fatigue, short of breath, and chills. Because of hypoxic effects upon the heart, tachycardia may also develop. Anemia can greatly impact quality of life, but can usually be corrected by a transfusion of RBCs. Chemotherapy-induced anemia is a relatively uncommon condition, since the bone marrow starts to recover prior to the amount of circulating RBCs becoming significantly decreased. While low levels of hemoglobin and hematocrit do not mean that chemotherapy must be withheld, they definitely affect the patient's health.

Anemia with chronic disease is related to **erythroid hypoplasia** of the bone marrow, in disease processes such as cancer, chronic infections, and rheumatoid arthritis. Erythroid hypoplasia causes a small decrease in **reticulocytosis, hypoferremia**, and a more significant decrease in serum **erythropoietin**. Also, chronic inflammation and cytokine release (such as interferon, interleukin-1, or tumor necrosis factor) suppresses the production of erythropoietin. This decreases the production of RBCs. The platinum-based chemotherapies can inhibit maturation of erythroid lineage cells within the bone marrow, and be toxic to the kidneys. Erythropoietin administration can correct chemotherapy-induced anemia. *Epoetin alfa (Epogen)* is a commonly used as a growth factor for RBCs. It is given subcutaneously three times per week, until a target level of hematocrit is achieved. It can also be given once per week over three weeks in larger doses with the same effectiveness.

Darbepoetin alfa (Aranesp) is another erythropoietin-stimulating agent, and has a long half-life with higher biologic activity. This means that dosing can be less frequent, which is more convenient and improves patient compliance while reducing office visits. It is given subcutaneously every week or in a higher dose every three weeks. Doses can be increased if no response appears in 4–6 weeks. Common adverse effects of darbepoetin alfa and epoetin alfa include hypertension and pain at the injection site. These agents are indicated to management chemotherapy-induced anemia, yet are of some controversy. There is disagreement as to their safety, since there is a risk of thrombosis and possible shorter survival.

Insomnia

As many as 90% of cancer patients, during or following treatment, report insomnia as an adverse outcome. Insomnia is difficult falling asleep or remaining asleep, or both, for at least three times per week over at least four weeks. Insomnia can greatly reduce quality of life and affect the morbidity of cancer. Insomnia may be caused by depression, so patients with insomnia must be referred for a complete evaluation. Medications may also cause insomnia or sleep disturbances. These include corticosteroids, stimulants, antidepressants, and antihistamines. Stimulants include caffeine, methylphenidate, and pseudoephedrine. For those experiencing insomnia, sleep hygiene may be extremely helpful. Sleep hygiene includes recommendations such as regular exercise, controlling times of exposure to bright light, avoiding eating and alcohol before bedtime, having a good sleep environment, going to bed and awakening at the same time every day, avoiding long naps, and turning of electronics and lights prior to bedtime. By optimizing sleep, cancer-related fatigue can be greatly improved. Specifics concerning exercise to relieve insomnia include use of newer activities such as yoga. Clinical trials on drugs that can be used for cancer-related insomnia are ongoing for alprazolam, lorazepam, mirtazapine, and zolpidem. Also, melatonin is an OTC agent used to help people fall asleep, but is not indicated by the FDA to be used for insomnia.

Cognitive Dysfunction

After cancer treatments, cognitive dysfunction affects many patients. There may be long-standing effects linked to chemotherapies, other treatments, and also to the cancer itself. Neuropsychologic evaluation must occur to rule out other causes of neurologic dysfunction. Occupational therapy may help some patients. Adequate treatment of patient depression, distress, fatigue, sleep disturbances, other medical conditions, and pain or other contributing symptoms must be given. Pharmacologic intentions are considered when non-pharmacologic interventions fail. There are controversial debates about using pharmacologic interventions for cognitive dysfunction in relation to cancer. Options include methylphenidate, and even more effective, modafinil.

Fatigue

Cancer patients often experience fatigue – not only from the disease itself, but also because of chemotherapy and other forms of therapy. Cancer-related fatigue is a distressing, continual, and subjective sense of tiredness or exhaustion. It affects the body, thought processes, and emotions, and is not in proportion to recent activity. Common activities of daily living are seriously impacted. A common cause of fatigue is anemia, with hemoglobin being less than 10 g/dL. This may be from the actual cancer or from the myelosuppression caused by anticancer treatments. The immune-mediated and immune checkpoint therapies as well as other anticancer agents may cause hypothyroidism, which can be signified by fatigue. The most common agents that cause hypothyroidism include cisplatin, dasatinib, aldesleukin, pazopanib, pembrolizumab, alemtuzumab, sorafenib, sunitinib, thalidomide, axitinib, imatinib, interferon, ipilimumab, lenalidomide, nilotinib, nivolumab, and vandetanib.

Cancer patients complaining of fatigue must be referred for further evaluation, since the condition may be caused by so many other factors.

These include antiemetics, analgesics, anemia, infection, depression, hypothyroidism, and hormonal deficiencies. Psychostimulants such as methylphenidate may be used to help treat fatigue once other causes are excluded. Non-pharmacologic interventions such as physical activity and psychosocial counseling provide some of the best results in the treatment of cancer-related fatigue.

Thrombocytopenia

Thrombocytopenia is a condition in which the number of circulating platelets is deficient, and causes spontaneous bleeding from small blood vessels all over the body. Even normal movement leads to wide-spread hemorrhage. Thrombocytopenia usually manifests 8–14 days after chemotherapy, usually along with neutropenia. Chemotherapy can be stopped if platelet counts drop below 50,000 per mm^3. The life span of platelets is about10 days. Thrombocytopenia is a dose-limiting toxicity that can be caused by carboplatin, gemcitabine, dacarbazine, fluorouracil, lomustine, mitomycin-C, thiotepa, and trimetrexate. Also, drugs that can cause cumulative, delayed onset of thrombocytopenia include carmustine, fludarabine, lomustine, mitomycin-C, omacetaxine, streptozocin, thiotepa, and vorinostat. If platelet levels drop below 50,000/mm^3, there is a moderate risk of bleeding. If they drop below 10,000 cells/mm^3, there is a severe risk of fatal hemorrhage in the GI and respiratory tracts, or CNS. Thrombocytopenia causes bleeding from the gums, nose, or body orifices; and **petechiae** on the elbows, palate, pressure points, and upper or lower. Platelet transfusion is often done if the count is lower than 10,000–20,000 cells /mm^3, but is often based on actual bleeding. Transfusions are limited by risks such as transfusion reactions, possibility of transmitting an infection, and alloimmunization that causes refractory platelets.

To minimize chemotherapy-induced thrombocytopenia, interleukin-11 (IL-11) has been approved as a **megakaryocyte** growth factor, for patients with non-myeloid cancers and for those receiving myelosuppressive chemotherapy. Interleukin-11 causes hematopoietic stem cells and megakaryocyte progenitors to proliferate, while inducing maturation of megakaryocytes. It accomplishes this independently of the effects of thrombopoietin. Interleukin-11 is given subcutaneously once per day until the platelets are more than 50,000 cells/mm^3. It is discontinued two days before the next chemotherapy session. Adverse effects are believed to be secondary to an increase in intravascular fluid from sodium retention in the kidneys and plasma volume expansions. Therefore, symptoms such as dyspnea, edema, and increased pleural effusions may occur. Patients with a history of coronary heart disease or congestive heart failure usually cannot receive IL-11. Newer agents have been approved to treat benign hematologic diseases such as immune thrombocytopenic purpura, but not for chemotherapy-induced thrombocytopenia. Such drugs include *eltrombopag (Promacta)* and *romiplostim (Nplate)*. They are thrombopoietin-receptor agonists, stimulating proliferation and differentiation of progenitor cells and megakaryocytes, to increase platelet production. Based on clinical studies, they are not recommended to be used prophylactically.

Neutropenia

Neutrophils survive for only 6–8 hours after being released from the bone marrow. When the **absolute neutrophil count** (ANC) decreases below 1,500 cells/mm^3, *neutropenia* develops, and there is a greatly increased risk of infections to occur. However, life-threatening grade 4 *severe neutropenia* is present if there are less than 500 cells/mm^3. Neutropenia usually develops 8–12 days after chemotherapy, and usually resolves in 3–4 weeks. Chemotherapy is usually not given if the WBC count is between 1,000 and 3,000 cells/mm^3 or if the ANC is less than 1,000–1,500 cells/mm^3. A neutropenic fever may be presented with neutropenia that is sustained for one hour. Neutropenic fevers are identified

when there are fewer than 500 neutrophils per microliter, or fewer than 1,000 neutrophils per microliter and a likelihood of decline to fewer than 500 neutrophils per microliter over the following 48 hours. Neutropenic fever is an oncologic emergency, and the patient may need to be treated on an outpatient basis with oral antibiotics, or be hospitalized and treated with IV antibiotics.

The treatment of neutropenia begins with appropriate cultures, followed by broad-spectrum antibiotics. These are continued until a culture shows that the causative organism has been eradicated, for a minimum of 7 days, or until the neutrophils have increased to more than 500/mm^3. For empiric monotherapy, the most commonly used drugs are cefepime or ceftazidime and imipenem or meropenem (carbapenems). Combination therapy using anti-pseudomonal third-generation cephalosporins and aminoglycosides or penicillin is often used. *Filgastrim* is also used to increase neutrophil counts. Additional combinations include:

- *Beta-lactam agents* – ticarcillin + clavulanate, piperacillin + tazobactam
- *Aminoglycosides* – gentamycin, tobramycin

Beta-lactam agents can be combined with other agents in the same class or with aminoglycosides. With gram-positive microorganisms becoming more common in neutropenic patients with fever, vancomycin has been used with an antipseudomonal beta-lactam agent effectively. However, this combination carries a chance of vancomycin-resistant organisms emerging. Empiric vancomycin is recommended when the patient is known to be colonized with methicillin-resistant organisms, if venous access devices are in place, or if the patient is on prophylactic quinolone and has severe mucositis while being at risk for streptococcal infections or positive blood cultures. For the patient to survive, effective antibiotics must be administered early.

Prophylactic antibiotics with agents such as fluoroquinolone are only considered if the patient is likely to have *profound neutropenia* with ANC being less than 100 cells/mm^3 for about one week. Antifungal prophylaxis with agents such as fluconazole is recommended only if the patient is on chemotherapy that is likely to cause profound neutropenia for about one week. If the patient has a 3.5% or higher risk for pneumonia due to pneumocystis (while receiving high doses of daily prednisone over one month, or if receiving purine analogs), prophylaxis with trimethoprim-sulfamethoxazole is considered. Antiviral prophylaxis is considered if the patient is at risk of reactivated hepatitis B virus infection, using lamivudine, or a reactivated herpes virus infection, using acyclovir. Influenza immunization should be given to any patient receiving chemotherapy.

For treatment of solid tumors, neutropenia usually lasts less than 10 days. If there is a hematologic malignancy, neutropenia often lasts 15–20 days. Patients at high risk include those with hematologic malignancies and those with prolonged neutropenia after a stem-cell transplant. Hospitalization is required, and broad-spectrum antibiotics are injected until fever and neutropenia subside and cultures show that the causative organism has been eradicated. Patients at moderate risk include those with comorbidities such as kidney failure or hypertension. They must be stabilized in a hospital, then discharged soon after the administration of oral or parenteral antibiotics. Patients at low risk can be treated on an outpatient basis, with oral ciprofloxacin or levofloxacin, or a combination therapy: ciprofloxacin + amoxicillin.

For a fever continuing past seven days without any infection site or organism being identified, it is likely due to an organism that is not a bacterium, antibiotic resistance, a secondary bacterial infection, drug fever, an abscess, or insufficient antibiotic serum and tissue levels. Antifungal therapy with fluconazole or voriconazole is then started. However, antiviral drugs are usually not indicated unless there is suspicion of viral disease or mucosal lesions. Recurring fever and infection are high risks for patients with neutropenia, or if there is poor bone marrow recovery, such as with disease-related dysfunction of the bone marrow. Protective isolation does not affect endogenous flora or organisms transmitted by food or water. This is why, even with careful hand washing and handling of supplies is done, adding protective isolation does not decrease infections in these patients. Hand washing is the best preventive method, however, for minimizing infections.

Clinical Case

1. What happens for neutropenia to develop?
2. After chemotherapy, when does neutropenia usually develop?
3. Is neutropenic fever a severe development?

A 62-year-old woman with stage III ovarian cancer underwent a total abdominal hysterectomy and bilateral salpingo-oophorectomy. She was referred to a medical oncologist, who recommended chemotherapy with IV carboplatin and paclitaxel to be administered every three weeks for six cycles. The patient agreed to the chemotherapy. After her first treatment, she only experienced fatigue and decreased appetite. However, after the fourth cycle, the patient was extremely fatigued and had seven pounds of weight loss, as well as a low-grade fever. The patient went for a follow-up consultation, and was diagnosed with chemotherapy-induced neutropenia. She was given *filgastrim*, which treats low neutrophil counts, and scheduled for another appointment the following day to receive an additional dose. The patient was counseled about the need to call immediately if any symptoms worsened or her fever increased. However, the drug was effective, and the patient recovered.

Answers:

1. **When the ANC decreases below 1,500 cells/mm^3, neutropenia develops. There is a greatly increased risk for infections to occur. Life-threatening grade 4 severe neutropenia is present if there are less than 500 cells/mm^3.**
2. **Neutropenia usually develops 8–12 days after chemotherapy and usually resolves in 3–4 weeks.**
3. **Neutropenic fever is an oncologic emergency. The patient may need to be treated on an outpatient basis with oral antibiotics, or be hospitalized and treated with IV antibiotics.**

Tumor Lysis Syndrome

Tumor lysis syndrome (TLS) is another oncologic emergency, occurring when cancer cells are destroyed by *lysis*. This can occur by using chemotherapy or can occur spontaneously. The lysed cells release uric acid, from DNA breakdown, along with intracellular potassium and phosphorus ions. Therefore, it causes *hyperuricemia, hyperkalemia*, and *hyperphosphatemia*. The resulting effects can include end-organ damage to the central nervous system, heart, and kidneys. Hyperphosphatemia may lead to *hypocalcemia*, from binding of calcium with phosphorus, which forms crystals. There is an increased risk of TLS with cancers such as ALL, AML, and very aggressive NHL. Generally, cancers with high proliferation rates and high responses to chemotherapy have an increased risk of TLS. Additional risk factors include acidic urine, dehydration, hypotension, and renal dysfunction.

Late effects of TLS include acute renal failure, cardiac arrhythmias, seizures, and sudden death. For high-risk patients, prophylactic efforts are extremely crucial, including normal saline to aggressively achieve hydration, diuresis, and the prevention of uric acid formation with *allopurinol*. This drug inhibits the enzyme, *xanthine oxidase*, which is required for the formation of uric acid. Allopurinol's inhibition decreases circulating uric acid. If a patient has low cardiac ejection fractions or congestive heart failure, hydration must be achieved carefully, since they accumulate fluid in the lungs and elsewhere. Excessive lung fluid causes shortness of breath and respiratory distress. Allopurinol cannot break down any previously formed uric acid. When the uric acid is elevated, the enzyme known as *rasburicase* is used, which is a form of *urate oxidase*. The uric acid is broken down into *allantoin* – a more soluble form in the urine that can be excreted comparatively easily. Rasburicase may be given in one IV dose or given intravenously over five days.

Management of electrolytes is also required. Quick-acting agents are needed since hyperkalemia can result in arrhythmias. Potassium can be removed via the gastrointestinal system by using a cation exchange resin known as *sodium polystyrene sulfonate*, but it can take hours to days for its effects. Quicker-acting agents include furosemide or other loop diuretics, which also help in diuresis, and regular insulin, since it moves potassium back into cells. Disadvantages in using regular insulin include possible hypoglycemia if dextrose 50% is not given immediately after insulin. Another problem is with the cells continuing to lyse, moving potassium back into them may not be completely effective. If cardiac changes are seen on the monitor, calcium gluconate may help stabilize the heart. Hyperphosphatemia is treated with aluminum hydroxide, calcium acetate, or sevelamer, as well as with the reduction of dietary calcium. Severe hyperkalemia and hyperphosphatemia are treated with emergent hemodialysis. For severe hypocalcemia, calcium can be supplemented with IV calcium gluconate.

Gastrointestinal Tract Toxicity

Treatment options to prevent chemotherapy-related nausea and vomiting must take into account different mechanisms of action, adverse effects, and routes of administration. Patients at a higher risk for nausea and vomiting include younger patients and females, people that expect they will experience these symptoms, and those with histories of morning sickness or motion sickness. Patients with a history of high alcohol consumption have lower risks for nausea and vomiting. There are also two primary therapy-related risk factors: chemotherapy dose and emetogenicity, which is related to the frequency that an agent causes vomiting (emesis). There is no universal classification system for emetogenicity, but in the United States, risks are usually divided into high, moderate, low, and minimal emetic classifications, which are based on percentages of patients that experience vomiting when antiemetics are not given. For chemotherapy, these emetogenicity categories are calculated as follows:

- High – more than 90% frequency of emesis
- Moderate – 30–90%
- Low – 10–30%
- Minimal – less than 10%

Vomiting is a motor-reflex response, and may or may not be preceded by nausea. Chemotherapy acts as the noxious stimuli and irritates the GI tract. This results in the release of serotonin (5-HT) from **enterochromaffin cells** of the GI tract, which bind to serotonin type 3 receptors (5-HT3) in the tract. This substance binds to neurokinin-1 (NK-1) receptors, and the central vomiting pathway is activated. Other neurotransmitters are also activated in the **chemoreceptor trigger zone** and vomiting center. These include cannabinoids, dopamine, acetylcholine, and histamine.

Antiemetics are usually used for three days after a day of chemotherapy. The National Comprehensive Cancer Network (NCCN) recommends multi-day regimens of antiemetics to combat the effects of oral chemotherapy agents.

However, with IV chemotherapy agents, recommendations for antiemetics are not as defined. For example, a five-day regimen using the highly emetogenic drug *cisplatin* each day requires a different amount of antiemetics than when cisplatin is given on day 1, plus *5-fluorouracil* (which has low emetogenicity) for the full five-day period. Many clinicians have an antiemetic regimen continue for two days following the last day of a chemotherapy drug being taken if the drug has a high level of emetogenicity. In the previous example, a high emetogenicity antiemetic regimen is used for all five days of the cisplatin regimen, and for two days after. In the second regimen, a highly emetogenic antiemetic regimen would be used for two days of cisplatin and also two days after, for a total of four days. This is followed by a low emetogenicity antiemetic for the fifth day.

Optional drugs to prevent nausea and vomiting include the serotonin (5-HT3) antagonists, neurokinin-1 (NK-1) antagonists, corticosteroids, dopamine antagonists, histamine antagonists, cannabinoids, and benzodiazepines.

Diarrhea and constipation are common adverse effects of chemotherapy. Diarrhea is caused by damage of the epithelial lining of the GI tract by chemotherapy drugs. Inflammation and irritation of the bowel lining occurs, decreasing the ability to absorb nutrients and fluids. If severe, diarrhea can result in dehydration, electrolyte abnormalities, and hospitalization. Treatment includes non-drug options such as eating small and frequent meals, avoiding lactose-containing products and alcohol, and drinking 8–10 glasses of clear fluids per day. Patients should keep symptom diaries. For drug-induced diarrhea, *loperamide (Diamode, Imodium A-D)* is the primary drug used. It inhibits GI motility via intestinal muscle opioid receptors. Dosing is every four hours or after every bowel movement. *Irinotecan (Camptosar)* is a chemotherapy drug that causes a different type of diarrhea – with two phases: acute and delayed. Acute diarrhea occurs within the first day of irinotecan being administered, since the drug acts as an acetylcholinesterase inhibitor. It increases acetylcholine to cause a cholinergic response, which is opposite to the intended effects of anticholinergic drugs used for nausea and vomiting. The symptoms are described with the abbreviation "SLUDGE" (excess <u>s</u>aliva, excess <u>lacrimation</u>, <u>urination</u>, <u>diaphoresis</u>, <u>GI upset</u> [diarrhea], and <u>e</u>mesis). To reverse irinotecan-induced diarrhea, *atropine (Atropen)* is given IV or subcutaneously. The delayed form of irinotecan-induced diarrhea begins after 24 hours have passed, since the active ingredient in the drug causes large and watery stools to be produced excessively. Loperamide can also be used to treat this, but larger quantities are required than would otherwise be recommended. It must be taken every 2 hours until the patient has had no diarrhea for 12 hours. The patient must be instructed about the doses of loperamide that are needed since they differ from the OTC packaging instructions.

Constipation often causes GI pain, bloating, nausea, and vomiting. Many medications causing constipation do this by inhibiting or slowing down motility. Severe, untreated constipation can cause ileus – an obstruction of the GI tract. It is best to use any method possible to prevent constipation, such as with scheduled stimulant laxatives – *bisacodyl (Alophen)* or *senna (Senokot)*. These laxatives are often given along with a stool softener such as *docusate (Colace)* to prevent straining during defecation – especially if the patient has low platelets – to avoid bleeding. *Methylnaltrexone (Relistor)*, an opioid receptor antagonist, only acts upon the opioid receptors of the GI tract. Therefore, it treats opioid-induced constipation, usually producing a bowel movement in four hours after being injected subcutaneously. Chemotherapy agents that commonly cause diarrhea or constipation are listed in Table 16.3.

Mucositis is defined as the inflammation, eroding, and ulceration of the mucosal barrier of the mouth or GI tract, which often occurs because of chemotherapy. This usually happens within 5–7 days, and is linked to a reduction in WBC counts. Mucositis usually improves as the neutrophils recover from chemotherapy. When the mucosal barrier breaks down, there is increased risk of infection, since bacteria can eventually move into the blood circulation. Mucositis can cause extreme pain and impair eating, resulting in problems with nutrition and hydration. Risk factors include the type and dose of a chemotherapy medication received. The alkylating agents and topoisomerase II inhibitors cause the highest rates of mucositis. Risk factors include poor dental hygiene, preexisting oral lesions, and dentures that do not fit well. Other risk factors include receiving chemotherapy along with radiation, and being Caucasian. There are five stages in which mucositis develops and resolves, as follows:

Table 16.3 Chemotherapy agents that commonly cause diarrhea or constipation.

Diarrhea	Constipation
Capecitabine (Xeloda, Xitabin, and others)	Anticholinergics (diphenhydramine [Benadryl, etc.])
5-Fluorouracil (Adrucil, Carac, and others) (used continuously)	Arsenic trioxide (Trisenox, etc.)
Immune checkpoint agents such as ipilimumab (Yervoy), nivolumab (Opdivo)	Opioids (pain medications)
Irinotecan (Camptosar, Campto, and others)	Serotonin type 3 (5HT3) antagonists such as ondansetron (Zofran, etc.)
Metoclopramide (Primperan, Reglan, and others)	Thalidomide (Contergan, etc.)
Tyrosine kinase inhibitors	Vincristine

- *Initiation* – chemotherapy or radiation causes the damage and death of GI cells and tissues
- *Up-regulation of messengers* – pro-inflammatory cytokines increase in number, then released; these cause more tissue damage and apoptosis
- *Signaling and amplification* – activation of positive feedback loops further increases the amount of pro-inflammatory cytokines
- *Ulceration* – the phase that signifies symptoms, with the development of sores, additional inflammation, pain, and infections
- *Healing* – since GI cells turnover usually within 7–14 days, healing involves new growth of epithelial cells in the GI tract

Anticancer agents that cause mucositis are summarized in Table 16.4.

There are only a few treatment options. Proper mouth hygiene is encouraged, but no specific regimen has been determined. Basically, daily teeth cleaning with topical fluoride, regular flossing, and frequent use of mouthwash is suggested. Cancer patients can be at risk for gum bleeding when their platelet counts are low. A soft bristle toothbrush is recommended, and they must monitor for any gum bleeding while brushing or flossing. There are many good mouthwashes available, and other options include normal saline, calcium phosphate, and sodium bicarbonate. The mouthwash called *chlorhexidine (generic only)* is not recommended for cancer patients because it contains alcohol, which can dry out the mouth and cause cracking of the mucosal lining. Other mouthwashes that contain alcohol should also be avoided.

The treatments for GI mucositis, not in the oral cavity, include amifostine (Ethyol), octreotide (Sandostatin), sucralfate (Carafate), sulfasalazine (Azulfidine), *lactobacillus*-containing probiotics, and hyperbaric oxygen. The treatments for oral mucositis include cryotherapy, palifermin (Kepivance), low-level laser therapy, morphine (Oramorph), benzydamine mouthwash (Tantum Verde), proper oral care, doxepin mouthwash (generic only), and oral zinc supplements.

Integumentary Toxicity

Chemotherapy agents have the potential to cause rashes because of varying mechanisms of

Table 16.4 Anticancer agents that cause mucositis.

Agents	Classifications
Actinomycin (Cosmegen), busulfan (Myleran), chlorambucil (Leukeran), cisplatin (Platinol), cyclophosphamide (Cytoxan), melphalan (Alkeran), mechlorethamine (Mustargen), mitomycin-C (Mitosol), oxaliplatin (Eloxatin), procarbazine (Matulane), thiotepa (Tepadina)	Alkylating agents
Capecitabine (Xeloda), cytarabine (Cytosar-U), fluorouracil (Adrucil), hydroxyurea (Droxia), mercaptopurine (Purinethol), methotrexate (Trexall), thioguanine (Lanvis)	Antimetabolites
Docetaxel (Taxotere), ixabepilone (Ixempra), paclitaxel (Taxol), vinblastine (Velban), vincristine (Oncovin), vinorelbine (Navelbine)	Microtubule inhibitors
Bortezomib (Velcade), everolimus (Afinitor), interferon beta-1b (Betaseron), interferon gamma-1b (Actimmune)	Miscellaneous
alemtuzumab (Campath), bevacizumab (Avastin), cetuximab (Erbitux), panitumumab (Vectibix), trastuzumab (Herceptin)	Monoclonal antibodies
Daunorubicin (Cerubidine), doxorubicin (Adriamycin), epirubicin, etoposide, idarubicin, irinotecan, mitoxantrone, topotecan	Topoisomerase II inhibitors
Erlotinib, imatinib, lapatinib, sunitinib	Tyrosine kinase inhibitors

action, such as with epidermal growth factor receptor inhibitors (EGFRIs). Many cancers are related to overexpression of EGFR, so EGFRIs can be monoclonal antibodies or tyrosine kinase inhibitors, utilized to target this situation. Erlotinib (Tarceva) is used as a single agent or as part of a multiple treatment regimen for lung and pancreatic cancers. Cetuximab (Erbitux) and panitumumab (Vectibix) are used to treat colorectal cancer, and cetuximab is additionally used for head and neck cancers. Lapatinib (Tykerb) is an option for breast cancer. The epidermal growth factor receptor is also involved with epidermal and other normal skin growth, so a primary adverse effect of the EGFRIs is in the upper skin layer, as the normal cell growth and turnover pathway becomes disrupted.

The rash caused by EGFRIs appears similar to acne, so it is referred to as an acneiform rash. It happens in as many as 80% of patients receiving these drugs, since EGFR inhibition causes arrested growth of keratinocytes in the skin, and cell death. The epidermis thins, and the skin is more likely to be damaged. Therefore, it recruits leukocytes and neutrophils, leading to an inflammatory reaction that appears as a papulo-pustular rash or acneiform rash. The rash does indicate that the drug is working and affecting its target. Patients often complain about the appearance of the rash, which often develops on the scalp, face, back, and upper chest. If severe, it can cause infections and scarring. Risk factors for the rash are varied between the causative agents. With erlotinib, the rash is more common in fair-skinned people, nonsmokers, and when the patient's age is under 70. The monoclonal antibodies usually cause more severe rashes that are more frequent (10–17% of patients) than the tyrosine kinase inhibitors (5–9%).

Prevention and treatment options for acneiform rash are good to consider because the therapy treating the cancer is causing the rash. The rash usually develops within 2–4 weeks of beginning chemotherapy. The inflammation of the skin usually decreases in severity after 6–8 weeks. So, preventive therapy should be given during this period. High-risk areas of the skin should be treated with *hydrocortisone 1% cream*, moisturizer, and sunscreen – two times per day. The doxycycline (Doryx) and minocycline (Minocin) antibiotics reduce the amount of lesions during the first eight weeks. If additional treatments are needed, stronger topical corticosteroids can be used, such as alclometasone 0.05% cream (Aclovate) or fluocinonide 0.05% cream (Lyderm). Topical antibiotics such as clindamycin (Cleocin T) 1% are also indicated. To improve quality of life during EGFRI therapy, isotretinoin (Accutane) can be used in low doses.

Cardiotoxicity

Cardiotoxicity is an acute or chronic process that may be caused by chemotherapy. The acute form is signified by temporary ECG changes, occurring in only about 10% of chemotherapy patients. They are immediate in their onset, resolving soon with no serious complications. Acute effects are not related to dose, and usually do not mean that the chemotherapy drug must be stopped. Less than 5% of patients develop chronic cardiotoxicity because of cumulative drug effects requiring immediate stoppage of the chemotherapy. Chronic effects manifest weeks or months after chemotherapy. There is non-reversible cardiomyopathy, with classic biventricular congestive heart failure and a low-voltage QRS complex. Signs and symptoms include dyspnea, non-productive cough, and edema of the feet. Chronic chemotherapy-related cardiomyopathy is usually not very responsive to diuretics or digitalis. It progressively worsens and is fatal in 60% of cases.

Cardiotoxicity is directly caused by the anthracyclines because they damage myocytes of the heart. After cumulative doses of anthracyclines, cardiotoxicity occurs in 10–26% of patients. Estimating incidence of anthracycline-caused cardiotoxicity is difficult. Long-term data are generally not available. The most cardiotoxic anthracyclines are: epirubicin, doxorubicin, and daunorubicin. Risks for cardiotoxicity are increased if these drugs are used along with mediastinal radiation or other cardiotoxic non-anthracycline agents, or if the patient has hypertension or preexisting cardiac disease. The patients most likely to develop cardiotoxicity from anthracyclines are children and the elderly.

To decrease cases of chemotherapy-related cardiotoxicity, doses and scheduling of doxorubicin can be changed so that more frequent but lower doses are given. This has reduced cardiotoxicity with no compromise of the effects of the drug upon tumors. Liposomal doxorubicin has been linked to reduced cardiotoxicity as well. *Chemoprotectants* may be able to block damage to myocytes, protecting cardiac tissues. *Dexrazoxane (Zinecard)* is approved for metastatic breast cancer patients who have received average doses of doxorubicin and are continuing to receive it, but when it was not the initial drug used. Patients can tolerate higher cumulative doses of doxorubicin as a result, with fewer cardiac events. Dexrazoxane is given 30 minutes before doxorubicin on a 10:1 dosage ratio, with 10 times more dexrazoxane being given than doxorubicin. This has allowed for extremely high doses of doxorubicin to be given without cardiotoxicity. Dexrazoxane is believed to interfere with intracellular processes that cause anthracycline-related cardiomyopathy. The drug has also been used in other types of adult cancers for which doxorubicin is the chemotherapeutic drug of choice.

Acute pericarditis has occurred with high doses of cyclophosphamide used in stem-cell-transplant patients, with later pericardial effusion and **cardiac tamponade**. Cyclophosphamide damages myocytes similarly to how the anthracyclines do, causing swelling and decreased contractility, as well as less effective heart pumping. Hemorrhagic myocardial necrosis has occurred, with blood leakage through the capillaries. Transient complete heart block has occurred, resulting in a temporary pacemaker being required. Toxicities may be minor, temporary ECG changes with elevated cardiac enzymes, to death from myopericarditis or myocardial necrosis. With infusion of fluorouracil in patients with or without preexisting heart disease, myocardial ischemia has occurred. There has also

been coronary vasospasm with angina pectoris, myocardial infarction, ST segment elevations, and ventricular ectopy. A direct toxic effect upon vascular endothelium has been identified, leading to coronary spasm and endothelial-independent vasoconstriction through interaction with **protein kinase C**. Angina in these cases may be a coronary artery spasm of the **Prinzmetal** variety, which could respond to nitrates. Stopping chemotherapy may not be required, since patients with this syndrome can be pretreated with calcium-channel blockers, preventing coronary artery spasm. Also, capecitabine has been linked to cases of myocardial infarction.

In about 30% of ovarian cancer patients being given paclitaxel, asymptomatic bradycardia has occurred. Other cardiac distrubances affect 5% of patients. They include atrioventricular conduction blocks, cardiac ischemia, left bundle branch blocks, and ventricular tachycardia. Paclitaxel-related cardiac abnormalities did not cause clinical symptoms, but were found incidentally during cardiac monitoring. Infusion of paclitaxel is not stopped unless there is progressive atrioventricular conduction disturbance. This may be due to the use of Cremophor EL, which activates cardiac histamine receptors. When the receptors are stimulated, there is increased myocardial oxygen demand, causing coronary vasoconstriction. *Trastuzumab (Herceptin)* has caused direct cardiac toxicity or potentiated anthracycline effects. There is a toxic effect of Erb B2 (tyrosine kinase 2) receptors upon the myocardium. These usually are protective of cardiac function.

Anti-vascular endothelial growth factor receptor agents have caused acute, systemic cardiovascular toxicities during administration or soon afterward. Symptoms include hypertension, left ventricle systolic dysfunction, heart failure, and myocardial infarction. Examples of these drugs include bevacizumab, pazopanib, sorafenib, sunitinib, and vandetanib. During their administration, the patient's BP must be carefully monitored and controlled. Cardiac function must be evaluated through the chemotherapy process if the patient is at high risk for cardiotoxicity, or requires high doses of paclitaxel, anthracyclines, or high-dose cyclophosphamide.

Lifelong cardiotoxicity of anthracyclines explains the need to monitor cardiac problems. Most often, radionuclide cardiography and echocardiograms are used, even though they are insensitive to early cardiotoxicity. Because of late-onset cardiac dysfunction risks, noninvasive long-term follow-up is indicated, based on the patient's cardiac symptoms and risk factors. Low-risk patients are those receiving low doses of anthracyclines and no mediastinal radiation, or that have no cardiac problems. High-risk patients are those receiving high doses of anthracyclines, with mediastinal radiation, or with abnormal cardiac findings. Detection of late toxicity can be done in a three-month follow-up echocardiogram or radionuclide angiography. Long-term follow-up varies based on the type of cancer and the treatment chosen. Generally, for asymptomatic patients, there should be one annual echocardiogram, and one cardiac scan every five years. A complete cardiac evaluation is needed if the patient complains of edema, fatigue, dyspnea, or pain during a routine follow-up session.

Neurotoxicity

Neurotoxicity that is caused by chemotherapy can directly or indirectly damage the CNS, cranial nerves, PNS, or combinations of these. Most chemotherapy patients have temporary neurotoxicity, but some have permanent neurotoxicity. Usually, the chemotherapy is suspended when the toxicity is severe, and time is allowed for the symptoms to resolve. Then, a 50% dose reduction may be tried, or the drug may have to be discontinued. Both the CNS and PNS are protected against neurotoxicity by the blood-brain barrier and blood-nerve barriers. These barriers normally exclude the majority of water-soluble chemotherapeutic drugs and comparatively large molecules from entering the nervous system. When nerves damaged by chemotherapy have been biopsied, they showed a slight decrease in large-diameter myelinated nerve fibers. Ultra-structural examination has revealed scattered, degenerated nerve fibers in axons as well as myelin sheaths. Neurotoxicity is usually dose-related. Symptoms are varied and unpredictable. *Peripheral neuropathy* is an injury, degeneration, or inflammation of the peripheral nerve fibers. Chemotherapy-induced peripheral neuropathy (CIPN) is caused by platinum agents, epothilones, taxanes, bortezomib, vinca alkaloids, and lenalidomide. The diagnosis of neurotoxicity is subjectively based on symptoms plus a neurological examination.

The CNS contains groupings of neurons with connections organized into brain and spinal cord regions. CNS damage most affects the cerebellum, causing altered reflexes, **ataxia**, confusion, and **unsteady gait**. The peripheral nervous system is mostly communication channels outside of the CNS, which consist of the cranial and spinal nerves. Damage causes paralysis or loss of sensation and movement to areas affected by a particular nerve. Common effects include numbness, **paresthesia**, hyperalgesia, burning, tingling, loss of tendon reflexes, **proprioception**, and vibration sensation. The effects begin in the toes and fingers, spreading progressively to the extremities, and is described as the typical "glove-and-stocking" distribution (see Figure 16.1). Peripheral neuropathy may start weeks to months after initial chemotherapy. In most cases, CIPN is only partly reversible and is often permanent. In rare cases, toxicity affects the cranial nerves.

The autonomic nervous system (ANS) includes peripheral nerves regulating functions that are "automatic" in the body. These include the functions of the cardiovascular, endocrine, and respiratory systems. Any ANS damage can cause impotence, ileus, or urinary retention. The severity of neurotoxicity is based on the actual chemotherapeutic drug used, length of therapy, cumulative dose, and any combinations of other neurotoxic agents. Some preexisting conditions cause nerve damage, such as diabetes mellitus, hypothyroidism, alcohol abuse, and

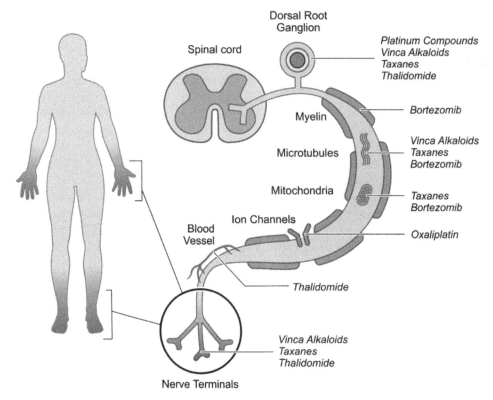

Figure 16.1 The typical "glove-and-stocking" distribution of chemotherapy-induced peripheral neuropathy. *Source*: Susanna B. Park. (2013).

vitamin B deficiency. Sometimes, these conditions increase risks of neurotoxicity. Risks are also increased by advanced age. Patient showing evidence of CIPN that improved greatly after discontinuance of chemotherapy have an increased risk for neurotoxicity if other neurotoxic syndromes are present.

Vincristine (Oncovin) has a strong potential for triggering peripheral neuropathy, with loss of deep tendon ankle reflexes, myalgia, and eventually, total areflexia, distal symmetric sensory loss, foot drop, motor weakness, and muscle atrophy. Autonomic neuropathy may be signified by constipation, ileus, impotence, postural hypotension, or urinary retention. Cranial nerve palsies sometimes occur. Vincristine is believed to disrupt microtubules of the neural tissues, inhibiting mitotic spindle movements needed for mitosis during cellular reproduction.

High doses of vincristine, as with other chemotherapies, are most harmful.

Cisplatin (Platinol) causes reversible neuropathy, but it also has caused continuing neuropathy. It affects large-diameter fibers of neural tissues, affecting sensation. An early sign is a decreased sense of vibration, which patients describe as hand–foot paresthesias in the classic stocking-glove distribution. Sensory loss occurs first. If doses are not modified, there is loss of the Achilles reflex, loss of deep tendon reflexes, and muscle weakness. With progressive neuropathy, sense of position is impaired and there is a significant sensory ataxia. Cisplatin combined with paclitaxel has also caused peripheral neuropathy. Sensory-motor neuropathy occurs within 21 weeks after initiating therapy. It is progressive with additional courses of chemotherapy, and much more extreme with high doses of paclitaxel. With cisplatin or carboplatin, hearing loss may occur. Loss of being able to hear higher frequencies may be due to loss of hairs in the **organ of Corti**. Ototoxicity is more likely with rapid drug delivery, dehydration, and simultaneous administration of aminoglycosides. Hearing loss may be reversed if cisplatin is discontinued, but permanent damage has occurred, requiring use of hearing aids.

With ifosfamide (Ifex), neurotoxicity may involve **metabolic encephalopathy**, causing blurred vision, motor system dysfunction, seizures, cranial nerve dysfunction, urinary incontinence, subclinical electroencephalographic changes, and irreversible coma. This has occurred in 10–20% of patients. In 48–72 hours of stopping infusion of ifosfamide, the majority of abnormalities resolve. Neurotoxic risk factors include length of administration, liver insufficiency, previous use of cisplatin, high serum creatinine, and low serum albumin. The encephalopathy may occur from accumulated metabolites (**chloracetaldehyde**), causing direct CNS damage. If the patient is disoriented or shows neurologic changes after ifosfamide is infused, additional doses must be withheld until the situation is adequately assessed.

High doses of methotrexate (Trexall), over several courses, have caused encephalopathy that is often transient and reversible. Intrathecal methotrexate has caused chemical meningitis: headache, fever, CSF leukocytosis, and muscle rigidity. While rare, this occurs within hours of an intrathecal injection, resolving on its own. Intrathecal chemotherapy may also cause direct toxic effects from methotrexate as well as cytarabine, causing cerebellar dysfunction, encephalopathy, and myelopathy.

Fluorouracil (Adrucil) can cause acute cerebellar dysfunction – mostly in elderly patients. There is a fast onset of **gait ataxia**, dysarthria, diplopia, **nystagmus**, lack of fine and coordinated movements, and limb incoordination. The effects are reversed with dose reduction or withdrawal of the drug. With fluorouracil + leucovorin, multifocal cerebral demyelination has occurred, causing acute confusion, ataxia, restlessness, and slurred speech. With discontinuance of chemotherapy and use of steroids, symptoms improve.

High doses of cytarabine (Cytosar) may cause encephalopathy, leukoencephalopathy, and occasionally, peripheral neuropathy in high doses. The drug, in these doses, has a higher transport rate over cell membranes. This enhances intracellular drug concentrations, lengthening cellular exposure to its metabolites. Toxicity in the CNS usually occurs in 5–7 days. Ocular toxicity plus cerebellar and cerebral dysfunction may occur. Ocular toxicity symptoms include conjunctivitis, burning, decreased acuity, and photophobia. Once cytarabine is stopped, neurological symptoms partially or totally resolve.

With docetaxel (Taxotere), arthralgia and myalgia sometimes occur. Symptoms usually last for up to four days. Discomfort can be relieved with prophylactic analgesics, including ibuprofen. Mild sensory neuropathy is common. With high doses, severe and disabling neuropathy may develop, with numbness, paresthesias, decreased deep tendon reflexes, and loss of sensation.

With paclitaxel (Taxol), similar symptoms may occur 2–3 days after administration, resolving in about one week. The most often affected areas include the shoulder and paraspinal muscles, and sometimes, the joints. Sensory neuropathy occurs with high doses of paclitaxel, causing numbness, burning, or tingling in the legs. Perioral numbness may occur, at first asymmetrically, and then symmetrically. A neurologic examination will show loss of proprioception and reduction or loss of deep tendon reflexes. Neurotoxicity is usually cumulative. Larger-fiber sensations involving vibration and proprioception are most often affected than small-fiber sensations of pain and temperature. After paclitaxel is discontinued, mild symptoms improve or resolve over several months. Autonomic neuropathy has occurred with higher doses, resulting in orthostatic hypotension and paralytic ileus. Diabetic patients are more often affected by autonomic neuropathy. Abraxene is a paclitaxel formulation that is an albumin-stabilized nanoparticle. It is given as a 30-minute infusion every 3 weeks, and causes much higher incidence or peripheral neuropathy than standard paclitaxel. Symptoms are similar, however.

Oral immunomodulatory agents such as lenalidomide, pomalidomide, and thalidomide can also cause sensory peripheral neuropathy because of antiangiogenic properties. These cause a reduction in the nerve blood supply along with metabolic changes of the dorsal root ganglia, resulting in numbness and tingling in the feet and hands. Symptoms usually resolve when these drugs are discontinued. Gemcitabine (Gemzar) causes a low-grade fever, fatigue, arthralgia with paresthesias, malaise, and myalgia in about 10% of patients.

Oxaliplatin (Eloxatin) is an example of a chemotherapeutic agent that can cause neurotoxicity. It can cause a syndrome of acute neuropathy. The condition can begin within hours to two days after treatment. It causes sensitivities to the touch of anything that is cold in temperature, muscle cramping, and throat discomfort. Patients receive oxaliplatin should avoid cold foods and drinks, use plastic eating utensils instead of metal utensils (since these are often cold), and wear appropriate protective clothing around the throat during cold, cool, or windy weather. Neuropathy often recurs with additional doses of oxaliplatin. Motor neuropathy may occur, with dysesthesia, hypoesthesia, and paresthesias.

Four drugs (bevacizumab, cisplatin, rituximab, and tacrolimus) are able to cause posterior reversible encephalopathy syndrome. There is headache, focal neurologic deficits, mental status changes, and visual changes. A brain MRI is the best imaging method to confirm PRES that presents as symmetrical, subcortical gray and white matter lesions. While reversible, PRES has high morbidity and mortality rates due to it often not being recognized. Treatment requires dose reduction or withholding the causative drug and then giving supporting care for symptoms.

Ixabepilone (Ixempra) may cause peripheral neuropathy since it induces tubulin polymerization into microtubules, and interferes with axonal transport. Neurotoxicity is due to higher doses and symptoms are mostly sensory related. Motor neuropathy is less common. Bortezomib (Velcade) causes peripheral neuropathy with morphological changes in the dorsal root ganglia, peripheral nerve fibers, and spinal cord. There is pain and paresthesias in the distal extremities. Distal sensory loss and changes in proprioception are found in neurological examinations. The deep tendon reflexes are absent or decreased. No treatments are able to prevent chronic adverse effects of this drug's peripheral neuropathy.

Prevention of neurotoxicity involves limiting cumulative drug dosing with thalidomide or vinca alkaloids and other agents, or reducing doses. Amifostine (Ethyol) was believed to decrease cisplatin- or paclitaxel-related neurotoxicity but it has now been found that the drug is not extremely effective. Venlafaxine (Effexor) has been studied to prevent neuropathy from oxaliplatin with some success. Other drugs studied to prevent chemotherapy-induced neuropathy include acetyl-L-carnitine, alpha-lipoic acid, infusions of calcium and magnesium, glutamine (GlutaSolve), glutathione, carbamazepine (Carbatrol), and vitamin E. Results have been mixed.

Chemotherapy often causes cognitive impairment and results in reduced short-term memory, poor attention, confusion, lack of concentration, and an inability to organize thoughts. Cancer patients often complain of difficulty in understanding what they read and in concentrating while driving. Cognitive changes may be worsened by fatigue and stress, and underlying conditions such as dementia or stroke also contribute. Chemotherapy-induced cognitive impairment has been called *chemo brain* and *chemo fog*. Cognitive problems start with the initial 1–2 cycles of chemotherapy and last for many years after chemotherapy is completed. Risk factors proposed as increasing these difficulties include higher doses and longer treatment times with chemotherapy. There are no current proven measures to prevent these impairments. The drug called modafinil (Provigil) may help reduce fatigue and improve attention. Mixed results have occurred in studies of methylphenidate (Ritalin) and dexmethylphenidate (Focalin).

Patients can also be encouraged to make lists of things they need to remember, or lists of household items to check such as locking doors and turning off the oven. Cognitive rehabilitation may be helpful in enhancing cognitive function. Rehabilitation training helps to maintain or restore cognitive function through repeated tasks that have been previously problematic. Neurologic assessment is crucial when neurotoxic agents are being administered. Baseline assessments include gait, motor and sensory function, cranial nerve function, range of motion, and reflexes. Liver and kidney function must be monitored. Agents such as cytarabine and ifosfamide have higher neurotoxicity when there is kidney dysfunction. CNS depressants such as antiemetics, sedatives, and tranquilizers must be limited since they can increase toxicities. Other causes of cognitive symptoms include electrolyte imbalances and cancer metastases. Electromyography (EMG) may be done if symptoms or neurologic presentation are abnormal.

Neurotoxicity decreases mobility performance of fine-motor skills, and the ability to care for oneself. Occupational therapists may help patients adapt to reduced motor skills. Balance and gait training, sometimes with gait aids, help prevent falling and aid in adaptation. Patients must be instructed about reporting any new numbness or tingling in the extremities, as well as any changes in status. Pain relief is another treatment goal. Medications used may include gabapentin (Neurontin), pregabalin (Lyrica), amitriptyline (Elavil), and duloxetine (Cymbalta). If the neurologic deficits are severe, safety measures may be needed to protect the patient.

Clinical Case

1. What can chemotherapy-induced neurotoxicity damage?
2. What is peripheral neuropathy defined as?
3. How can a dose of chemotherapy cause damage to the peripheral nervous system?

A 59-year-old man who had been treated with chemotherapy for colorectal cancer developed CIPN. As his symptoms worsened, the patient became worried about being unable to continue working. The neuropathy had begun on the sole of his left foot, with numbness and tingling, eventually affecting his left hand. Over time, the left hand became numb and very weak. Physical examination revealed that both hands and feet felt colder to the touch than other areas of the patient's body. It was discovered that the patient's kidneys were also affected by the chemotherapy, and hemodialysis was indicated, which helped to reverse but not fully resolve his neuropathy.

Answers:

1. **Neurotoxicity that is caused by chemotherapy can directly or indirectly damage the CNS, cranial nerves, PNS, or combinations of these. Most chemotherapy patients have temporary neurotoxicity, but some have permanent neurotoxicity.**
2. **Peripheral neuropathy is an injury, degeneration, or inflammation of the peripheral nerve fibers. Chemotherapy-induced peripheral neuropathy (CIPN) is caused by platinum agents, epothilones, taxanes, bortezomib, vinca alkaloids, and lenalidomide.**
3. **Damage to the peripheral nervous system from a large dose of chemotherapy**

causes paralysis or loss of sensation and movement to areas affected by a particular nerve. Common effects include numbness, paresthesia, hyperalgesia, burning, tingling, loss of tendon reflexes, proprioception, and vibration sensation. The effects begin in the toes and fingers, spreading progressively to the extremities. Peripheral neuropathy may start weeks to months after initial chemotherapy.

Pulmonary Toxicity

Usually, chemotherapy-induced pulmonary toxicity is irreversible and progressive, occurring many years after chemotherapy is completed. The endothelial cells are often the first site of damage, with an inflammatory-type reaction. This causes pneumonitis. Another form of damage occurs from an immunologic mechanism. Chronic chemotherapy causes significant changes in the pulmonary parenchyma. There are alterations of the connection tissues, dilatation of air spaces, and obliteration of the alveoli – collectively known as *honeycombing*. Continual injury and repair cause restrictive lung disease. It is harder to breathe, and the lung volume is functionally reduced, causing impaired gas exchange. Hypoxemia occurs since oxygen cannot diffuse in the areas of damage as perfusion continues.

Clinically, pulmonary toxicity is signified as mild to progressive dyspnea, bilateral basial rales, an unproductive cough, low-grade fever, and tachypnea. Chest X-rays may be normal, but there might be diffuse interstitial markings. The arterial blood gases show hypoxia with hypocapnia and respiratory alkalosis. The carbon monoxide diffusion capacity test is highly sensitive, indicating abnormalities before any clinical symptoms present. Other pulmonary function tests can reveal restrictive patterns if pulmonary fibrosis has already developed. An open-lung biopsy or a fiberoptic bronchoscopy is indicated for diagnosis and exclusion of infections. Bacterial or fungal infections and metastasis can be ruled out as a result.

Bleomycin (Blenoxane) causes pulmonary toxicity in 5% of patients receiving smaller doses and up to 46% with larger doses. Risk factors predisposing patients to bleomycin-induced toxicity include advanced age, kidney dysfunction, smoking history, administration of supplemental oxygen, and mediastinal radiation. The drug is concentrated mostly in the lungs, and inactivated by a **hydrolase enzyme** that is relatively deficient in the lung tissues compared with areas such as the liver. This may explain why bleomycin, in the lungs, causes early endothelial cell damage, decreased type I pneumocytes with proliferation, and migration of type II pneumocytes into the alveolar spaces, causing interstitial changes. When the type I cells are destroyed, repair involves hyperplasia and dysplasia of the type II pneumocytes. Irreversible changes may be caused by proliferation of fibroblasts that lead to **pulmonary fibrosis**. The first symptom of pulmonary toxicity is dyspnea, and fine rales may be revealed during examination. With more lung parenchyma affected, there is more reduction of respiratory function. In severe cases, acute respiratory failure and acute respiratory distress syndrome (ARDS) develop. In early stages, pulmonary function tests are altered, showing reduction in diffuse lung capacity of carbon monoxide. There is a decrease in lung volume that indicates a typical restrictive syndrome. In chest X-rays, there may be bilateral consolidation with alveolar and interstitial infiltrates. Once infection is excluded, steroids are the best form of treatment.

Cytarabine has direct toxic effects upon the pneumocytes and capillary endothelial cells. It reduces integrity of cell membranes and increases capillary permeability. Capillary leak syndrome, mostly in the lungs, occurs in up to 21 days after dosing. Pulmonary edema and respiratory failure follow, with components of acute respiratory disease (ARD). Cytarabine in high doses and continuous administration appear to be more causative. High doses of corticosteroids have been successful for treatment. If the lungs are damaged by mitomycin-C (Mutamycin), there is diffuse alveolar damage, capillary leakage, and pulmonary edema. This occurs in 3–36% of patients, from 6 to 12 months after therapy starts. Sometimes, only a short exposure will cause damage. If dyspnea develops while chest X-rays are normal, mitomycin-C may need to be permanently discontinued. High-dose cyclophosphamide causes pulmonary fibrosis in less than 1% of patients. There may be endothelial swelling, edema, pneumocyte dysplasia, fibrosis, and proliferation of fibroblasts. Eventually, there is alveolar hemorrhage and deposition of fibrin.

Carmustine (Gliadel) inhibits lung glutathione disulfide reductase, mediating the cellular injury that occurs. Damage happens after a long period of about three years, but can occur after only six weeks of chemotherapy. High-dose carmustine causes pulmonary toxicity in 20–30% of cases. There is an insidious cough, dyspnea, or sudden respiratory failure. Chest X-rays and CT scans show upper-zone fibrosis in many cases. This may be more common if other chemotherapy or radiation therapy was administered, or if there was preexisting pulmonary disease. Glucocorticoid administration has been beneficial, but a small number of patients die. Methotrexate can also cause an acute or chronic process that is related to endothelial injury. Diffuse alveolar damage is indicated by lack of type I pneumocytes, formation of a hyaline membrane, and inflammatory cells found in the alveoli and interstitium. Incidence ranges from 2% to 8%. An acute onset of pulmonary edema produces ARD or more gradual systemic toxicity (with fever or chills). Malaise may precede actual pulmonary symptoms. In a chest X-ray, there is a diffuse interstitial pattern that may be accompanied by peripheral consolidations, pulmonary infiltrates, or chronic eosinophilic pneumonia. Nonspecific symptoms are common, including progressive dry cough and dyspnea that may or may not be accompanied by fever. Pulmonary function tests will reveal restrictive lung disease.

Docetaxel uncommonly causes fluid retention that is related to the cumulative dose. It may become disabling and worse with higher doses. The fluid retention occurs peripherally as abdominal ascites or pleural effusion, or a combination of both. The condition is reversible and may be controlled with diuretics. Docetaxel has caused dyspnea and bronchospasm. All-*trans*-retinoic acid may cause a syndrome of high fever, pulmonary infiltrates, pericardial or pleural effusion, and respiratory distress. This manifests within two days to three weeks after chemotherapy. Corticosteroids usually reverse the condition. Irinotecan (Camptosar) may cause exertion-related dyspnea and pneumonitis with pulmonary infiltrates. These toxicities are not dose-related. Busulfan (Myleran) may cause pulmonary fibrosis in high doses. Lung toxicity usually occurs within three years, but can occur after only six weeks. The drugs called erlotinib (Tarceva) and gefitinib (Iressa) can cause interstitial lung disease.

Gemcitabine causes pulmonary symptoms that range from mild and self-limiting dyspnea to toxicities that can be fatal, appearing to be due to hypersensitivity pneumonitis. Signs and symptoms include significant hypoxemia, tachypnea, and interstitial infiltrates seen on chest X-rays that are consistent with pulmonary edema. The toxicity appears to be reversed by corticosteroids and diuretics. Pemetrexed (Alimta) can cause pneumonitis, with dyspnea and dry cough. The mechanism of action of the lung injury is not understood. Fludarabine can cause interstitial pulmonary toxicity that is well-treated with corticosteroids. There is a non-productive cough, dyspnea, and fever usually beginning two weeks after the last course of the drug. Chlorambucil (Leukeran) may cause interstitial pneumonitis that usually develops later on. The pneumonitis may be acute to chronic, and rarely is a fatal lung fibrosis. Pneumonitis usually occurs weeks to months after chlorambucil is discontinued. There is no clear dose–response relationship.

Pulmonary toxicity must be detected as early as possible since lung damage is usually irreversible and progressive. The causative drug can be discontinued or its dose reduced. High concentrations of inspired oxygen are toxic, so concurrent administration of various chemotherapies may cause lung damage. The patient's oxygen saturation and breath sounds must be monitored closely for early pulmonary toxicity. If oxygen saturation is compromised by restrictive lung damage, there is dyspnea upon exertion or at rest. The patient can be taught breathing techniques such as pursed lip breathing to reduce effects of dyspnea. Supplemental oxygen therapy may help relieve dyspnea. The family and patient are instructed about the use of oxygen and its safety precautions. Corticosteroids usually reduce pulmonary symptoms. Preventive measures include routine vaccinations against influenza and streptococcal pneumonia. If the patient smokes, he or she is strongly advised to stop. Adequate fluid intake, cough techniques, and deep-breathing techniques may also be indicated.

Nephrotoxicity

Nephrotoxicity is a dose-limited adverse effect of chemotherapeutic agents. Direct and indirect effects may cause serious fluid and electrolyte imbalances and even renal failure. Many drugs are metabolized and excreted by the kidneys. Others are excreted unchanged. These include cisplatin, high-dose methotrexate, ifosfamide, mithramycin, mitomycin, and streptozocin. The kidneys may be damaged by chemotherapies via direct renal cell damage to obstructive nephropathy caused by the formation of precipitate. TLS or uric acid nephropathy may cause acid-based disorders, electrolyte abnormalities, and kidney failure. Chronic renal disease may eventually occur because of reversible acute kidney injury. If the renal clearance rate for a chemotherapeutic with linear pharmacokinetics is 35–40%, and there is moderate to severe kidney dysfunction, there can be a large increase in the drug's area under the plasma concentration curve. With preexisting kidney disease or early signs of toxicity, dosages may need to be reduced or stopped entirely. Older patients have a higher risk for

nephrotoxicity. This is because they have decreased total body water and an unknown depressed GFR.

Mild to severe nephrotoxicity may be caused by cisplatin, with damage of the proximal and distal tubules. Platinum metal chelates within the kidney tubules directly damage the proximal tubular cells. This injures the tubular basement membranes, and may lead to focal tubular necrosis. Acute damage may happen in 4–21 hours, proven by renal enzyme changes if precautions are not taken. This renal dysfunction can continue for years after cisplatin therapy, and can be irreversible. The damage involves the degeneration of renal tubular epithelium, a thickened basement membrane, and slight interstitial fibrosis. Prevention of toxicity involves saline hydration of 1–2 liters and diuresis during therapy, based on the dose of cisplatin.

Mannitol (Osmitrol) may assist with diuresis, and can prevent immediate binding of cisplatin to the renal tubules. Cautious use of loop diuretics such as furosemide (Lasix) is advised since there have been increases in cisplatin toxicity. Renal function must be closely monitored. If creatinine clearance is less than 50 mg/mL, the chemotherapy should be stopped until kidney function improves. If serum creatinine is elevated, cisplatin must be stopped. Almost 50% of all patients receiving cisplatin develop hypomagnesemia. Up to 75% have persistent hypomagnesemia. Daily magnesium supplements may be indicated. Electrolyte levels are monitored often. Carboplatin nephrotoxicity is similar but usually milder and less common.

Amifostine, an organic thiophosphate, may reduce cumulative renal toxicity from continual cisplatin-based chemotherapy. Amifostine can protect normal tissues without affecting tumor cell death, because it has higher capillary alkaline phosphatase activity, higher pH, and a better bed of normal vascular tissue. The drug is dephosphorylated at the tissue location by alkaline phosphatase, and free thiol is formed. In the cells, thiol neutralizes reactive cisplatin components before there can be any normal cell DNA or RNA damage. Thiol is a strong scavenger of reed radicals and superoxide anions. This is important since free radicals can damage cell membranes, DNA, and other important components of cells. Amifostine is given over 15 minutes following antiemetics and adequate hydration. Cisplatin is administered 15 minutes after that. The most common adverse effect is transient systolic hypotension, nausea, and vomiting. Therefore, amifostine should be administered with the patient in a supine position, with continuous BP monitoring. If the BP drops below the threshold level from the baseline, the infusion is interrupted. It can be restarted if the BP returns to the threshold in five minutes and the patient has no symptoms. If not, the infusion is discontinued, and the next dose is reduced by about 25%.

Methotrexate in standard doses does not cause renal toxicity unless there is preexisting renal dysfunction. However, high doses cause obstructive nephropathy due to precipitation of the drug or its metabolites in the renal tubules. Risk factors include dehydration, low urine pH, decreased urine output, low methotrexate clearance, intravascular volume depletion, and underlying kidney disease. Risk of nephrotoxicity is increased with exposure to contrast media within one week of cisplatin administration. Generally, urinary alkalization to maintain urine pH higher than 7, with the administration of sodium bicarbonate or acetazolamide (Diamox) will prevent the formation of precipitates, allowing a high-dose therapy to occur. High doses of methotrexate are given with leucovorin to counteract the folic acid antagonists. Delayed methotrexate clearance can cause extreme toxicity. Glucarpidase, a recombinant bacterial enzyme, quickly hydrolyzes methotrexate to an inactive metabolite. This clears the drug during high-dose treatment if hydration and leucovorin fail.

Ifosfamide may cause acute subclinical tubular nephrotoxicity. Though at first reversible, the effect can become chronic with additional treatments. Chloracetaldehyde is a metabolite produced by ifosfamide that damages the kidneys. Mesna is a drug used to counteract this, but is not extremely effective. Ifosfamide nephrotoxicity is signified by amino aciduria, glucosuria,

phosphaturia, bicarbonaturia, and proteinuria. Pemetrexed may cause acute interstitial nephritis, acute tubular necrosis, and nephrogenic diabetes insipidus. It is excreted unchanged by the kidneys. If nephrotoxicity develops with this drug, there is usually acute kidney insufficiency that reverses when the drug is discontinued. Sometimes, chronic renal disease has developed.

Streptozocin in high doses causes renal dysfunction in over 65% of cases. It usually causes tubulointerstitial nephritis and tubular atrophy, from direct tubule damage. Signs include hypokalemia, increased blood urea nitrogen (BUN), proteinuria, and increased creatinine. Renal function tests and creatinine clearance tests are required before using streptozocin. If elevated serum creatinine develops, even with resolution, the patient should not receive additional streptozocin since severe toxicity is likely. Carmustine and lomustine may cause delayed kidney failure, months to years after therapy. Azotemia and proteinuria occur, followed by progressive renal failure that often requires dialysis. Incidence of renal failure may increase significantly with high doses of these drugs. Mitomycin-C has caused renal failure with microangiopathic hemolytic anemia in about 20% of patients receiving high doses. The development usually happens about six months after therapy, with fast onset of the anemia, thrombocytopenia, azotemia, hematuria, and proteinuria. Hemolytic-uremic syndrome is fatal in about 50% of cases.

Preventive management of nephrotoxicity includes aggressive hydration with hypertonic saline, diuresis, careful monitoring of urine output, and urinary alkalinization. Renal function tests – primarily to measure creatinine clearance and serum creatinine – should occur before and after nephrotoxic drugs are administered. If the patient must receive aminoglycosides or contrast dyes, which are also nephrotoxic, there must be close monitoring for early signs of toxicity. Renal function tests continue throughout treatment, and occasionally after therapy is completed. Treatment of nephrotoxicity is mostly supportive. There are no effective therapies to reverse nephrotoxicity.

Clinical Case

1. How is nephrotoxicity caused by chemotherapy?
2. How can chemotherapy damage the kidneys?
3. What is the relationship between high doses of methotrexate and kidney damage?

A 19-year-old man experienced pain and swelling in his right leg after playing soccer. An X-ray revealed a destructive lesion, which was later confirmed to be a non-metastatic osteosarcoma of the tibia. The patient was started on high-dose methotrexate (four cycles), with leucovorin rescue, plus two cycles of cisplatin + doxorubicin. The tumor was soon surgically resected. Chemotherapy was resumed, and two more cycles of cisplatin + doxorubicin were given, as well as one more cycle of methotrexate with leucovorin rescue. Over time, the patient developed acute nephrotoxicity, with significant kidney dysfunction and delayed methotrexate clearance. The patient was given aggressive hydration, diuresis, and IV leucovorin for several days. Eventually, his condition was brought under control, and there was no tumor recurrence.

Answers:

1. **Nephrotoxicity is a dose-limited adverse effect of chemotherapeutic agents. Direct and indirect effects may cause serious fluid and electrolyte imbalances and even renal failure.**
2. **Chemotherapy can damage the kidneys via direct cell damage to obstructive nephropathy caused by the formation of precipitate. TLS or uric acid nephropathy may cause acid-based disorders, electrolyte abnormalities, and kidney failure. Chronic renal disease may eventually occur because of reversible acute kidney injury.**
3. **High doses of methotrexate cause obstructive nephropathy due to precipitation of the drug or its metabolites in the renal tubules. Risk factors include dehydration, low urine pH, decreased urine output, low methotrexate clearance, intravascular volume depletion, and underlying kidney disease.**

Hepatotoxicity

Hepatotoxicity from chemotherapy usually occurs because of an **idiosyncratic reaction**. Incidence is rare, not related to dose, and usually occurs 1–4 weeks after chemotherapy administration, often after multiple treatments. The parenchymal cells of the liver are the first site of damage. If there is obstructed hepatic blood flow, developments include fatty changes, **cholestasis**, hepatocellular necrosis, and hepatitis. Diagnosis of hepatoxicity begins with transient elevations of hepatic enzymes during chemotherapy. This can progress to abdominal pain, hepatomegaly, and jaundice. Liver biopsy is the best method of diagnosis, but is related to high risks and is often not practical. Hepatotoxicity is reversible and not fatal unless there is extensive fibrosis or necrosis. Liver toxicity from high-dose methotrexate is temporary, usually not causing chronic liver disease. Elevation of hepatic enzymes is common. Levels increase with additional courses of chemotherapy and are usually high in patients treated daily rather than intermittently. There may be chronic inflammatory infiltrates in the portal tracts, fibrosis, focal liver cell necrosis, and cirrhosis. The abnormalities resolve in about one month once methotrexate is stopped.

High doses of cytarabine can cause intrahepatic cholestasis, which may be due to hepatocyte transport system injury. The changes can be reversed and do not appear to limit use of cytarabine. Fluorouracil also causes liver damage and an increase in hepatocyte steatosis. In CT studies, liver fat content has increased 30–47% after 5-fluorouracil treatments. Capecitabine has also caused similar hepatic steatosis. When treatments are discontinued, the liver changes resolve. Transient increase in hepatic enzymes is also linked to antitumor antibiotics, gemcitabine, oxaliplatin, topotecan, and trimetrexate.

Fluorodeoxyuridine (Floxuridine) is usually given as a continuous arterial dose, and may cause chemical hepatitis. There are increases in alkaline phosphatase, transaminases, and serum bilirubin. Stricture of the intrahepatic or extrahepatic bile ducts may occur. Toxicity is dependent upon timing and dosing. Liver function usually returns to normal when the drug is discontinued, but if biliary sclerosis occurs, it is irreversible. Hepatic failure has occurred with erlotinib, gefitinib, imatinib (Gleevec), pazopanib (Votrient), and sorafenib (NexAVAR). If liver dysfunction is present, clearance has been reduced of erlotinib, gefitinib, and imatinib. These drugs are metabolized by the liver's P450 system. The tyrosine kinase inhibitors cause liver toxicity, with a slight increase in liver enzymes. In most cases, this toxicity takes 2–8 weeks after starting chemotherapy. Hepatotoxicity is usually reversible with dose reduction or drug discontinuation. The drugs everolimus (Zortress) and temsirolimus (Torisel) are mostly metabolized in the liver, and reduced clearance has occurred if liver dysfunction was present. Irinotecan causes steatohepatitis in 20% of patients, and is more common in obese patients. Oxaliplatin causes increased sinusoidal dilation, which may resolve over time after the drug is discontinued.

Hepatocellular disease is caused by 6-mercaptopurine in high doses, signified by intrahepatic cholestasis and parenchymal cell necrosis. There are slight elevations of alkaline phosphatase, serum bilirubin, and transaminases. Jaundice occurs 30 days after therapy is started. If the patient has concurrent hepatitis B or C infection, there may be a reactivation of these viruses during or following chemotherapy. Once the immune system recovers, viral replication can be enhanced, increasing severity of viral hepatitis. The hepatitis B virus is linked to a higher risk of hepatotoxicity. Chemotherapies linked to hepatitis reactivation include the antitumor antibiotics, alkylating agents, antimetabolites, docetaxel, etoposide, and plant alkaloids. For patients with underlying hepatitis, prior to chemotherapy, prophylactic antivirals may be given, but this is an area lacking definition.

If liver dysfunction is present, many hepatotoxic drugs must be avoided. Reduced liver function slows excretion, and causes increased accumulation of the chemotherapeutic agents in the plasma and tissues. This is especially true for daunorubicin, doxorubicin, docetaxel, paclitaxel, vinblastine, vincristine, and the tyrosine kinase inhibitors. All of these are mostly excreted by the liver into the bile. If serum bilirubin is 1.5–3 mg/dL, these agents should be avoided or reduced in dosage. Doses should be reduced by 50% if the serum glutamic pyruvic transaminase (SGOT) is between 60 and 180 international units. Liver toxicity can be a serious outcome and even lead to permanent cirrhosis. Therefore, during chemotherapy, liver function tests are monitored closely. The shift of fluid from the vascular space to the interstitial space is known as *third spacing*. This can occur because of hepatotoxicity. Signs include decreased BP, increased pulse rate, decreased urine output, low central venous pressure, increased specific gravity, hemoconcentration, and low levels of serum albumin. Therefore, albumin is given to replace the plasma protein and help fluid to be absorbed. Fluid restriction reduces third spacing, enhances renal blood flow, reduces systemic congestion, and improves the comfort of the patient. Additional supportive techniques include decreased protein intake, diuretics, emotional support, and lactulose.

Significant Point

The selection of chemotherapy is first based on the available and effective drugs, and then how to balance possible treatment-related hepatoxicity. Liver function abnormalities are often seen after chemotherapy. Conditions that can worsen the situation include immunosuppression, infections, paraneoplastic conditions, metastases, and polypharmacy. Dose modifications must often rely on clinical evaluation.

Key Terms

Absolute neutrophil count
Adducts
Affinity
Ataxia
Cardiac tamponade
Chemical aquation
Chemoreceptor trigger zone
Chloracetaldehyde
Cholestasis
Clearance
Emetogenic
Emetogenicity
Enterochromaffin cells
Erythroid hypoplasia
Erythropoietin
Esterolysis
Folate antagonists
Gait ataxia
Gynecomastia
Half-life
Hydrolase enzyme
Hypoferremia
Idiosyncratic reaction
Inducibility
Intercalation
Interstrand cross-links
Megakaryocyte

Metabolic encephalopathy
MOPP chemotherapy
Mucositis
Nadir
Nystagmus
Object drug
Oophorectomy
Organ of Corti
Paresthesia
Petechiae
P-gp efflux pump
Pharmacogenomics
Pharmacokinetics
Precipitating drug
Prinzmetal
Proprioception
Protein kinase C
Pulmonary fibrosis
Purine analogs
Pyrimidine analogs
Reticulocytosis
Taxus brevifolia
Tumor lysis syndrome
Unsteady gait
Vinca alkaloids
Volume of distribution
Yew tree needles

Bibliography

1 American Cancer Society (ACS) Journals. (2013). *CA: A cancer journal for clinicians – Chemotherapy-induced peripheral neurotoxicity: A critical analysis*. John Wiley & Sons, Inc. https://acsjournals.onlinelibrary.wiley.com/ doi/10.3322/caac.21204. Volume 63, Issue 6, p. 419–437, Figure 1. Accessed 2021.

2 Aronson, J.K. (2010). *Meyler's Side Effects of Drugs in Cancer and Immunology*. Amsterdam: Elsevier Science.

3 Baron-Esquivias, G. and Asteggiano, R. (2015). *Cardiac Management of Oncology Patients: Clinical Handbook for Cardio-Oncology*. New York: Springer.

4 Bhushan, B. (2021). *Platinum Analogs: Chemotherapy Comprehensive Review Series, Book Two*. Jaipur: Bhushan.

5 Boyiadzis, M.M., Frame, J.N., Kohler, D.R., and Fojo, T. (2014). *Hematology-Oncology Therapy*, 2nd Edition. New York: McGraw-Hill Education/Medical.

6 Chabner, B.A. and Longo, D.L. (2018). *Cancer Chemotherapy, Immunotherapy and Biotherapy: Principles and Practice*, 6th Edition. Philadelphia: Lippincott, Williams, and Wilkins.

7 Chen, J. (2010). *Tumor-Targeting Taxane-Based Anticancer Agents: Designs, Synthesis and*

Biological Evaluation. Riga (Latvia): VDM Verlag / Dr. Muller.

8 Chu, C.K. (2002). *Recent Advances in Nucleosides: Chemistry and Chemotherapy*. Amsterdam: Elsevier Science.

9 Chu, E. and DeVita, V.T., Jr. (2021). *Physicians' Cancer Chemotherapy Drug Manual 2021*, 21st Edition. Burlington: Jones & Bartlett Learning.

10 Denis, L. (2012). *Antiandrogens in Prostate Cancer: A Key to Tailored Endocrine Treatment (European School of Oncology Monographs)*. New York: Springer.

11 Dillion, I., Cavalcanti, L., Cleberson, J., and Soares, S. (2021). *Advances in Cancer Treatment: From Systemic Chemotherapy to Targeted Therapy*. New York: Springer.

12 Elgemeie, G. and Mohamed, R. (2016). *New Anticancer Pyrimidine Nucleoside Analogs*. New Delhi: Lap Lambert Academic Publishing.

13 Emadi, A. and Karp, J.E. (2019). *Cancer Pharmacology: An Illustrated Manual of Anticancer Drugs*. New York: Demos Medical.

14 Fish, J.D., Lipton, J.M., and Lanzkowsky, P. (2021). *Lanzkowsky's Manual of Pediatric Hematology and Oncology*, 7th Edition. Cambridge: Academic Press.

15 Foon, K.A. and Muss, H.B. (2012). *Biological and Hormonal Therapies of Cancer (Treatment and Research, Book 94)*. New York: Springer Science.

16 Galea, A. (2011). *Investigating the Chemotherapeutic Mechanism of Action of Cisplatin: Drug-DNA Interactions in Reconstituted Chromatin and Human Gene Expression Profiling*. New Delhi: Lap Lambert Academic Publishing.

17 Gullatte, M.M., Schwartz, R., Spinks, R., and Kirk Walker, D. (2020). *Clinical Guide to Antineoplastic Therapy: A Chemotherapy Handbook*, 4th Edition. Pittsburgh: Oncology Nursing Society.

18 Hacker, M.P., Lazo, J.S., and Tritton, T.R. (2012). *Organ Directed Toxicities of Anticancer Drugs (Developments in Oncology Book 53)*. Leiden: Martinus Nijhoff Publishing.

19 Ignoffo, R., Viele, C., and Ngo, Z. (2007). *Mosby's Oncology Drug Reference*. Maryland Heights: Mosby.

20 Imre, G. (2008). *Anti-apoptotic and Pro-inflammatory Signaling in Cancer Cells: Status and Modulation by Chemotherapeutic Drugs*. Riga (Latvia): VDM Verlag.

21 Larionov, A. (2015). *Resistance to Aromatase Inhibitors in Breast Cancer (Resistance to Targeted Anti-Cancer Therapeutics, 8)*. New York: Springer.

22 Lednicer, D. (2015). *Antineoplastic Drugs: Organic Syntheses*. Hoboken: Wiley.

23 Lee, M., Arya, D.P., Brown, T., Daneshtalab, M., Gupton, J.T., Holt, H., Jr., Kamalesh Babu, R.P., Love, B.E., Maiti, S.N., and Shan, R. (2006). *Heterocyclic Antitumor Antibiotics (Topics in Heterocyclic Chemistry, 2)*. New York: Springer.

24. Li, R. and Stafford, J.A. (2011). *Kinase Inhibitor Drugs (Series in Drug Discovery and Development, Book 11)*. Hoboken: Wiley.

25 Maximov, P.Y., McDaniel, R.E., and Jordan, V.C. (2013). *Tamoxifen: Pioneering Medicine in Breast Cancer (Milestones in Drug Therapy)*. New York: Springer.

26 Navari, R.M. (2016). *Management of Chemotherapy-Induced Nausea and Vomiting: New Agents and New Uses of Current Agents*. Auckland: Adis.

27 Olsen, M.M., LeFebvre, K.B., and Brassil, K.J. (2018). *Chemotherapy and Immunotherapy Guidelines and Recommendations for Practice*. Pittsburgh: Oncology Nursing Society.

28 Pasha, I., Naik, R., and Banu Ternikar, S. (2017). *Neutropenia and Its Management in Cancer Patients on Chemotherapy*. New Delhi: Lap Lambert Academic Publishing.

29 Polk, A. (2008). *Platinum-Based Chemotherapeutic Drugs*. Boston: Boston University Academy/Lulu Enterprises, Inc.

30 Raffa, R.B., Langford, R., Pergolizzi, J.V., Jr., Porreca, F., and Tallarida, R.J. (2012). *Chemotherapy-Induced Neuropathic Pain*. Boca Raton: CRC Press.

31. Raffa, R.B. and Tallarida, R.J. (2010). *Chemo Fog: Cancer Chemotherapy-Related Cognitive*

Impairment (*Advances in Experimental Medicine and Biology, Volume 678*). New York: Springer.

32 Refaie, M. (2019). *Cancer Chemotherapy and Nephrotoxicity*. New Delhi: Lap Lambert Academic Publishing.

33 Staritz, M., Schmiegel, W., Adler, G., Schmoll, H.J., and Knuth, A. (2003). *Side-effects of Cancer Chemotherapy on the Gastrointestinal Tract: Pathophysiology, Prophylaxis and Therapy (Falk Symposium, 132A)*, 2nd Edition. New York: Springer.

34 Sunil, D., Kamath, P.R., and Raghu Chandrashekhar, R. (2017). *In Vitro Bioassay Techniques for Anticancer Drug Discovery and Development*. Boca Raton: CRC Press.

35 Tolstoouhov, A.V. and Green, D.M. (2013). *Ionic Interpretation of Drug Action in Chemotherapeutic Research*. Whitefish: Literary Licensing, LLC.

36 U.S. Department of Health and Human Services/National Institutes of Health/National Cancer Institute. (2017). *Common Terminology Criteria for Adverse Events (CTCAE), version 5.0*. https://ctep.cancer.gov/protocoldevelopment/ electronic_applications/docs/CTCAE_v5_ Quick_Reference_8.5x11.pdf Accessed 2021.

37 Yuan, D. and Wong, Q. (2018). *Rethinking Platinum Anticancer Drug Design: Towards Targeted and Immunochemotherapeutic Approaches (Theses – Recognizing Outstanding Ph.D. Research)*. New York: Springer.

17

Immunotherapy

Immunology Overview

It is very important to understand immunology as part of the treatment of cancer. The immune system basically consists of *humoral* and *cellular* components. The humoral immune system is antibody-mediated, and based on the actions of B-cells. The cellular immune system is based on the actions of T-cells. For cancer, cell-mediated immunity provides the main immune response that results in tumor regression. The immune response to cancer also involves two types of cellular responses: *innate* and *adaptive* immunity.

Innate Immunity

Innate immunity is nonspecific. The body can distinguish cells and tissues as being "self" or "nonself." Anything considered "self" is normal, but anything considered "nonself" may be a malignancy, an infection, or transplanted tissue. The ability to distinguish between "self" and "nonself" is the first line of defense of the immune system. Innate immunity is not specific to antigens and does not develop **immunological memory** or protect the body when a similar threat occurs again. The physical barriers of innate immunity include the skin and mucous

Global Epidemiology of Cancer: Diagnosis and Treatment, First Edition. Jahangir Moini,
Nicholas G. Avgeropoulos, and Craig Badolato.
© 2022 John Wiley & Sons Ltd. Published 2022 by John Wiley & Sons Ltd.

membranes. The mechanical barriers include blinking of the eyes, coughing, and sneezing. Chemical barriers include the **lysozyme** and phospholipases in saliva, sweat, and tears. This type of immunity induces inflammatory responses that require the production of macrophages, monocytes, polymorphonuclear cells, and large granular lymphocytes such as **natural killer cells** (NK cells). Innate immunity activates the **complement cascade** and causes acute-phase proteins to be produced. An example of an acute-phase protein is *interleukin-2 (IL-2)*.

Adaptive Immunity

Adaptive immunity is the second line of immune defense and is specific. It depends upon antigens and becomes activated when a phagocytized antigen is present to either B- or T-cells. Adaptive immunity utilizes specificity as well as immunological memory. B-cells and T-cells work together. T-cells recognize antigens when they are processed and presented by **antigen-presenting cells** (APCs). T-cells then signal B-cells to produce antibodies that have specificity against that foreign substance. Out of all the cells that combat tumor activities, T-cells are the most important. The three types of adaptive immunity are as follows:

- *Humoral immunity* – B lymphocytes, memory B-cells, and plasma cells mediate this via the production of antibodies that recognize an antigen's challenge. Therefore, **immunoglobulins** are produced.
- *Cell-mediated immunity* – regulated by T-cells and the cytokines they produce. This involves cytotoxic T-cells (TC, which are usually positive for *cluster of differentiation 8 [CD8]*) and helper T-cells (TH$_1$ or TH$_2$, which are usually positive for *CD4*).
- *T regulatory cell immunity* – these T$_{reg}$ cells are also called *suppressor T-cells (TS)*. They show markers CD4, CD25, and *forkhead box P3 (foxp3)*, and limit the activity of other immune effector cells. The main role of T$_{reg}$ cells is thought to be prevention of activation of immunity against normal body tissues, while

limiting the inflammatory response that occurs due to infections. Without T$_{reg}$ cells, many inflammatory disorders can develop – mostly of the intestines, liver, and skin.

> **Significant Point**
>
> Innate immunity consists of neutrophils, dendritic cells, NK cells, macrophages, complement, and physical barriers. Adaptive immunity consists of T-cells, B-cells, and antibodies to protect against viruses, bacteria, and other pathogens. Innate immunity responds more quickly than adaptive immunity, but the adaptive response "understands" exactly how to destroy a pathogen by "remembering" it from a previous encounter.

Cytokines

Cytokines are glycoproteins produced by lymphocytes and macrophages. They are not usually cytotoxic, but mediate effector defense functions. Examples of cytokines include *colony-stimulating factors, interferons (IFNs), interleukins (ILs)*, and *tumor necrosis factor (TNF)*. The activities of cytokines are based on the following two factors:

- Cytokines can act on various types of cells and affect many immune functions; one example is how interleukin-2 (IL-2) affects B-cells, T-cells, macrophages, and NK cells; it induces the activation of lymphocytes and macrophages, while stimulating lymphokine secretion
- Various cytokines may have similar effects; for example, both interleukin-1 (IL-1) and tumor necrosis factor alpha (TNF-α) are inflammatory mediators

Antigen Presentation Cells

The immune pathway is activated by the antigen presentation cells, resulting in a tumor-specific

T-cell response. Also called *APCs*, they engulf antigens that contact them. The cells present antigen fragments on their own surfaces so that T-cells can recognize them. **Naïve T-cells** are only activated by antigens presented to them on **major histocompatibility complex** (MHC) proteins. Types of APCs include dendritic cells, macrophages, and B lymphocytes.

The **dendritic cells** are extremely involved in the initiation of primary T-cell immunity, and are located in areas such as the skin. Dendritic cells have long, thin extensions. After phagocytizing antigens, dendritic cells enter adjacent lymphatics to reach a lymph node so that they can present the antigens to T-cells. Migration of dendritic cells to secondary lymphoid organs ensures that lymphocytes encounter the antigens – presentation of antigens is their only function and prevents large amounts of tissue damage. This is a link between innate and adaptive immunity. Dendritic cells trigger adaptive immune responses focused on the type of pathogen that is found.

The CD4 + helper T-cells and CD8 + cytotoxic T-cells use a T-cell receptor (TCR) to recognize antigens upon the target cell surface. The CD8 + cytotoxic T-cells recognize the antigen along with class I MHC molecules. The CD4 + helper T-cells (TH) recognize the antigen along with class II MHC molecules. All of this usually occurs at the same time. A co-stimulatory signal resulting from interaction between CD28 + molecules on the T-cell surface with ligand B7 on the APCs is required so that complete T-cell activation can occur. Interleukin-2 and IFN gamma (IFN-γ) are secreted from the activated CD4 + cells, helping activated CD8 + cells to mature and then differentiate into cytotoxic T-cells. The cytotoxic T-cells kill target cells that express the antigen that originally caused this response.

Macrophages are present throughout lymphoid organs and connective tissues. Though they can activate naïve T-cells, they often present antigens to T-cells so that they themselves can be activated. Some effector T-cells release chemicals that induce macrophages to become activated. The activated macrophages are actual killers of tumor cells that trigger strong inflammatory responses and attract other defenses. **B lymphocytes** do not activate naïve T-cells, but present antigens to helper T-cells, which aids in B lymphocyte activation.

Tumor Escape Mechanisms

Tumors can escape being detected by the immune system. This may involve variable expression of antigen by the tumor, inadequate antigen processing, loss or presentation of antigen expression, and suppressor T-cell induction. Poor immune recognition of tumors may also involve factors related to disease such as apoptosis of T-cells, defective signaling of T-cells, and immunological aging. This type of aging involves altered T-cell functions, resulting in the reduction of T-cell proliferation, cytotoxic T-cell generation, IL-2 production, lymphocytic signal transduction, and a decline in overall function of B-cells, dendritic cells, and NK cells.

With infections, inflammation triggers the innate immune response. This activates dendritic cells, macrophages, and monocytes. Tumors are different because they do not send out inflammatory "warning" signals known as *danger signals* that stimulate an immune response. Without the danger signals, the immune system may not be completely stimulated. The **genomes** of tumors are unstable, resulting in the development of heterogeneous expression of *tumor-associated antigens (TAAs)*. When tumors acquire more mutations over time, they may continually escape immune recognition. Another therapy is that the mutations of TAAs can let the immune system recognize tumor cells, potentially resulting in their destruction. Often, the immune response is insufficient because of tolerance, since differences between normal self-antigens on healthy cells and TAAs on tumor cells are so small. It may also be possible that the immune recognition process may eventually be selective for tumor variants that are not as easily identifiable.

The immunosuppressive mechanisms produced by tumors inhibit growth factors that normally would stimulate an immune response. Production of interleukins 10 and 18 by tumors can reduce the effectiveness of immune surveillance, including antigen presentation that is mediated by macrophages. Another possible escape mechanism is the expression of the **Fas ligand** by a tumor. This may cause lymphocytes expression Fas receptors to undergo apoptosis, allowing tumors to avoid immune recognition. Also, tumors may be able to inhibit the functions of T-cells via the expression of ligands on the tumor cell surface that bind to T-cell inhibitor co-receptors. One example is *programmed death ligand 1 (PD-L1)*, which is expressed by some tumors. It binds to the *programmed death receptor 1 (PD-1)* on T-cells. When PD-1 finds PD-L1, the interaction may reduce the activation signaling pathway within T-cells. Many tumors express PD-L1 on their cell surfaces. Also, significant expression of PD-L1 by tumors has been linked to poor prognosis in various cancers. These include bladder, ovarian, and pancreatic cancers, as well as renal cell carcinoma.

Significant Point

Regulatory B-cells, also called *bregs* or B_{reg} *cells*, are a small population of B-cells involved in the immunomodulation and suppression of immune responses. They regulate the immune system in various ways, but mostly by producing the anti-inflammatory cytokine called interleukin 10 (IL-10). Cancerous proliferation may utilize regulatory B-cells to "leak out" from the immune system. However, with metastatic cancer, patients with higher numbers of CD20 positive B lymphocytes in the lymph nodes are more likely to survive.

Interleukin-2

Interleukins (ILs) are cytokines synthesized by lymphocytes, monocytes, and macrophages, as a response to the exposure to antigens. They are signaling molecules that allow immune cells to communicate. The ILs work differently from the IFBs and have many effects upon immune function, including:

- Stimulating cytotoxic T-cells to attack tumor cells
- Activating and increasing the production of NK cells
- Increasing the production of B-cells and plasma cells
- Increasing the chemotaxis of neutrophils
- Promoting inflammation

There are over 30 different interleukins, yet only a small amount can be used as medications. Interleukin-2 is produced by activated helper T-cells, and promotes the proliferation of T-cells and activated B-cells. This cytokine was originally thought of as a T-cell growth factor. It has been used in cancer treatment for more than 40 years since their discovery in 1976. Originally, natural IL-2 was derived from stimulated normal lymphocytes in melanoma patients. Widespread use of IL-2 was not possible until *recombinant IL-2 (rIL-2)* became available. The IL-2 gene was discovered to have expressed in *Escherichia coli (E. coli)*. This led to the production of a new molecule that had similar properties to natural IL-2. Next to the interferons, IL-2 has been a primary biological therapy against cancer. Over many phase II trials, IL-2 has shown to cause extreme tumor responses in metastatic melanoma and renal cell carcinoma. This resulted in the Food and Drug Administration's (FDA) approval of IL-2 for the treatment of these cancers.

Biological Activity

Interleukins basically function via communicating with or signaling various lymphocytes. Each interleukin is given a number using the order of its approval by the *International Congress of Immunology*. Interleukins stimulate various immune system components in complicated ways that are still not fully understood. The production of IL-2 is via the activation of T helper cells. Two signals are required. There must be T helper cell recognition of an antigen along with the MHC antigens on an antigen-presenting cell. T helper cells must also interact with co-stimulatory molecules on the antigen-presenting cell. IL-2 is a strong immunomodulator. It is also a chemical messenger that mediates the response of other cytokines. It activates macrophages and lymphocytes while stimulating the secretion of lymphokine. Mostly, IL-2 induces the proliferation of antigen-stimulated T-cells, activates NK cells and cytotoxic T lymphocytes (CTLs) such as CD8 +, and acts as a cofactor for B-cell growth and differentiation. With the stimulation of B-cells, immunoglobulins are produced. Release of other cytokines is induced by IL-2 from activated T-cells. These cytokines include interferon-α, granulocyte-macrophage colony-stimulating factor (GM-CSF), and TNF.

Indications of Interleukin-2

High-dose intravenous interleukin-2 was approved by the FDA in 1992 for metastatic renal cell carcinoma. It was approved in 1998 for metastatic melanoma. Other dosages and routes of administration have been studied for various cancers, with various degrees of effectiveness. A variety of IL-2 regimens are prescribed so that toxicities can be limited, since some toxicities are severe. Since IL-2 stimulates the patient's cytotoxic immunological response, it is an excellent cytokine to test for other cancers or immune disorders.

Significant Point

Interleukins are not stored inside cells, but are secreted quickly in response to a stimulus, with short-lived effects. Interleukins travel to target cells and bind via receptor molecules on the cells' surfaces. This triggers a cascade of signals in the target cells, altering their behavior. The administration of interleukin-2 (IL-2), for example, affects tumor cells significantly, and can result in long-term regressions as well as cures.

Clinical Case

1. How important is interleukin-2 in cancer therapy?
2. How is interleukin-2 produced?
3. Why is interleukin-2 used to test for other cancers or immune disorders?

A 57-year-old man was evaluated by his physician because of right flank pain and hematuria. An abdominal ultrasound revealed a mass on his right kidney, and the patient was referred to a urologist, who ordered blood tests and CT scans of the patient's chest and abdomen. The disease was found to only affect the right kidney, which was surgically resected. The tumor was found to be a renal cell carcinoma. The patient was started on therapy with IL-2 so that the likelihood of any further cancer would be reduced. Over 18 months of follow-up, the patient remained cancer free.

Answers:

1. **Interleukin-2 has been used in cancer treatment for more than 40 years. Widespread use was not possible until recombinant IL-2 (rIL-2) became available. Next to the interferons, IL-2 has been a primary biological therapy against cancer. It causes extreme tumor responses in metastatic melanoma and renal cell carcinoma.**
2. **The production of IL-2 is via activation of T helper cells. Two signals are required. There must be T helper cell recognition of an antigen along with the MHC antigens on an antigen-presenting cell. T helper cells must also interact with co-stimulatory molecules on the antigen-presenting cell.**
3. **Since interleukin-2 stimulates the cytological immunological response, it is an excellent cytokine to test for other cancers or immune disorders.**

Interferons

Interferons were the first cytokines to be discovered. They occur naturally, and have antiviral effects. They were named because they interfere with the replication of viruses. There are three interferons (IFNs) with clinical indications: alpha (α), beta (ß), and gamma (γ). In humans, the two other IFNs known as tau (τ) and omega (ω) are not approved for therapeutic use. Interferon-α was first derived from human blood in the 1970s. Initially, impurity with the prepared substance was a problem, but it was still usable as an anticancer treatment. Like IL-2, interferons could not be produced in enough quantity until recombinant DNA technology became available. Interferon-α (Intron A) is the only type of interferon used to treat cancer.

Interferons are produced by body cells in reaction to tumor cells, viruses, bacteria, or parasites. They bind to cell surface receptors, activating downstream signal transduction pathways. Signaling reaches the cell nuclei, and the activities of genes regulating cellular activities such as apoptosis are regulated. Interaction occurs between interferons, hormones, and growth-factor signaling pathways, blocking RNA development. Endogenous interferons regulate **angiogenesis**. They inhibit endothelial cell migration and the production of basic fibroblast growth factor and interleukin-8, both of which promote tumor angiogenesis.

Clinical trials have occurred to study IFN-α on its own and along with other drugs to treat melanoma, chronic myeloid leukemia (CML), follicular non-Hodgkin lymphoma, Kaposi sarcoma, hepatocellular carcinoma, superficial bladder cancer, and renal cell carcinoma. High-dose IFN-α2b was approved in the 1990s for adjuvant treatment of stage II or III melanoma if there is a high risk of recurrence. Lower doses of interferon have not improved survival rates. There are significant toxicities and costs related to the use of interferons. Toxicities result in influenza-like symptoms, fatigue, mood disorders, depression, suicidal thoughts, cognitive changes, behavioral changes, sleep disturbances, anorexia, weight loss, psoriasis, urticaria, rash, photosensitivity, alopecia, pruritus, skin dryness and erythema, worsening of herpes labialis, cutaneous vascular lesions, dry mouth, **sarcoidosis**, granuloma annulare, injection site reactions, taste alterations, and sexual dysfunction.

IFN-α, when used alone, has an approximate 15% response rate when used to treat renal cell carcinoma. The response is only of short duration. The interferon may be beneficial after nephrectomy if the patient has minimal symptoms and metastases at the time of diagnosis. Intravesical IFN-α has been studied for superficial bladder cancer, but is not as effective as bacillus Calmette-Guérin (BCG). In high doses, it is beneficial as a second-line treatment if the patient does not respond to previous intravesical chemotherapy or BCG. It may also be used along with BCG.

Pegylated IFN-α (Pegasys) is made when polyethylene glycol is added to the interferon. This allows for a slower release into the cells and extends the half-life of the interferon. Other benefits include less frequent administration, better drug solubility, and reduced toxicity. Pegylated IFN-α2b has been approved as adjuvant therapy for high-risk melanoma, and also investigated for CML and renal cell carcinoma. Fatigue is common (96% of patients), so doses are limited for treatment of solid tumors. Additional studies are ongoing. Interferon-induced fatigue can greatly affect the quality of life, and may be the result of CNS toxicity or frontal lobe neurotoxicity. Influenza-like symptoms include chills, fevers, headaches, malaise, and myalgias. Myalgias involve generalized muscle aches and weakness that do not improve with rest.

Significant Point

In 1995, interferon became the first adjuvant therapy approved by the FDA to treat patients that previously had surgery to remove advanced melanomas. Interferon can stop the growth as well as the spread of any melanoma cells that may not have been removed. It can also delay the recurrence of melanoma.

Bacillus Calmette-Guérin

Bacillus Calmette-Guérin (BCG) is an attenuated strain of the *Mycobacterium* virus. It was first developed to treat tuberculosis but was found that it had antineoplastic capabilities. While its actual antitumor mechanism is unknown, BCG activates B lymphocytes, T lymphocytes, macrophages, and NK cells. Intravesical BCG has been approved as an instillation to treat carcinoma in situ of the bladder. For an optimal response, the tumor must be localized, there must be a minimal tumor burden, and the BCG must directly contact the tumor cells. The agent enters bladder epithelial cells by using a fibronectin attachment protein, resulting in a mucosal infection that can last for a few months. Interleukins 1, 2, 6, and 12, as well as interferon-γ and TNF-α are stimulated. A T-cell-mediated immune response occurs, and the tumor cells are attacked. Continual contact with the bladder and the immune stimulation allows for a longer duration of action than with chemotherapy agents. Chemotherapeutic drugs are eliminated from the body when the patient urinates. The BCG penetrates deeply into the bladder wall and can be found in the pelvic lymph nodes after its instillation.

However, BCG cannot be used for immunocompromised patients, those with liver disease, or if there is a history of tuberculosis. The therapy is also contraindicated if there is acute febrile illness, active tuberculosis, hypersensitivity to the agent, urinary tract infection, hematuria, and for 7–14 days after biopsy, transurethral resection, or traumatic catheterization (because there is a higher risk for a systemic BCG infection). Instillation of BCG usually occurs two weeks after a bladder tumor is resected via the transurethral route, or seven days after traumatic catheterization has occurred. Adverse effects include lower urinary tract symptoms (in 90% of patients), as well as painful and frequent urination, and influenza-like symptoms. Lower urinary tract symptoms include dysuria and hematuria. Doses of BCG can be reduced if needed.

> **Significant Point**
>
> Topical biotherapy with the drug called *imiquimod* is indicated for superficial basal cell carcinoma. It has also been studied for lentigo melanoma and squamous cell carcinoma. Another agent called *ipilimumab* has been approved to treat surgically unresectable or metastatic melanoma.

Cancer Vaccines

Cancer vaccines are different from traditional vaccines. With a common vaccine, an immune-stimulating agent is administered, which causes an immune reaction against the foreign antigens contained in the vaccine. An initial immune response is stimulated, and later exposures to the antigen cause the immune system to destroy it. Examples include polio and smallpox vaccines. However, cancer vaccines are not generally preventative – instead, they are therapeutic. They can prevent viruses such as the human papillomavirus, which has known links to cervical cancer, and the hepatitis virus, since hepatitis infection is linked to liver cancer.

Cancer vaccines ready the immune system so that it can attack existing cancer cells. They do this by causing an immune response against TAAs. The TAAs are present on tumor cells but are either absent or only slightly present on normal cells. The TAAs can be enzymes, carbohydrates, or proteins. They create a target for the recognition and destruction of tumor cells, and are summarized as follows.

- *Cancer testis antigen* – expressed in the testis but not in other normal tissues; melanoma-associated antigens (MAGEs) are expressed in the placenta, and are not perceived as "foreign"; neoplasia includes melanoma and cancers of the bladder, breast, lung, and stomach
- *Overexpressed antigens* – shared by normal tissues, yet overexpressed or changed on tumor cells; the mutations cause altered protein sequences in tumor cells, and the immune

system recognizes them; neoplasia includes breast, colorectal, lung, ovarian, and pancreatic cancers

- *Tissue-specific antigen and differentiation antigens* – found on the tumor's tissue of origin, such as the melanocytes of the eyes; neoplasia includes colon, breast, liver, pancreatic, and prostate cancers as well as melanoma
- *Tumor-specific antigen* – unique for individual tumors, they are normal proteins that contain mutations or gene fusions, causing unique proteins to be generated; neoplasia includes B-cell non-Hodgkin lymphoma, CML, myeloma, T-cell non-Hodgkin lymphoma, and cancers of the bladder, colon, lung, head, neck, and rectum
- *Viral antigens* – strongly related in some cases of cancer; viral antigens expressed on tumor cells can be specific immune system targets; they may be prophylactic cancer vaccines in the future; neoplasia includes Burkitt's lymphoma, and cervical or hepatocellular cancers

Melanoma is a highly immunogenic tumor and has been the prototype for many other tumor vaccines. The high immunogenicity had led to malignant melanoma being an initial target for the development of a cancer vaccine. MAGEs are often expressed on normal melanocytes. They include *glycoprotein 100, MAGE recognized by T-cells 1*, and *tyrosinase*. The MAGEs are also expressed in the testis and placenta, not being perceived as foreign.

Cancer vaccines are developed to cause an immune response that leads to the recognition and destruction of tumor cells. When the immune system recognizes a TAA as foreign, the specific T-cells for that TAA proliferate. They circulate, locate the tumor that expresses that TAA, and work together to destroy it. Major obstacles in cancer vaccine development include finding antigens that can be targeted safely, and the generation of a strong immune response against TAAs to which the immune system is already tolerant because of previous exposure.

Major Histocompatibility Complex

For cancer vaccines to be effective, T-cells must be stimulated to distinguish "self" from "nonself." They can only do this if the antigens are presented in association with MHC molecules. These are also called *human leukocyte antigens (HLAs)*. They are unique to each individual and are found on most body cells. On the surface of a T-cell, the TCR specifically interacts with a peptide. For example, there is a TAA/MHC complex on tumor cell surfaces. If the desired TAA is not presented for recognition as a peptide/MHC complex, the needed immune response does not occur. This is called *MHC restriction*.

There are three classes of human MHC molecules. Only classes I and II are active in antigen presentation. The MHC class I molecules are on almost all nucleated cells, as well as platelets. They restrict the presentation of antigens to cytotoxic T-cells through interactions with CD8 molecules. The MHC class II molecules are located on certain APCs, such as B-cells, dendritic cells, macrophages, and monocytes. They restrict the presentation of antigens to T helper cells, through interactions with the CD4 molecule.

Clinical Case

1. Why are cancer vaccines generally therapeutic instead of preventative?
2. How do cancer vaccines ready the immune system to attack existing cancer cells?
3. When a cancer vaccine causes an immune response, what occurs next?

A 62-year-old woman was hospitalized because of bloody diarrhea, left lower abdominal cramping, and pain. A CT scan revealed masses in her colon and liver, and the diagnosis was of stage IV colorectal cancer that had metastasized to the liver. A new clinical trial was occurring, so the oncology team decided to use immunotherapy in combination with chemotherapy prior to surgery. The investigational CV301 vaccine was combined with nivolumab (a monoclonal antibody chemotherapeutic agent). When CV301 is combined with nivolumab, the effect is that the chemotherapy becomes more targeted to two protein markers of colorectal cancer. Four months later, the patient had surgery to remove the colon and liver tumors. However, when the areas surrounding the location of the tumors were removed, there was no evidence of any remaining tumor tissue. The patient has had no recurrence over two years of follow-up.

Answers:

1. **Cancer vaccines are generally therapeutic because they can prevent viruses such as the human papillomavirus (which has known links to cervical cancer) and the hepatitis virus (since hepatitis infection is linked to liver cancer).**

2. **Cancer vaccines ready the immune system to attack existing cancer cells by causing an immune response against TAAs. These TAAs are present on tumor cells, but are either absent or only slightly present on normal cells. They can be enzymes, carbohydrates, or proteins.**

3. **When a cancer vaccine causes an immune response, it leads to the recognition and destruction of tumor cells. When the immune system recognizes a TAA as being foreign, the specific T-cells for that TAA proliferate. They circulate, locate the tumor that expresses that TAA, and work together to destroy it.**

Immunoadjuvants

Immunoadjuvants are co-stimulatory molecules that include chemokines and cytokines. When immunoadjuvants are added to cancer vaccines, pro-inflammatory cytokines can be generated. Tumor cells do not produce the pro-inflammatory chemokines or cytokines needed to develop a strong immune response. Chemokines are a type of cytokines that act as chemoattractants, and are produced by local tissues – usually when a pathogen is present. They act upon leukocytes, causing immune cell activation. Cytokines are needed to mediate T-cell activation and proliferation.

Immunoadjuvants affect the immune responses to a cancer vaccine. They recruit APCs, begin nonspecific immune responses, activate the reticuloendothelial system, and recruit innate immune responses. When T-cells interact with tumor cells, there is an increased chance that the cancer vaccine will destroy tumor cells. Responses to immunoadjuvants are not specific to chemokines and cytokines. The immune effect is strengthened by the stimulation of macrophages, T-cells, and NK cells. Immunoadjuvants in clinical trials are of various types, as follows:

- *Bacterial origin* – such as BCG
- *Cytokines* – such as IL-12 (activating T-cells and NK cells)
- *Growth factors* – such as GM-CSF
- *Gel-like materials* – such as aluminum hydroxide (enhancing the humoral response)

Human Papillomavirus

The human papillomavirus (HPV) infection is sexually transmitted. It is related to genital warts and cancers of the cervix, vulva, vagina, penis, and anus. Though infection is widespread, HPV is usually undetected, yet there may be 25 times more HPV infections in the United States alone than human immunodeficiency virus (HIV) infections. The FDA-approved Gardasil is a quadrivalent vaccine against HPV types 6, 11, 16, and 18 – the types most often linked with cervical cancer. It is approved for preventing cervical pre-cancer and cancer, as well as genital warts, in females between 9 and 26 years of age. A second approved drug called Cervarix, is a bivalent vaccine against HPV types 16 and 18.

About 70% of cervical cancers are related to HPV 16 and 18. Genital warts are highly related to HPV 6 and 11.

Gardasil and Cervarix were created from extremely purified virus-like particles of HPV. The particles cause a humoral immune response, followed by high titers of neutralizing antibodies. Gardasil is administered in three doses, at zero, two, and six months. Cervarix also requires three doses, but at months 0, 1, and 6. In clinical studies, booster doses given later have been shown to increase antibody titers, and have an acceptable safety profile. The vaccines are indicated to be initially given before puberty since they do not cause regression of an established HPV infection. They are given IM in the deltoid or gluteus muscles. The vaccines must be well agitated prior to administration.

Significant Point

The vaccine that helps prevent HPV infection is safe and effective, and the American Cancer Society recommends the vaccine to reduce cervical cancer. Studies have shown that the vaccine provides nearly 100% protection against infections and pre-cancers caused by HPV. It works best when given between ages 9 and 12. Both girls and boys should receive it. The vaccine contains no harmful ingredients, lasts for a long time, and can also protect fertility.

Prostate Cancer

In 2010, the FDA approved a therapeutic autologous cellular vaccine against prostate cancer called sipuleucel-T (Provenge). It is indicated for the treatment of asymptomatic or slightly symptomatic metastatic hormone-refractory prostate cancer. It contains autologous peripheral-blood mononuclear cells (PBMCs). These cells are activated ex vivo with a recombinant fusion protein called PA2024. This is made of a prostate antigen (prostatic acid phosphatase or PAP), fused to GM-CSF, which activates the immune system. Every dose contains PBMCs obtained by using leukapheresis, and contains at least 50 million CD54 + cells activated with PAP-GM-CSF. The cells are suspended in lactated Ringers injection solution, and every infusion bag is specific to the individual patient.

Sipuleucel-T is administered in three doses, once every two weeks. The patient receives pre-medication with acetaminophen and diphenhydramine (or another antihistamine). The patient's identity must be verified with the identifiers printed on the medication bag. The drug is given IV, as an infusion, with no cell filter, and takes 60 minutes to be infused. Infusion can be slowed or stopped if a severe, acute infusion reaction occurs. Adverse effects are temporary, usually within one day, and disappear in two days. They usually include chills, fever, fatigue, back pain, arthralgia, headache, and nausea.

Significant Point

The sipuleucel-T prostate cancer vaccine boosts the immune system to help it attack tumor cells. It is best used for advanced prostate cancer that has stopped responding to hormonal therapy. The vaccine is developed individually for each patient by removing some of the patient's white blood cells and mixing them with prostatic acid phosphatase. The mixture is reinfused into the patient, and increases survival time by at least a few months. While not yet completely curative, its effects appear to be promising.

Clinical Studies of New Vaccines

New cancer vaccines are continually being tested in clinical studies. A vaccine currently called *PGV-001* is under study for patients with solid tumors or multiple myeloma, with a high risk of recurrence following surgery or stem cell transplant. The vaccine effectively cured the cancers in 60% of test patients. The PGV-001 vaccine is a personalized treatment, formulated for each individual patient. It consists of customized peptides that target neoantigens identified from patient tumor samples. The vaccine is designed as part of a new protocol called the **personalized genomic vaccine** (PGV) pipeline. The tested patients had a variety of different malignancies that included head, neck, lung, breast, and bladder cancers, as well as multiple myeloma. The vaccine was broken up into 10 separate doses. It is well tolerated by patients, with about 50% experiencing only mild injection site reactions or low-grade fevers. The vaccine is most effective for lung, breast, and bladder cancers as well as multiple myeloma.

Immune stimulants are another new option, and are also referred to as *immunostimulants*. They are injected directly into tumors. They "teach" the immune system to recognize and destroy similar cancer cells throughout the body. Focusing on lymphomas, two different immune stimulants are being injected into a single tumor. What follows is very amazing – all other tumors that may be present shrink and disappear. The immune stimulants have caused more than 70% of patients to experience partial or complete tumor destruction after the first injections. The vaccines stopped overall cancer progression in almost 55% of test patients for 3–18 months. As a result of this lymphoma trial, the study is being expanded to include breast, head, and neck cancer patients. The immune stimulants focus on the dendritic cells, which guide the responses of T cells to fight off tumor cells. Examples of immune stimulants include elapegademase (Revcovi), glatiramer (Copaxone), pegademase bovine (Adagen), plerixafor (Mozobil), and trilaciclib (Cosela).

Duke University established another way to destroy brain tumor cells by directly injecting a modified form of the poliovirus. It quickly killed tumor cells of primary malignancies as well as cells derived from breast and colon cancer metastases within 4–6 hours. Polio destroys infected host cells quickly, so the researchers used this ability therapeutically. The ability of polio to kill normal brain cells was stopped by changing out a critical genetic element from the *rhinovirus* that causes the common cold with the corresponding genetic element of the polio virus. This genetic element is called an *internal ribosomal entry site (IRES)*. It allows a virus to express its genetic information inside an invaded host cell. The rhinovirus was selected since it usually does not infect the brain. Within brain tumor cells, the rhinovirus IRES activates gene expression, but the genes being expressed come only from the poliovirus. The polio proteins kill the tumor cells quickly, in large numbers. Polio has a natural affinity for invading the brain by binding to a receptor called *CD155* on the surface of motor neurons. Brain tumors overproduce this receptor, so their cells are highly vulnerable to the poliovirus. Though this virus can still enter normal motor neurons, it can no longer grow in normal cells. The poliovirus does not carry the toxic side effects of chemotherapy or radiation. Infusing the poliovirus directly into brain tumors is the most effective method of killing the cells.

In 2021, the technology that was used in designing the Pfizer vaccine against COVID-19 (coronavirus) began to be tested for the development of new cancer vaccines. Both the coronavirus and cancer vaccines use messenger RNA (mRNA) to carry instructions for making proteins that combat these diseases. It is anticipated that the new cancer vaccines will be available within a few years. They will work by targeting tumor antigens that are recognized by T-cells, which are unique in every cancer patient. The vaccines are based on analyses of a patient's tumor and determining which antigens would be suitable, then producing each vaccine based on this information. New technology could allow each vaccine to be manufactured within only a few weeks – potentially saving the lives of many patients. Since mRNA is expressed in the dendritic cells, the researchers quickly determined that mRNA is a prime target in cancer vaccine therapy.

Key Terms

Adaptive immunity
Angiogenesis
Antigen-presenting cells
B lymphocytes
Burkitt's lymphoma
Complement cascade
Cytokines
Dendritic cells
Fas ligand
Genomes
Immune stimulants
Immunoadjuvants

Immunoglobulins
Immunological memory
Interleukins
Innate immunity
Interferons
Lysozyme
Macrophages
Major histocompatibility complex
Naïve T-cells
Natural killer cells
Personalized genomic vaccine
Sarcoidosis

Bibliography

1 Abbas, A.K., Lichtman, A.H., and Pillai, S. (2017). *Cellular and Molecular Immunology*, 9th Edition. Amsterdam: Elsevier.

2 AP News. (2021). *Scientist behind coronavirus shot says next target is cancer.* The Associated Press. https://apnews.com/article/covid-vaccine-scientist-fight-cancerd6fd143e9fd9b4bd50d0c1cb697b6dab Accessed 2021.

3 Bonavida, B. and Jewett, A. (2021). *Successes and Challenges of NK Immunotherapy: Breaking Tolerance to Cancer Resistance.* Cambridge: Academic Press.

4 Bot, A., Obrocea, M., and Marincola, F. (2015). *Cancer Vaccines: From Research to Clinical Practice.* London: Informa Healthcare.

5 Butterfield, L.H., Kaufman, H.L., and Marincola, F.W. (2017). *Cancer Immunotherapy Principles and Practice.* New York: Demos Medical.

6 Chabner, B.A. and Longo, D.L. (2018). *Cancer Chemotherapy, Immunotherapy and Biotherapy – Principles and Practice*, 6th Edition. Philadelphia: Lippincott, Williams, and Wilkins.

7 Delves, P.J., Martin, S.J., Burton, D.R., and Roitt, I.M. (2021). *Roitt's Essential Immunology (Essentials)*, 12th Edition. Hoboken: Wiley-Blackwell.

8 Doan, T., Lievano, F., Swanson-Mungerson, M., and Viselli, S.M. (2021). *Immunology*, 3rd Edition. *(Illustrated Reviews).* Philadelphia: Lippincott, Williams, and Wilkins.

9 Dong, H. and Markovic, S.N. (2018). *The Basics of Cancer Immunotherapy.* New York: Springer.

10 Drugs.com. (2021). *Other immunostimulants – What are other immunostimulants?* Drugs.com. https://www.drugs.com/drug-class/other-immunostimulants.html Accessed 2021.

11 DukeHealth – News & Media. (2016). *Researchers use crippled poliovirus to attack brain cancer.* Duke University Health System. https://corporate.dukehealth.org/news/researchers-use-crippled-poliovirus-attack-brain-cancer Accessed 2021.

12 Dumke, N.M. (2007). *The Low Dose Immunotherapy Handbook: Recipes and Lifestyle Advice for Patients on LDA and EPD Treatment.* Louisville: Allergy Adapt, Inc.

13 Ernstoff, M.S., Puzanov, I., Robert, C., Diab, A., and Hersey, P. (2019). *SITC's Guide to Managing Immunotherapy Toxicity.* New York: Demos Medical.

14 Faustman, D.L. (2014). *The Value of BCG and TNF in Autoimmunity*. Cambridge: Academic Press.

15 Graeber, C. (2018). *The Breakthrough: Immunotherapy and the Race to Cure Cancer*. New York: Hachette.

16 Greiner, J. (2020). *Immunotherapies for Acute Myeloid Leukemia (Journal of Clinical Medicine)*. Basel: MDPI Ag.

17 Horizon – The European Union Research & Innovation Magazine. (2021). *Q&A: BioNTech vaccine is only 'mRNA 1.0'. This is just the beginning, say co-founders*. European Commission. https://horizon-magazine.eu/content/about-horizon.html Accessed 2021.

18 Karp, D.D., Falchook, G.S., and Lim, J. (2018). *Handbook of Targeted Cancer Therapy and Immunotherapy*, 2nd Edition. Philadelphia: Lippincott, Williams, and Wilkins.

19 Katz, S.G. and Rabinovich, P.M. (2020). *Cell Reprogramming for Immunotherapy: Methods and Protocols (Methods in Molecular Biology, 2097)*. Totowa: Humana Press.

20 Lasek, W. and Zagozdzon, R. (2016). *Interleukin 12: Antitumor Activity and Immunotherapeutic Potential in Oncology (Briefs in Immunology)*. New York: Springer.

21 Lawman, M.J.P. and Lawman, P.D. (2014). *Cancer Vaccines: Methods and Protocols (Methods in Molecular Biology, 1139)*. Totowa: Humana Press.

22 Male, D., Peebles, R.S., Jr., and Male, V. (2021). *Immunology*, 9th Edition. Amsterdam: Elsevier.

23. Naing, A. and Hajjar, J. (2020). *Immunotherapy (Advances in Experimental Medicine and Biology, 1244)*, 3rd Edition. New York: Springer.

24 Nair, S.S. and Tewari, A. (2020). *Cancer Immunotherapy in Urology (Clinics Review Articles – Urologic Clinics – 47*. Amsterdam: Elsevier.

25 National Library of Medicine – National Center for Biotechnology Information. (2018). *Computational pipeline for the PGV-001 neoantigen vaccine trial*. National Library of Medicine. https://pubmed.ncbi.nlm.nih.gov/29403468 Accessed 2021.

26 Olsen, M.M. (2018). *Chemotherapy and Immunotherapy Guidelines and Recommendations for Practice*. Pittsburgh: Oncology Nursing Society.

27 Rezaei, N. (2020). *Cancer Immunology: Cancer Immunotherapy for Organ-Specific Tumors*, 2nd Edition. New York: Springer.

28 Rezaei, N. and Keshavarz-Fathi, M. (2018). *Vaccines for Cancer Immunotherapy: An Evidence-Based Review on Current Status and Future Perspectives*. Cambridge: Academic Press.

29 Rich, R.R., Fleisher, T.A., Shearer, W.T., Schroeder, H.W., Jr., Frew, A.J., and Weyand, C.M. (2021). *Clinical Immunology: Principles and Practice*, 5th Edition. Amsterdam: Elsevier.

30 Savalyeva, N. and Ottensmeier, C. (2017). *Cancer Vaccines (Current Topics in Microbiology and Immunology)*. New York: Springer.

31 Singh, M. and Salnikova, M. (2014). *Novel Approaches and Strategies for Biologics, Vaccines and Cancer Therapies*. Cambridge: Academic Press.

32 Sofer, W. (2020). *Cancer Immunotherapy: Basic Biology*. Wichita: Sofer.

33 Thomas, J.H. and Roberts, A. (2012). *Interferons: Characterization, Mechanism of Action and Clinical Applications (Protein Biochemistry, Synthesis, Structure and Cellular Functions: Immunology and Immune System Disorders)*. Waltham: Nova Biomedical.

34 Thurin, M., Cesano, A., and Marincola, F.M. (2020). *Biomarkers for Immunotherapy of Cancer: Methods and Protocols (Methods in Molecular Biology, 2055)*. Totowa: Humana Press.

35 WebMD Cancer Center. (2021). *Cancer vaccine shows early promise across tumor types*. WebMD LLC. https://www.webmd.com/cancer/multiple-myeloma/news/20210416/cancer-vaccine-shows-early-promise-across-tumor-types Accessed 2021.

36 WebMD Cancer Center. (2019). *New 'Cancer Vaccine' attacks tumors from within.* WebMD LLC. https://www.webmd.com/cancer/news/20190409/new-cancer-vaccine-attacks-tumors-from-within Accessed 2021.

37 Williams, J.R. (2019). *The Immunotherapy Revolution: The Best New Hope for Saving Cancer Patients' Lives.* Fort Lauderdale: Williams.

38 Zitvogel, L. and Kroemer, G. (2017). *Oncoimmunology: A Practical Guide for Cancer Immunotherapy.* New York: Springer.

18

Gene Therapy

Gene Therapy Regulation

Thousands of gene therapy clinical trials have occurred throughout the world, and they are continuing. The guidelines for gene therapy protocols were created by the National Institutes of Health (NIH), as part of their publication entitled *Points to Consider in the Design and Submission of Human Somatic Cell Gene Therapy Protocols*. This is periodically updated as an appendix to the NIH guidelines on recombinant DNA research. As a result, proposals for human gene therapy must be reviewed at a variety of levels. Each new protocol must be reviewed initially by local biosafety and bioethics boards, and must follow the standards of conventional research. The protocol is next reviewed by the Human Gene Therapy Research Subcommittee and the Recombinant DNA Advisory Committee (RAC). These committees advise the director of the NIH, who approves every gene transfer and gene therapy proposal. Since the Food and Drug Administration (FDA) addresses the scientific methodology that is used as well as preclinical safety testing, it created guidelines for starting gene therapy. These guidelines are distinct from those of the previously discussed groups. They focus on the biological substances used for gene

Global Epidemiology of Cancer: Diagnosis and Treatment, First Edition. Jahangir Moini,
Nicholas G. Avgeropoulos, and Craig Badolato.
© 2022 John Wiley & Sons Ltd. Published 2022 by John Wiley & Sons Ltd.

transfer, and their characteristics, production, and certification. In the United States, most gene therapy clinical trials have focused on cancer indications.

Cancer Gene Therapy

The use of gene therapy to treat cancer focuses on the inhibition of oncogene function and the restoration of tumor-suppressor function. The normal cellular genes essential for cell growth and development are called **proto-oncogenes**. They activate **oncogenes** by encoding a growth factor or another protein, disturbing normal cell development as well as regulation. Oncogenes stimulate neoplastic growth. **Anti-oncogenes** block the action of growth-inducing proteins, and are also called *tumor-suppressor genes*. This reveals their ability to block actions of oncogenes. During normal functions, tumor-suppressor genes work with proto-oncogenes to allow the body to conduct vital functions. This includes the replacement of dead cells and the repair of defective cells.

Gene marking is the labeling of cells for identification in the future. A genetically marked gene is introduced into cells. This is usually done by using a retrovirus as a vector. It is used to determine the reasons for relapse in people having autologous bone marrow transplantation procedures. Gene-marking studies have been used to treat leukemia, melanoma, neuroblastoma, and the effects of stem-cell transplantation. **Gene therapy** studies involve modifying expression or content of altered genes within somatic ells. This is done by transferring the enhanced or function genes. Both gene marking and gene therapy are used in clinical trials investigating gene therapy for cancer.

Cancer Gene Therapy Protocols

Many protocols investigate gene transfer to correct an error, known as **gene alteration**, or to add a new function, known as **gene addition**. The following two general approaches are used:

- *The tumor-directed approach* – the therapeutic gene is brought into tumor cells, destroying them
- *The immunotherapy approach* – involves active and adoptive immunotherapy. In *active immunotherapy*, there is the introduction of cytokines, tumor-associated antigens, or tumor antigens. These stimulate the immune system, and an antitumor response occurs. In *adoptive immunotherapy*, there is a transfer of a genetically modified tumor lymphocyte. This mediates regression of the tumor.

These studies are based on previous gene-marking studies that revealed that a new gene was able to be safely inserted into patients and then monitored.

Tumor-Directed Gene Therapy Protocols

Tumor-directed gene therapy protocols include those that utilize "suicide genes," tumor-suppressor gene therapy, antisense oligonucleotides, and oncolytic viral gene therapy.

Suicide Gene Therapy

A **suicide gene** is the toxic form of a nontoxic prodrug. It is converted from nontoxic to toxic by an enzyme. This enzyme is produced by the transfer of a specific gene during a *suicide gene therapy protocol*. The gene transfer is targeted to tumor cells. The gene makes the cells susceptible to a substance that does not harm the normal cells, yet kills the malignant cells. The suicide is only toxic to cells that are dividing. Therefore, it does not harm the normal cells or any nondividing tumor cells. The gene that is usually used is the *herpes simplex virus thymidine kinase gene (HSV-TK)*. A cell that incorporates this gene then becomes sensitive to the antiviral drug called *ganciclovir (GCV)*. When exposed to this drug, the sensitive cell dies. Genes are transferred to actively dividing cells by retroviral vectors. This means that this gene therapy is indicated for treating brain tumors, since in the brain, only the malignant cells divide and replicate. The ganciclovir easily kills brain tumor cells. Additional changes of the promoter region of the vector results in organ or tissue specificity. The suicide gene is only expressed in cell types that are restricted by that specific promotor.

More recently, suicide gene therapy has involved the use of ultrasound and nano/microbubbles (NBs). It delivers exogenous molecules in a noninvasive manner, into a certain target site. Low-intensity pulsed ultrasound and NBs are used to transduce the HSV-TK gene in vitro. This leads to gene transfer. When ganciclovir is added to transduced cells, there is HSV-TK/GCV-dependent cell death due to apoptosis. For subcutaneous tumors, there is a significant reduction in tumor size. This shows the potential for using ultrasound with NBs for physical gene delivery and cancer gene therapy.

Since the use of intravenous chemotherapy for lymph node metastasis is impeded as far as access to the lymphatic system, there have been recent studies about combining intralymphatic chemotherapy with ultrasound and nano/microbubbles. This was found to have an extreme antitumor effect compared with IV administration alone. The addition of ultrasound and nano/microbubbles enhance the effect of chemotherapy, but only when it is given intralymphatically. Decreases in the volumes and blood vessel densities of lymph nodes that contain tumors accurately measure the effect of therapy. This can be confirmed in histopathology.

Significant Point

Suicide gene therapy is an experimental treatment option that has the potential to be a targeted therapy for mesothelioma, though it is currently only available via clinical trials. Trials for prostate cancer have also shown positive results. Suicide gene therapy has also been tested for glioma and ovarian cancer.

Tumor-Suppressor Gene Therapy

About 50% of all cancers contain the *p53 tumor-suppressor gene*. In clinical trials, a normal copy of the gene was introduced, restoring its function in lung cancer patients, as well as individuals with breast, colorectal, and other cancers. The treatments have been somewhat successful, and tumor-suppressor gene therapy is being combined with chemotherapy in clinical studies. Phase I clinical trials show that p53 replacement therapy, using retroviral and adenoviral vectors, is safe. This therapy induces tumor regression in patients with advances in non-small cell lung cancer and in recurrent head and neck cancers.

There are many tumor-suppressor genes (TSGs) involved in resistance to chemotherapy agents. These include *adenomatosis polyposis coli (APC), BCL2 associated X (Bax), BLU (also called zinc finger MYND-type containing 10 or ZMYND10), breast cancer 1 (BRCA1), cyclin-dependent kinase inhibitor (CDKN) 1A and 2A, Fas associated via death domain (FADD), F-box and WD repeat domain containing 7 (FBW7), hexosaminidase (hEx), high-in-normal-1 (HIN-1), inhibitor of growth family (ING) members 1 and 4, leucine zipper tumor-suppressor 1 (LZTS1), programmed cell death 4 (PDCD4), PIN2/TRF1-interacting telomerase inhibitor 1 (PinX1), polo-like kinase 2 (PLK2), phosphatase and tensin homolog (PTEN), Ras association domain family member 1 (RASSF1), RE1 silencing transcription factor (REST), transforming growth factor beta induced (TGFBI),* and *Yes1 associated protein (YAP).* These genes have direct and indirect relationships with each other. Therefore, they may work "as a group" to contribute to resistance to chemotherapy. Various expression status and regulation function upon the cell cycle in different tumors may play a strong role in chemotherapy resistance.

Antisense Oligonucleotides

Genetic therapies have been developed that specifically target DNA and RNA. Specific DNA segments are used called **antisense**

oligonucleotides. These are nucleic binding agents – short lengths of nucleotides that join with other nucleotides predictably. Therefore, drugs can be designed that recognize particular sites on target genes. Oligonucleotides are inserted into cells, interfering with RNA translation into oncogene proteins. In the patient, oligonucleotides stop the RNA message of oncogenes from being translated into functional oncogene proteins. This method is used for the antiepidermal growth factor receptor to treat head and neck squamous cell carcinomas.

Oncolytic Viral Gene Therapy

Oncolytic viruses reproduce within tumor cells and cause lysis to occur. They can be used in cancer treatment if the patient has a defective p53 pathway. Normally, p53 is destroyed by an adenovirus since it produces the *E1B 55 K protein*. The protein binds with p53. Along with another viral protein, E1B 55 K directs p53 to be destroyed. Researchers have modified an adenovirus strain so that it cannot encode the E1B 55 K protein. Therefore, p53 is not destroyed. Normally, activity of p53 causes an event cascade resulting the death of affected cells. Viral replication cannot occur. In a cancer cell lacking p53, the normal features leading to the death of infected cells is stopped. Only the modified adenovirus can replicate, and tumor cells die. This is being used for head and neck cancers, sometimes in combination with chemotherapy.

The first FDA-approved oncolytic virus for immunotherapy was *Talimogene laherparepvec [T-VEC]* (Imlygic), for melanoma. The approval occurred in 2015. The treatment utilizes a herpes virus that has been engineered so that it is unlikely to infect healthy cells, while causing infected cancer cells to produce *granulocyte-macrophage colony stimulating factor (GM-CSF)*, and immune-stimulating protein. Adverse effects may include chills, fatigue, flu-like symptoms, fever, injection site pain, and nausea. Another example, from 2018, revealed that treating triple-negative breast cancer patients with oncolytic virus therapy before surgery offered

higher likelihood of a response to checkpoint immunotherapy. There is also a phase I/II clinical trial that is combining an oncolytic virus with a checkpoint inhibitor to treat advanced appendiceal, colorectal, and ovarian cancers.

Significant Point

Oncolytic viruses tend to infect and kill tumor cells. They include viruses found in nature and viruses modified in the laboratory, to reproduce cancer-killing effects without harming healthy cells. Some research suggests that oncolytic viruses may partly work by triggering an immune response against cancer.

Active Immunotherapy

Active immunotherapy focuses on stimulating the immune system or a specific immune response, and is often used in cancer treatment. Direct immune system stimulation occurs, and generic or specific immune responses can be controlled. Active immunotherapy utilizes tumor-infiltrating lymphocytes, cytokine genes, DNA vaccines, adoptive immunotherapy, chimeric receptors, and tumor-specific T cells.

Tumor-Infiltrating Lymphocytes

A patient's immunological responses can be used to change the course of malignant melanomas and some other cancers. Tumor-infiltrating lymphocytes (TILs) have been identified that mediate tumor regression in melanoma patients. Researchers have mapped and cloned genes that encode shared melanoma antigens and antigenic epitopes. If an epitope is administered with IV high-dose interleukin-2 (IL-2), there can be regression of malignant melanoma. Clinical trials have used melanoma antigen genes to strengthen the immune system. Ongoing clinical trials related to TILs include the following:

- Lifileucel (LN-144) – for cervical carcinoma and solid tumors
- Modified immune cells (LN-145) – for metastatic non-small cell lung cancer and pretreated metastatic triple-negative breast cancer
- LN-145 or LN-145-S1 (a modified version that chooses a specific portion of T cells) – for relapsed or refractory ovarian cancer, anaplastic thyroid cancer, osteosarcoma, or other bone and soft tissue sarcomas
- Autologous TILs with high-dose interleukin-2 – for recurrent or metastatic head and neck squamous cell cancer, or stage III or IV cutaneous or mucosal melanoma
- Cell therapy with TILs – for locally advanced, metastatic, or recurrent solid cancers
- Cyclophosphamide/fludarabine/tumor-infiltrating lymphocytes/aldesleukin – for metastatic uveal melanoma
- Genetically modified T cells followed by aldesleukin – for stage III or IV melanoma
- Genetically modified therapeutic autologous lymphocytes followed by aldesleukin – for stage III or metastatic melanoma
- TILs and high-dose aldesleukin, with or without autologous dendritic cells – for metastatic melanoma
- Autologous TILs MDA-TIL (melanocyte differentiation antigens-TILs) – for recurrent or refractory ovarian cancer, colorectal cancer, or pancreatic ductal adenocarcinoma

---

Significant Point

TILs have been described in many cases of solid tumors. They are emerging as important biomarkers to predict the efficacy and outcome of cancer treatment. The TILs consist of all types of lymphocytic cells that have invaded tumor tissue. They mostly comprise cytotoxic (CD8 +) and helper (CD4 +) T cells, and a small amount of B and NK cells.

Cytokine Genes

Cytokines enhance the immune response to tumor antigens. Cytokine genes can be used to improve the ability to generate an immune response to tumor cells. The two most commonly used cytokine genes are IL-2 and tumor necrosis factor (TNF). They are modified, and can no longer proliferate yet still support expression of introduced gene products. The altered cells are injected into the patient via the intradermal, intramuscular, or subcutaneous routes.

DNA Vaccines

Cancer vaccines have become more common and effective. They avoid the use of adenoviruses as vectors or cellular immunity against gene products derived from vectors. The DNA vaccines containing tumor-associated antigen genes or cytokine genes are used since pure DNA encodes just the tumor-associated antigen gene. The DNA vaccines are usually given IM, with or without coadministration of cytokine genes. Metastatic renal cell carcinoma is one type of cancer that is highly responsive, and DNA vaccines are also used for prostate cancer. In clinical trials, a recombinant vaccine of prostatic acid antigen was given – an antigen expressed in nearly all (95%) of prostate cancers. The recombinant vaccine results in circulating immune cells to recognize the antigen. This boosts the tumor response rate. Tumor-specific vaccines that use antigen-presenting cells such as the dendritic cells are being studied regarding the induction of T-cell tumor responses.

Adoptive Immunotherapy

Adoptive immunotherapy utilizes the patient's own peripheral blood lymphocytes or TILs. These are modified after being removed from the body, using genes to increase their antitumor activities. The modified genes are reinfused back into the patient. The anti-Epstein–Barr virus (anti-EBV) has been studied for a variety of cancers. The EBV infection is linked with Hodgkin disease, lymphoproliferation, Burkitt's lymphoma, and nasopharyngeal carcinoma. In vitro generation and expansion of virus-specific cytotoxic lymphocytes has been studied. They are now used both as treatment and for prophylaxis. Adoptive immunotherapy with EBV-specific cytotoxic T lymphocytes has been effective against immunogenic tumors. One example is their effectiveness for lymphoproliferative disease following a transplant. Clinical trials have revealed a lot about adoptive immunotherapy. It has been used in melanoma cases, with patient-derived immune cells targeting tumor antigens with specificity. In 2014, it was found that regional delivery of mesothelin-targeting **chimeric antigen receptor (CAR) T cells** improved their activities against cancers.

Chimeric Receptors

Chimeric receptors are part of adoptive immunotherapy. They contain two molecules joined to form a functional molecule: an extracellular antibody molecule that is linked to the intracellular signal domains of T-cell receptors. Autologous T cells of the patient are a vector for inserted chimeric antibody molecules. The molecules have specificity for a tumor antigen. Once transferred into the patient, the altered T cells are able to recognize the tumor from the specific surface antibody. T cells are activated by the signaling chain and regulate antitumor activity. Chimeric receptor therapy is being used for kidney cancer, metastatic ovarian cancer, and neuroblastoma. Examples of FDA-approved chimeric receptors include the following:

- *Axicabtagene ciloleucel (Yescarta)* – for adults with relapsed or refractory large B-cell lymphoma, after two or more lines of systemic therapy, including diffuse large B-cell lymphoma (DLBCL) not otherwise specified, primary mediastinal large B-cell lymphoma, high-grade B-cell lymphoma, and DLBCL arising from follicular lymphoma. Yescarta is also indicated for adults with relapsed or refractor follicular lymphoma after two or more lines of systemic therapy

- *Brexucabtagene autoleucel (Tecartus)* – for adults with relapsed or refractory mantle cell lymphoma
- *Idecabtagene vicleucel (Abecma)* – for adults with relapsed or refractory multiple myeloma after four or more lines of therapy including an immunomodulatory agent, a proteasome inhibitor, and an anti-CD38 monoclonal antibody
- *Tisagenlecleucel (Kymriah)* – for patients up to 25 years of age with B-cell precursor acute lymphoblastic leukemia that is refractory or in the second or later relapse; also approved for adults with relapsed or refractory large B-cell lymphoma after two or more lines of systemic therapy, including DLBCL not otherwise specified, high-grade B-cell lymphoma, and DLBCL arising from follicular lymphoma
- *Tocilizumab (Actemra)* – for adults and children (two years of age and older) with chimeric antigen receptor (CAR) T-cell-induced severe or life-threatening cytokine release syndrome (CRS)

Significant Point

Autologous CAR T-cell therapy for hematologic malignancies is actively being studied. This type of therapy equips T cells with an ability to detect and destroy malignant cells by combining specificity of the monoclonal antibodies with the cytotoxic and memory abilities of the endogenous T cells.

Clinical Case

1. What does active immunotherapy such as the use of chimeric receptors focus on?
2. How are chimeric receptors used in cancer treatment?
3. Which chimeric receptor therapies are available?

A 57-year-old woman, previously diagnosed with follicular lymphoma, suddenly developed extreme fatigue and hypercalcemia. A PET scan and bone marrow biopsy revealed that she had a DLBCL. Over 18 months, the patient was treated with three different chemotherapy regimens, with a mixed response. Her disease progressed, and she was considered for CAR T-cell therapy. After much discussion, the procedure was performed. Within four weeks, the patient's follow-up PET scan revealed that she had a complete response. At one-year of follow-up, she is still in remission with no signs of any recurrence.

Answers:

1. **Active immunotherapy, including chimeric receptors, focuses on stimulating the immune system or a specific immune response. It is often used in cancer treatment. Direct immune system stimulation occurs. Generic or specific immune responses are able to be controlled.**
2. **Chimeric receptors are a part of adoptive immunotherapy. Their functional molecule contains an extracellular antibody molecule linked to the intracellular signal domains of T-cell receptors. Autologous T cells of the patient are a vector for inserted chimeric antibody molecules, since they have specificity for a tumor antigen. Altered T cells can recognize the tumor from the specific surface antibody, and are activated by the signaling chain, regulating antitumor activity.**
3. **Chimeric receptor therapies include axicabtagene ciloleucel (Yescarta) for lymphoma, brexucabtagene autoleucel (Tecartus) for lymphoma, Idecabtagene vicleucel (Abecma) for multiple myeloma, tisagenlecleucel (Kymriah) for leukemia and lymphoma, and tocilizumab (Actemra) for CAR T-cell-induced cytokine release syndrome.**

Tumor-Specific T Cells

Transduction of the IL-2 gene into antitumor T lymphocytes is under study as part of adoptive immunotherapy. It can overcome limitations of toxicity after lengthy in vivo administration of IL-2. The IL-2 gene has been transduced into a TIL to treat patients with melanoma and renal cell carcinoma.

Pharmacogenetics and Pharmacogenomics

Pharmacogenetics focuses on the differences in drug responses between individual patients. It attempts to identify the inherited basis for these differences, while translating this information into molecular diagnostics. The goal is to achieve more individualized drug effects. Human genes related to pharmacogenetics have been widely identified on a molecular basis, and can be used with more accuracy today. **Pharmacogenomics** researches genetic variants related to the effectiveness of drugs. It combines the areas of pharmacology and genomics. Pharmacogenomics results in drugs being developed that are adapted to the genetic makeup of each patient. A good example is the genetic polymorphism of *thiopurine methyltransferase (TPMT)*. This is linked to altered drug metabolism and a higher risk for severe toxicity when *6-meraptopurine* is used in cancer therapy. The testing for TPMT genotypes has become the basis for dose modification of this agent as well as *azathioprine*, used to treat acute lymphoblastic leukemia. If TPMT activity is of deficient or intermediate activity, the patient is at risk for toxicity. This can include fatal myelosuppression, even at standard drug doses. Testing for the low-activity TPMT gene variant has been done for decades in the United States. Caucasians have been tested because the specific variant alleles are understood in this population. Additional study is ongoing for other patient populations. Similarly, pharmacogenetics has studied *5-fluorouracil*. If the enzyme called *dihydropyrimidine dehydrogenase* is deficient, severe toxicity results even when 5-fluorouracil is given in standard doses. Doses must be adjusted based on the DNA sequence of enzyme genes involved in drug metabolism.

Pharmacogenetics in clinical practice may be illustrated by use of *trastuzumab (Herceptin)*. The *human epidermal growth factor receptor 2 (HER2)* protein is located on cell surface. When it is overexpressed, cancers become more aggressive. The HER2 oncogene is overexpressed in 20–30% of all breast cancers. The tumors are more aggressive and more resistant to chemotherapy than tumors that do not overexpress the oncogene. In clinical trials, gene therapy has delivered an antibody against HER2. This led to Herceptin being created. It is a humanized monoclonal antibody that acts against overexpression of HER2. Today, women with breast cancer are tested for HER2 before drug therapy begins. Herceptin benefits those with overexpression of HER2, and the drug may be combined with chemotherapy, improving response and lengthening overall survival. Different therapy is used for patients that do not have HER2 overexpression.

A molecular defect known as *breakpoint cluster region-Abelson murine leukemia (BCR-ABL)* occurs because of the Philadelphia chromosome being translocated. This can be used as part of treatment for Philadelphia chromosome-positive leukemias. The translocation is found in over 90% of patients with chronic myelogenous leukemia (CML). The BCR and ABL genes are moved beside each other. This causes the BCR-ABL *tyrosine* to remain active. This activity blocks apoptotic cell death. The drug called *imatinib (Gleevec)* was formulated to target the BCR-ABL defect. The medication has resulted in an 88% response in cases of CML that are positive for the Philadelphia chromosome.

Significant Point

Pharmacogenomics studies how medicine interacts with inherited genes. This includes how the inherited genes affect the effects of medications for each patient. A drug can be safe for one person, but harmful to another. Some people experience severe adverse effects while others do not, even with similar doses.

Ethical, Social, and Legal Issues

The ethical, social, and legal issues concerning human gene therapy are controversial. The ethical issues in particular have brought about discussion between scientists, ethicists, and religious theologians. Regulations have been established based on these discussions, in an attempt to protect against breaches of ethics. There is a *Biomedical Technology Assessment Program* that is part of the NIH and its Office of Science Policy. The program oversees human gene transfer research, focusing on ethical, scientific, medical, and social factors.

The director of the NIH, in 1995, assembled a panel for the assessment of the institution's investment in research on gene therapy. It was decided that gene therapy and its extensive publicity was resulting in some patient avoiding conventional medical therapies. Further research was greatly needed to develop a better understanding of genetic diseases and their causative mechanisms. The first fatality from gene therapy occurred in 1999. Additional investigations found that six more people died after gene therapy. In 2000, the U.S. Senate held hearings, increasing the investigation into and awareness of the outcomes of gene therapy. There is now better reporting of adverse effects and more in-depth oversight of gene therapy trials by the FDA and NIH.

Potential research subjects must be able to freely choose to participate in gene therapy. Choice of test subjects must be equitable. Candidates for gene therapy research must be fairly chosen from different patient populations, which are considered vulnerable. For example, prisoners must not be used as test subjects. The choice of test subjects also concerns the emergency or compassionate use of gene therapy, such as for a patient with a limited life expectancy. If a patient is granted permission, how is it that others are not granted permission to have gene therapy? How is research data maintained, as to its integrity, if emergency-use patients are accepted into the study, even if they do not meet the clinical trial research criteria?

Clinical research involves an informed consent process. This ensures that participants are making free choices about gene therapy on a voluntary basis. They must be completely informed about the benefits and risks. This does not mean that protocols must be totally risk-free, or that benefits must be totally established. For informed consent, risks must be described honestly. Patients considered gene therapy research participation must decide the value of the possible benefits against the possible risks. For patients that are under the age of 18, the NIH's *Points to Consider* document stresses the need for informed consent, by both the minor and his or her parents. Informed consent must also include discussion of how follow-up will occur with primary care providers, geneticists, psychologists, and social workers – as well as with the clinical investigators. This team of professionals ensures that support will be provided in all health-care disciplines. This includes reproduction and psychological development.

Regarding **germline therapy**, informed consent is of more controversy. Germline gene therapy alters the genes of future generations of people. This could create unknown consequences that last throughout lifetimes. This type of therapy may be ethically undesirable since future unborn individuals cannot give informed consent before the gene therapy causes changes in their genetic coding. Therefore, the U.S.

government does not allow any federal funds to be used for germline therapy research in humans. Another area of concern is based on the short- and long-term adverse effects and toxicities of gene therapy. Human clinical gene therapy trials must utilize expert staff members, trained professional support staff members, and counseling of patients and their families. These factors help ensure safety and proper implementation of gene therapy research.

Along with the reported deaths from gene therapy, children receiving therapy for *severe combined immunodeficiency (SCID)* have developed an illness that resembles leukemia. As a result, there are stricter safety measures in place. During administration, the patient is monitored and evaluated for allergic reactions to foreign proteins. Common adverse effects have included chills, fever, fatigue, headache, myalgia, nausea, and vomiting. Less common effects include anorexia, anemia, extremity weakness, and leukopenia, as well as diarrhea. Adverse effects reported in clinical trials for cancer gene therapy are summarized in Table 18.1.

Long-term risks to patients receiving gene therapy, or to their offspring, are unpredictable. Some adverse effects require years to manifest. Close follow-up is required to identify, diagnose, and prevent adverse effects. Unfortunately, long-term follow-up is often not part of gene therapy protocols. It is important to develop a plan for adequate patient follow-up and monitoring. Another area of concern is the safety of the clinical investigators, as well as involved providers, families, and the public. There can be infectious transmission of recombinant genes that have viral vectors. Though infectious spreading of recombinant viruses has not been seen, it still may occur in the future. Retroviral vectors are not used in all gene therapy protocols. However, when they are used, universal precautions are implemented as a safety measure.

It is important to also consider ethical implications of treatments designed for people with end-stage disease in comparison with research focused on preventing disease. Gene therapy is

Table 18.1 Adverse effects in clinical trials for cancer gene therapy.

Adverse effect	Vector
Erythema and induration, pain, pruritus, elevation of liver function tests, fever, abdominal pain, peritumor edema, diarrhea, nausea, increased local edema, paresis, seizures abducens, confusion, intratumoral hemorrhage, mild worsening of graft-versus-host disease	Retrovirus
Abnormal liver function, fever, fatigue, pulmonary infiltrate, transient abnormal lung function	Adenovirus
Injection site pain, transient pneumothorax	Liposome
Fever	Plasmid

expensive. Access may only be given to a selected few test subject. These studies are only done at medical centers, often requiring patients to have to pay for travel and lodging, since insurance companies do not cover these. Unless research funding covers these costs, patients may be unable to receive gene therapy. Other ethical concerns are also in place. Genetic testing and gene therapies reveal information about test subjects and their families, which could label individuals that are currently healthy as being "at risk patients." Also, personal and family genetic information could accidently become publicized.

In 2008, the federal *Genetic Information Nondiscrimination Act (GINA)* was implemented, prohibiting individual and group health insurers and employers from discriminating against people based on genetic information. The act prohibits insurers from using genetic information to determine eligibility or premiums. It also prohibits insurers from requiring that potential test subjects undergo any genetic tests. The act stops employers from using genetic information in relation to hiring or firing employees, assigning jobs, or in relation to any other terms of employment. Employers cannot request, require, or purchase genetic information of individuals or their family members. The act does not mandate coverage for any test or treatment, and does not prohibit medical underwriting based on an individual's current health status. The act does not cover disability, long-term care, or life insurance. Active-duty military personnel are an exception to the protections against employment and insurance discrimination based on genetic information; however, the act does not extend to genetic testing of active-duty military personnel or genetic data obtained from them. Confidentiality must be enforced in all areas of genetic testing and research.

Emerging ethical issues are focusing on fetal gene therapy. Possible candidates are individuals with the serious, life-threatening genetic disorders known as *adenosine deaminase (ADA) deficiency* and *alpha-thalassemia*. The ADA deficiency is a metabolic disorder that causes immunodeficiency. Alpha-thalassemia is an inherited blood disorder that reduces the body's ability to produce healthy red blood cells and normal hemoglobin. Is it better to treat ADA deficiency, which has other therapies that are effective? Is it better to continue with gene therapy for alpha-thalassemia, since it is often fatal to fetuses? Most experts agree that additional information is needed about safety, efficacy, and costs of fetal gene therapy.

Significant Point

Since gene therapy involves changing the body's "basic instructions," there are many ethical issues surrounding its use. Who decides which traits are normal or abnormal? Will the extreme costs of gene therapy mean that only wealthy patients can have access to it? Though germline therapy has the potential to cure future cases of cancer, what are the unknown effects that could harm future generations.

Key Terms

Active immunotherapy
Adoptive immunotherapy
Anti-oncogenes
Antisense oligonucleotides
CAR T cells
Chimeric receptors
Gene addition
Gene alteration

Gene marking
Gene therapy
Germline therapy
Oncogenes
Pharmacogenomics
Proto-oncogenes
Suicide gene

Bibliography

1 Altman, R.B., Flockhart, D., and Goldstein, D.B. (2012). *Principles of Pharmacogenetics and Pharmacogenomics*. Cambridge: Cambridge University Press.

2 Balkhi, M.Y. (2019). *Basics of Chimeric Antigen Receptor (CAR) Immunotherapy*. Cambridge: Academic Press.

3 Brenner, M.K. and Hung, M.C. (2014). *Cancer Gene Therapy by Viral and Non-viral Vectors (Translational Oncology, Book 4)*. Hoboken: Wiley Blackwell.

4 Cancer Network. (1999). p53 tumor suppressor gene therapy for cancer. Cranbury: *Cancer Network – "Oncology"* 13 (10).

5 Cancer Research Institute. (2021). *Oncolytic virus therapy – Immunotherapy with engineered viruses to fight cancer – How oncolytic virus therapy is changing cancer treatment*. Cancer Research Institute. https://www.cancerresearch.org/immunotherapy/treatment-types/oncolytic-virus-therapy Accessed 2021.

6 Cancer Research Institute. (2021). *Adoptive cell therapy – TIL, TCR, CAR T, and NK cell therapies – How cellular immunotherapies are changing the outlook for cancer patients*. Cancer Research Institute. https://www.cancerresearch.org/immunotherapy/treatment-types/adoptive-cell-therapy Accessed 2021.

7 Colavito, M.C. and Palladino, M.A. (2006). *Gene Therapy*. London: Pearson.

8 Curiel, D.T. (2016). *Adenoviral Vectors for Gene Therapy*. Cambridge: Academic Press.

9 Curiel, D.T. and Douglas, J.T. (2004). *Cancer Gene Therapy (Contemporary Cancer Research)*. Totowa: Humana Press.

10 Duzgunes, N. (2018). *Suicide Gene Therapy: Methods and Protocols (Methods in Molecular Biology, 1895)*. Totowa: Humana Press.

11 Galli, M.C. and Serabian, M. (2015). *Regulatory Aspects of Gene Therapy and Cell Therapy Products: A Global Perspective (Advances in Experimental Medicine and Biology, 871 – American Society of Gene & Cell Therapy)*. New York: Springer.

12 Giacca, M. (2010). *Gene Therapy*. New York: Springer.

13 Harrington, K.J., Vile, R.G., and Pandha, H.S. (2008). *Viral Therapy of Cancer*. Hoboken: Wiley.

14 Herzog, R.W. and Zolotukhin, S. (2010). *A Guide to Human Gene Therapy*. Singapore: World Scientific.

15 Kelley, M.R. (2011). *DNA Repair in Cancer Therapy: Molecular Targets and Clinical Applications*. Cambridge: Academic Press.

16 Kunt, K.K., Vorburger, S.A., and Swisher, S.G. (2007). *Gene Therapy for Cancer (Cancer Drug Discovery and Development)*. Totowa: Humana Press.

17 Leukemia & Lymphoma Society. (2021). *Chimeric Antigen Receptor (CAR) T-Cell Therapy*. The Leukemia & Lymphoma Society (LLS). https://www.lls.org/treatment/types-of-treatment/immunotherapy/chimeric-antigen-receptor-car-t-cell-therapy Accessed 2021.

18 Merten, O.W. and Al-Rubeai, M. (2016). *Viral Vectors for Gene Therapy: Methods and Protocols (Methods in Molecular Biology, 737).* Totowa: Humana Press.

19 Mukhopadhyay, T., Maxwell, S.A., and Roth, J.A. (2013). *P53 Suppressor Gene (Molecular Biology Intelligence Unit).* Georgetown: R.G. Landes Company/Springer.

20 National Institutes of Health – National Cancer Institute. (2021). *Clinical trials using tumor infiltrating lymphocyte therapy.* National Cancer Institute at the National Institutes of Health. https://www.cancer.gov/about-cancer/treatment/clinical-trials/intervention/tumor-infiltrating-lymphocyte-therapy Accessed 2021.

21 National Library of Medicine – National Center for Biotechnology Information. (2014). *The combination of intralymphatic chemotherapy with ultrasound and nano-/microbubbles is efficient in the treatment of experimental tumors in mouse lymph nodes.* National Library of Medicine. https://pubmed.ncbi.nlm.nih.gov/24656719 Accessed 2021.

22 National Library of Medicine – National Center for Biotechnology Information. (2016). *Tumor suppressor genes and their underlying interactions in paclitaxel resistance in cancer therapy.* National Library of Medicine. https://pubmed.ncbi.nlm.nih.gov/26900348 Accessed 2021.

23 Nobrega, C., Mendonca, L., and Matos, C.A. (2020). *A Handbook of Gene and Cell Therapy.* New York: Springer.

24 Rak, J.W. (2002). *Oncogene-Directed Therapies (Cancer Drug Discovery and Development).* Totowa: Humana Press.

25 Rezaei, N. and Keshavarz-Fathi, M. (2018). *Vaccines for Cancer Immunotherapy: An Evidence-Based Review on Current Status and Future Perspectives.* Cambridge: Academic Press.

26 Rinaldi, M., Fioretti, D., and Iurescia, S. (2014). *DNA Vaccines: Methods and Protocols,* 3rd Edition. *(Methods in Molecular Biology, 1143).* Totowa: Humana Press.

27 Saboowala, H. (2020). *A Glance at Advances in the Techniques and Methodologies of Cancer Gene Therapy.* Mumbai: Saboowala.

28 Saboowala, H. (2019). *Understanding the Basic Concept, Mechanism & Therapeutic Applications of Antisense Oligonucleotide (ASO) Technology.* Mumbai: Saboowala.

29 Scherman, D. (2019). *Advanced Textbook on Gene Transfer, Gene Therapy and Genetic Pharmacology,* 2nd Edition. Singapore: World Scientific.

30 Smyth Templeton, N. (2015). *Gene and Cell Therapy: Therapeutic Mechanisms and Strategies,* 4th Edition. Boca Raton: CRC Press.

31 Stevenson, H.C. (2021). *Adoptive Cellular Immunotherapy of Cancer (Immunology Series Volume 48).* Boca Raton: CRC Press.

32 Vertes, A.A., Smith, D.M., Qureshi, N., and Dowden, N.J. (2019). *Second Generation Cell and Gene-based Therapies: Biological Advances, Clinical Outcomes and Strategies for Capitalisation.* Cambridge: Academic Press.

33 Walther, W. (2016). *Current Strategies in Cancer Gene Therapy (Recent Results in Cancer Research, 209).* New York: Springer.

34 Walther, W. and Stein, U. (2015). *Gene Therapy of Solid Cancers: Methods and Protocols (Methods in Molecular Biology, 1317).* Totowa: Humana Press.

35 Zdanowicz, M.M. (2017). *Concepts in Pharmacogenomics,* 2nd Edition. Bethesda: American Society of Health-System Pharmacists.

Glossary

Abdominal gutters the paracolic gutters (paracolic sulci, paracolic recesses) are spaces between the colon and the abdominal wall. For example, fluid from an infected appendix can track up the right paracolic gutter to the hepatorenal recess.

Abducens nerves (VI) either of the sixth pair of cranial nerves, which are motor nerves, arising beneath the floor of the fourth ventricle and supplying the lateral rectus muscle of each eye.

Absolute neutrophil count the number of neutrophils in one ml of blood.

Acantholytic referring to acantholysis – a rare, temporary skin condition. It causes sudden red, raised, blistery, and sometimes very itchy spots that form around the middle of the body. The rash is most often seen in middle-aged men. Another name for this condition is *Grover's disease*.

Acanthosis nigricans a skin condition that is marked by dark discoloration and velvety thickening of the skin, especially of body folds or creases (as of the armpit, groin, or neck) and that is often associated with obesity, insulin resistance, hormonal irregularity, or medication use.

Achalasia a disorder characterized by the constriction of the lower portion of the esophagus, preventing normal swallowing.

Acrochordon a skin tag.

Acromegaly excessive enlargement of the limbs due to thickening of bones and soft tissues, caused by hypersecretion of growth hormone, usually from a tumor of the pituitary gland.

Active surveillance a treatment plan that involves closely watching a patient's condition but not giving any treatment unless there are changes in test results that show the condition is getting worse. Active surveillance may be used to avoid or delay the need for treatments such as radiation therapy or surgery, which can cause side effects or other problems.

Acute lymphoblastic leukemia a cancer of the lymphoid blood cells involving large numbers of immature lymphocytes.

Acute myeloid leukemia a malignant neoplasm of blood-forming tissues characterized by the uncontrolled proliferation of immature granular leukocytes that usually have azurophilic Auer rods.

Adenoma a benign tumor of epithelial tissue with glandular origin, glandular characteristics, or both.

Adnexal torsion an uncommon but serious condition called *ovarian torsion* occurs when the ovary, and sometimes the fallopian tube, twist on the tissues that support them. This cuts off the blood supply to the ovary, which, if not treated promptly, can cause tissue in the organ to die.

Adoptive immunotherapy the transfer of immune cells with antitumor activity into a patient to mediate tumor regression, especially a treatment typically for cancer in

Global Epidemiology of Cancer: Diagnosis and Treatment, First Edition. Jahangir Moini, Nicholas G. Avgeropoulos, and Craig Badolato.
© 2022 John Wiley & Sons Ltd. Published 2022 by John Wiley & Sons Ltd.

which lymphocytes removed from a patient are cultured with interleukin-2 and are returned to the patient's body.

Adrenal cortical carcinoma a malignant neoplasm emerging from the cells that comprise the adrenal cortex.

Advance directive a written statement of a person's wishes regarding medical treatment, often including a living will, made to ensure those wishes are carried out should the person be unable to communicate them to a doctor.

Affinity the measure of the binding strength of the antigen-antibody reaction.

Aflatoxins any of a class of toxic compounds that are produced by certain molds found in food and can cause liver damage and cancer.

Age-specific death rates the amount of deaths based on certain age groups.

Alopecia areata a disease of unknown cause in which sudden well-defined bald patches occur. The bald areas are usually round or oval and located on the head.

Alpha-fetoprotein a blood test used to assist in diagnosing certain neoplastic conditions, such as hepatoma, teratomas, Hodgkin's disease, lymphoma, and renal cell carcinoma. Increased AFP concentration also may indicate cirrhosis, active chronic hepatitis, and neural tube defects in the fetus.

Amyloidosis a progressive, incurable metabolic disease in which a waxy, starchlike glycoprotein (amyloid) accumulates in tissues and organs, impairing their function.

Anal verge the area between the anal canal and the perianal skin.

Anaplastic ependymoma a rare type of brain tumor that is often fatal.

Anaplastic carcinoma a malignant neoplasm arising from the transformed cells of epithelial origin, or showing some epithelial characteristics.

Anaplastic ependymoma a rare type of brain tumor that is often fatal.

Anaplastic oligodendroglioma a grade III neuroepithelial tumor believed to originate from oligodendrocytes.

Anetodermic referring to anetoderma, a benign condition with focal loss of dermal elastic tissue, resulting in localized areas of flaccid or herniated saclike skin.

Aneuploidy the presence of an abnormal number of cellular chromosomes.

Angiogenesis the formation of new blood vessels, a process controlled by chemicals produced in the body that stimulate blood vessels or form new ones.

Angiomyolipomas the most common benign tumors of the kidneys.

Angiosarcoma a cancer of the endothelial cells lining the walls of blood or lymphatic vessels.

Aniridia an absence of the iris, a usually bilateral, hereditary anomaly.

Anode the electrode at which oxidation occurs.

Apoptosis necrosis of keratinocytes in which the nuclei of the necrotic cells dissolve and the cytoplasm shrinks, rounds up, and is subsequently phagocytized.

Arteriosclerosis the thickening and hardening of the walls of the arteries, occurring typically in old age.

Asterixis a hand-flapping tremor, often accompanying metabolic disorders. The tremor is usually induced by extending the arm and dorsiflexing the wrist. Asterixis is seen frequently in hepatic encephalopathy.

Astrocytes star-shaped glial cells in the CNS.

Astrocytoma a primary tumor of the brain composed of astrocytes and characterized by slow growth, cyst formation, invasion of surrounding structures, and often the development of a highly malignant glioblastoma within the tumor mass.

Ataxia an impaired ability to coordinate movement, often characterized by a staggering gait and postural imbalance.

Ataxia-telangiectasia a rare, neurodegenerative, autosomal recessive disease that impairs movement and coordination, weakens the immune system, and predisposes to cancer.

Atelectasis an abnormal condition characterized by the collapse of alveoli, preventing the respiratory exchange of carbon dioxide and oxygen in a part of the lungs.

Atherosclerosis a condition in which a thrombus originates in an atheromatous blood vessel.

Atomic number the number of protons in the nucleus of an atom of a particular element.

Atretic cells the cells of the atretic follicles, which degenerate before coming to maturity, located within the ovary.

Atypia a condition of being irregular.

Auer rods pink or red-stained, needle-shaped structures seen in the cytoplasm of myeloid cells.

Autosomal dominant a pattern of inheritance in which the transmission of a dominant allele on an autosome causes a trait to be expressed.

Azurophilic staining with azure or similar blue aniline dyes.

B lymphocytes white blood cells that function in the humoral immunity component of the adaptive immune system, by secreting antibodies.

Bannayan-Zonana syndrome a genetic condition characterized by a large head size (macrocephaly), multiple noncancerous tumors and tumor-like growths called *hamartomas*, and dark freckles on the penis in males.

Barrett esophagus a disorder of the lower esophagus marked by a benign ulcer-like lesion in columnar epithelium, resulting most often from chronic irritation of the esophagus by gastric reflux of acidic digestive juices.

Bartholin's gland one of two small mucous-secreting glands located on the posterior and lateral aspect of the vestibule of the vagina.

Basal cell carcinoma a malignant epithelial cell tumor that begins as a pearly-appearing papule and enlarges peripherally, developing a central crater that erodes, crusts, and bleeds.

Bazex syndrome the presence of hyperkeratotic lesions on the nose, ears, palms, and soles that appear in association with malignancies of the upper aerodigestive tract, most often a squamous cell carcinoma.

Beam Radiation Therapy treatment by radiation emitted from a source located at a distance from the body; also called *external beam radiotherapy* or *beam therapy*.

Beckwith-Wiedemann syndrome an overgrowth disorder with an increased risk of childhood cancer and congenital abnormalities.

Benign prostatic hyperplasia a histological diagnosis associated with nonmalignant, noninflammatory enlargement of the prostate. It is most common among men over 50 years of age.

Beta particle an electron emitted from the nucleus of an atom during radioactive decay of the atom. These particles form beta rays.

Betel quid a type of smokeless tobacco that is made in India and is widely used throughout Asia. It is a mixture of tobacco, crushed areca nut (also called *betel nut*), spices, and other ingredients. It is used like chewing tobacco and is placed in the mouth, usually between the gum and cheek. Betel quid with tobacco contains nicotine and many harmful, cancer-causing chemicals. Using it can lead to nicotine addiction and can cause cancers of the lip, mouth, tongue, throat, and esophagus. Also called *gutka*.

Biopsy gun a hand-held, single-use device to obtain a tissue sample.

Bipolar resectoscope in bipolar electrosurgery, the current flow through the tissue is restricted to the area between the two electrode's loops that are under the visual control of the surgeon.

Bitemporal hemianopsia partial blindness in which vision is missing in the outer half of the right and left visual fields.

Bloom syndrome congenital telangiectatic erythema, usually in butterfly distribution, on the face and sometimes the hands and forearms, with sun sensitivity of skin lesions and dwarfism with normal body proportions except for a narrow face and altered skull; it is a predisposition to malignancy.

Boswellia a standardized extract derived from the plant *Boswellia* serrata of the family Burseraceae, with anti-inflammatory activity.

Bowen disease a skin disease marked by scaly or thickened patches on the skin and often caused by prolonged exposure to arsenic. The patches often occur on sun-exposed areas of the skin and in older white men. These patches may become malignant. Also called *precancerous dermatitis* and *precancerous dermatosis*.

Brachytherapy a form of radiotherapy where a sealed radiation source is placed inside or next to the area requiring treatment.

Breast tomosynthesis a new type of digital x-ray mammogram which creates 2D- and 3D-like pictures of the breasts.

Breslow thickness the greatest thickness of a primary cutaneous melanoma, measured in millimeters in a biopsy specimen from the granular layer of the epidermis down to the deepest point of invasion.

Bruit an abnormal blowing or swishing sound or murmur heard while auscultating a carotid artery, the aorta, an organ, or a gland.

Burkitt lymphoma a cancer of the lymphatic system, mostly the lymphocytes in the germinal center; mostly occurring in children.

Buschke-Lowenstein tumor (BLT) a solid tumor that usually develops around the external genitals or anus. BLT grows slowly into a bulky, cauliflower-shaped mass.

Cachexia general ill health and malnutrition, marked by weakness and emaciation, usually associated with severe disease such as advanced malignancy or AIDS.

Calcimimetic a pharmaceutical drug that mimics the action of calcium on tissues, by allosteric activation of the calcium-sensing receptor that is expressed in various organ tissues; used to treat secondary hyperparathyroidism.

Caldesmon a calmodulin binding protein, involved in the regulation of smooth muscle and non-muscle contraction.

Canalicular related to small passageways known as *canaliculi*.

Carcinoid syndrome occurs when a rare cancerous tumor called a *carcinoid tumor* secretes certain chemicals into the bloodstream, causing a variety of signs and symptoms. A carcinoid tumor, a type of neuroendocrine tumor, occurs most often in the gastrointestinal tract or the lungs.

Cardiac angioplasty a procedure used to open blocked coronary arteries caused by coronary artery disease. It restores blood flow to the heart muscle.

Cardiac tamponade compression of the heart produced by the accumulation of blood or other fluids in the pericardial sac.

Carina any structure shaped like a ridge, such as the carina of the trachea, which projects from the lowest tracheal cartilage.

Cathode the electrode at which reduction occurs. It is also known as the *negative side* of the x-ray tube, which consists of the focusing cup and the filament.

Cavography angiography of a vena cava.

Cell sterilization a technique that results in complete inhibition of a cell, so that it cannot divide.

Cell-free DNA refers to all non-encapsulated DNA in the bloodstream.

Cell-pellets prepared from early passage human primary cells. Each pellet contains 5 million cells and can be used for a variety of applications, including genomic DNA library construction and gene expression profiling.

Cellular plasticity the ability of cells to change their phenotypes without genetic mutations in response to environmental cues.

Centigray a unit of radioactivity used in radiotherapy that is 1/100 of a gray.

Cerebellopontine relating to the cerebellum and pons; especially denoting the cerebellopontine recess or angle between these two structures.

Chamberlain procedure a procedure in which a tube is inserted into the chest to view the tissues and organs in the area between the lungs and between the breastbone and heart. The tube is inserted through an incision next to the breastbone.

Charged particle EBRT a type of external radiation therapy that uses a special machine to make invisible, high-energy particles (protons or helium ions) that kill cancer cells.

Chédiak-Higashi syndrome a rare, inherited, complex, immune disorder that usually occurs in childhood, characterized by reduced pigment in the skin and eyes (oculocutaneous albinism), immune deficiency with an increased susceptibility to infections, and a tendency to bruise and bleed easily.

Chemical aquation the formation of a complex with water molecules, on an intracellular level.

Chemoresistance the resistance of bacteria or a cancer cell to a chemical designed to treat the disorder.

Chloracetaldehyde an organic compound that is a highly electrophilic reagent.

Cholestasis interruption in the bile flow through any part of the biliary system, from the liver to the duodenum.

Cholesterolosis a condition that most often affects the gallbladder. It occurs when there is a buildup of cholesteryl esters and they stick to the wall of the gallbladder, forming polyps.

Choriocarcinoma a malignant, trophoblastic cancer, usually of the placenta.

Chorion the outermost membrane surrounding an embryo of humans that contributes to the formation of the placenta.

Chromatin the material of which the chromosomes of organisms other than bacteria (such as eukaryotes) are composed. It consists of protein, RNA, and DNA.

Chromogranin A also called *parathyroid secretory protein 1*, located in secretory vesicles of neurons and endocrine cells.

Chronic lymphocytic leukemia a type of cancer in which the bone marrow makes too many lymphocytes, usually worsening slowly over years.

Chronic myelogenous leukemia a cancer of the white blood cells, with increased, unregulated growth of myeloid cells in the bone marrow, and their accumulation in the blood.

Clearance removal of a substance from the blood; usually expressed in the context of the rate of removal of a drug by the kidneys.

Clival related to the clivus.

Cloacogenic carcinoma a rare tumor of the anorectal region originating from a persistent remnant of the cloacal membrane of the embryo. The tumor accounts for 2–3% of anorectal carcinomas and occurs more than twice as often in women.

Codman triangle an area of new subperiosteal bone created when a tumor or other lesion raises the periosteum away from the bone.

Complement cascade a biochemical process in the blood that helps or "complements" cells of the immune system to eliminate invading pathogens.

Conformal Radiation Therapy a procedure that uses computers to create a 3D picture of the tumor in order to target the cancer cells.

Core-needle biopsy a procedure to remove a small amount of suspicious tissue, using a large hollow "core" needle.

Costophrenic angles the places where the diaphragm meets the ribs. Each costophrenic angle can normally be seen as on chest x-ray as a sharply-pointed, downward indentation (dark) between each hemi-diaphragm (white) and the adjacent chest wall (white).

Crypt stem cells an intestinal stem cell, similar to stem cells of the mouse hematopoietic system and the hair follicle; they are maintained for long periods of time.

Cushing's disease a cause of Cushing's syndrome that involves increased secretion of adrenocorticotropic hormone (ACTH) from the anterior pituitary.

Cushing's syndrome signs and symptoms caused by prolonged exposure to glucocorticoids such as cortisol; also called *hypercortisolism*.

Cutaneous adnexae any functional anomaly of the skin appendages, which are specialized skin structures located within the dermis and focally within the subcutaneous fatty tissue, comprising hair follicle, sebaceous glands and the eccrine sweat.

Cyberknife a radiation therapy device used to deliver radiosurgery with gamma radiation, for treating tumors and other medical conditions.

Cytokines small proteins that are important in cell signaling.

Deletion the loss of a piece of a chromosome.

Dendritic cells specialized cells of the hematopoietic system with branch-like extensions that present antigens to T cells.

Denys-Drash syndrome a rare disorder that causes kidney failure before age 3, abnormal development of the sexual organs, and Wilms tumor (a type of kidney cancer).

Dermabrasion a treatment for the removal of superficial scars on the skin by the use of revolving wire brushes or sandpaper.

Dermatofibroma a cutaneous nodule that is painless, round, firm, gray or red, elevated, and commonly found on the extremities.

Diffusion-weighted imaging a form of MR imaging based upon measuring the random Brownian motion of water molecules within a voxel of tissue.

DiGeorge syndrome a condition caused by the deletion of a small segment of chromosome 22, with heart problems, distinct facial features, infections, developmental delays, learning problems, and cleft palate.

Disability-adjusted life years measures of overall disease burden, as the number of years lost due to ill-health, disability, or early death.

Disomies also called *aneuploidies*; abnormal numbers of chromosomes in cells.

Discoid dermatitis a common type of eczema/dermatitis defined by scattered, well-defined, coin-shaped, and coin-sized plaques of eczema.

DNA fragments the separation or breaking of DNA strands into pieces. It can be done intentionally by laboratory personnel or by cells, or can occur spontaneously.

Doppler effect an increase (or decrease) in the frequency of sound, light, or other waves as the source and observer move toward each other. The effect causes the sudden change in pitch noticeable in a passing siren.

Doppler ultrasonography a Doppler ultrasound is an imaging test that uses sound waves to show blood moving through blood vessels.

Dosimeter a device that measures exposure to ionizing radiation.

Double minutes small fragments of extrachromosomal DNA that have been observed in a large number of human tumors such as those of the breast, lung, and ovary.

Driver mutations mutations of genes increasing net cell growth under certain microenvironmental conditions existing in the cell, in vivo.

Drop metastasis when a tumor metastasizes down to the cauda equina.

Dumping syndrome a condition that can develop after surgery to remove all or part of the stomach or after surgery to bypass the stomach to aid in weight loss.

Duplex ultrasonography the generation of diagnostic images called *sonograms* based on differences in the acoustic impedance of tissues.

Dysarthria a disturbance of speech due to paralysis, incoordination, or spasticity of the muscles used for speaking.

Dysgerminomas malignant germ cell cancers that derive from cells that give rise to egg cells, usually occurring in the ovaries.

Dyskeratosis congenita a rare, inherited disorder that can affect many parts of the body, especially the nails, skin, and mouth. It is marked by abnormally shaped fingernails and toenails that may grow poorly; changes in skin color, especially on the neck and chest; and white patches inside the mouth.

Dysphagia difficulty swallowing or the inability to swallow.

Eaton-Lambert syndrome a rare autoimmune disorder characterized by muscle weakness of the limbs.

Echogram the visual output from echocardiography, of the structures of the heart and major blood vessels.

Ectasia the distension or dilation of a duct, vessel, or hollow viscus.

Ectoderm the most exterior of the three primary germ layers in a new embryo.

Electrocoagulation the coagulation of blood or other tissues by the local application of an electric current to produce concentrated heat.

Electrodesiccation the drying up of tissue by a high-frequency electric current applied with a needle-shaped electrode – also called *fulguration*.

Electrophoresis the movement of charged particles in a fluid or gel under the influence of an electric field.

Electrosurgery surgery using a high-frequency electric current to heat and cut tissue with great precision.

Electrovaporization a procedure used to treat benign prostatic hypertrophy (BPH). An instrument is inserted through the urethra into the prostate. A ball or special wire loop on the instrument heats the prostate tissue and turns it to vapor. This relieves pressure and improves urine flow.

Elephantiasis neuromatosa enlargement of a limb due to diffuse neurofibromatosis of the skin and subcutaneous tissue.

Embryonal carcinoma an uncommon germ cell tumor of the ovaries and testes.

Emergent surgery nonelective surgery performed when the patient's life or well-being is in direct jeopardy.

Emetogenic having the capacity to induce emesis (vomiting), a common property of some drugs.

En bloc resection removal of a large bulky tumor virtually without dissection.

End replication problem where all organisms with linear chromosomes show loss of telomeric DNA with each cell division.

Endoderm the inner of the three primary germ layers of a new embryo.

Endonasal within the nose.

Endoscopy examination of an interior structure by means of a flexible fiber tube. An endoscope may be used to examine the esophagus and stomach, colon, lungs, and other areas.

Endothoracic fascia the layer of loose connective tissue deep to the intercostal spaces and ribs, separating these structures from the underlying pleura.

Enterochromaffin cells an enteroendocrine cell that produces serotonin and is found in the small intestine.

Enteroclysis an imaging test of the small intestine. The test looks at how a liquid called *contrast material* moves through the small intestine.

Epigenetic the study of changes in gene function that are heritable and which are not attributed to alterations of the DNA sequence.

Erythroid hypoplasia a condition in which immature red blood cells (erythroid cells) in the bone marrow are abnormal in size, shape, organization, and/or number.

Erythroplakia an abnormal reddened patch with a velvety surface that is found in the mouth.

Erythroplasia of Queyrat an early form of skin cancer found on the penis. The cancer is called *squamous cell carcinoma in situ*, and can occur on any part of the body.

Erythropoietin a glycoprotein hormone that acts on stem cells of the bone marrow to stimulate red blood cell production.

Euchromatin a lightly packed form of chromatin enriched in genes, and often under active transcription.

Ewing sarcoma a malignant neoplasm that usually occurs before age 20, usually involving bones of the extremities, with a predilection for the metaphysis.

Excrescence an abnormal outgrowth, especially of this skin.

Exophytic an abnormal growth that protrudes from the surface of a tissue.

Expressivity the degree to which a phenotype is expressed by individuals having a particular genotype.

Extravasate to force the flow of blood or lymph from a vessel into surrounding tissue.

Fanconi anemia a rare genetic disease resulting in impaired response to DNA damage.

Fas ligand a molecule on the surface of cytotoxic T cells that binds to the FasL receptor.

Field carcinogenesis increased susceptibility of an entire area to carcinogenesis.

Fine-needle aspiration a diagnostic procedure to investigate lumps, masses, and body fluids, in which a 23–25 gauge hollow needle is inserted to sample cells.

Fluoroscopy a study of moving body structures, similar to an x-ray "movie." A continuous x-ray beam is passed through the body part being examined.

Foley catheter a thin, flexible catheter used especially to drain urine from the bladder by way of the urethra.

Follicular carcinoma a malignant thyroid neoplasm consisting of differentiated follicular cells.

Fractionation the process of dividing or separating into parts; breaking up. The division of a total therapeutic dose of radiation into small doses to be administered over a period of time.

Frasier syndrome a condition that affects the kidneys and genitalia. It is characterized by kidney disease that begins in early childhood.

Freckle a small patch of light brown color on the skin, often becoming more pronounced through exposure to the sun.

Free radical an uncharged molecule (typically highly reactive and short-lived) having an unpaired valence electron.

Fulguration a procedure that uses heat from an electric current to destroy abnormal tissue, such as a tumor or other lesion. The tip of the electrode is heated by the electric current to burn or destroy the tissue.

Fungate to assume a fungal form or grow rapidly like a fungus.

Gadolinium a metal or salt that absorbs neutrons and is sometimes used for shielding in neutron radiography and as a contrast agent.

Gadolinium contrast a combination of agents used for contrast in an MRI, to aid in the imaging of blood vessels, tissues, and intracranial lesions.

Gait ataxia a failure of muscle coordination, characterized by irregular foot placement, wide base, and instability.

Gamma knife radiosurgery a treatment that uses Gamma radiation to treat tumor cells, especially in the brain.

Gamma radiation the rays that arise from the radioactive decay of atomic nuclei.

Gantry a device that holds radiation detectors and/or a radiation source, to diagnose or treat an illness.

Gardner's syndrome also called *familial polyposis* of the colon; characterized by multiple colon polyps along with osteomas of the skull, thyroid cancer, epidermoid cysts, fibromas, and desmoid tumors.

Gastrin a hormone that stimulates secretion of gastric juice and is secreted into the bloodstream by the stomach wall in response to the presence of food.

Gastroenterostomy the surgical formation of a passage between the stomach and small intestine.

Gene addition the insertion of a gene by non-homologous recombination.

Gene alteration permanent changes in the DNA sequence of a gene.

Gene amplification an increase in the number of copies of a gene. There may also be an increase in the RNA and protein made from that gene.

Gene marking a specific sequence of DNA at a known location on a chromosome. There are many genetic markers on each chromosome.

Gene rearrangement a phenomenon in which a programmed DNA recombination event occurs during cellular differentiation to reconstitute a functional gene from gene segments separated in the genome.

Gene therapy a type of experimental treatment in which foreign genetic material (DNA or RNA) is inserted into cells to prevent or fight disease. It is designed to introduce genetic material to compensate for abnormal genes or to make a beneficial protein.

Genodermatosis an inherited genetic skin condition, including epidermolysis bullosa, ichthyosis, palmoplantar keratoderma, and neurofibromatosis.

Genomes the complete set of genes on a chromosome or group of chromosomes.

Genotype the genetic constitution of an individual organism.

Germ disc a flattened round bilaminar plate of cells in the blastocyst of a mammal, where the first traces of the embryo are seen; also called *embryonic* or *germinal area*.

Germline mutations gene changes in a reproductive cell (egg or sperm) that become incorporated into the DNA of every cell in the body of the offspring.

Germline therapy the process of DNA being transferred into the cells that produce the body's reproductive cells.

Gerota fascia a fibrous envelope of tissue that surrounds the kidney. Also called *Gerota's capsule* and *renal fascia*.

Giant cell tumor a relatively uncommon bone tumor characterized by multinucleated osteoclast-like cells.

Glucosinolates a natural class of organic compounds that contain sulfur and nitrogen and are derived from glucose and an amino acid.

Goiter an enlargement of the thyroid gland visible as a swelling of the front of the neck.

Gorlin's syndrome a complex genetic disorder or multiple tumors, including multiple schwannomas.

Grayscale image a range of shades of gray without apparent color. The darkest possible shade is black, which is the total absence of transmitted or reflected light.

Growth factors a naturally occurring substance capable of stimulating cell proliferation, wound healing, and, occasionally, cellular differentiation.

Gutka bacteria and other organisms that live inside the intestines. They help digest food. Vitamins such as biotin and vitamin K are made.

Gynecomastia the development of abnormally large mammary glands in males, causing breast enlargement.

Hailey-Hailey disease a rare genetic disorder that is characterized by blisters and erosions most often affecting the neck, armpits, skin folds, and genitals. The lesions may come and go and usually heal without scarring. Sunlight, heat, sweating, and friction often aggravate the disorder.

Half-life the time it takes for the plasma concentration of a drug to be reduced by 50%.

Happle-Tinschert syndrome a disorder causing unilateral segmentally arranged basaloid follicular hamartomas of the skin associated with ipsilateral osseous, dental, and cerebral abnormalities, including tumors.

Harmonic scalpel a surgical instrument used to simultaneously cut and cauterize tissue.

Hashimoto's thyroiditis an autoimmune disease in which the thyroid gland is destroyed by various immune processes; it often results in either hypo- or hyperthyroidism.

Hassall's corpuscles also called *thymic corpuscles*; structures in the medulla of the thymus, formed from eosinophilic epithelial reticular cells that are arranged concentrically.

Helical CT a procedure that uses a computer linked to an x-ray machine to make a series of detailed pictures of areas inside the body.

Helicobacter pylori a gram-negative microaerophylic bacterium usually found in the stomach that has been associated with mucosa-associated lymphoid tissue, extranodal marginal zone B-cell lymphoma, and diffuse large B-cell lymphoma.

Hemangioma a usually benign vascular tumor derived from blood vessel cell types; usually called a *strawberry mark*, seen soon after birth.

Hematogones the normal bone marrow precursors of mature B-lymphocytes with morphologic and immunophenotypic properties that overlap those of lymphoblasts.

Hemihypertrophy a condition in which one side of the body or a part of one side is larger than the other. Children with hemihypertrophy have an increased risk of developing certain types of cancer, including Wilms tumor (a kidney cancer) and liver cancer.

Hepatocellular carcinoma a primary malignancy of the liver that is now the third leading cause of cancer deaths.

Heterozygosity the state of being heterozygous, which is having two alleles at corresponding loci on homologous chromosomes different for one or more loci.

Hidradenitis suppurativa a chronic condition characterized by swollen, painful lesions, occurring in the armpit, groin, anal, and breast regions.

Hirschsprung disease a congenital disorder of the digestive system, in which nerves are missing from parts of the intestine.

Hodgkin's lymphoma a condition marked by chronic lymph node enlargement, usually local at first and then generalized, with spleen and liver enlargement, anemia, and fever; a malignant neoplasm of lymphoid Reed-Sternberg cells, with infiltration of lymphocytes, eosinophilic leukocytes, and fibrosis.

Hydatidiform mole a rare mass or growth that forms inside the uterus at the beginning of a pregnancy. It contains many cysts and is usually benign, but it may spread to nearby tissues as an invasive mole.

Hypoferremia a deficiency of iron in the circulating blood.

Hypospadias a congenital condition in males in which the opening of the urethra is on the underside of the penis.

Hysterectomy surgical removal of the uterus; in most cases, the ovaries are left intact to prevent the sudden onset of menopausal symptoms.

Idiosyncratic reaction a unique, strange, or unpredicted reaction to a drug.

Ileostomy a surgically implanted passageway that connects the ileum to an opening on the outside of the body.

Immortalization a change in a eukaryotic cell line that confers the ability to go on dividing and reproducing indefinitely.

Immune stimulants naturally occurring compounds that modulate the immune system by increasing the host's resistance to disease.

Immunoadjuvants a nonspecific substance acting to enhance the immune response to an antigen with which it is administered.

Immunoglobulin a group of proteins in the blood that function as part of the immune system. All antibodies are immunoglobulins.

Immunological memory the ability of the immune system to recognize an antigen that the body has previously encountered, and initiate a corresponding immune response.

Incidence the number of new cases of a disorder or problem that occur in a specified period of time.

Inducibility the quality or condition of being inducible, as when an enzyme is formed by a cell in response to the presence of its substrate.

Indurated a soft tissue or organ that has become firm or hard.

Infantile hemangiomas benign vascular tumors in infants that appear as red or blue raised lesions.

Innate immunity defense responses mediated by germline encoded components that directly recognize components of potential pathogens.

Intercalation the reversible inclusion or insertion of a molecule (or ion) into layered materials with layered structures.

Interferons proteins made and released by host cells in response to the presence of pathogens.

Interleukins cytokines expressed by white blood cells that mediate communication between cells, and regulate cell growth, differentiation, and motility.

Interstitial pneumonitis a heterogeneous group of diffuse parenchymal lung diseases characterized by specific clinical, radiologic, and pathologic features.

Interstrand cross-links lesions that are a covalent linkage between opposite strands of double-stranded DNA.

Intramural situated or occurring within the substance of the walls of an organ.

Intravasate to enter into a vessel of the body, especially a blood vessel, such as by a foreign pathogen.

Intravasation the entrance of foreign matter into a vessel of the body, especially a blood vessel.

Invasive carcinoma cancer that has spread beyond the layer of tissue in which it developed and is growing into surrounding, healthy tissues.

Isotopes each of two or more forms of the same element that contain equal numbers of protons but different numbers of neutrons in their nuclei, and hence differ in relative atomic mass but not in chemical properties; in particular, a radioactive form of an element. Some elements have only one stable isotope.

Ivory vertebrae one or more vertebrae has been affected by a density increase without any changes in the opacity or size of the adjacent intervertebral discs.

Kaposi sarcoma a cancer that may form masses in the skin, lymph nodes, and other organs, with the lesions usually being purple in color.

Keloids an area of irregular fibrous tissue formed at the site of a scar or injury.

Keratoacanthoma a rapidly growing skin tumor that occurs especially in elderly individuals; resembles a carcinoma of squamous epithelium.

Keratohyalin a colorless translucent protein that occurs especially in granules of the stratum granulosum of the epidermis and stains deeply.

Kilobase pairs a unit of measurement in molecular biology equal to 1,000 base pairs of DNA or RNA.

Kinetic energy the energy of a body or a system with respect to the motion of the body or of the particles in the system.

Klinefelter syndrome the set of symptoms resulting from 2 or more X chromosomes in males; common features include infertility and small testicles.

Lentigo maligna a point at which melanocyte cells have become malignant and grow continuously along the stratum basale of the skin, but have not invaded below the epidermis.

Leptomeninges the pia mater and the arachnoid considered together as investing the brain and spinal cord.

Leukemia a cancer of the blood or bone marrow characterized by an abnormal increase of white blood cells.

Leukoplakia a firmly attached white patch on a mucous membrane, associated with an increased risk of cancer.

Li-Fraumeni syndrome a rare, autosomal dominant disorder that predisposes carriers to cancer development.

Lichen planus a condition that can cause swelling and irritation in the skin, hair, nails, and mucous membranes.

Lichenoid dermatoses a chronic skin eruption characterized by hardening and thickening of the skin with the accentuation of normal skin markings.

Life expectancy a statistical measure of the average time a person is expected to live, based on birth year, current age, gender, and demographic factors.

Life table a graphical depiction of the probability for a person of a specific age to die before their next birthday.

Linear accelerator also called a *linear particle accelerator*, a device that accelerates charged subatomic particles or ions to a high speed by subjecting them to a series of oscillating electric potentials along a linear beamline.

Lipofuscin yellow-brown pigment granules made up of lipid-containing residues of lysosomal digestion.

Lipoma a benign tumor made of fat tissue.

Liquid biopsies also known as *fluid biopsies* or *fluid phase biopsies*; the sampling and analysis of non-solid biological tissue, primarily blood.

Lucent during x-ray, an area that is marked by clarity of translucence.

Lumbar puncture spinal tap; the insertion of a needle into the spinal canal, usually to collect CSF for diagnostic testing.

Lupus vulgaris painful cutaneous tuberculosis skin lesions with nodular appearance, most often on the face around the nose, eyelids, lips, cheeks, ears, and neck.

Lymphedema localized swelling of the body caused by an abnormal accumulation of lymph.

Lymphogranuloma venereum an ulcerative disease of the genital area. It is a contagious venereal disease caused by various strains of a chlamydia (such as *Chlamydia trachomatis*).

Lymphomas cancer of the lymph nodes; usually malignant tumor of lymphoid tissue.

Lynch syndrome hereditary nonpolyposis colorectal cancer.

Lysozyme an enzyme that destroys bacteria and functions as an antiseptic; found in tears, leukocytes, and mucus.

Macrophages white blood cells of the immune system that engulf and digest cellular debris, foreign substances, microbes, and cancer cells.

Maffucci syndrome a rare disorder with multiple benign tumors of cartilage within bones, usually in the hands, feet, and limbs.

Major histocompatibility complex a genetic system that allows large proteins in immune system cells to identify compatible or foreign proteins. It allows the matching of potential organ or bone marrow donors with recipients.

Mammary duct ectasia a benign condition in which a milk duct under the nipple widens and thickens. This can cause the milk duct to become blocked and fluid to build up inside it.

Marfanoid body habitus the body characteristics resembling those of Marfan syndrome, including long limbs, crowded oral maxilla sometimes with a high arch in the palate, arachnodactyly, and hyperlaxity.

Matrix metalloproteases endopeptidases that hydrolyze extracellular proteins, especially collagens and elastin.

Meckel's cave the trigeminal cave, a dura mater pouch containing CSF.

Median furrow midline longitudinal depression in the surface of the back; it begins superiorly in the cervical region and is continuous inferiorly with the gluteal cleft, diminishing at the base of the neck and over the sacral base.

Mediastinoscopy examination of the mediastinum through an incision above the sternum.

Medullary carcinoma the type of thyroid cancer that originates from the parafollicular cells, which produce calcitonin.

Megakaryocyte a large cell normally found in the bone marrow and rarely in circulating blood that serves as a precursor cell for platelets.

Meigs syndrome a rare condition affecting females that is characterized by pleural effusion, ascites, and non-malignant ovarian neoplasms – usually benign.

Melanoma a malignant skin cancer developing from melanocytes, usually caused by ultraviolet light exposure.

Meningioma a slow-growing tumor that forms from the meninges; it is linked to family history, ionizing radiation, and neurofibromatosis type 2.

Menometrorrhagia excessive uterine bleeding, during menstruation and in between menstrual periods.

Menorrhagia an increased amount and duration of menstrual flow.

Merkel cell skin cancer a rare type of skin cancer that usually appears as a flesh-colored or bluish-red nodule, often on the face, head, or neck. Also called *neuroendocrine carcinoma* of the skin.

Mesenchymal refers to cells that develop into connective tissue, blood vessels, and lymphatic tissue.

Mesoderm the middle layer of the three primary germ layers in a new embryo.

Mesothelioma a type of cancer that develops from the thin layer of tissue covering many internal organs – usually in the lining of the lungs and chest wall.

Metabolic encephalopathy an alteration in consciousness caused by diffuse or global brain dysfunction, from impaired cerebral metabolism.

Metanephrines catabolites of epinephrine in the urine and some tissues.

Metaplasia the transformation of one differentiated cell type into another.

Metastasis the spread of a disease process such as cancer from one part of the body to another due to dissemination of tumor cells.

Microinvasive microscopic extension of malignant cells into adjacent tissue in carcinoma, in situ.

Microsatellite instability a change that occurs in certain cells (such as cancer cells) in which the number of repeated DNA bases in a microsatellite (a short, repeated sequence of DNA) is different from what it was when the microsatellite was inherited.

Mohs surgery a procedure to remove a visible lesion on the skin in several steps. First, a thin layer of cancerous tissue is removed.

Molar pregnancy also known as *hydatidiform mole*; a rare complication of pregnancy characterized by the abnormal growth of trophoblast.

Molluscum contagiosum a mild chronic disease of the skin caused by a poxvirus that results in small, raised, pink lesions with a dimple in the center.

Monoclonal antibody one that is made by identical immune cells that are all clones of a unique parent cell; it can be used to detect antigens in fixed tissue sections; in cancer treatment, it binds only to cancer-cell-specific antigens to induce an immune response.

Monoclonal proteins those by identical immune cells that are all clones of a unique parent cell; they can be used to detect antigens in fixed tissue sections; in cancer treatment, they bind only to cancer-cell-specific antigens to induce an immune response.

Multidetector row CT the latest advancement in CT technology. The use of multiple detector rows allows faster scanning and thinner collimation. These improvements allow routine scans to be performed faster with higher z-axis resolution.

Multioculated having or comprising several small cavities or compartments.

Multiple myeloma abnormal plasma cells (a type of white blood cell) that build up in the bone marrow and form tumors in many bones of the body.

Myelography radiographic visualization of the spinal cord after injection of a contrast medium into the spinal subarachnoid space.

Myomectomy the surgical removal of a myoma, especially the excision of a fibroid tumor from the uterus.

Myxoid foci the type of connective tissue that usually shows *myxoid* type change is called *stroma*.

Myxomatous referring to a benign myxoma, most often found in the heart, composed of connective tissue embedded in mucus.

Naïve T cells those that have matured and been released by the thymus but that have not yet encountered their corresponding antigens.

Nasopharyngeal angiofibromas also known as *juvenile nasal angiofibromas*, histologically benign but locally aggressive vascular tumors of the nasopharynx that arise from the superior margin of the sphenopalatine foramen and grow in the back of the nasal cavity.

Nasopharyngeal hemangiomas benign tumors originating from vascular structures in the body. Cavernous hemangiomas in the nasal cavity usually originate from the lateral nasal wall.

Natural killer cells large, granular lymphocytes critical to the innate immune system that play a similar role to that of the cytotoxic T cells in adaptive immune response.

Neurasthenia a condition that is characterized especially by physical and mental exhaustion, usually with accompanying headache and irritability; of unknown cause, it is often associated with depression or emotional stress, and is sometimes considered similar to or identical with chronic fatigue syndrome.

Neurofibroma a benign tumor that develops from the cells and tissues that cover nerves.

Neurofibromatosis type 1 a complex multi-system disorder involving tumors along the nervous system that can grow anywhere on the body, and also includes changes in skin pigmentation.

Neurofibromatosis type 2 a rare genetic disorder that is primarily characterized by noncancerous tumors of the nerves that transmit balance and sound impulses from the inner ears to the brain.

Neurofibrosarcomas malignant tumors that form in the soft tissues surrounding the peripheral nerves.

Nevus a benign growth on the skin that is formed by a cluster of melanocytes.

Nevus sebaceous a rare type of birthmark that can be found on the face, neck, forehead, or scalp. While it can appear anywhere on the head, it most often occurs on the scalp. Though technically classified as a hair follicle tumor and associated with other conditions, a nevus sebaceous is benign.

Nidus the point of origin or focus of a disease process.

Nitrosation a chemical reaction in which organic compounds are converted into nitroso compounds.

Non-Hodgkin's lymphoma actually a group of blood cancers that includes all types of lymphomas except Hodgkin's lymphomas.

Normetanephrine a metabolite of norepinephrine created by the action of catechol-O-methyl transferase on norepinephrine.

Nuclear medicine the use of radioactive substances in research, diagnosis, and treatment.

Nystagmus a spasmodic, backward movement of the eyeball during attempts to move the eye – a sign of midbrain disease.

Object drug the medication that has its therapeutic effect modified by the drug interaction process.

Odynophagia pain on swallowing food and fluids, a symptom often due to disease of the esophagus.

Ollier disease a rare disorder that causes benign growths of cartilage in the bones. These growths usually occur in the bones of the hands and feet, but they may also occur in the skull, ribs, and spine. They may cause bones to break, to be deformed, or to be shorter than normal.

Oncogenes genes that contribute to cancerous changes in cells.

Oncolytic virotherapy treatment using an oncolytic virus (that infects and breaks down cancer cells but not normal cells).

Oncoprotein antibodies proteins encoded by an oncogene that can cause the transformation of a cell into a tumor cell if introduced into it.

Oophorectomy the surgical removal of one or both ovaries. If both ovaries are removed, the procedure causes immediate infertility and menopause.

Open biopsy a surgical procedure in which an incision is made through the skin to expose a tumor and allow for a sample of tissue to be cut or scraped away.

Organ of Corti an organ of the inner ear located within the cochlea that contributes to hearing. It includes three rows of outer hair cells and one row of inner hair cells. Vibrations caused by sound waves bend the stereocilia on these hair cells via an electromechanical force.

Osteitis fibrosa cystica a skeletal disorder due to loss of bone mass, weakening of bones, and cyst-like tumors in and around bones; based on hyperparathyroidism.

Osteoradionecrosis a condition of nonvital bone in a site of radiation injury. It can be spontaneous, but it most commonly results from tissue injury. The absence of reserve reparative capacity is a result of the prior radiation injury.

Osteosarcoma a cancerous bone tumor also known as *osteogenic sarcoma*.

Oxidative stress an imbalance between systemic manifestation of reactive oxygen species and a system's ability to detoxify reactive intermediates or repair damage.

Oxygen tension the partial pressure of oxygen (PO2); the activity of the molecules of oxygen dissolved in the plasma.

P450 enzyme actually a group of enzymes involved in drug metabolism and found in high levels in the liver; these enzymes are necessary for the detoxification of foreign chemicals and the metabolism of drugs.

Pancoast tumor a type of lung cancer that begins in the upper part of a lung and spreads to nearby tissues such as the ribs and vertebrae. Most are non-small-cell cancers. Also called *pulmonary sulcus tumor*.

Pancytopenia an abnormal reduction in the number of all circulating blood cells.

Papillary carcinoma the most common type of thyroid cancer, characterized by the small mushroom shape of the tumor, with a stem attached to the epithelial layer.

Paraneoplastic syndrome a group of rare disorders that are triggered by an abnormal immune system response to a cancerous tumor; causes difficulty in walking or swallowing, loss of muscle tone, loss of fine motor coordination, slurred speech, memory loss, and vision problems.

Paresthesia an abnormal sensation, typically tingling or pricking, caused chiefly by pressure on or damage to peripheral nerves.

Parturition the process of delivering a baby and placenta from the uterus to the vagina to the outside world; commonly referred to as *labor*.

Passenger mutations those that do not directly drive cancer initiation and progression, as opposed to driver mutations.

Pathognomic a sign or symptom that is so characteristic of a disease that it can be used to make a diagnosis. For example, Koplik spots present on the buccal mucosa are considered a diagnostic feature of measles or rubeola.

Pedicle a stub of bone that connects the lamina to the vertebral body to form the vertebral arch. Two short, stout processes extend from the sides of the vertebral body and join with broad flat plates of bone (laminae) to form a hollow archway that protects the spinal cord.

Pel-Ebstein fever a cyclic fever occasionally seen in Hodgkin's disease and other diseases, characterized by irregular episodes of fever of several days' duration.

Penetrance the frequency with which a heritable trait is manifested by people carrying the principal gene or genes conditioning it.

Percussible able to be tapped (percussed) in order to determine abnormalities.

Perforin a protein in the cytoplasmic granules of T-cytotoxic lymphocytes and natural killer cells, implicated in target cell lysis.

Pericardiocentesis surgical puncture of the pericardium, especially to aspirate pericardial fluid.

Pericytes elongated, contractile cells wrapped around precapillary arterioles outside the basement membrane.

Perlman syndrome characterized principally by polyhydramnios, neonatal macrosomia, bilateral renal tumors (hamartomas with or without nephroblastomatosis), hypertrophy of the islets of Langerhans, and facial dysmorphism.

Personalized genomic vaccine the injection of multiple patient-specific tumor peptides that are immunogenic and unique to the patient's tumor.

Petechiae a small red or purple spot caused by bleeding into the skin.

Peutz-Jeghers syndrome an autosomal dominant genetic disorder, with development of benign hamartomatous polyps in the gastrointestinal tract and hyperpigmented macules on the lips and oral mucosa.

Pharmacogenetics the branch of pharmacology concerned with the effect of genetic factors on drug responses.

Pharmacogenomics the study of the role of the genome in drug responses.

Pharmacokinetics the study of the movement of drugs in the body, including the processes of absorption, distribution, tissue localization, biotransformation, and excretion.

Phenotype the complete observable characteristics of an organism or group, including anatomic, physiologic, biochemical, and behavioral traits.

Pheochromocytoma a rare tumor arising from chromaffin cells of the adrenal medulla, causing excessive sweating, headaches, and elevated heart rate.

Philadelphia chromosome also called *Philadelphia translocation*, a specific chromosomal abnormality associated with chronic myelogenous leukemia.

Photodynamic therapy a two-stage treatment that combines light energy with a drug (photosensitizer) designed to destroy cancerous tumors.

Phyllodes tumor a type of tumor found in breast or prostate tissue. It is often large and bulky and grows quickly. It may be benign or malignant and may spread to other parts of the body.

Pineoblastoma a malignant pineal gland neoplasm in the brain.

Pituitary adenoma a benign neoplasm of the anterior pituitary gland that may be secretory or non-secretory.

Pituitary apoplexy a stroke occurring in the pituitary area.

Pituitary carcinoma a malignant tumor of the pituitary gland, made of epithelial cells.

Plasma cells antibody-secreting cells in lymphoid tissue, derived from B-cells via lymphokine stimulation, reacting with specific antigens.

Plasmacytoid resembling or derived from a plasma cell.

Pleomorphic referring to a variable appearance or morphology.

Pleomorphism the ability of some microorganisms to alter their morphology, biological functions, or reproductive modes in response to environmental conditions.

Pleurodesis a procedure that is sometimes performed to relieve pleural effusions – a build-up of fluid between the membranes surrounding the lungs that recur due to lung cancer and other conditions.

Plummer-Vinson syndrome a disorder marked by anemia caused by iron deficiency, and a web-like growth of membranes in the throat that makes swallowing difficult.

Pluripotent cells those that have the capacity to self-renew by dividing and developing into the three primary germ cell layers of the early embryo, and, therefore, into all cells of the adult body, but not extra-embryonic tissues such as the placenta.

Pneumothorax the presence of air or gas in the cavity between the lungs and the chest wall, causing collapse of the lung.

Pocket ion chambers dosimeters that did not have self-reading capabilities, widely used in World War II and in postwar government and military projects, consisting of simple ionization chambers with an electrode running down the center – read by plugging them into electrometers/chargers.

Point mutation one that affects only one or very few nucleotides in a gene sequence.

Polycystic ovary syndrome a condition marked by infertility, enlarged ovaries, menstrual problems, high levels of male hormones, excess hair on the face and body, acne, and obesity. Women with polycystic ovary syndrome have an increased risk of diabetes, high blood pressure, heart disease, and endometrial cancer.

Polycythemia an abnormal increase in the production of blood cells. It is a serious condition that can be controlled by removing blood and by chemotherapy that reduces the activity of bone marrow cells.

Port cannula a small medical appliance that is installed beneath the skin and used for repeated required injections.

Positron emission tomography an imaging technology in which substances containing positron-emitting isotopes are introduced into the body, allowing the precise location of physiological processes by detection of the gamma rays produced by the isotopes.

Precipitating drug a chemotherapeutic drug used before the primary object drug; there are often therapeutic or drug interactions that occur between them.

Preosteoblast a mesenchymal cell that differentiates into an osteoblast.

Prevalence the number of people in a population who have a disease at a given time.

Prinzmetal angina a variant form that is characterized by chest pain during rest and by an elevated ST segment during pain; typically caused by an obstructive lesion in the coronary artery.

Prolactinoma a noncancerous tumor of the pituitary gland. This tumor causes the pituitary to make too much of a hormone called *prolactin*.

Proprioception perception or awareness of the position and movement of the body.

Prostate Health Index a mathematical formula that provides a probability of prostate cancer.

Proto-oncogenes normal genes that, with slight alterations by mutations or other mechanisms, become oncogenes.

Proton therapy a type of particle therapy using a beam of protons to irradiate diseased tissue – most often in the treatment of cancer.

Psammoma bodies round collections of calcium that appear microscopically.

Pseudofolliculitis barbae a common condition of the beard area occurring in up to 60% African American men and other people with curly hair.

Pseudoinvasion resembling actual invasion of cells or tumors.

Pulmonary fibrosis a serious lung disease that occurs when lung tissue becomes damaged and scarred.

Punctate having or marked with minute spots, holes, or depressions.

Purulent containing or composed of pus.

Pyloroplasty the surgical alteration of the pylorus, usually a widening to facilitate the passage of food from the stomach to the duodenum.

Pyogenic granulomas benign blood vessel tumors that usually form on the skin; they may also form on mucous membranes and inside capillaries or other body sites.

Pyrimidine dimers molecular lesions formed from thymine or cytosine bases in DNA via photochemical reactions.

Radical trachelectomy surgery to remove the cervix, nearby tissue and lymph nodes, and the upper part of the vagina.

Radicular pain also called *radiculitis*; pain radiated along the sensory distribution of a nerve due to inflammation or irritation of the nerve root.

Radiofrequency ablation the use of electrodes to generate heat and destroy abnormal tissue.

Radiopharmaceutical a radioactive drug used for diagnostic or therapeutic purposes.

Reed-Sternberg cells also called *lacunar histiocytes*, they are distinctive, giant cells found with light microscopy in biopsies from people with Hodgkin's lymphoma.

Renal cell carcinoma the most common type of kidney cancer. It begins in the lining of the renal tubules in the kidney.

Renal sarcoma a rare type of kidney cancer that begins in the blood vessels or connective tissue of the kidney. It makes up less than 1% of all kidney cancers.

Rete testis a network of small tubes in the testicle that helps move sperm cells from the testicle to the epididymis, where the sperm mature and are stored.

Reticulocytosis increased number of reticulocytes in the blood. Reticulocytosis occurs when the body is recovering from blood loss or anemia.

Reticuloendothelial relating to a diverse system of fixed and circulating phagocytic cells (macrophages and monocytes) involved in the immune response. They are spread throughout the body, and are especially common in the liver, spleen, and lymphatic system.

Richter's transformation a rare condition in which chronic lymphocytic leukemia changes into a fast-growing type of lymphoma. Symptoms include fever, loss of weight and muscle mass, and other health problems.

Ring badge a device worn on a finger that contains a radiation-sensitive lithium fluoride crystal.

Robotic surgery procedures done using robotic assistance systems; instead of directly moving the instruments, extremely precise robotic arms carry out the movements needed, as guided by a surgeon and computer technology.

Roentgenogram a photograph of internal structures made by passing x-rays through the body to produce a shadow image on specially sensitized film.

Rombo syndrome a very rare, inherited disorder that causes a bluish-red skin color on the lips, hands, and feet. It also causes skin lesions that leave pitted scars, usually on the cheeks.

Rosenthal fibers thick, elongated, worm-like bundles found on staining of brain tissue, accompanying gliosis, occasional tumors, and some metabolic disorders.

Rotationplasty a surgical procedure that can be used to treat malignant bone tumors occurring near a child's knee. It preserves the lower leg, attaches it to the thighbone, then uses the ankle as a knee joint.

Rubinstein-Taybi syndrome a condition characterized by short stature, learning difficulties, distinctive facial features, and broad thumbs and first toes.

Salvage radiation a treatment using radiation, given after recurrence of a tumor.

Sarcoidosis a chronic disease of unknown cause characterized by the enlargement of lymph nodes in many parts of the body and the widespread appearance of granulomas derived from the reticuloendothelial system.

Sarcoma botryoides a subtype of embryonal rhabdomyosarcoma that can be observed in the walls of hollow, mucosa-lined structures such as the nasopharynx, common bile duct, urinary bladder of infants and young children, or the vagina in females, typically younger than age 8.

Sarcopenia a progressive and generalized skeletal muscle disorder involving the accelerated loss of muscle mass and function that is associated with increased adverse outcomes including falls, functional decline, frailty, and mortality.

Schwannoma a usually benign nerve sheath tumor made up of Schwann cells.

Scintigraphy a technique in which a scintillation counter or similar detector is used with a radioactive tracer to obtain an image of a bodily organ or a record of its functioning.

Scintiscan a 2D representation of radioisotope radiation from an organ such as the spleen or kidney.

Seborrheic keratoses a benign hyperkeratotic tumor that occurs singly or in clusters on the surface of the skin, is usually light to dark brown or black in color, and typically has a warty texture often with a waxy appearance.

Sedimentation rate the distance that red blood cells travel in one hour in a sample of blood as they settle to the bottom of a test tube. The rate is increased in inflammation, infection, cancer, rheumatic diseases, and diseases of the blood and bone marrow. Also called *erythrocyte sedimentation rate* (ESR).

Sentinel lymph node biopsy a procedure that takes a sample of a sentinel lymph node, the first node or group of nodes that drain a tumor.

Sestamibi protein a small protein which is labeled with the radio-pharmaceutical technetium99. This mild, safe radioactive agent is injected into the veins of a patient with hyperparathyroidism (parathyroid disease) and is absorbed by the overactive parathyroid gland.

Shear stress the external force acting on an object or surface parallel to the slope or plane in which it lies; the stress tending to produce shear.

Sigmoidoscopy examination of the sigmoid colon by means of a flexible tube inserted through the anus.

Sipple syndrome a rare, genetic disorder that affects the endocrine glands and causes medullary thyroid cancer, pheochromocytoma, or parathyroid gland cancer.

Sjögren syndrome a chronic autoimmune disease of the lacrimal and salivary glands, and often of the lungs, kidneys, and nervous system.

Solar lentigo a harmless patch of darkened skin. It results from exposure to ultraviolet (UV) radiation, which causes local proliferation of melanocytes and accumulation of melanin within the skin cells (keratinocytes).

Somatic mutation genetic alteration acquired by a cell that can be passed to the progeny of the mutated cell in the course of cell division.

Somatic tissue the body tissues that do not contribute to the production of gametes; mutations in these tissues, therefore, are not heritable.

Sonohysterography also known as *saline infusion sonography*, a minimally invasive ultrasound technique. It provides pictures of the inside of the uterus and helps diagnose unexplained vaginal bleeding.

Spectroscopy the study of interactions between matter and electromagnetic radiation, as a function of wavelengths or frequency.

Squamocolumnar junction the junction between the squamous epithelium and the columnar epithelium. Its location on the cervix is variable.

Squamous cell carcinoma also called *epidermoid carcinoma*, a malignant cancer that is derived from squamous epithelial cells.

Stauffer syndrome a paraneoplastic condition characterized by biochemical changes: increased alkaline phosphatase, cholesterol and prothrombin time, cholestatic jaundice, hepatosplenomegaly (associated with and regressing after successful treatment of renal cell carcinoma and, less commonly, malignant schwannoma and other cancers).

Stereotactic radiosurgery a minimally invasive surgery using a 3D coordinate system to locate small target lesions.

Stokes-collar a tumorous outbreak into the upper mediastinum with the relocation of the superior vena cava. This results in upper inflow congestion.

Strawberry hemangiomas hyperproliferation of immature capillary vessels, usually on the head and neck, present at birth or within the first 2–3 months postnatally, which commonly regresses without scar formation.

Stromal cells connective tissue cells of any organ, such as fibroblasts.

Sturge-Weber syndrome a rare, congenital disorder that affects the brain, skin, and eyes. Abnormal blood vessel growth occurs in the trigeminal nerve in the face and the meninges of the brain.

Suicide gene one that will cause a cell to kill itself through apoptosis.

Superior vena cava syndrome a group of symptoms caused by obstruction of the superior vena cava, usually due to malignant tumors within the mediastinum such as lung cancer and non-Hodgkin's lymphoma.

Supratentorial referring to the area of the brain above the tentorium cerebelli.

Synchronous cancer two or more malignancies identified simultaneously or within 6 months of initial diagnosis.

Syncytiotrophoblast large cells within a syncytiotrophoblast, the epithelial covering of the embryonic placental villi.

Target theory the concept that the biological effects of radiation result from formation of electrically charged particles absorbed at targets in cells.

Tectal plate the junction of gray and white matter in an embryo.

Telangiectasia an abnormal dilation of red, blue, or purple superficial capillaries, arterioles, or venules typically localized just below the skin's surface.

Telomeres the sections of DNA that form the natural end of a chromosome.

Tenesmus cramping rectal pain.

Teratoma a tumor made up of different tissues, such as hair, muscle, teeth, or bone.

Therapeutic index the margin of safety that exists between the dose of a drug that produces the desired effect and the dose that produces unwanted and possibly dangerous side effects.

Thrombocytopenia deficiency of platelets in the blood. This causes bleeding into the tissues, bruising, and slow blood clotting after injury.

Thymolipoma a rare, benign anterior mediastinal mass of thymic origin, with both thymic and mature adipose tissue.

Thymoliposarcoma an extremely rare malignant thymic neoplasm, with features of well-differentiated or dedifferentiated liposarcoma and intervening thymic tissue.

Thymoma a rare type of tumor that is the most common tumor type located in the area in the center of the chest between the lungs (the anterior mediastinum).

Tomographic images those produced by motion of the x-ray tube and film or by motion of the patient that blurs the image except in a single plane.

Tonofibrils one of the fine fibrils in epithelial cells, thought to give a supporting framework to the cell.

Transitional cell carcinoma cancer that develops in the lining of the renal pelvis, ureter, or bladder.

Transoral laser microsurgery an emerging technique for the management of laryngeal and other head and neck malignancies.

Transoral robotic surgery a procedure to remove mouth and throat cancers in which a surgeon uses a sophisticated, computer-enhanced system to guide the surgical tools.

Transrectal ultrasonography a method of creating an image of organs in the pelvis, most commonly used to perform an ultrasound-guided needle biopsy evaluation of the prostate gland.

Transsphenoidal referring to a surgical approach that goes through or across the sphenoid bone.

Transvaginal ultrasound a procedure used to examine the vagina, *uterus*, fallopian tubes, ovaries, and bladder. An instrument is inserted into the vagina that causes sound waves to bounce off organs inside the pelvis. These sound waves create echoes that are sent to a computer, which creates a picture called a *sonogram*.

Trimorphic the occurrence of three forms distinct in structure and coloration.

Trismus refers to the restriction of the range of motion of the jaws. Commonly referred to as "lockjaw," trismus typically stems from a sustained, tetanic spasm of the muscles of mastication.

Trophoblasts cells that form the outer layer of a blastocyst. They are present four days post-fertilization in humans. They provide nutrients to the embryo and develop into a large part of the placenta.

Trousseau syndrome an acquired blood clotting disorder that results in migratory thrombophlebitis. Although not always associated with an internal malignancy, many cases do show an underlying cancer.

Tuberous sclerosis a rare multisystem autosomal dominant genetic disease, with non-cancerous tumors growing in the brain and other vital organs.

Tumor DNA sequencing sequencing of somatic tissue, such as tumors, refers to looking for variants in DNA that typically occur after conception.

Tumor lysis syndrome metabolic disturbances that occur when large numbers of neoplastic cells are killed rapidly, leading to the release of intracellular ions and metabolic byproducts into systemic circulation. It is characterized by the rapid development of hyperuricemia, hyperkalemia, hyperphosphatemia, hypocalcemia, and acute kidney injury.

Tumor margin the edge or border of the tissue removed in cancer surgery.

Tumor neovasculature the development of new blood vessels at a tissue site; angiogenesis.

Turcot syndrome a rare form of multiple intestinal polyposis associated with brain tumors.

Tylosis a genetic disorder characterized by thickening of the palms and soles, white patches in the mouth (oral leukoplakia), and a very high risk of esophageal cancer. This is the only genetic syndrome known to predispose to squamous cell carcinoma of the esophagus.

Type II pneumocytes the cells responsible for the production and secretion of surfactant (which reduces the surface tension of pulmonary fluids, contributing to the elastic properties of the lungs).

Tyrosinemia a genetic disorder involving the metabolism of the amino acid tyrosine, characterized by abnormally high levels of tyrosine in the blood. It causes cirrhosis of the liver before 6 months of age and, untreated, leads to death from liver failure.

Unopposed estrogen an imbalance of estrogen, dominating over the levels of progesterone; also called *estrogen dominance* and linked to endometrial cancer.

Unsteady gait an abnormality in walking that can be caused by diseases of or damage to the legs and feet (including the bones, joints, blood vessels, muscles, and other soft tissues) or to the nervous system that controls the movements necessary for walking.

Urachus a canal that connects the urinary bladder to the during fetal development. The urachus is normally obliterated, so it is usually a solid cord.

Uroflowmetry timed measurement of the rate of urination. Uroflowmetry is used to diagnose conditions that result in slow urinary output.

Urostomy a surgically created opening in the abdominal wall through which urine passes. A urostomy may be performed when the bladder is either not functioning or has to be removed.

Uterine sarcoma a cancer of the smooth muscle and supporting tissues of the uterus.

Vagotomy a surgical operation in which one or more branches of the vagus nerve are cut, typically to reduce rates of gastric secretion (such as when treating peptic ulcers).

Vasovagal syncope fainting due to a sudden drop in blood pressure, when vessels open too wide and/or the heartbeat slows down, causing a temporary lack of blood flow to the brain.

Venous lakes small, dark blue to purple, slightly elevated papules. These papules are soft and compressible. They commonly appear on sun-exposed areas such as the face, lips, ears, neck, and back of the hands of elderly people. They are benign, but are often confused with melanoma.

Vermillion border also called a *margin* or *zone*; the normally sharp demarcation between the lip and the adjacent normal skin.

Vimentin a structural protein encoded by the VIM gene. Its name comes from the Latin *vimentum*, which refers to an array of flexible rods.

Volume of distribution the amount of a drug in the blood as compared to the concentration measured in a body fluid.

Von Hippel-Lindau disease a rare genetic disorder with visceral cysts and benign tumors that can become malignant.

Von Recklinghausen disease neurofibromatosis type 1.

Vulvar cancer a rare cancer of the labia or skin of a woman's genitals. Having HPV is a risk factor.

Waldeyer ring a partial *ring* of tonsillar or adenoid tissue formed by the two palatine tonsils, the pharyngeal tonsil, and the lingual tonsil.

Werner syndrome a fatal autosomal recessive disorder, also called *adult progeria*, characterized by the appearance of premature aging.

Whipple procedure also called *pancreaticoduodenectomy*, to remove the head of the pancreas, duodenum, gallbladder, and bile duct.

Wilms' tumor a rare kidney cancer that primarily affects children. Also known as *nephroblastoma*, it is the most common cancer of the kidneys in children. Wilms' tumor most often affects children of ages 3–4 and becomes much less common after age 5.

Wilson's disease a rare inherited disorder that causes copper to accumulate in the liver, brain, and other vital organs. Most people are diagnosed between the ages of 5 and 35, but it can affect younger and older people as well.

Wiskott-Aldrich syndrome a rare X-linked recessive disease, with eczema, thrombocytopenia, immune deficiency, and bloody diarrhea.

Xeroderma pigmentosum a rare inherited disorder marked by extreme sensitivity to ultraviolet light, and a high risk of developing cancer. Signs and symptoms are usually seen in children by age 2 years.

Xerostomia a genetic disease characterized by such extraordinary sensitivity to sunlight that it results in the development of skin cancer at a very early age.

XY gonadal dysgenesis also known as *Swyer syndrome*, is a type of hypogonadism in a person whose karyotype is 46,XY. The gonads are typically surgically removed (as they have a significant risk of developing cancer).

Years of life lived with a disability the number of years that a person lives with some type of disabling disease; it is a component of the disability-adjusted life year (DALY).

Years of life lost a calculation of the age at which deaths occur by giving more weight to deaths at a younger age and less weight to deaths at an older age.

Zeolites one of a group of minerals consisting of hydrated aluminosilicates of sodium, potassium, calcium, and barium. They can be readily dehydrated and rehydrated, and are used as cation exchangers and molecular sieves.

Zollinger-Ellison syndrome a condition in which tumors of the pancreas stimulate excessive gastric acid production.

Index

Note: Page numbers are followed by *f* indicates figure and *t* indicates table respectively.

Global Epidemiology of Cancer: Diagnosis and Treatment, First Edition. Jahangir Moini, Nicholas G. Avgeropoulos, and Craig Badolato.
© 2022 John Wiley & Sons Ltd. Published 2022 by John Wiley & Sons Ltd.

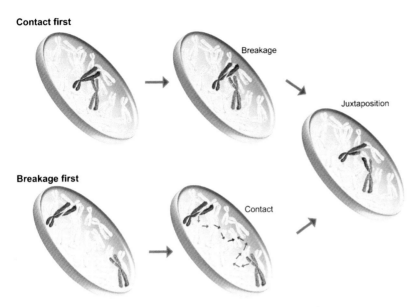

Contact first

Breakage

Juxtaposition

Breakage first

Contact

Plate 1 The two modes of alteration in chromosomal translocations. *Source:* Javadekar and Raghavan [19].

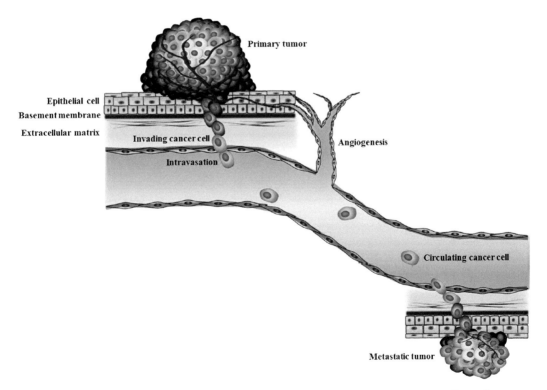

Primary tumor

Epithelial cell

Basement membrane

Extracellular matrix

Invading cancer cell

Angiogenesis

Intravasation

Circulating cancer cell

Metastatic tumor

Plate 2 Biological processes linked to cancer spread from a primary site to other body organs. *Source:* Courtesy: "From Invasion to Metastasis".

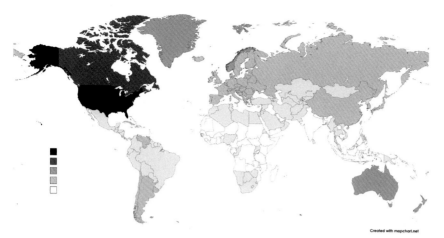

Plate 3 The varying prevalence of cancer throughout the world, 2017.

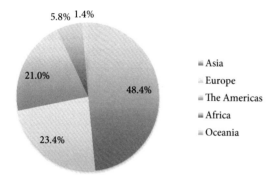

5.8% 1.4%

21.0%

48.4%

23.4%

- Asia
- Europe
- The Americas
- Africa
- Oceania

Plate 4 Cancer prevalence throughout the world.

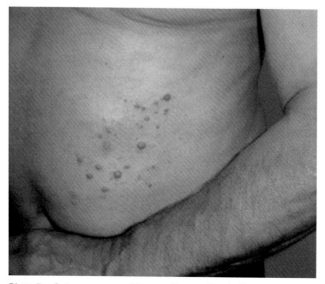

Plate 5 Cutaneous neurofibroma. *Source:* García-Romero et al. (2015).

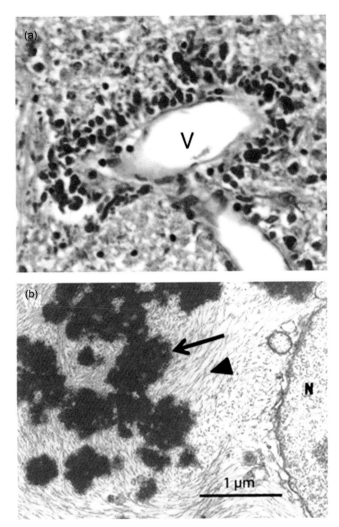

Plate 6 Rosenthal fibers, (a) among the astrocytes surrounding a blood vessel (labeled "V"); (b) an arrow indicating the Rosenthal fibers surrounded by intermediate filaments (arrowhead). *Source:* Messing et al. (2012).

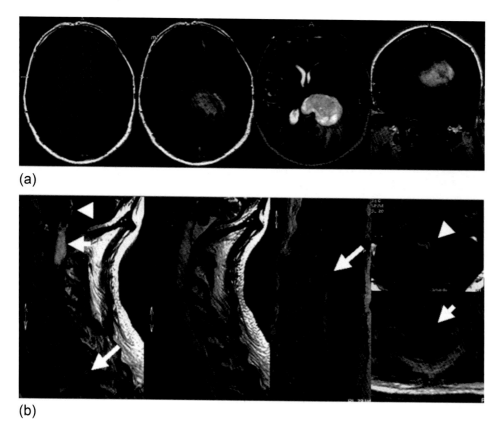

(a)

(b)

Plate 7 Pilocytic astrocytoma, (a) from left to right: T1-weighted axial MRI before and after administration of contrast medium, plus T2-weighted images showing perifocal edema; (b) from left to right: T1-weighted sagittal MRI with contrast of the craniocervical junction and cervical spine, with arrowhead indicating subarachnoid spread in the fourth ventricle; the small arrow indicates intramedullary tumor growth in the upper cervical cord; the large arrow indicates leptomeningeal metastasis at the level of the first thoracic segment. In the third image, the large arrow indicates another leptomeningeal metastasis at the level of the first and second lumbar segments. In the fourth image, the arrowhead indicates subependymal growth in the fourth ventricle, and the small arrow indicates the intramedullary tumor. *Source*: Stüer et al. (2007).

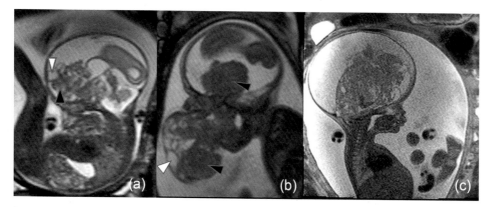

Plate 8 Teratomas within the brain. (a) Heterogeneous tumor with cystic (white arrowhead) and solid (black arrowhead) components; (b) Intracranial component (upper black arrowhead), cystic components (white arrowhead), and solid components (lower black arrowhead); (c) Large teratoma causing distortion and enlargement of the head. *Source:* Feygin et al. (2020.

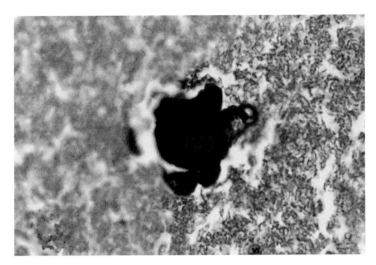

Plate 9 Psammoma bodies in a papillary carcinoma of the thyroid. *Source:* Ellison et al. (1998).

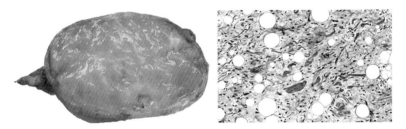

Plate 10 Spindle cell thymoliposarcoma. (a) Macroscopy of resected specimen; (b) histology of fat cells with variations of vacuole size, hyperchromatic stromal cells, and broad short coarse collagen fibers. *Source:* Courtesy: Dr. Margaret Burke, Harefield Hospital, Royal Brompton & Harefield NHS Trust, London, UK. den Bakker and Oosterhuis.

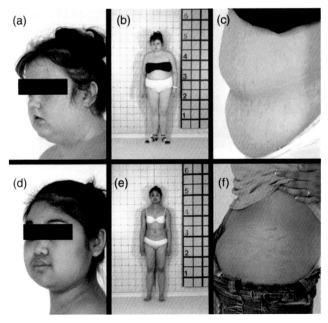

Plate 11 Manifestations of Cushing's syndrome. (a) Caucasian female face changes; (b) overall body shape; (c) fat distribution; (d) Asian female face changes; (e) overall body shape; (f) fat distribution. *Source:* Hsiao et al. (2007).

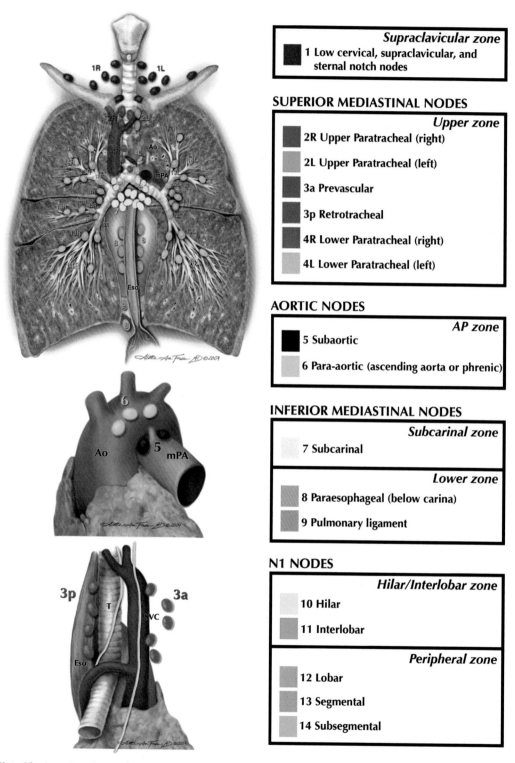

Plate 12 Lymph node map, including groupings of lymph node stations into zones for prognostic analysis (from the International Association for the Study of Lung Cancer, IASLC). *Source:* Rusch, V. W., Asamura, H., Watanabe, H., Giroux, D. J., Rami-Porta, R., & Goldstraw, P. (2009). The IASLC Lung Cancer Staging Project: A Proposal for a New International Lymph Node Map in the Forthcoming Seventh Edition of the TNM Classification for Lung Cancer. Journal of Thoracic Oncology, 4(5), 568–577. Reproduced with permission of Elsevier.

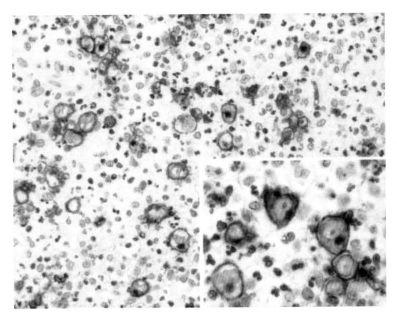

Plate 13 Cluster of Reed–Sternberg cells and variants. Original magnification 400×, with inset showing 600× magnification. *Source:* Portlock et al. (2004).

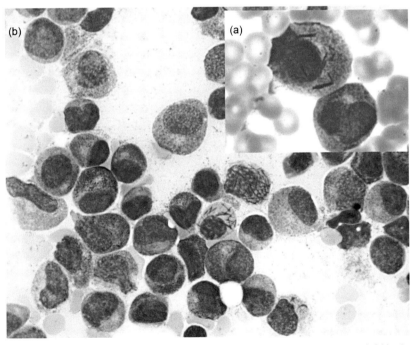

Plate 14 (a) Peripheral blood; (b) bone marrow in a patient with acute myeloid leukemia, showing cells that contain multiple splinters known as Auer rods. *Source:* Merino et al. (2018).

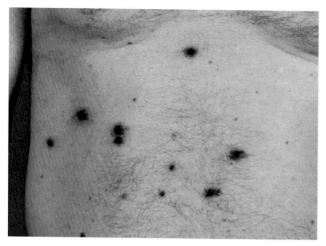

Plate 15 Leukemia cutis on the trunk, of the hemorrhagic subtype. *Source:* Wagner et al. (2011).

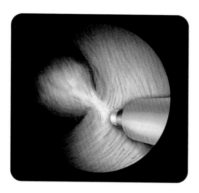

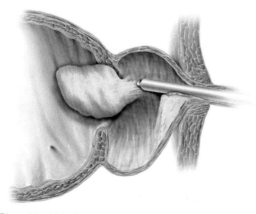

Plate 16 Holmium laser enucleation of the prostate (HoLEP) showing (a) the laser close to the prostate; (b) a lateral view. *Source:* Peter Gilling et al. (2007) / with permission of John Wiley & Sons, Inc.

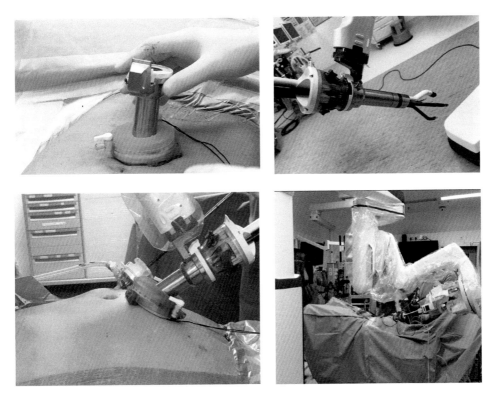

Plate 17 Robotic laparoscopic radical prostatectomy procedure. (a) Port cannula covering incisions; (b) the robotic arms, instruments, and camera; (c) placement of the robotic components through the port cannula; (d) the position of the patient during the robotic surgery. *Source:* Figure 02 from Ng et al. (2019).

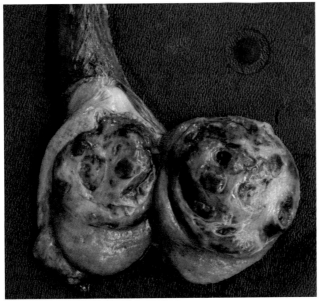

Plate 18 A resected testicle that has been cut partially through (bivalved), showing a mixed nonseminoma replacing most of the testicular parenchyma. *Source:* Stein and Luebbers [48]. with permission of John Wiley & Sons.

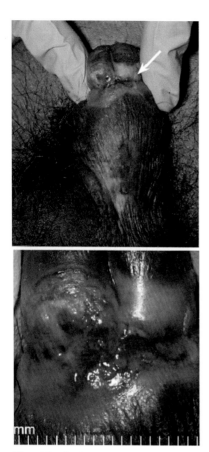

Plate 19 Penile squamous cell carcinoma in late stages. *Source:* Kravvas et al. (2017). With permission of John Wiley & Sons, Inc.

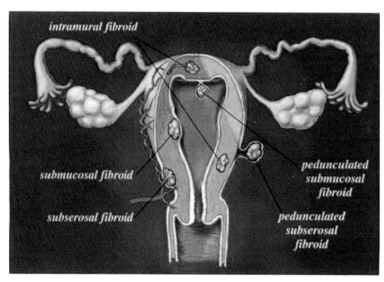

Plate 20 Locations of uterine fibroids. *Source:* AORN Journal – Clinical [9].

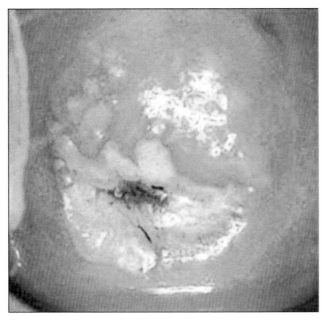

Plate 21 Acetowhite changes on the cervix, indicating high-grade cervical intraepithelial neoplasia. *Source:* Courtesy: Mr. John Tidy, Royal Hallamshire Hospital, Sheffield. AORN Journal – Clinical [9].

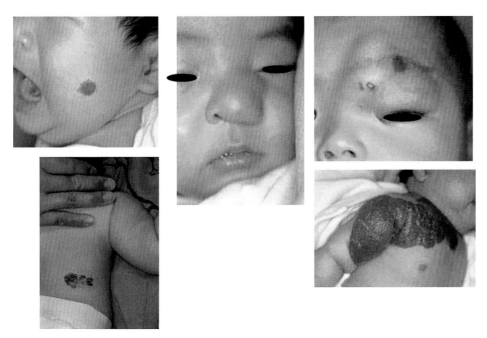

Plate 22 Strawberry hemangiomas. (a) Cheek; (b) nose; (c) forehead and eyebrow; (d) back; (e) shoulder and neck. *Source*: https://onlinelibrary.wiley.com/doi/10.1111/j.1346-8138.2010.00927.x. Journal of Dermatology [20].

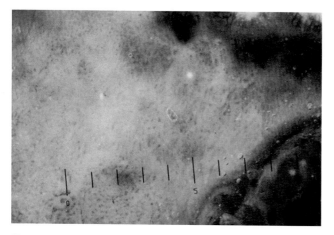

Plate 23 Melanoma viewed with immersion contact dermoscopy, revealing many dotted vessels in the depigmented area. *Source:* Figure 5 from https://onlinelibrary.wiley.com/doi/full/10.1111/1346-8138.13686. Journal of Dermatology [21].

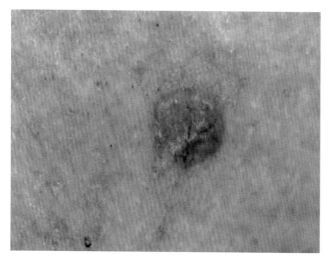

Plate 24 A nodular basal cell carcinoma. *Source:* Burns et al. (2013), Figure 141.3 from Page 3634. With permission of John Wiley & Sons.

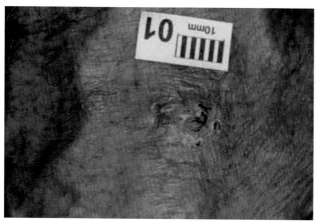

Plate 25 Squamous cell carcinoma showing hyperkeratosis with a raised nodule. *Source:* Burns et al. (2013), Figure 142.6 from Page 3646. With permission of John Wiley & Sons.

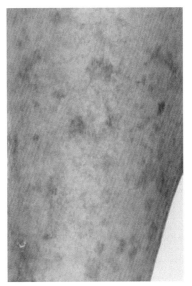

Plate 26 Multiple areas of Bowen disease on the lower leg. *Source:* Burns et al. (2013), Figure 142.23 from Page 3655. With permission of John Wiley & Sons.

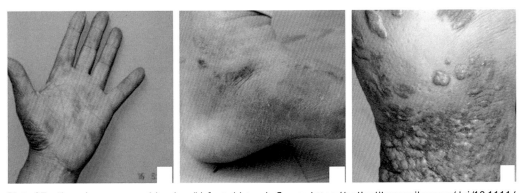

Plate 27 Kaposi sarcoma on (a) palm; (b) foot; (c) trunk. *Source:* https://onlinelibrary.wiley.com/doi/10.1111/jdv.12349. Journal of the European Academy of Dermatology and Venereology [22].

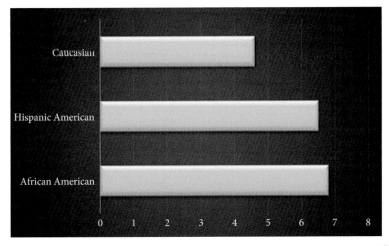

Plate 28 Rates of various children and adolescents with osteosarcomas, per million.

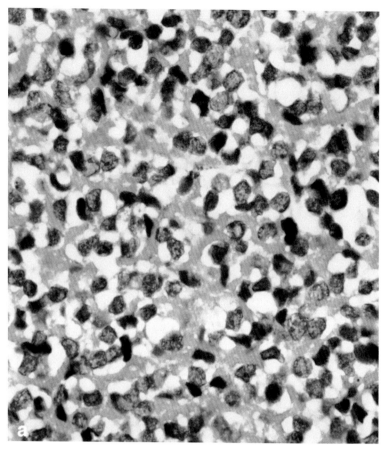

Plate 29 Lace-like osteoid and multinuclear giant cells of an osteosarcoma, in large areas of round cells that have medium-sized nuclei. *Source:* American Cancer Society (ACS) Journals – Cancer [12].

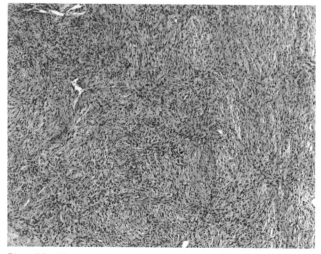

Plate 30 Histopathology of renal sarcoma, with spindle cells in an interlacing, fascicular pattern, plus elongated hyperchromatic nuclei and eosinophilic cytoplasm. *Source:* Figure 1 from Wiley Online Library – Clinical Case Reports [58].

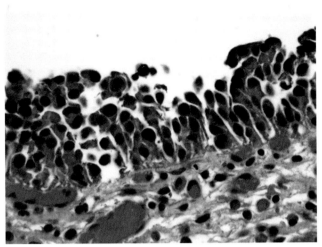

Plate 31 Transitional cell carcinoma of the bladder, in situ. *Source:* Figure 18.1 from Page 238 of the American Cancer Society's Oncology in Practice [9].

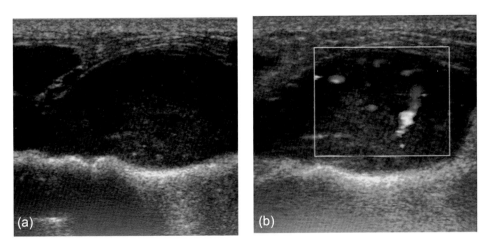

Plate 32 (a) Doppler ultrasonography of a desmoid tumor of the right foot, showing a homogeneous mass; (b) duplex Doppler ultrasonography showing substantial blood flow to the tumor. *Source:* Figure 3 from Wiley Online Library – Journal of Ultrasound in Medicine – Case Series [54].

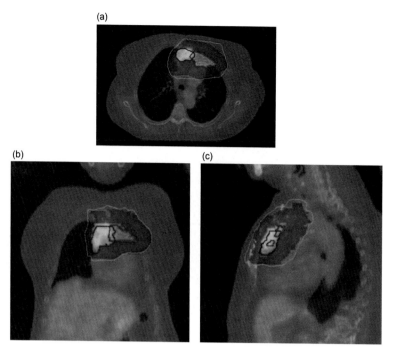

Plate 33 Three-dimensional intensity-modulated radiation therapy (IMRT) for stage IIB thymic carcinoma after thymectomy with a positive margin in (a) axial, (b) coronal, and (c) sagittal planes. The preoperative PET scan has been fused to the CT simulation scan for target delineation purposes. The red line shows the preoperative gross tumor volume. The pink line shows the postoperative tumor bed. The clinical target volume is green, and the planning target volume is blue. The orange line indicates the total irradiated area. *Source:* Figure 2.1 from Page 24 of The American Cancer Society's Oncology in Practice [1].

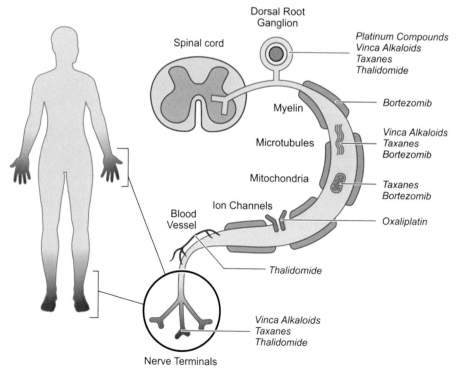

Plate 34 The typical "glove-and-stocking" distribution of chemotherapy-induced peripheral neuropathy. *Source:* Susanna B. Park. (2013).